Differential Diagnoses in Surgical Pathology:
Genitourinary System

DIFFERENTIAL DIAGNOSES IN SURGICAL PATHOLOGY SERIES

Series Editor: Jonathan I. Epstein

Differential Diagnoses in Surgical Pathology: Genitourinary System
Jonathan I. Epstein and George J. Netto, 2014

Differential Diagnoses in Surgical Pathology: Gastrointestinal System
Elizabeth Montgomery and Whitney Green, 2014

Differential Diagnoses in Surgical Pathology:
Genitourinary System

Jonathan I. Epstein, MD

Professor of Pathology, Urology and Oncology
The Reinhard Professor of Urological Pathology
Director of Surgical Pathology
The Johns Hopkins Medical Institutions
Baltimore, Maryland

George J. Netto, MD

Professor of Pathology, Urology and Oncology
Director of Surgical Pathology Molecular Diagnostics
Johns Hopkins University
Baltimore, Maryland

SERIES EDITOR

Jonathan I. Epstein, MD

Professor of Pathology, Urology and Oncology
The Reinhard Professor of Urological Pathology
Director of Surgical Pathology
The Johns Hopkins Medical Institutions
Baltimore, Maryland

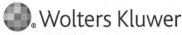

Wolters Kluwer
Health

Philadelphia • Baltimore • New York • London
Buenos Aires • Hong Kong • Sydney • Tokyo

Acquisitions Editor: Ryan Shaw
Product Development Editor: Kate Marshall
Production Project Manager: David Saltzberg
Senior Manufacturing Coordinator: Beth Welsh
Designer: Stephen Druding
Production Service: SPi Global

Library of Congress Cataloging-in-Publication Data
Epstein, Jonathan I., author.
  Differential diagnoses in surgical pathology: genitourinary system / Jonathan I. Epstein, George J. Netto.
     p. ; cm.
  Includes bibliographical references and index.
  ISBN 978-1-4511-8958-2 (hardback : alk. paper)
I. Netto, George J., author. II. Title.
  [DNLM: 1. Male Urogenital Diseases—diagnosis. 2. Diagnosis, Differential. 3. Male Urogenital Diseases—surgery.
4. Pathology, Surgical—methods. 5. Urologic Diseases—diagnosis. 6. Urologic Diseases—surgery. WJ 141]
RC900.9
616.6'075—dc23
                                                                                       2013041073

PREFACE

How often in surgical pathology, when confronted with a difficult case, do we arrive at a differential diagnosis between two or three entities? After turning to one of the many excellent general surgical pathology books or specialty texts, we read about each entity and still are unsure of the diagnosis. In part, this situation arises from these books' all encompassing nature. By having to include both the very common "classic" lesions which pose no diagnostic difficulty, as well as rare entities which are unlikely to be seen by most pathologists, these books devote less text and photographs to specific differential diagnoses. Also, because these books are arranged in a standard format where each entity is discussed and illustrated in its own section, the text and photographs are not directed toward differentiating between entities.

This book hopes to fill this niche in urologic pathology. By arranging the book according to differential diagnoses, the text and illustrations have been specifically tailored to helping the pathologist differentiate between entities that are commonly confused with each other. In addition to illustrating and discussing the "classical" features of these entities, atypical features, which can "sandbag" the pathologist have been stressed.

It is hoped that this book will supplement existing general and subspecialty books, and provide diagnostic aid for pathologists who must contend with an ever increasing number of urologic pathology specimens.

ACKNOWLEDGMENTS

Dr. Epstein's Acknowledgment

With great affection, I dedicate this book to my former and current Genitourinary Pathology Fellows spanning the last 21 years. It is a life cycle event when each academic year brings a new group of enthusiastic pathologists eager to tackle our challenging consult service and participate in multiple research projects. Without the fellows, I would not be able to handle the heavy consult load nor would I be able to be as productive academically. Although initially, they often dread the "unknowns" portion of my teaching sessions, they soon appreciate its value. Knowledge of which lesions cause the fellows difficulty is a major source of the differential diagnoses that comprises this book.

But it is not just about the Pathology! The fellows have been a fantastic group of very diverse individuals from the United States and over 10 countries. They bring their unique personalities to each daily sign-out making the review of approximately 50 cases an experience that I look forward to each day. Each year, one of the four fellows is sponsored from an institution from another country. Having these fellows from around the world has expanded all of our cultural horizons. I thoroughly enjoy subsequently lecturing at their institutions and seeing how they have become leaders in Genitourinary (GU) Pathology in their country. As a bonus, I am hosted by my former fellows who provide a local's view of their country. How else would I have been able to see a Sumo match in Japan, visit an Eastern Medicine Pharmacy in China, or attend the Camel Market in Saudi Arabia?

It also gives me great pleasure to see my former fellows thrive in their subsequent practice. Many of the fellows have risen over the years to leadership positions in academics, private practice, or laboratories. However, what unifies them is that they all provide the best and most up-to-date knowledge of Urological Pathology in helping patients, which ultimately is what is most important. Our GU fellows and faculty are truly a big family that gathers together every year for a lively dinner at USCAP. Everyone gets to know the new fellows and has fun catching up with former ones. My fellows are not just my mentees but are friends who I feel incredibly fortunate to have had the opportunity to know and keep up with over the ensuing years. Not only do all the fellows and I share a common strong bond but we also have our own unique language. "Backslash flyaway time."

Dr. Netto's Acknowledgment

I would like to acknowledge the great efforts contributed by his two Urologic Pathology Fellows, Dr. Sheila Friedrich Faraj and Dr. Enrico Munari in obtaining some of the photomicrographs and references.

CONTENTS

CONTENTS

1

Prostate

	Nonspecific Granulomatous Prostatitis (NSGP)	Infectious Granulomas
Age	Teens to elderly, typically older men	Typically adults
Location	Peripheral = transition zone	Transition > peripheral zone
Symptoms	Variable irritative and obstructive symptoms, fever, chills. Most with h/o recent urinary tract infection	Fungal and systemic TB with systemic symptoms. BCG granulomas typically asymptomatic unless rare cases where attenuated bacilli of BCG become active and result in systemic symptoms
Signs	Pyuria frequent. About 50% with indurated rectal exam, hematuria. PSA can be markedly elevated	Can result in indurated nodular rectal exam. PSA typically not elevated
Etiology	Reaction to bacterial toxins, secretions from ruptured acini	Fungal and systemic TB granulomas in immunocompromised hosts. BCG granulomas in men treated for superficial bladder cancer
Histology	1. Early lesion with dilated ducts and acini filled with neutrophils, debris, foamy histiocytes, and desquamated epithelial cells *(Fig. 1.1.1)* 2. Rupture of ducts and acini leads to localized destruction of acini *(Fig. 1.1.2)*. 3. Lacks central caseation but may have central microabscess formation *(Fig. 1.1.3)* 4. Extension of infiltrate into surrounding ductal and acinar units gives rise to lobular dense infiltrate of histiocytes, lymphocytes, plasma cells, and some neutrophils. Older lesions more fibrous *(Fig. 1.1.4)*. Some lesions can have more histiocytes more closely mimicking an infectious granuloma *(Fig. 1.1.5)*	1. Early lesions show nonnecrotizing granulomas adjacent to intact glands *(Figs. 1.1.6–1.1.8)* 2. Later lesions show larger granulomas, which can destroy glands *(Fig. 1.1.9)*. 3. Later lesions develop caseation with granulomatous and mixed inflammatory reaction *(Fig. 1.1.10)* 4. Typically not as polymorphous inflammation as NSGP. Mostly lymphocytes/plasma cells with neutrophils also seen in fungal granulomas *(Fig. 1.1.6)*
Special studies	• In classic NSGP, no organism stains needed unless if unsure if infectious	• If no prior BCG, fungal and acid-fast stains should be performed. If h/o of BCG, no need for organism stains
Treatment	Warm sitz baths, fluids, and antibiotics if urinary tract infection is documented	Infectious granulomas in immunocompromised hosts treated with systemic therapy. BCG prostatitis requires no therapy unless a rare case of systemic BCG infection
Prognosis	Most symptoms resolve within a few months	Infectious and systemic granulomas in immunocompromised hosts have a poor prognosis. BCG granulomas unless systemic have no clinical significance

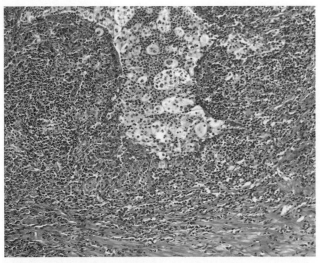

Figure 1.1.1 Early lesion of NSGP.

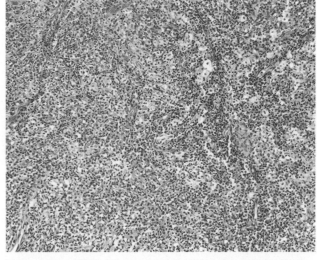

Figure 1.1.2 NSGP with destruction of acini by polymorphous infiltrate.

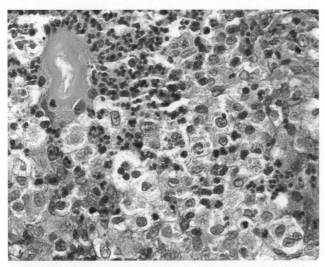

Figure 1.1.3 Central area of NSGP with microabscess formation, yet lacking caseation. In addition to neutrophils, there are histiocytes, lymphocytes, and eosinophils.

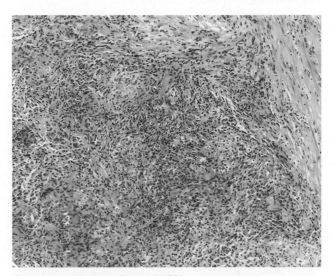

Figure 1.1.4 Lobular infiltrate of NSGP.

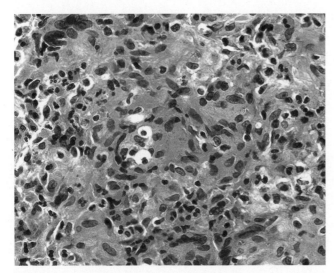

Figure 1.1.5 NSGP with more histiocytes, yet admixed eosinophils and neutrophils more typical of NSGP than of infectious granuloma.

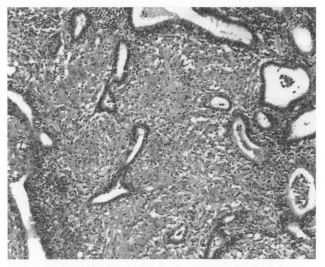

Figure 1.1.6 Infectious granuloma with periglandular granulomas consisting of histiocytes and lymphocytes without admixed plasma cells, neutrophils, or eosinophils.

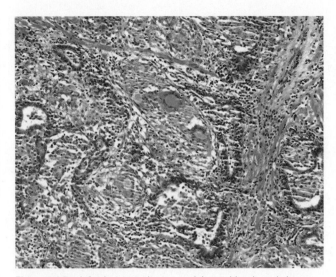

Figure 1.1.7   Infectious granuloma containing multinucleated giant cells surrounding intact glands.

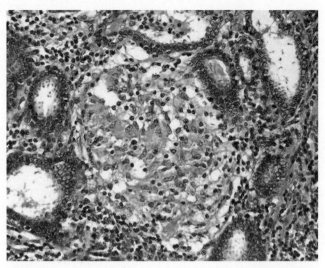

Figure 1.1.8   Higher magnification of infectious granuloma with intact glands.

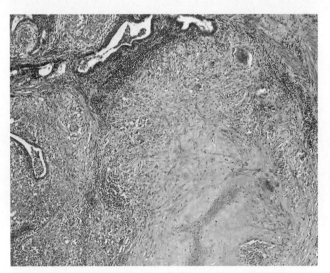

Figure 1.1.9   Infectious granuloma with focal intact glands (*left*) and larger granulomas (*center*) that have destroyed glands.

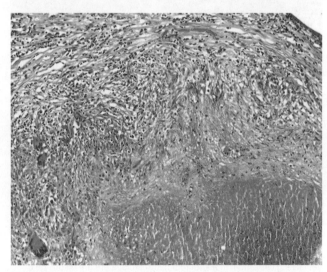

Figure 1.1.10   Infectious granuloma with caseous necrosis (*bottom*).

	Infectious Granuloma	Postbiopsy Granuloma
Age	Typically adults	Typically adults after prostate TURP
Location	Transition > peripheral zone	Transition > peripheral zone
Symptoms	Fungal and systemic TB with systemic symptoms. BCG granulomas typically asymptomatic unless rare cases where attenuated bacilli of BCG become active, resulting in systemic symptoms	Asymptomatic
Signs	Can result in indurated nodular rectal exam. PSA typically not elevated	None
Etiology	Fungal granulomas in immunocompromised hosts. BCG granulomas in men treated for superficial bladder cancer	Typically results from cautery injury of prior TURP. Rarely can be seen following needle biopsy. Can be seen from 9 d to 52 mo after TURP
Histology	1. Early lesions show nonnecrotizing granulomas adjacent to intact glands. Later lesions develop caseation with destruction of acini *(Fig. 1.2.1)* 2. Necrosis consists of fine granular debris lacking visible structures *(Figs. 1.2.2 and 1.2.3)* 3. Granulomas tend to be round and relatively regular *(Fig. 1.2.1)* 4. Lymphocytes/plasma cells predominate with neutrophils also seen in fungal granulomas. Scattered multinucleated giant cells seen *(Fig. 1.2.3)*	1. Early and late granulomas show central necrosis and tend to be near urethra and can destroy glands. Nonspecific foreign body giant cell granulomas also seen *(Fig. 1.2.4)* 2. Central region of fibrinoid necrosis surrounded by palisading epithelioid histiocytes. Necrosis often contains ghost-like structures of vessels, acini, and stroma *(Fig. 1.2.5)* 3. Irregular shapes including wedge-shaped, ovoid, and sinuous *(Fig. 1.2.6)* 4. With recent TURP, abundant eosinophils may be identified. Older granulomas are most lymphocytes and plasma cells *(Figs. 1.2.7 and 1.2.8)*
Special studies	If h/o of BCG, no need for organism stains. If no prior BCG, fungal and acid-fast stains should be performed	None
Treatment	Infectious granulomas in immunocompromised hosts treated with systemic therapy. BCG prostatitis requires no therapy unless a rare case of systemic BCG infection	None
Prognosis	Infectious and systemic granulomas in immunocompromised hosts have a poor prognosis. BCG granulomas unless systemic have no clinical significance	Lesions fibrose over time

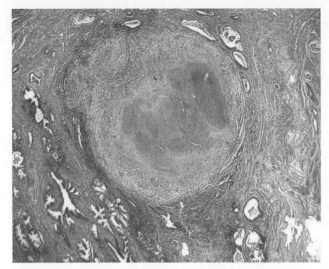

Figure 1.2.1 Infectious necrotizing granuloma with relative sparing of glands.

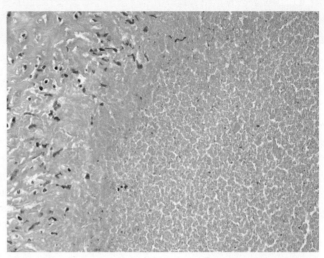

Figure 1.2.2 Caseous necrosis with fine granular debris surrounded by histiocytes.

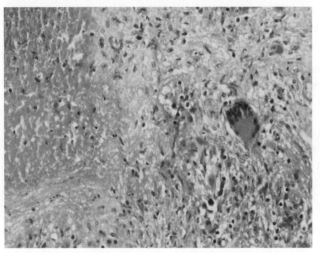

Figure 1.2.3 Caseous necrosis (*left*) with adjacent multinucleated histiocytes.

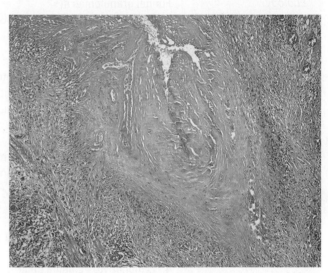

Figure 1.2.4 Oval-shaped postbiopsy granuloma with central necrosis.

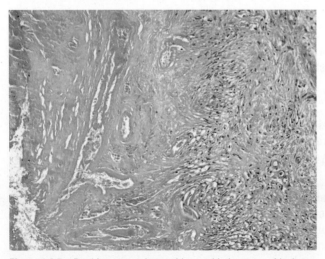

Figure 1.2.5 Postbiopsy granuloma with necrobiotic center with ghosts of necrotic vessels.

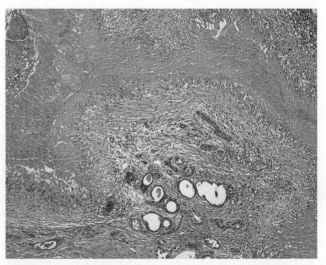

Figure 1.2.6 Irregular linear necrobiotic granuloma of postbiopsy granuloma.

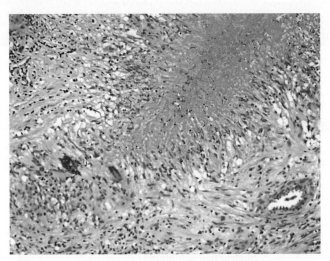

Figure 1.2.7   Postbiopsy ovoid granuloma mimicking an infectious granuloma with palisading histiocytes and scattered multinucleated histiocytes.

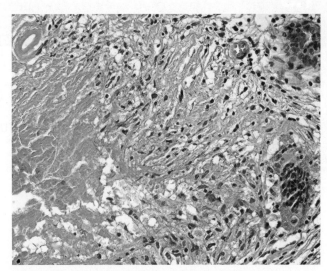

Figure 1.2.8   Higher magnification of Figure 1.2.7 with central necrosis lacking the fine granular amorphous appearance of infectious granulomas.

	Postbiopsy Granuloma	Allergic Granuloma
Age	Typically adults after prostate TURP	Typically adults
Location	Transition > peripheral zone	Transition > peripheral zone
Symptoms	Asymptomatic	Almost all with either asthma or evidence of systemic allergic reaction at the time of diagnosis of their prostatic lesions. Severity of the asthmatic symptoms may fluctuate synchronously with the severity of urinary obstructive symptoms
Signs	None	Majority have increased blood eosinophil counts
Etiology	Typically results from cautery injury of prior TURP. Rarely can be seen following needle biopsy. Can be seen from 9 d to 52 mo after TURP	Allergic granulomatous prostatitis and Churg-Strauss syndrome
Histology	1. Variably sized, irregular shapes including wedge-shaped, ovoid, and sinuous *(Fig. 1.3.1)* 2. Central region of fibrinoid necrosis surrounded by palisading epithelioid histiocytes *(Fig. 1.3.1)* 3. Necrosis often contains ghost-like structures of vessels, acini, and stroma *(Fig. 1.3.2)* 4. With recent TURP, abundant eosinophils may be identified immediately around the granulomas *(Fig. 1.3.3)*. Later granulomas with lymphocytes/plasma cells 5. Nonspecific foreign body giant cell granulomas also seen	1. Multiple ovoid granulomas of uniform small size *(Fig. 1.3.4)* 2. Central eosinophilic necrosis surrounded by histiocytes with less palisading *(Fig. 1.3.5)* 3. No visible prostatic structures within necrosis *(Fig. 1.3.6)* 4. Granulomas surrounded by numerous eosinophils and extensive eosinophils throughout the stroma *(Figs. 1.3.7 and 1.3.8)* 5. Churg-Strauss syndrome may also have necrotizing vasculitis
Special studies	None	Clinically workup for increased peripheral blood eosinophilia and rule out Wegener's
Treatment	None	Allergic granulomatous prostatitis treated with steroids
Prognosis	Lesions fibrose over time	Systemic granulomas may be seen, possibly contributing to death

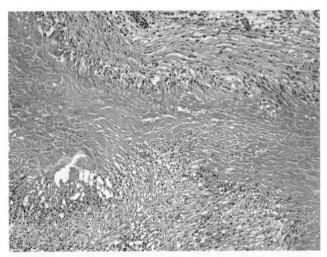

Figure 1.3.1   Linear necrobiotic postbiopsy granuloma with palisading histiocytes.

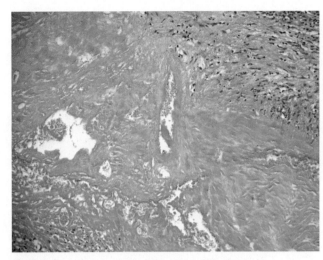

Figure 1.3.2   Postbiopsy granuloma ghost of blood vessels.

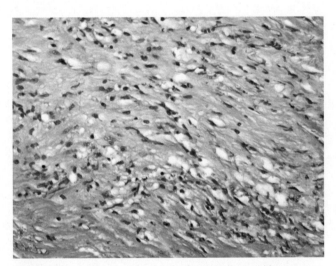

Figure 1.3.3   Scattered eosinophils (*top*) surrounding postbiopsy granuloma.

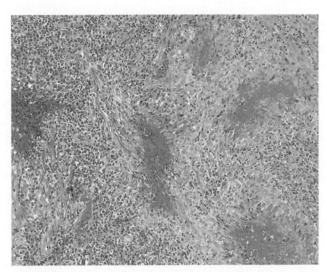

Figure 1.3.4   Allergic granuloma with multiple relatively uniformly sized and shaped ovoid necrotic granulomas.

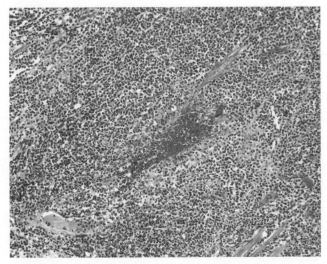

Figure 1.3.5   Allergic granuloma central eosinophilic necrosis surrounded by histiocytes and numerous eosinophils.

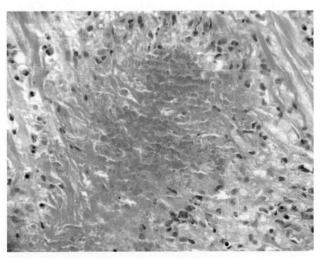

Figure 1.3.6   Central necrosis of allergic granuloma lacking necrotic prostate structures.

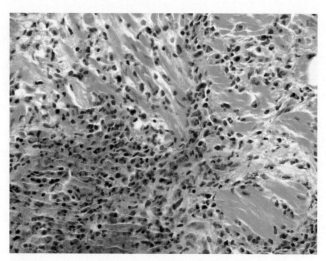

Figure 1.3.7   Allergic granuloma necrosis surrounded by numerous eosinophils.

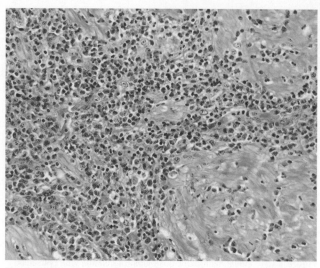

Figure 1.3.8   Numerous eosinophils of allergic granuloma infiltrating prostatic stroma.

	Acute/Chronic Prostatitis	Prostatic Acute/Chronic Inflammation
Age	Typically adults	Typically adults seen on needle biopsy, TURP, or radical prostatectomy
Location	Transition = peripheral zone	Transition = peripheral zone
Symptoms	Acute bacterial prostatitis associated with fever, chills, and dysuria. Chronic bacterial prostatitis usually associated with recurrent urinary tract infections (asymptomatic periods). Chronic prostatitis may present with low back pain, dysuria, and perineal and suprapubic discomfort	Asymptomatic
Signs	Acute bacterial prostatitis with an exquisitely tender and boggy prostate on rectal examination. Diagnosis of chronic nonbacterial prostatitis (chronic pelvic pain syndrome) is difficult and requires completion of the NIH Chronic Prostatitis Symptom Index survey by the patient, digital rectal exam, urinalysis, and sequential collection of urine and prostatic fluid specimens, before, during, and after prostatic massage	Conflicting data as to whether either focal acute inflammation or chronic inflammation associated with elevated serum PSA levels
Etiology	Urinary tract infection source of acute and chronic bacterial prostatitis. Unknown for pelvic pain syndrome, which accounts for 90%–95% of prostatitis cases	Nonspecific, unrelated to infections. Almost ubiquitously found in prostates unrelated to clinical prostatitis
Histology	1. Clinical chronic prostatitis not associated with specific histologic findings 2. Clinical acute prostatitis consists of numerous neutrophils within acini associated with extensive neutrophils throughout stroma. Microabscess formation can be seen *(Figs. 1.4.1–1.4.6)* 3. Typically, biopsy of acute prostatitis contraindicated due to increased risk of sepsis. Clinically no need to biopsy chronic prostatitis	1. Focal nonspecific periglandular lymphocytes and plasma cells *(Fig. 1.4.7)* 2. Focal nonspecific acute inflammation in acini *(Fig. 1.4.8)* 3. Inflammation should not be commented on in pathology reports unless prominent. Can mislead urologists that elevated serum PSA levels result from the inflammation, when in some cases, unsampled carcinoma is the source of the elevated PSA
Special studies	None	None
Treatment	Both acute and chronic bacterial prostatitis treated with antibiotics. No proven therapies for chronic pelvic pain syndrome	None
Prognosis	Favorable for bacterial prostatitis, although acute bacterial prostatitis may be accompanied by sepsis	Inflammation on biopsy is not associated with an increased risk of cancer on subsequent biopsy

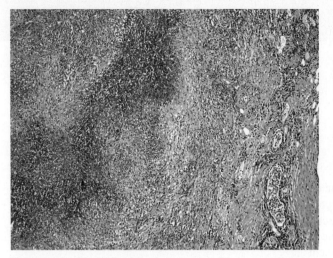

Figure 1.4.1 Abscess formation in acute prostatitis.

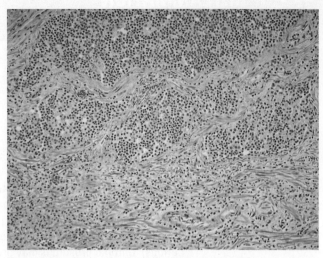

Figure 1.4.2 Sheets of neutrophils with acute prostatitis.

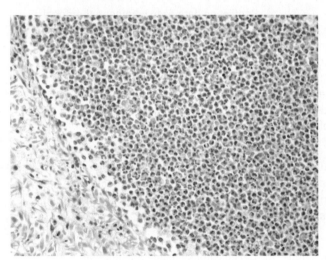

Figure 1.4.3 Higher magnification of Figure 1.4.2 with abscess formation.

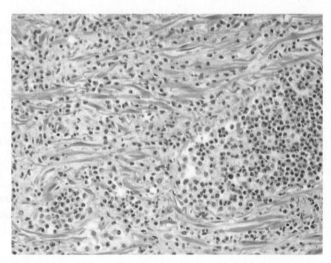

Figure 1.4.4 Diffuse infiltration of stroma by neutrophils in acute prostatitis.

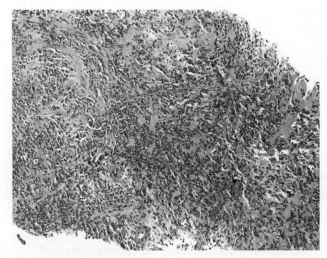

Figure 1.4.5 Low magnification of acute prostatitis with heavily inflamed prostatic stroma.

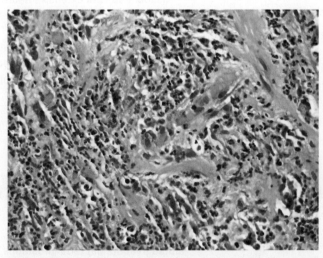

Figure 1.4.6 Higher magnification of Figure 1.4.5 showing numerous neutrophils infiltrating prostatic stroma.

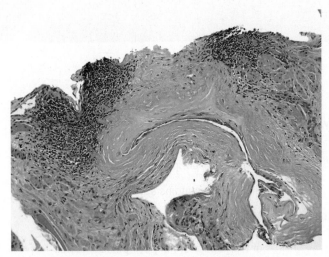

Figure 1.4.7　Nonspecific periglandular chronic inflammation.

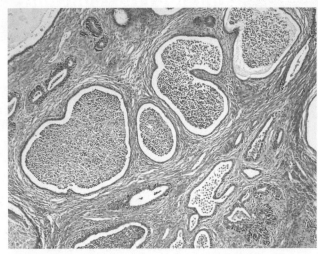

Figure 1.4.8　Nonspecific acute inflammation in prostate glands.

1.5 PROSTATIC CHRONIC INFLAMMATION VS. CHRONIC LYMPHOCYTIC LEUKEMIA

	Prostatic Chronic Inflammation	Chronic Lymphocytic Leukemia
Age	Typically adults seen on needle biopsy, TURP, or radical prostatectomy	Most > 60 years old
Location	Transition = peripheral zone	Transition = peripheral zone
Symptoms	Asymptomatic	Prostatic symptoms asymptomatic
Signs	Conflicting data as to whether either focal chronic inflammation associated with elevated serum PSA levels	Most patients are known leukemics or have their diagnosis established at the time of workup for urinary symptoms. May be associated with lymphadenopathy (small lymphocytic lymphoma), eventually anemia and infections. Initial diagnosis may be made on a histologic specimen
Etiology	Nonspecific, unrelated to infections	Unknown
Histology	1. Inflammation periglandular *(Fig. 1.5.1)* 2. Focal inflammation with lymphocytes and plasma cells *(Fig. 1.5.2)* 3. Inflammation should not be commented on in pathology reports unless prominent. Can mislead urologists that elevated serum PSA levels result from the inflammation, when in some cases, unsampled carcinoma is the source of the elevated PSA	1. Infiltrate not restricted to periglandular location. Dense infiltrate of small, mature, round lymphocytes extensively infiltrating the prostatic stroma with preservation of prostatic glands *(Figs. 1.5.3–1.5.7)* 2. Infiltrates with monotonous collection of lymphocytes, lacking admixed plasma cells *(Fig. 1.5.8)*
Special studies	None	None
Treatment	None	Early disease not treated. Late disease is treated with chemotherapy and monoclonal antibodies
Prognosis	Inflammation on biopsy is not associated with an increased risk of cancer on subsequent biopsy	Low-grade lymphoma in the prostate does not impact the therapy or prognosis of prostate cancer, due to its indolent course

1.5 Prostatic Chronic Inflammation vs. Chronic Lymphocytic Leukemia **15**

PROSTATE

1

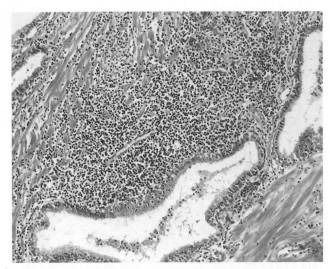

Figure 1.5.1 Focal periglandular nonspecific chronic inflammation.

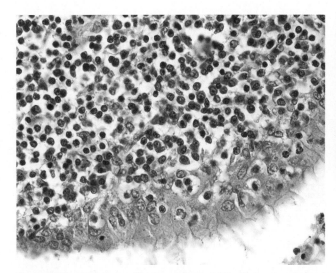

Figure 1.5.2 Higher magnification of Figure 1.5.1 with lymphocytes and plasma cells.

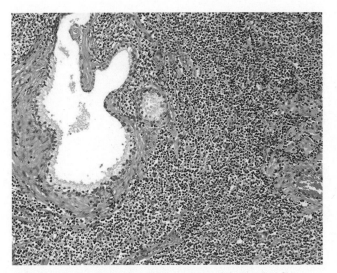

Figure 1.5.3 Extensive periglandular lymphocytic infiltrate of CLL.

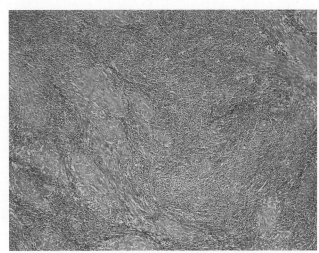

Figure 1.5.4 Moderately dense lymphocytic infiltrate of CLL extending into stroma.

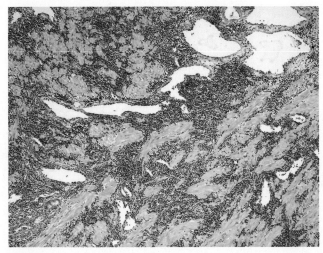

Figure 1.5.5 CLL with dense infiltrate extensively involving prostatic stroma.

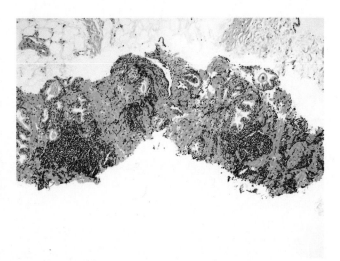

Figure 1.5.6 Needle biopsy with scattered dense infiltrates of CLL not in a periglandular distribution.

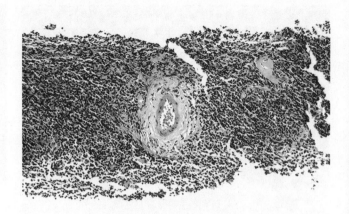

Figure 1.5.7 CLL with effacement of prostate by dense lymphoid infiltrate.

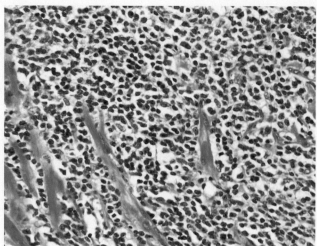

Figure 1.5.8 Monotonous CLL lymphocytic infiltrate.

	Epithelioid Nonspecific Granulomatous Prostatitis	High-Grade Prostatic Adenocarcinoma
Age	Teens to elderly, typically older men	Typically 50 to elderly, although not rare in 40s
Location	Transition = peripheral zone	Peripheral > transition zone
Symptoms	Variable irritative and obstructive symptoms, fever, chills. Most with h/o recent urinary tract infection	Typically asymptomatic. Advanced disease with urinary obstructive symptoms and/or hematuria or from distant metastases
Signs	Pyuria frequent. About 50% with indurated rectal exam, hematuria. PSA can be markedly elevated	Serum PSA levels typically elevated, yet occasionally not increased significantly as poorly differentiated cancers not effectively produce PSA
Etiology	Reaction to bacterial toxins, secretions from ruptured acini	Genetic with differences in the incidence of prostate cancer between countries and ethnicity. Family history with degree of risk related to the age of the relatives at diagnosis and the number of relatives affected. Diet with strongest link with high-fat intake and lower risk with consumption of fruits and vegetables, especially tomatoes. Testosterone and its derivative, dihydrotestosterone, important in prostate cancer growth, yet serum levels of these androgens not consistently associated with prostate cancer risk
Histology	1. Can be extensive, replacing and effacing the normal architecture of an entire core (Fig. 1.6.1) 2. Epithelioid histiocytes with prominent nucleoli (Figs. 1.6.2 and 1.6.3) 3. Admixed lymphocytes, plasma cells, neutrophils, and eosinophils (Figs. 1.6.4–1.6.7) 4. Multinucleated giant cell in only 50% of cases 5. Earlier lesions localized around ruptured ducts and acini (Fig. 1.6.8)	1. Can extensively involve a core 2. Sheets or individual cells with enlarged nuclei and prominent nucleoli. Mitoses vary from scattered to more frequent. Cancers mimicking NSGP tend to be relatively uniform without marked pleomorphism (Fig. 1.6.9) 3. Typically lacks associated inflammation (Figs. 1.6.9 and 1.6.10) 4. Lacks multinucleated giant cells 5. Not localized around ruptured acini
Special studies	• Epithelioid histiocytes CD68 positive • Negative for keratins and prostate markers. Entrapped, disrupted reactive glands are keratin positive (see Section 1.8)	• CD68 negative • Immunohistochemically, high-grade cancers may not express PSA. Best markers to differentiate cancer vs. inflammation/histiocytes are keratins such as CAM5.2 or AE1/AE3, which are not decreased in higher-grade tumors

	Epithelioid Nonspecific Granulomatous Prostatitis	High-Grade Prostatic Adenocarcinoma
Treatment	Warm sitz baths, fluids, and antibiotics if urinary tract infection is documented	Stage and age dependent with localized disease treated with either radical prostatectomy or combination hormone therapy/radiation; the latter the best option in men >70 years old. Advanced disease initially treated with hormone therapy
Prognosis	Most symptoms resolve within a few months	Stage dependent

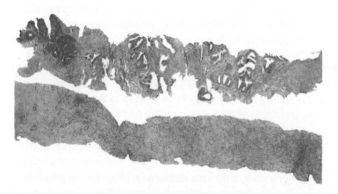

Figure 1.6.1   NSGP at low magnification (*bottom core*) can extensively involve a core destroying underlying benign glands and stroma, mimicking carcinoma.

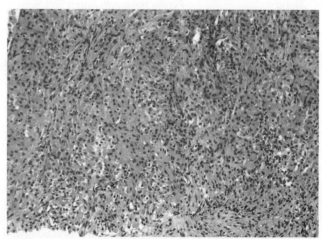

Figure 1.6.2   Low magnification of NSGP with sheets of epithelioid cells.

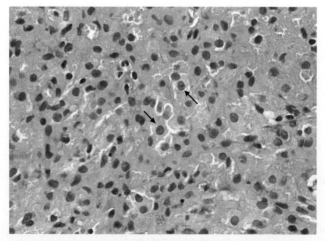

Figure 1.6.3   Higher magnification of Figure 1.6.2 with epithelioid histiocytes having prominent nucleoli (*arrows*).

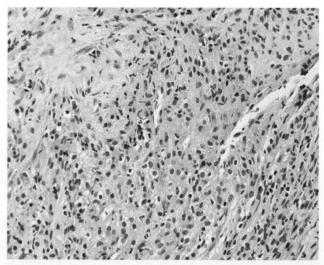

Figure 1.6.4   Low magnification of NSGP with sheets of epithelioid cells.

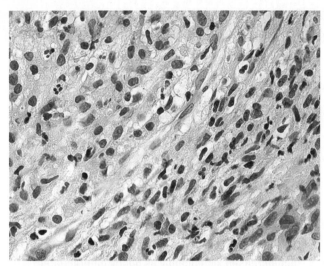

Figure 1.6.5   Higher magnification of Figure 1.6.4 with epithelioid histiocytes and admixed neutrophils and lymphocytes.

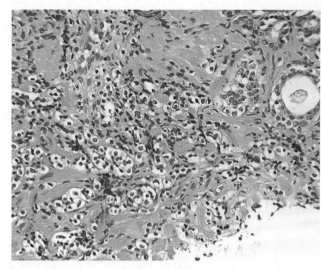

Figure 1.6.6   Low magnification of NSGP with cords of epithelioid cells.

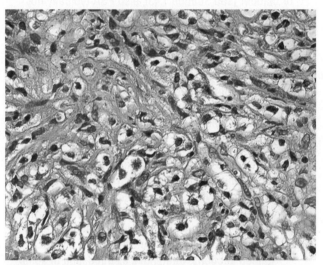

Figure 1.6.7   Higher magnification of Figure 1.6.6 with epithelioid histiocytes and admixed neutrophils and lymphocytes.

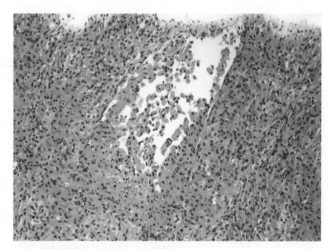

Figure 1.6.8   Partially ruptured dilated prostatic gland with intraluminal and periglandular epithelioid histiocytes.

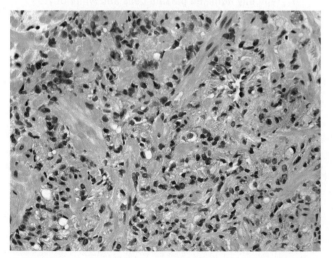

Figure 1.6.9   Cords of infiltrating relatively bland Gleason score 10 adenocarcinoma without admixed inflammation.

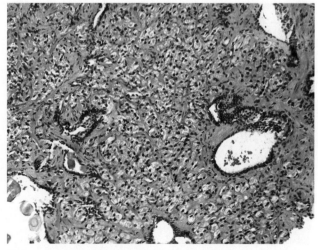

Figure 1.6.10   Gleason score 10 adenocarcinoma with foamy cytoplasm mimicking histiocytes, yet lacking interspersed inflammation.

	Signet-Ring Cell Lymphocytes	Prostate Adenocarcinoma with Signet-Ring Cell Features
Age	Any age	Typically 50 to elderly, although not rare in 40s
Location	Peripheral > transition zone	Peripheral > transition zone
Symptoms	Asymptomatic	Typically asymptomatic. Advanced disease with urinary obstructive symptoms and/or hematuria or from distant metastases
Signs	Conflicting data as to whether either focal chronic inflammation associated with elevated serum PSA levels	Serum PSA levels typically elevated, yet occasionally not increased significantly as poorly differentiated cancers not effectively produce PSA. If extension from signet-ring cell adenocarcinoma from the colon or bladder (see Section 1.43), also PSA typically not elevated
Etiology	Nonspecific, unrelated to infections. Benign lymphocytes can assume the appearance of signet ring cells, due to thermal injury	Signet-ring cell–like adenocarcinomas can be primary in the prostate and are typically high grade although Gleason pattern 3 cancers can also occasionally have signet ring features. True mucin-positive signet-ring cell adenocarcinomas involving the prostate, with rare exception, represent spread from the intestinal tract or the urinary bladder
Histology	1. Cluster of lymphocytes with scant cytoplasm with small, dark, bland nuclei *(Fig. 1.7.1)* 2. Most cells have a central nucleus surrounded by clear space with occasional cells having an eccentric nucleus and clear vacuole *(Fig. 1.7.2)* 3. Often admixed with plasma cells and other nonvacuolated lymphocytes	1. A greater degree of nuclear atypia, nucleomegaly, and prominent nucleoli compared to signet-ring cell lymphocytes *(Figs. 1.7.5 and 1.7.6)* 2. Signet-ring cell–like adenocarcinomas of the prostate contain a clear eccentric vacuole. True signet-ring cell adenocarcinoma, even on H&E-stained sections, often have a suggestion of some substance within the vacuoles; in some cases, blue-tinged mucin is visible 3. Typically admixed plasma cells and lymphocytes absent
Special studies	• Keratin stains negative • Positive for CD45 *(Figs. 1.7.3 and 1.7.4)* • Negative for mucin stains	• Immunohistochemically, high-grade cancers may not express PSA. Best markers to label high-grade prostate adenocarcinoma are keratins, such as CAM5.2 and AE1/AE3, which are not decreased in higher-grade tumors • CD45 negative • Prostatic signet-ring cell–like carcinomas are mucin negative. Secondary spread from other sites with true signet-ring cell carcinomas are mucin positive

	Signet-Ring Cell Lymphocytes	**Prostate Adenocarcinoma with Signet-Ring Cell Features**
Treatment	None	High-grade prostate adenocarcinoma stage and age dependent with localized disease treated with either radical prostatectomy or combination hormone therapy/radiation, the latter the best option in men >70 years old. Advanced disease initially treated with hormone therapy. Secondary involvement by bladder or colon signet-ring cell adenocarcinoma and only treated with chemotherapy
Prognosis	Inflammation on biopsy is not associated with an increased risk of cancer on subsequent biopsy	High-grade prostate adenocarcinoma stage dependent. Secondary involvement by bladder or colon signet-ring cell adenocarcinoma associated with a dismal prognosis

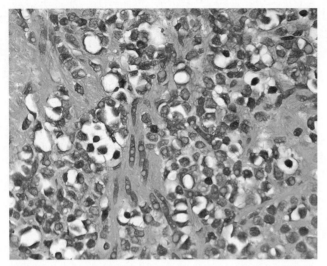

Figure 1.7.1 Bland lymphocytes with some having eccentric vacuoles.

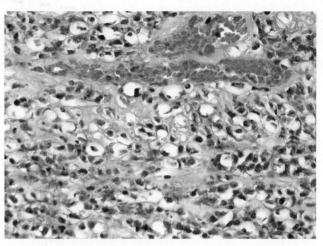

Figure 1.7.2 Lymphocytes with most having a centrally located nucleus surrounded by a clear space.

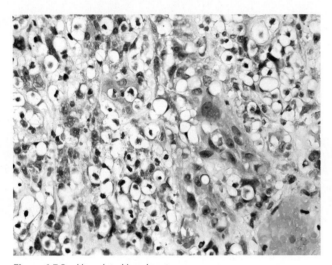

Figure 1.7.3 Vacuolated lymphocytes.

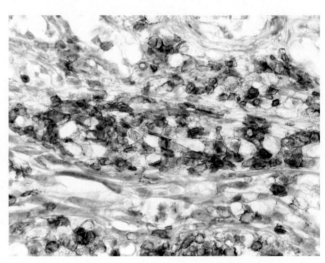

Figure 1.7.4 CD20 staining of signet-ring cell lymphocytes (same case as Fig. 1.7.3).

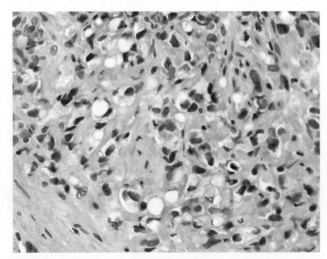

Figure 1.7.5 Gleason score 10 adenocarcinoma with vacuoles. Nuclei are more variably shaped, hyperchromatic, and larger than of lymphocytes.

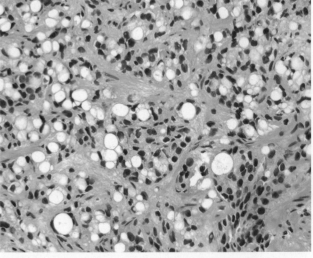

Figure 1.7.6 Extensive signet-ring cell–like change in adenocarcinoma with hyperchromatic nuclei.

	Reactive Noncribriform Prostate Glands	Prostatic Adenocarcinoma with Inflammation
Age	Any age	Typically 50 to elderly, although not rare in 40s
Location	Peripheral = transition zone	Peripheral > transition zone
Symptoms	Typically asymptomatic	Typically asymptomatic. Advanced disease with urinary obstructive symptoms and/or hematuria or from distant metastases
Signs	Conflicting data as to whether either focal acute or chronic inflammation associated with elevated serum PSA levels	Serum PSA levels variably elevated, no data if different from cancer without inflammation
Etiology	Even a few lymphocytes or neutrophils within epithelium or within acini can result in reactive atypia	Same as usual adenocarcinoma of the prostate (see Section 1.6)
Histology	1. Reactive glands can be increased in number and crowded, mimicking cancer *(Figs. 1.8.1 and 1.8.2)* 2. Nuclear enlargement, prominent nucleoli, and occasional mitotic figures *(Fig. 1.8.3)*. In some small foci, the diagnosis is "atypical inflamed glands" where cannot be distinguished reactive benign glands from carcinoma *(Fig. 1.8.4)* 3. Lacks perineural invasion	1. Cancer with inflammation has numerous crowded small glands infiltrating in between larger benign glands *(Fig. 1.8.5)* and atypical glands that extend away from inflammation *(Fig. 1.8.6)* 2. Degree of cytologic atypia in the small atypical glands is significantly greater than the adjacent benign glands even though both are associated with the same inflammation *(Fig. 1.8.7)* 3. May show perineural invasion *(Fig. 1.8.8)*
Special studies	• Immunohistochemistry for basal cell markers p63 and high molecular weight cytokeratin (HMWCK) is positive • AMACR negative *(Fig. 1.8.2)*	• Since benign glands with inflammation can mimic cancer, caution should be exercised in diagnosing cancer in the setting of inflammation. Typically, immunohistochemistry for basal cell markers (p63 and HMWCK) should be performed and entirely negative in the atypical inflamed glands *(Figs. 1.8.9 and 1.8.10)*. If only a few inflamed atypical glands present and negative for basal cell markers, may not be definitive for diagnosis of carcinoma • If positive for AMACR also helpful, yet not as critical for the diagnosis as absence of basal cells
Treatment	None	Most are Gleason score 3 + 3 = 6 with no unique treatment compared to usual carcinoma
Prognosis	No affect	Most are Gleason score 3 + 3 = 6 with no unique prognosis compared to usual carcinoma

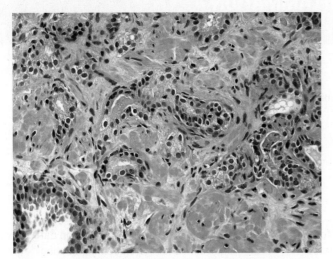

Figure 1.8.1 Crowded benign glands with intraluminal acute inflammation (*right*).

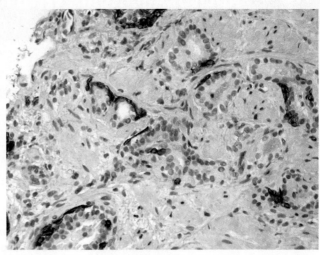

Figure 1.8.2 Same case as Figure 1.8.1 with a patchy basal cell layer for high molecular weight cytokeratin ruling out carcinoma.

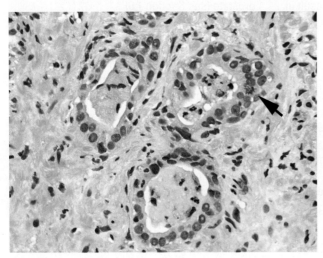

Figure 1.8.3 Benign atrophic glands with acute inflammation, nucleoli, and mitotic figure (*arrow*).

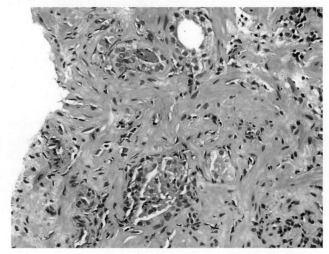

Figure 1.8.4 Cluster of crowded glands suspicious for carcinoma, yet a definitive diagnosis cannot be made due to associated inflammation.

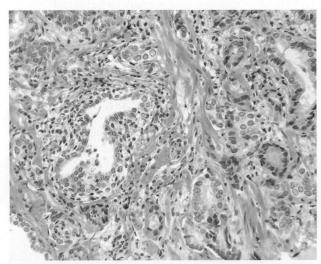

Figure 1.8.5 Small atypical glands of carcinoma associated with a lymphocytic infiltrate around benign gland (*left*).

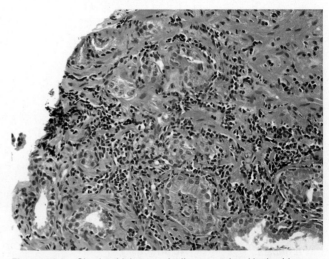

Figure 1.8.6 Glands with huge nucleoli are associated both with heavily inflamed glands (*lower*) as well as similarly atypical glands (*upper*) with less inflammation, the latter diagnostic of carcinoma.

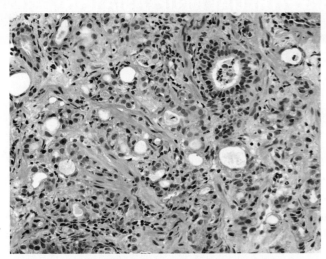

Figure 1.8.7 Inflamed cancer with greater degree of cytologically atypia compared to adjacent benign inflamed gland (*upper right*).

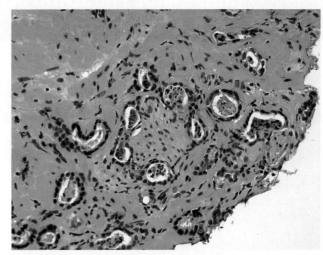

Figure 1.8.8 Perineural invasion by inflamed carcinoma glands.

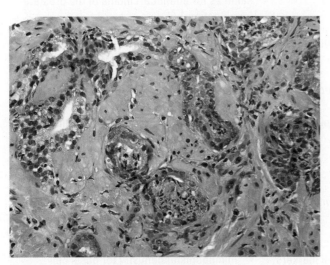

Figure 1.8.9 Adenocarcinoma with inflammation.

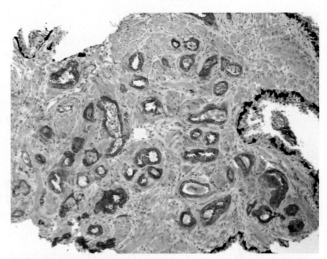

Figure 1.8.10 Same case as Figure 1.8.9 with numerous inflamed atypical glands negative for p63 and high molecular weight cytokeratin (*brown*) and positive for AMACR (*red*), consistent with carcinoma.

	Reactive Cribriform Prostate Glands	Cribriform High-Grade Prostatic Intraepithelial Neoplasia (PIN)
Age	Any age	Typically adults
Location	Peripheral = transition zone	Peripheral = transition zone
Symptoms	Typically asymptomatic	Typically asymptomatic
Signs	Conflicting data as to whether either focal acute or chronic inflammation associated with elevated serum PSA levels	None. Usually, incidentally detected on prostate needle biopsy performed for elevated serum PSA levels
Etiology	Even a few lymphocytes or neutrophils within epithelium or within acini can result in reactive atypia	As a precursor to some adenocarcinomas of the prostate, etiology assumed to be the same as for adenocarcinoma of the prostate (see Section 1.6)
Histology	1. Reactive cribriform glands have rounded contours that fit within the normal architecture of benign glands *(Fig. 1.9.1)* 2. Nuclear enlargement, prominent nucleoli, and occasional mitotic figures *(Fig. 1.9.2)* 3. Epithelium may have a streaming spindled pattern *(Fig. 1.9.1)* 4. Variable extent of acute or chronic inflammation present around and within the cribriform glands *(Fig. 1.9.3)*	1. Cribriform high-grade PIN glands have rounded contours that fit within the normal architecture of benign glands *(Fig. 1.9.4)* 2. Nuclear enlargement, prominent nucleoli, and occasional mitotic figures 3. Cribriform high-grade PIN has rigid bridges with epithelium unoriented relative to the basement membrane (i.e., no streaming) *(Fig. 1.9.4)* 4. Inflammation rarely present *(Fig. 1.9.4)*. Difficult to diagnose high-grade PIN in the setting of inflammation as it is very difficult to distinguish from reactive atypia
Special studies	• Immunohistochemistry for basal cell markers p63 and HMWCK is positive • AMACR typically negative	• Immunohistochemistry for basal cell markers p63 and HMWCK is positive, yet p63/HMWCK can be patchy or negative in occasional glands • AMACR typically positive, yet can be negative
Treatment	None	None
Prognosis	No affect	Rebiopsy depends on extent of PIN (see Section 1.33)

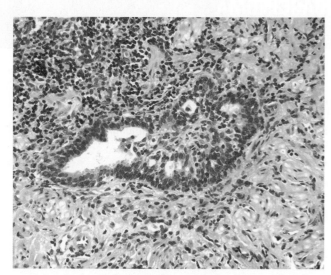

Figure 1.9.1   Partially involved inflamed benign gland with cribriform pattern. Nuclei have a slightly spindled appearance.

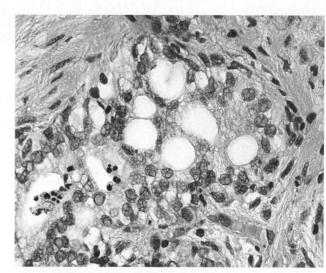

Figure 1.9.2   Inflamed benign cribriform gland with intraluminal acute inflammation. Nuclei are enlarged with visible nucleoli yet lack nuclear hyperchromasia.

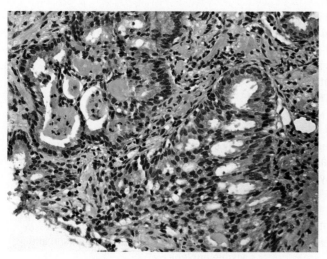

Figure 1.9.3   Inflamed benign cribriform gland with intraluminal acute inflammation.

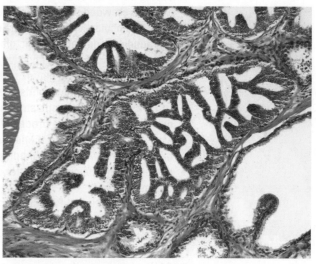

Figure 1.9.4   Cribriform high-grade PIN with rigid transluminal bridges, lacking associated inflammation.

	Post–atrophic Hyperplasia of the Prostate (PAH)	Atrophic Prostatic Adenocarcinoma
Age	Typically 50 to elderly, yet can even occur in children	Typically 50 to elderly, although not rare in 40s
Location	Peripheral > transition zone	Peripheral > transition zone
Symptoms	Asymptomatic	Same as usual adenocarcinoma of the prostate
Signs	Usually none	Same as usual adenocarcinoma of the prostate
Etiology	None	In minority of cases, associated with antiandrogen therapy
Histology	1. Very basophilic at low power due to glands' scant cytoplasm and crowded nuclei *(Fig. 1.10.1)*; at low magnification one is merely seeing a nuclear outline of the gland 2. Multiple crowded small round atrophic acini 3. Typically lobular. May see small acini surrounding a dilated atrophic gland *(Figs. 1.10.2 and 1.10.3)*. Appears invasive as a patch not as individual glands infiltrating in between larger benign glands *(Fig. 1.10.4)* 4. Often associated sclerotic stroma, mimicking an infiltrative process *(Fig. 1.10.4)* 5. May show enlarged nuclei and nucleoli with mitotic figures *(Fig. 1.10.5)*. Although larger nucleoli with inflammation, latter may be absent or scant 6. Tangential section of PAH shows multilayered cords of cells with scant cytoplasm and small bland nuclei *(Fig. 1.10.6)* 7. PAH not associated with carcinoma. In some cases, diagnosis is atypical glands, cannot rule out atrophic adenocarcinoma	1. Very basophilic at low power due to glands' scant cytoplasm and crowded nuclei 2. Multiple crowded small round atrophic acini 3. Truly infiltrative process with individual small atrophic glands situated between larger benign glands *(Figs. 1.10.7–1.10.10)* 4. Typically not associated with sclerotic stroma 5. May show enlarged nuclei and prominent nucleoli, sometimes accompanied by mitotic figures. May see more prominent nucleoli than PAH *(Fig. 1.10.11)* 6. Cords of adenocarcinoma composed of short single row of cells typically with enlarged nuclei, abundant cytoplasm, and visible nucleoli 7. May be intimately associated with less atrophic carcinoma *(Fig. 1.10.12)*
Special studies	• Immunohistochemistry for basal cell markers (p63 and HMWCK) typically strongly and diffusely positive • AMACR usually negative	• Basal cell markers entirely negative in the atypical atrophic glands *(Fig. 1.10.10)*. If only a few atypical glands present and negative for basal cell markers, may not be definitive for diagnosis of carcinoma • AMACR variably positive
Treatment	None	Same as usual adenocarcinoma
Prognosis	Not a risk factor for cancer on repeat biopsy	Same as usual adenocarcinoma

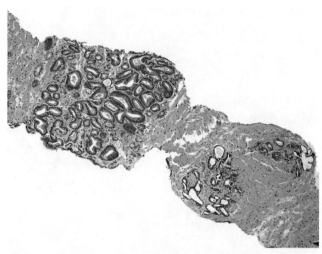

Figure 1.10.1 Benign atrophic glands (*lower right*) with very basophilic appearance compared to adenocarcinoma with amphophilic cytoplasm (*upper left*).

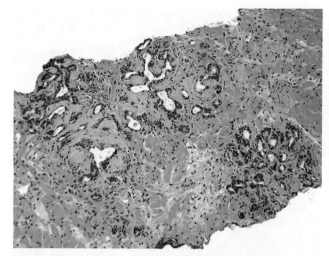

Figure 1.10.2 Lobular collections of rounded basophilic glands.

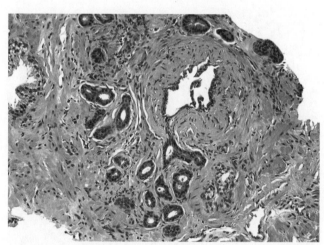

Figure 1.10.3 Post–atrophic hyperplasia with central dilated glands and surrounding smaller atrophic glands.

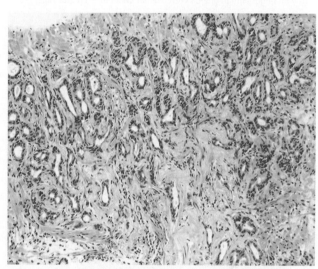

Figure 1.10.4 Post–atrophic hyperplasia with sclerosis imparting an infiltrative pattern on needle biopsy where the entire lesion is not visualized.

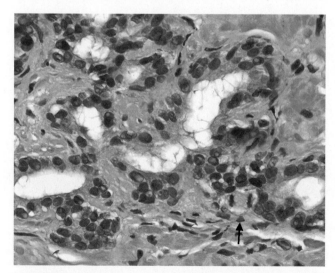

Figure 1.10.5 Post–atrophic hyperplasia showing occasional nucleoli and mitotic figure (*arrow*).

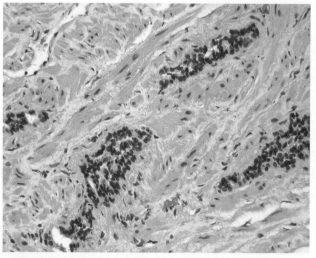

Figure 1.10.6 Tangential section of PAH with columns composed of cells with bland, small nuclei and scant cytoplasm.

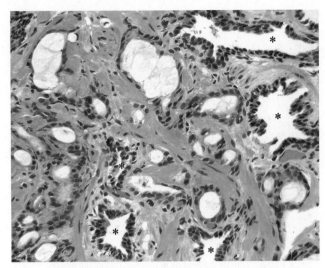

Figure 1.10.7   Small glands of atrophic adenocarcinoma infiltrating between larger benign glands with luminal undulations (*asterisk*).

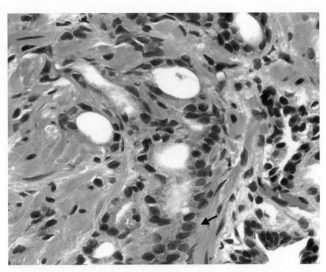

Figure 1.10.8   Higher magnification of Figure 1.10.7 showing some of the small atrophic glands of adenocarcinoma with prominent nucleoli (*arrow*).

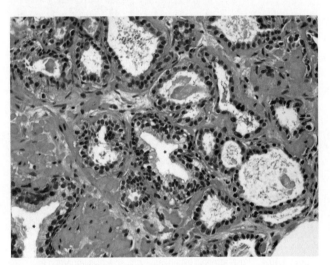

Figure 1.10.9   Atrophic adenocarcinoma infiltrating between two benign glands (*asterisk*).

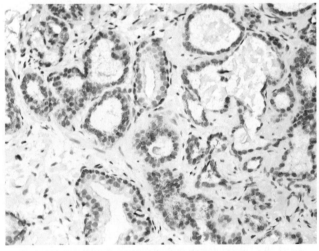

Figure 1.10.10   Triple stain of Figure 1.10.9 with atrophic adenocarcinoma lacking basal cells (*brown*) and positive for AMACR (*red*).

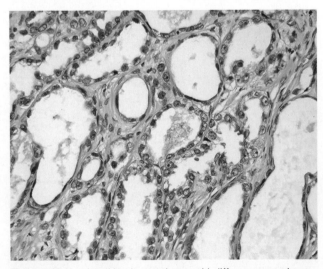

Figure 1.10.11   Atrophic adenocarcinoma with diffuse very prominent nucleoli.

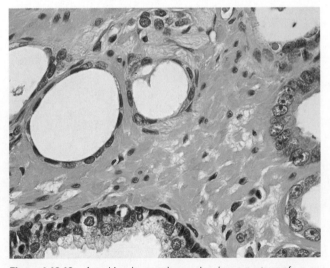

Figure 1.10.12   Atrophic adenocarcinoma showing a spectrum of nuclear atypia from none (*left*) to focal moderate (*center*) to marked (*right*) where the glands begin having slightly more cytoplasm.

	Partial Atrophy	Prostatic Adenocarcinoma
Age	Typically 50 to elderly, although not rare in 40s	Typically 50 to elderly, although not rare in 40s
Location	Peripheral > transition zone	Peripheral > transition zone
Symptoms	None	Typically, asymptomatic. Advanced disease with urinary obstructive symptoms and/or hematuria or from distant metastases
Signs	None	Serum PSA levels variably elevated, no data if different from cancer without inflammation
Etiology	None known	Same as usual adenocarcinoma of the prostate (see Section 1.6)
Histology	Most common mimicker of prostate cancer. Typically more disorganized pattern and lacks the low-magnification basophilic appearance than PAH, although can merge with glands of PAH	
	1. Crowded small/medium glands *(Figs. 1.11.1 and 1.11.2)* 2. Noninfiltrative but often multifocal *(Figs. 1.11.1 and 1.11.2)* 3. Slight undulations of luminal surface *(Figs. 1.11.3–1.11.5)* 4. Pale, lightly eosinophilic cytoplasm 5. Apical cytoplasm partially strophic with nuclei extending almost to top of the cell. Abundant lateral cytoplasm *(Figs. 1.11.3–1.11.8)* 6. Nuclei at most slightly enlarged *(Fig. 1.11.5)* 7. At most small nucleoli 8. Mitoses and apoptosis absent 9. Lumen typically lacks crystalloids, blue mucin, pink secretions	1. Crowded small/medium glands 2. May show small atypical glands on both sides of benign glands 3. Often straight luminal border *(Fig. 1.11.10)* 4. Cytoplasm may be pale or amphophilic 5. Typically more abundant apical cytoplasm 6. Nuclei may be significantly enlarged 7. May have prominent nucleoli *(Fig. 1.11.10)* 8. Occasional mitoses and apoptosis 9. Lumen may have crystalloids, blue mucin, pink secretions
Special Studies	• Immunohistochemical studies for basal cell markers (p63 and HMWCK) shows patchy positive cells in some glands and no staining in other glands *(Figs. 1.11.4 and 1.11.7)*. In some clusters of PTAT, the entire focus is negative for basal cell markers *(Fig. 1.11.9)* • AMACR can be positive in a significant minority of cases *(Fig. 1.11.4)*	• Negative for basal cell markers (p63 and HMWCK) • On biopsy, about 80% positive for AMACR
Treatment	None	Stage and age dependent
Prognosis	Not a risk factor for cancer on repeat biopsy	Cancers in the differential diagnosis with PTAT are Gleason score 3 + 3 = 6 and typically have an excellent prognosis

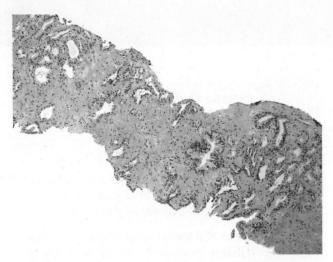

Figure 1.11.1   Multiple foci of partial atrophy on needle biopsy.

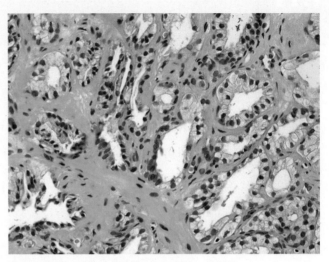

Figure 1.11.2   Higher magnification of Figure 1.11.1.

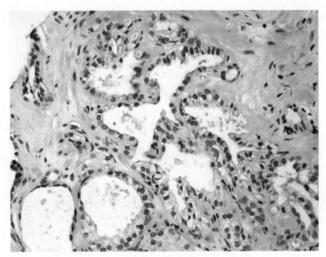

Figure 1.11.3   Partial atrophy with several glands having luminal undulation.

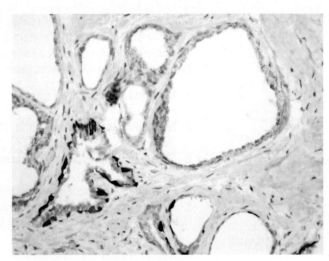

Figure 1.11.4   Triple stain of Figure 1.11.3 with several glands of partial atrophy having a patchy basal cell layer (*bottom*) with others negative for basal cells and positive for AMACR (*top*).

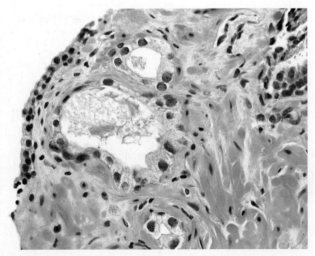

Figure 1.11.5   Partial atrophy with slightly enlarged nuclei.

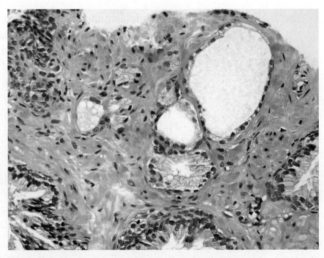

Figure 1.11.6   Partial atrophic glands admixed with some benign glands having more abundant cytoplasm.

1.11 Partial Atrophy vs. Prostatic Adenocarcinoma **33**

1 PROSTATE

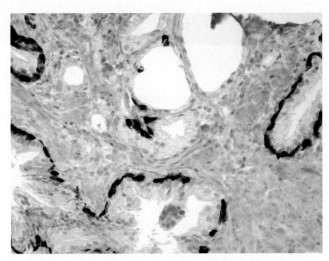

Figure 1.11.7 Some of the partially atrophic glands have patchy basal cells with others lacking high molecular weight cytokeratin staining.

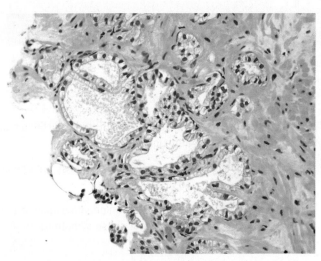

Figure 1.11.8 Classic example of partial atrophy.

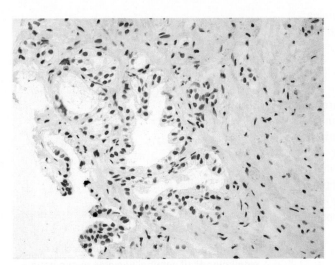

Figure 1.11.9 Partial atrophy negative for high molecular weight cytokeratin.

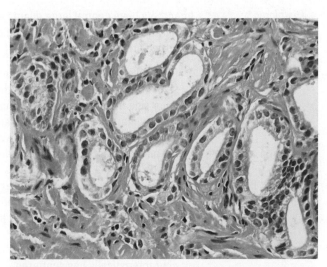

Figure 1.11.10 Adenocarcioma where malignant glands have straight luminal borders, slightly more apical cytoplasm, and numerous prominent nucleoli.

	Seminal Vesicles	Prostatic Adenocarcinoma
Age	On biopsy or TURP, typically 50 to elderly, although not rare in 40s	Typically 50 to elderly, although not rare in 40s
Location	More commonly on biopsy but can be seen on TURP	Peripheral > transition zone
Symptoms	SVs sampled on needle biopsy or TURP typically not cause symptoms	Typically asymptomatic. Advanced disease with urinary obstructive symptoms and/or hematuria or from distant metastases
Signs	Occasionally, seminal vesicle targeted for biopsy in patients with advanced cancer toward the base on imaging or rectal exam	Serum PSA levels variably elevated, no data if different from cancer without inflammation
Histology	Intact SVs have central large dilated lumina with numerous small glands budding off and clustered around the periphery *(Fig. 1.12.1)*	
	1. On needle biopsy, the dilated lumen is seen as a flat epithelial lining on the tip or side of the core, where the core has fragmented as it enters the seminal vesicle lumen. Surrounding these strips of epithelium are clusters of smaller glands *(Figs. 1.12.2–1.12.4)*. In cases when the needle biopsy does not transect the central lumen, only crowded glands are seen, which more closely mimics prostatic carcinoma *(Figs. 1.12.5–1.12.8)* 2. Epithelium in strips and small glands characteristically has scattered atypical cells with markedly enlarged, hyperchromatic, and pleomorphic nuclei. Atypia is degenerative in nature with smudgy chromatin, lacking mitotic activity *(Figs. 1.12.8 and 1.12.9)* 3. Prominent, globular, golden brown lipofuscin granules within the epithelium *(Figs. 1.12.6 and 1.12.8)*	1. Adenocarcinoma glands do not cluster around a strip of epithelium at the tip or edge of the core 2. Gleason score 6 carcinomas, which the small glands of seminal vesicles mimic have only slight to moderate nuclear atypia that is uniform throughout the gland 3. Benign prostate tissue, high-grade PIN, and rarely carcinoma may contain lipofuscin pigment, but it differs in that the granules are smaller and more red-orange or blue *(Fig. 1.12.10)*
Special studies	• Basal cell markers (p63 and HMWCK) are positive around SVs • AMACR negative • MUC6 positive • Prostatic markers (PSA, PSAP, PSMA, P501s, NKX3.1) negative	• Basal cell markers (p63 and HMWCK) are negative in carcinoma • Usually positive for AMACR • MUC6 negative • Prostatic markers (PSA, PSAP, PSMA, P501s, NKX3.1) uniformly positive in Gleason score 6 carcinomas
Treatment	None	Grade and stage dependent
Prognosis	Does not cause morbidity if biopsied	Grade and stage dependent

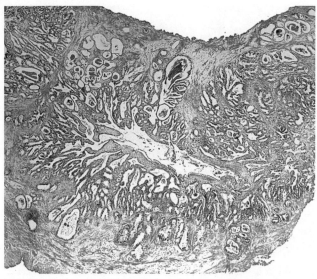

Figure 1.12.1 Seminal vesicle on a TURP showing central lumen surrounded by small glands.

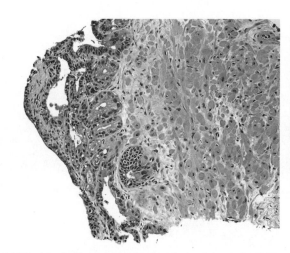

Figure 1.12.2 Needle biopsy with strip of seminal vesicle at edge (**left**) surrounded by small crowded glands.

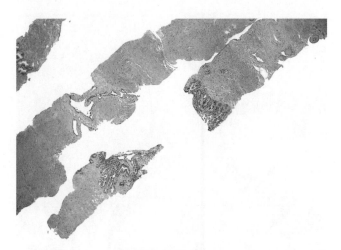

Figure 1.12.3 Needle biopsy with seminal vesicle epithelium on each side of break in tissue representing seminal vesicle lumen (*bottom core*).

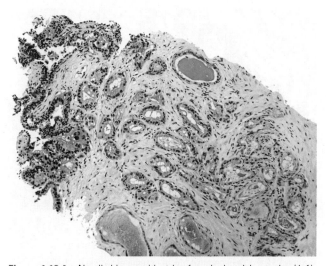

Figure 1.12.4 Needle biopsy with strip of seminal vesicle at edge (*left*) surrounded by small crowded glands.

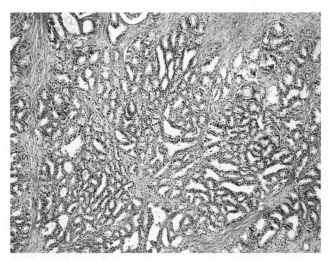

Figure 1.12.5 Crowded glands of seminal vesicle mimicking prostatic adenocarcinoma.

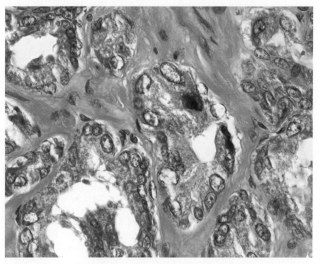

Figure 1.12.6 Higher magnification of Figure 1.12.5 where glands have degenerative atypia and golden brown lipofuscin pigment.

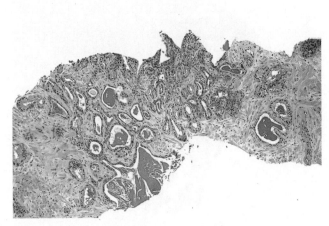

Figure 1.12.7   Crowded glands of seminal vesicle.

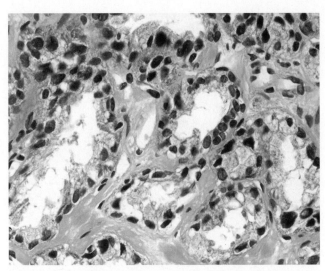

Figure 1.12.8   Same case as Figure 1.12.7 with glands showing degenerative atypia and *golden brown* lipofuscin pigment.

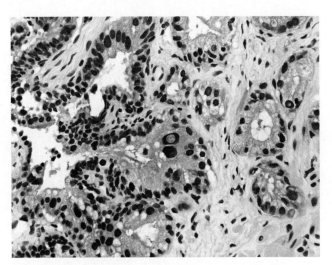

Figure 1.12.9   Degenerative atypia in seminal vesicle epithelium.

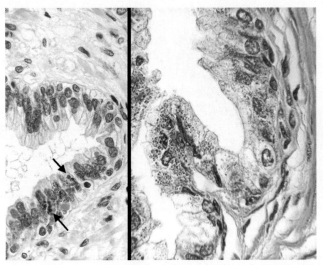

Figure 1.12.10   Benign prostate epithelium with small cytoplasmic blue (**left**, *arrows*) or red-orange (**right**) lipofuscin granules.

	Benign Prostate Tissue with Radiation Affect	Prostatic Adenocarcinoma with Radiation Affect
Age	Typically 50 to elderly, although not rare in 40s	Typically 50 to elderly, although not rare in 40s
Location	Peripheral = transition zone	Peripheral > transition zone
Symptoms	Typically asymptomatic unless bleeding from sloughed benign tissue with radiation necrosis	Typically asymptomatic unless bleeding from sloughed cancer with radiation necrosis. Advanced disease with urinary obstructive symptoms and/or hematuria or from distant metastases
Signs	Typically, following radiotherapy, serum PSA level decreases to a nadir level in men without cancer. Occasional bleeding or obstruction due to sloughed tissue with radiation necrosis within the urethra	In some men, PSA rises following radiation (nadir PSA + 2 defines radiation failure). Recommended that biopsies be performed 30–36 mo after radiotherapy
Etiology	Degree of cytologic atypia in nonneoplastic glands and degree of stromal fibrosis higher after brachytherapy compared to external beam radiation. Marked epithelial atypia tends to persist for a longer time (up to 6 y) following brachytherapy	Quiescent cancer with radiation affect or cancer without radiation affect resistant to radiation therapy
Histology	1. Glands maintain their normal architectural configuration. Nonneoplastic glands are separated by a modest amount of prostatic stroma (*Fig. 1.13.1*) 2. Typically atrophic (*Fig. 1.13.2*) 3. Multilayered with epithelium streaming parallel to the basement membrane (*Fig. 1.13.3*) 4. Scattered markedly atypical nuclei within well-formed acini (*Fig. 1.13.3*). Scattered atypical nuclei often lack apparent nucleoli and are either large with bizarre shapes or pyknotic with smudged chromatin. Occasionally nucleoli can be seen (*Fig. 1.13.2*) 5. Diagnosis is benign prostate tissue with radiation affect	1. Architecturally, inconsistent with benign glands. Cancers with radiation affect show numerous infiltrating individual epithelial cells or poorly formed glands. Usual morphology of adenocarcinoma without radiation affect (*Figs. 1.13.4–1.13.10*) 2. With radiation affect, individual cells have abundant vacuolated cytoplasm or single cells with indistinct cytoplasm (*Figs. 1.13.4–1.13.8, and 1.13.10*). Abundant cytoplasm typically in cancers without radiation affect (*Fig. 1.13.9*) 3. Cancer with radiation affect typically lacks well-formed glands vs. gland-forming cancer without radiation affect shows a single cell layer without streaming 4. Nuclei in cancer with radiation affect often benign appearing, lacking nucleoli (*Figs. 1.13.5 and 1.13.8*). Occasionally can appear pleomorphic with degenerative atypia (*Fig. 1.13.10*). In cancer without radiation affect, nuclei often have prominent nucleoli 5. Cancers with significant radiation affect are not graded. Cancers without significant radiation affect are graded the same as cancers that have not been radiated

	Benign Prostate Tissue with Radiation Affect	**Prostatic Adenocarcinoma with Radiation Affect**
Special Studies	• HMWCK and p63 show multilayered positive staining • AMACR negative	• HMWCK and p63 are negative • Often positive AMACR in both cancers with and without radiation affect
Treatment	None	Cancer with radiation affect not further treated. Cancer without radiation affect may be treated depending on age and comorbidity with salvage therapies (cryosurgery, HIFU, radical prostatectomy) and/or hormonal therapy
Prognosis	If postradiation serum PSA levels keep rising, a negative biopsy probably reflects sampling error	Cancers with radiation affect have a favorable prognosis. Cancer without radiation affect ultimately will progress

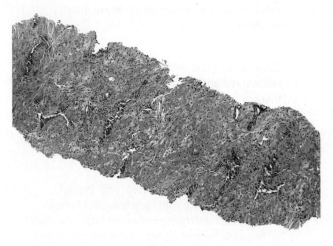

Figure 1.13.1   Benign prostate tissue with radiation atypia. At low magnification, glands are separated by a modest amount of stroma and are the size of normal benign prostate glands. Glands appear very blue due to atrophic cytoplasm.

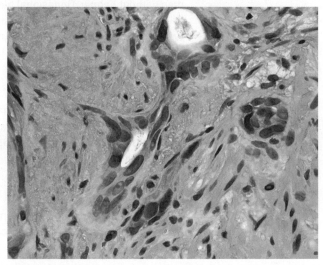

Figure 1.13.2   Atrophic benign-radiated glands. Scattered nuclei are enlarged and hyperchromatic.

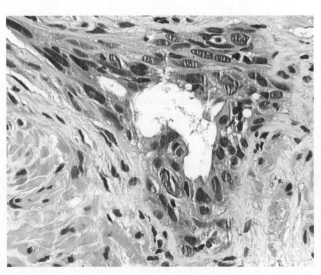

Figure 1.13.3   Multilayered benign-radiated gland with cells streaming parallel to the basement membrane.

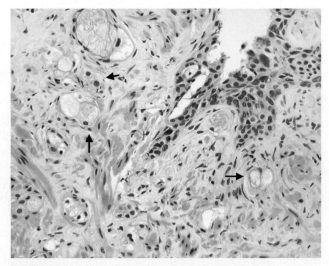

Figure 1.13.4   Scattered crowded smaller glands with vacuolated cytoplasm diagnostic of adenocarcinoma with treatment affect (*arrows*) adjacent to a larger multilayered benign gland with radiation atypia (*upper right*).

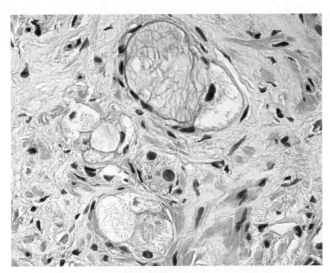

Figure 1.13.5   Higher magnification of Figure 1.13.4 with vacuolated crowded glands lined by bland nuclei.

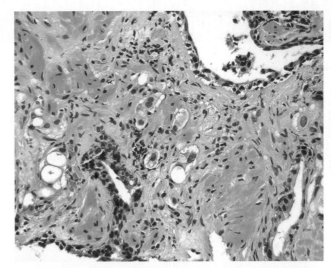

Figure 1.13.6   Radiated carcinoma with clusters of vacuolated cells invading between larger benign atrophic glands with radiation atypia.

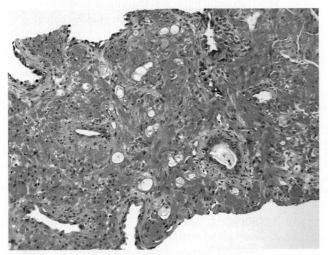

Figure 1.13.7   Crowded smaller glands with vacuolated cytoplasm diagnostic of adenocarcinoma with treatment affect in between darker, larger, more evenly spaced benign glands.

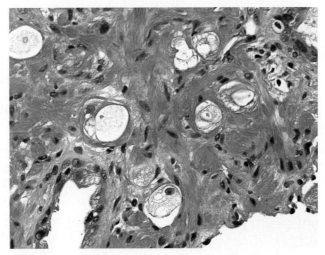

Figure 1.13.8   Higher magnification of Figure 1.13.7 with small vacuolated cancer glands (*center*) lacking prominent atypia invading between benign glands (*lower left* and *upper right*).

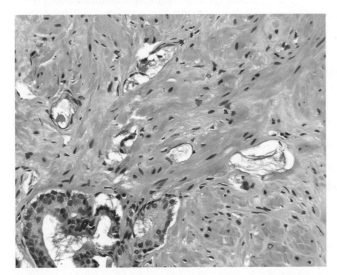

Figure 1.13.9   Atrophic glands of adenocarcinoma with abundant mucin showing treatment affect (*top*) adjacent to adenocarcinoma without treatment affect (*lower left*).

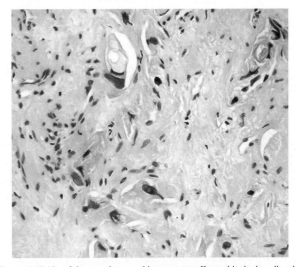

Figure 1.13.10   Adenocarcinoma with treatment affect with single cells with vacuolated cytoplasm. There is more prominent nuclear atypia, yet still with a degenerative appearance, than is typically seen in cancer with radiation affect.

	Xanthoma	Prostatic Adenocarcinoma with Hormone Therapy Affect and High-Grade Foamy Gland Carcinoma
Age	Typically, adults seen on needle biopsy, TURP, or radical prostatectomy	Typically, adults seen on needle biopsy, TURP, or radical prostatectomy
Location	Transition = peripheral zone	Transition < peripheral zone
Symptoms	Asymptomatic	May be asymptomatic or advanced disease with urinary obstructive symptoms and/or hematuria or from distant metastases
Signs	None	Serum PSA levels variably elevated
Etiology	Xanthomas unrelated to serum lipid levels	High-grade cancer mimicking xanthoma can be seen following hormonal therapy. High-grade foamy gland cancer of unknown etiology can also mimic xanthoma
Histology	1. Background may reveal stroma that is unremarkable or elastotic, yet typically not fibrotic *(Fig. 1.14.1)* 2. Collections of histiocytes in clusters *(Figs. 1.14.1 and 1.14.2)* 3. Nuclei are bland *(Figs. 1.14.1 and 1.14.3)* 4. In some cases can form cords *(Fig. 1.14.4)* 5. Foci are typically small, yet occasionally can occupy larger areas *(Fig. 1.14.5)*	1. Hormone-treated patients with typically fibrotic stroma *(Fig. 1.14.8)*. High-grade foamy gland cancer has variably fibrotic stroma 2. Neoplastic glands can develop pyknotic nuclei and abundant xanthomatous cytoplasm resembling histiocytes *(Figs. 1.14.8 and 1.14.9)*. Histiocytic-appearing cancer cells can be seen as desquamated cells in cancer lumina or as scattered cells in the stroma. Xanthomatous cytoplasm also seen in high-grade foamy gland cancer *(Fig. 1.14.10)* 3. Small bland nuclei can be seen in cancers following hormonal therapy and in foamy gland cancer *(Figs. 1.14.9–1.14.12)* 4. Can form cords and single cells 5. Typically Gleason score 10 adenocarcinoma is extensive on TURP and needle biopsy, although uncommon cases exist with small foci of high-grade cancer
Special studies	• Negative for keratins such as CAM5.2 and AE1/AE3 • Positive for CD68 *(Figs. 1.14.6 and 1.14.7)*	• Positive for keratins, such as CAM5.2 or AE1/Ae3. Prostate markers may be negative in Gleason score 10 adenocarcinoma • CD68 negative
Treatment	None	High-grade foamy gland cancer same treatment as usual high-grade cancer
Prognosis	Inflammation on biopsy is not associated with an increased risk of cancer on subsequent biopsy	Following a response to combination endocrine therapy, the grade of the tumor appears artifactually higher and should not be assigned a Gleason score. High-grade foamy gland cancer same poor prognosis as usual high-grade cancer

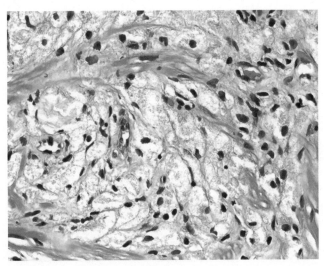

Figure 1.14.1   Xanthoma with bland cells.

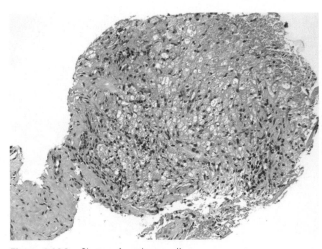

Figure 1.14.2   Cluster of xanthoma cells.

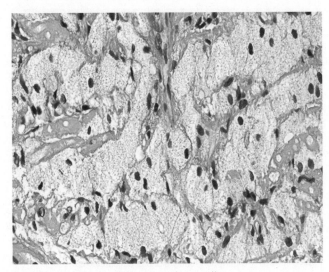

Figure 1.14.3   Bland cytology of xanthoma cells.

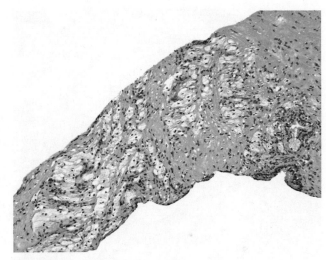

Figure 1.14.4   Cords of xanthoma cells.

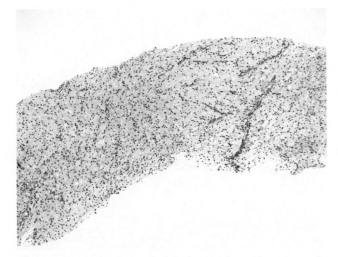

Figure 1.14.5   Unusual case of relatively extensive xanthoma on needle biopsy.

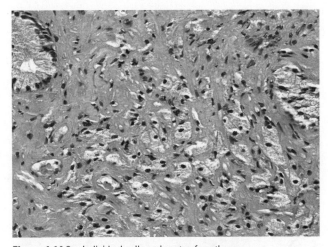

Figure 1.14.6   Individual cells and nests of xanthoma.

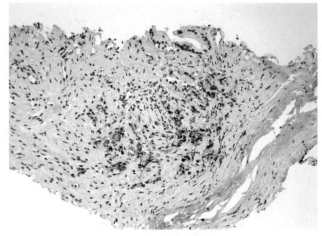

Figure 1.14.7   Same case as Figure 1.14.6 with positive staining for CD68.

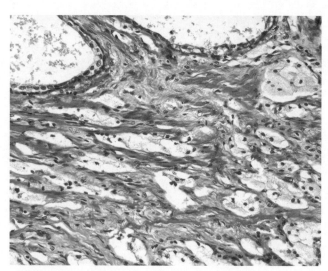

Figure 1.14.8   Adenocarcinoma with hormone treatment affect consisting of nests of cells with foamy cytoplasm in a slightly fibrotic stroma.

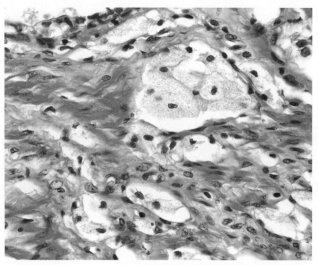

Figure 1.14.9   Higher magnification of Figure 1.14.8 showing cords of cells resembling xanthoma. Focal glandular differentiation is noted (*top*).

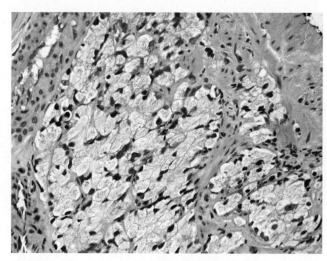

Figure 1.14.10   High-grade foamy gland adenocarcinoma.

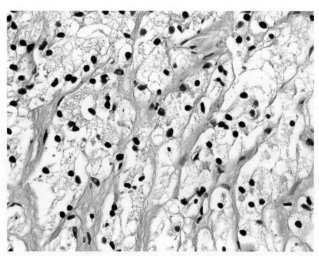

Figure 1.14.11   Hormone-treated prostate cancer with pyknotic hyperchromatic nuclei and abundant xanthomatous cytoplasm.

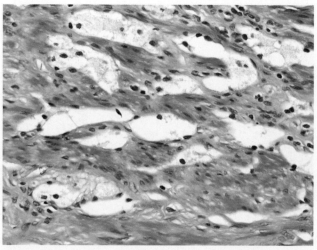

Figure 1.14.12   Adenocarcinoma of the prostate with hormone therapy affect with small nuclei, xanthomatous cytoplasm, and clear cleft-like spaces lined by pyknotic tumor nuclei resembling lymphocytes.

	Basal Cell Hyperplasia with Nucleoli	High-Grade Prostatic Intraepithelial Neoplasia
Age	Typically, adults seen on needle biopsy, TURP, or radical prostatectomy	Typically adults
Location	Transition > peripheral zone	Peripheral = transition zone
Symptoms	Asymptomatic	Typically asymptomatic
Signs	None	Usually incidentally detected on biopsy performed for elevated serum PSA levels
Etiology	Usually nonspecific and focal. If diffuse, usually associated with antiandrogen therapy. Basal cells with nucleoli can be seen as a component of normal glands as either single or multiple rows of cells underlying secretory cells or as a hyperplastic process	See Section 1.6
Histology	1. Basal cells with blue nuclei having prominent nucleoli undermining secretory cells with red/violet nuclei lacking prominent nucleoli *(Fig. 1.15.1)*. Basal cells in normal glands or in basal cell hyperplasia may have prominent nucleoli *(Figs. 1.15.1 and 1.15.2)* 2. May consist of proliferation of small crowded glands *(Fig. 1.15.2)* 3. Basal cell nuclei tend to be round *(Figs. 1.15.2 and 1.15.3)* 4. Occasional solid nests *(Figs. 1.15.2 and 1.15.3)* 5. May have coarse calcifications *(Fig. 1.15.4)* 6. Glandular lumina have atrophic cytoplasm *(Fig. 1.15.3)* 7. Pseudocribriform glands with back to back to individual glands maintaining their own identity *(Figs. 1.15.5 and 1.15.6)*	1. Basal cells are often indistinct and lack prominent nucleoli with overlying high-grade PIN nuclei having prominent nucleoli *(Figs. 1.15.8–1.15.10)*. May show maturation of high-grade PIN nuclei with more benign-appearing nuclei toward the center of the gland *(Fig. 1.15.10)* 2. Large architecturally benign glands without much crowding 3. High-grade PIN nuclei are columnar *(Figs. 1.15.8 and 1.15.9)* 4. Lacks solid nests; has well-formed lumina *(Figs. 1.15.8 and 1.15.9)* 5. Lacks calcifications 6. Glandular lumina have nonatrophic cytoplasm *(Figs. 1.15.9 and 1.15.10)* 7. True cribriform glands with rounded sheet of cells having punched out lumina and more benign-appearing nuclei in the center *(Fig. 1.15.11)*
Special Studies	• Atypical nuclei positive for HMWCK/p63 although staining not present in all cells; within a nest or gland, centrally located cells may not be immunoreactive *(Fig. 1.15.7)* • AMACR negative	• Atypical nuclei negative for HMWCK/p63 with often a patchy basal cell layer positive for HMWCK/p63 *(Fig. 1.15.12)* • AMACR frequently positive
Treatment	None	None
Prognosis	Basal cells with prominent nucleoli were in the past called "atypical basal cell hyperplasia." As no worse prognosis than basal cell hyperplasia without nucleoli should merely be called basal cells or basal cell hyperplasia with prominent nucleoli	Rebiopsy depends on the extent of PIN (see Section 1.33)

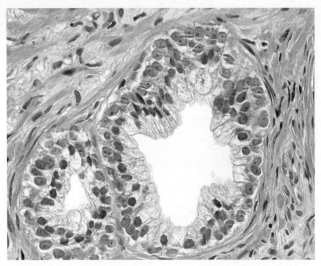

Figure 1.15.1   Basal cells with blue-gray nuclei containing prominent nucleoli undermine secretory cells with red-violet nuclei.

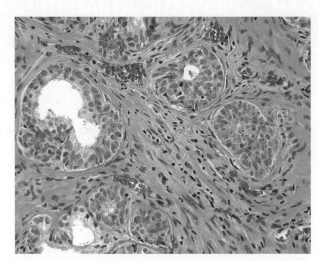

Figure 1.15.2   Proliferation of small glands of basal cell hyperplasia with prominent nucleoli. While one gland is larger resembling high-grade PIN (*upper left*), others are small with either a small central lumen with atrophic cytoplasm or composed of solid nests.

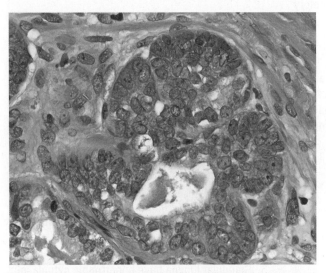

Figure 1.15.3   Basal cell hyperplasia with prominent nucleoli composed of solid nests surrounding the central lumen with atrophic cytoplasm.

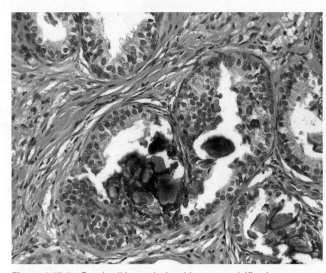

Figure 1.15.4   Basal cell hyperplasia with coarse calcifications.

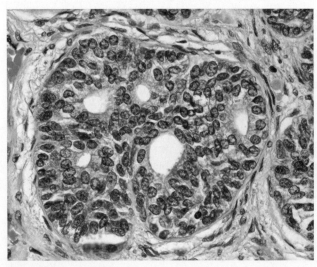

Figure 1.15.5   Pseudocribriform hyperplasia back-to-back glands of basal cell hyperplasia.

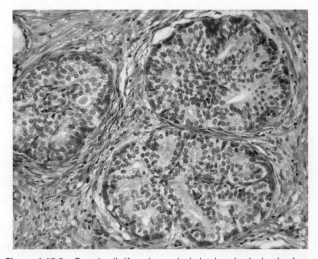

Figure 1.15.6   Pseudocribriform hyperplasia back-to-back glands of basal cell hyperplasia. Each gland maintains its integrity, where one can still identify each gland surrounding a lumen.

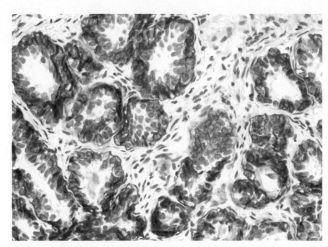

Figure 1.15.7 High molecular weight cytokeratin stain of basal cell hyperplasia labeling multilayered peripheral cells with prominent nucleoli.

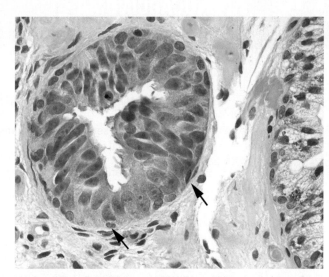

Figure 1.15.8 Tufted high-grade PIN with small basal cells (*arrows*) and overlying columnar PIN nuclei with prominent nucleoli.

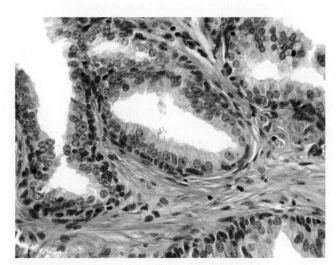

Figure 1.15.9 Flat high-grade PIN with small bland basal cells undermines columnar cells with nuclei containing prominent nucleoli.

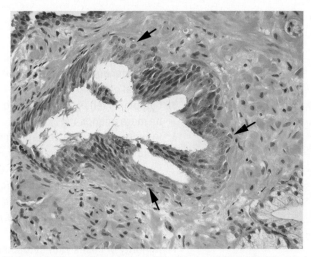

Figure 1.15.10 Tufted high-grade PIN with maturation of nuclei toward the center of the gland. However, note the presence of a distinct bland basal cell layer (*arrows*) with an abrupt transition to overlying atypical high-grade PIN nuclei.

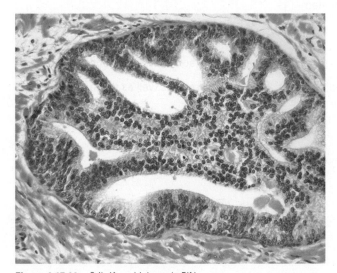

Figure 1.15.11 Cribriform high grade PIN.

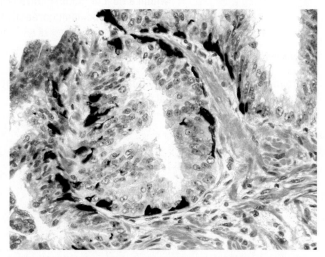

Figure 1.15.12 Patchy basal cell staining with p63 and high molecular weight cytokeratin. Overlying atypical PIN nuclei are negative.

	Basal Cell Hyperplasia with Nucleoli	Prostatic Adenocarcinoma
Age	Typically adults seen on needle biopsy, TURP, or radical prostatectomy	Typically 50 to elderly, although not rare in 40s
Location	Transition > peripheral zone	Peripheral > transition zone
Symptoms	Asymptomatic	Typically asymptomatic. Advanced disease with urinary obstructive symptoms and/or hematuria or from distant metastases
Signs	None	Serum PSA levels variably elevated
Etiology	If focal, none known. If diffuse, usually associated with antiandrogen therapy	Cases mimicking basal cell hyperplasia consist of either individual glands of Gleason pattern 3 or cribriform glands of Gleason pattern 4
Histology	1. May have solid nests of cells (Fig. 1.16.1) 2. Cases that most closely mimic carcinoma have retention of lumina with only a couple of basal cell layers (Figs. 1.16.2–1.16.5) 3. Cytoplasm tends to be atrophic, yet can be more abundant (Fig. 1.16.3) 4. Glands can be crowded and in between acini appearing infiltrative (Fig. 1.16.3) 5. Very prominent nucleoli with occasional mitotic figures can be seen (Fig. 1.16.5) 6. Often with calcifications (Fig. 1.16.6) 7. Minority of cases with cytoplasmic eosinophilic globules (Fig. 1.16.7)	1. Solid cell nests not a pattern of adenocarcinoma 2. Typically, there is only a single cell layer, yet occasionally cancers can appear multilayered (Fig. 1.16.9) 3. Cytoplasm tends to be abundant (Fig. 1.16.9) 4. Glands can be crowded and situated between benign with an infiltrative appearance 5. Very prominent nucleoli with occasional mitotic figures can be seen 6. Rare carcinomas can have calcifications (Fig. 1.16.10) 7. Cancers lack cytoplasmic eosinophilic globules
Special Studies	• Atypical nuclei positive for HMWCK/p63 although staining not present in all cells; within a nest or gland, centrally located cells may not be immunoreactive • AMACR negative (Fig. 1.16.8)	• Cancer glands negative for HMWCK/p63 • AMACR variably positive
Treatment	None	Depends on grade as well as stage
Prognosis	Benign. Should not use the term "atypical basal cell hyperplasia"	Depends on grade as well as stage

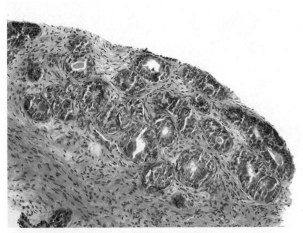

Figure 1.16.1   Basal cell hyperplasia on needle biopsy consisting of multilayered glands and solid nests.

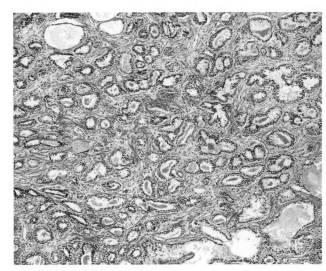

Figure 1.16.2   Basal cell hyperplasia.

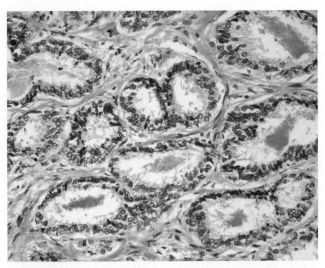

Figure 1.16.3   Same case as Figure 1.16.2 with two rows of basal cells and scant cytoplasm.

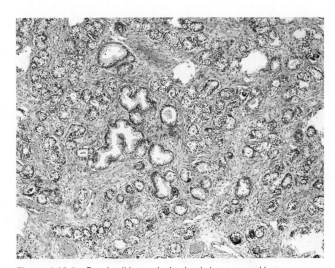

Figure 1.16.4   Basal cell hyperplasia glands interspersed between usual prostate glands.

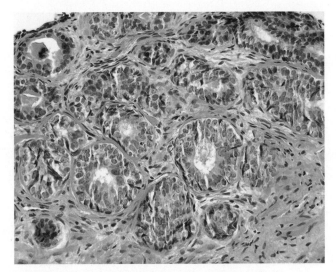

Figure 1.16.5   Basal cell hyperplasia with prominent nucleoli.

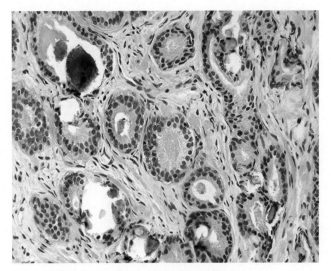

Figure 1.16.6   Basal cell hyperplasia with calcification.

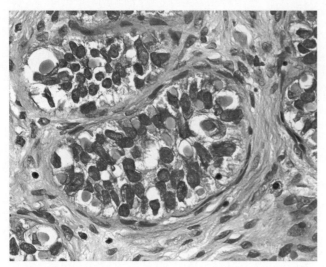

Figure 1.16.7   Same case as Figure 1.16.6 with numerous intracytoplasmic globules.

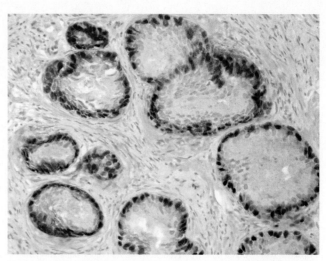

Figure 1.16.8   HMWCK and p63 staining of basal cell hyperplasia.

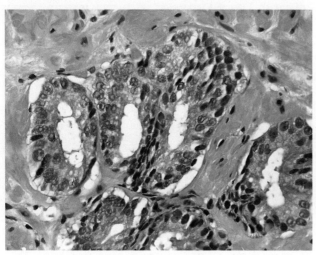

Figure 1.16.9   Adenocarcinoma with multilayered nuclei.

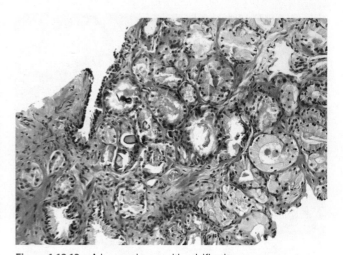

Figure 1.16.10   Adenocarcinoma with calcifications.

	Basal Cell Hyperplasia	Basal Cell Carcinoma
Age	Typically adults, more commonly on TURP or radical prostatectomy compared to needle biopsy	Typically adults seen on needle biopsy, TURP, or radical prostatectomy
Location	Transition > peripheral zone	Transition > peripheral zone
Symptoms	Asymptomatic	Typically urinary obstructive symptoms
Signs	None	None. Serum PSA levels not elevated as a result of basal cell carcinoma
Etiology	Usually nonspecific and focal. If diffuse, usually associated with antiandrogen therapy. In cases mimicking carcinoma, seen as a hyperplastic process	No risk factors known. Basal cell hyperplasia does not progress to basal cell carcinoma
Histology	1. Uniformly sized small glands or nests with multilayered basal cells *(Fig. 1.17.1)*. May be extensive and appear diffusely as opposed to nodular *(Fig. 1.17.2)* 2. Pseudocribriform or cribriform glands *(Fig. 1.17.3)* 3. Lack of large nests and absence of necrosis 4. Lack of central eosinophilic cells 5. May have prominent nucleoli yet not pleomorphic *(Fig. 1.17.4)* 6. Confined to the prostate. Lacks perineural invasion 7. Lack of prominent stromal reaction, although occasionally slightly myxoid *(Fig. 1.17.1)*	1. Variably small/medium-sized nests with irregular shapes with multilayered basal cells *(Figs. 1.17.5 and 1.17.6)* 2. Adenoid cystic pattern *(Fig. 1.17.7)* 3. Large basaloid nests with necrosis *(Fig. 1.17.8)* 4. Anastomosing basaloid nests and tubules centrally lined by eosinophilic cells *(Fig. 1.17.9)* 5. Indistinguishable from basal cell hyperplasia *(Fig. 1.17.10)* 6. Extension into periprostatic adipose tissue, seminal vesicles, or bladder neck muscle *(Fig. 1.17.10)*. May show perineural invasion 7. Occasional dense or myxoid stromal reaction *(Fig. 1.17.11)*
Special Studies	• Lack of diffuse strong BCL2 staining • Ki-67 typically <5% and should not be >20% • Basal cell markers (p63 and HMWCK) may highlight multiple cell layers, just the outermost layers or only a few scattered cells with some negative for HMWCK	• Strong diffuse strong BCL2 staining • May show Ki-67 >20% *(Fig. 1.17.12)* • Basal cell markers (p63 and HMWCK) may highlight multiple cell layers, just the outermost layers or only a few scattered cells with some negative for HMWCK
Treatment	None	Radical prostatectomy depending on stage, age, and comorbidity
Prognosis	Basal cells with prominent nucleoli were in the past called "atypical basal cell hyperplasia." As no worse prognosis than basal cell hyperplasia without nucleoli should merely be called basal cells or basal cell hyperplasia with prominent nucleoli	Can locally recur. Distant metastases most commonly seen with large solid nests with central necrosis, high Ki-67 rate, and less staining with basal cell markers

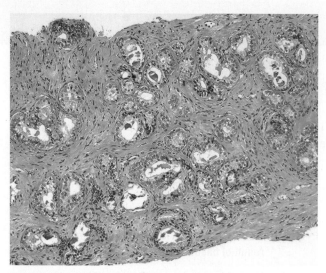

Figure 1.17.1 Basal cell hyperplasia on needle biopsy consisting of crowded, uniformly sized, and distributed small glands in prostatic stroma without a desmoplastic reaction.

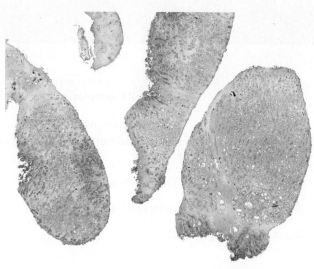

Figure 1.17.2 Extensive basal cell hyperplasia on TURP.

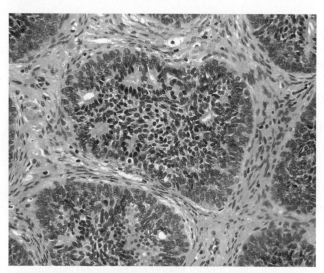

Figure 1.17.3 Pseudocribriform structure with individual well-defined glands surrounded by solid cells.

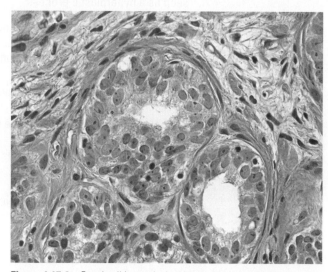

Figure 1.17.4 Basal cell hyperplasia with prominent nucleoli.

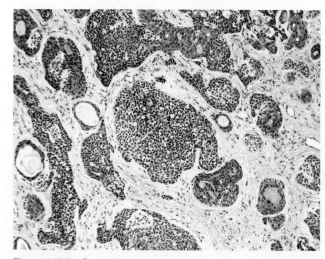

Figure 1.17.5 Basal cell carcinoma with irregular variably sized glands and nests in a desmoplastic stroma. Within inner aspect of some nests are tubules lined by eosinophilic cytoplasm.

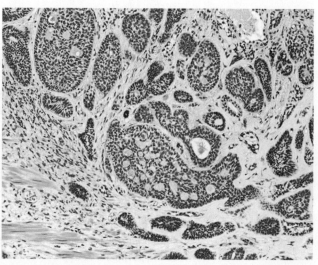

Figure 1.17.6 Small and medium nests of basal cell carcinoma in a desmoplastic stroma.

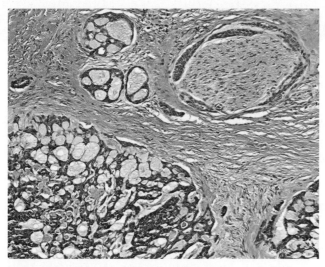

Figure 1.17.7 Adenoid cystic pattern of basal cell carcinoma with perineural invasion.

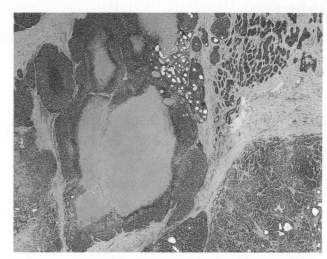

Figure 1.17.8 Basal cell carcinoma with solid nests with necrosis.

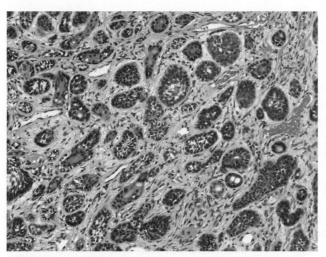

Figure 1.17.9 Small nests of basal cell carcinoma with tubules lined by eosinophilic cytoplasm.

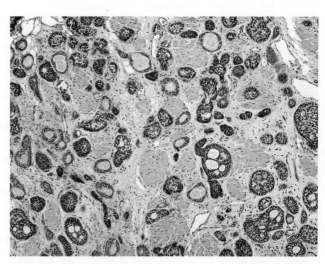

Figure 1.17.10 Basal cell carcinoma resembling basal cell hyperplasia. Nests and tubules infiltrated thick bladder neck muscle diagnostic of carcinoma.

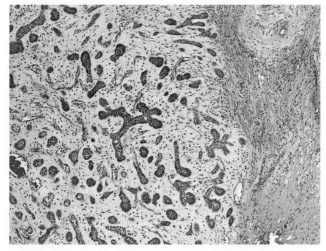

Figure 1.17.11 Basal cell carcinoma with prominent myxoid stromal reaction.

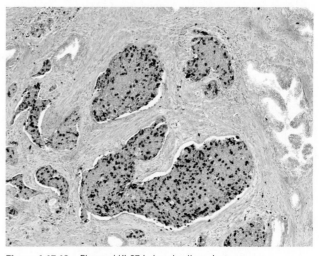

Figure 1.17.12 Elevated Ki-67 in basal cell carcinoma.

	Cowper Glands	Foamy Gland Prostatic Adenocarcinoma
Age	Typically adults seen on needle biopsy, uncommonly on TURP	Same as usual prostate adenocarcinoma
Location	Located just distal to the prostate in skeletal muscle of the urogenital diaphragm	Same as usual prostate adenocarcinoma
Symptoms	Normal anatomical structure. No symptoms	Typically asymptomatic
Signs	Normal anatomical structure. No signs	Detected as a result of abnormal digital rectal examination or elevated serum PSA level
Etiology	Typically not biopsied since external to the prostate but occasionally sampled on apical biopsy	Same as usual prostate adenocarcinoma
Histology	1. Crowded Cowper glands in skeletal muscle *(Fig. 1.18.1)*. No prostate tissue in core with Cowper glands 2. Lobular pattern *(Fig. 1.18.2)* 3. Dimorphic population of nonmucinous ducts and mucinous acini *(Figs. 1.18.2 and 1.18.3)*. Lacks dense pink intraluminal secretions 4. Distended rounded cells with distinct cell borders *(Fig. 1.18.3)* 5. Small, round, bland, basally situated nuclei *(Fig. 1.18.3)* 6. Glandular lumina are often totally or subtotally occluded *(Fig. 1.18.2)*	1. Crowded well-formed glands in prostate tissue *(Fig. 1.18.6)* 2. Diffuse growth pattern *(Fig. 1.18.7)* 3. Uniform population of mucinous acini *(Fig. 1.18.8)* 4. Columnar cells lacking the distended ovoid cytoplasm *(Figs. 1.18.9 and 1.18.10)* 5. Small, round, bland, basally situated nuclei, uncommon to see prominent nucleoli *(Figs. 1.18.9–1.18.11)* 6. Glandular lumina well developed with dense pink amorphous secretions *(Fig. 1.18.8)*
Special Studies	• Acini positive for neutral mucin *(Fig. 1.18.4)* • PSA negative • HMWCK and p63 outline the peripheral of acini *(Fig. 1.18.5)*	• Negative for neutral mucin • PSA positive • Lacks HMWCK and p63 *(Fig. 1.18.12)*
Treatment	None	Same as usual prostate adenocarcinoma
Prognosis	Normal structures that only very rarely develop neoplasia	Patients with differential diagnosis of Cowper glands are Gleason score 3 + 3 = 6. Less frequently, foamy gland cancer can be higher grade with cribriform or poorly formed glands (Gleason pattern 4) or lack of gland formation (Gleason pattern 5)

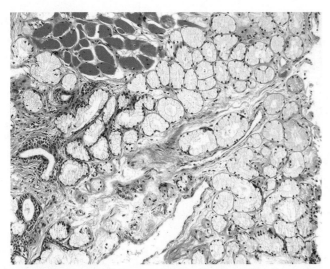

Figure 1.18.1   Cowper glands in skeletal muscle.

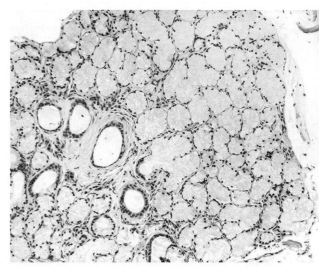

Figure 1.18.2   Lobular Cowper glands with mucinous glands and atrophic ducts lined by cuboidal nonmucinous epithelium. Distended cytoplasm results in small central lumina.

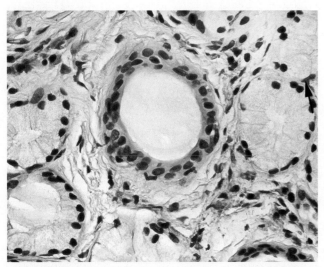

Figure 1.18.3   Higher magnification of Figure 1.18.2 with central duct and surrounding mucinous glands. Some cells have rounded distended appearance (*arrow*).

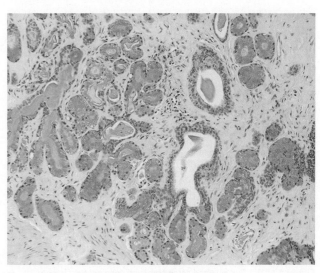

Figure 1.18.4   Mucicarmine-positive Cowper glands.

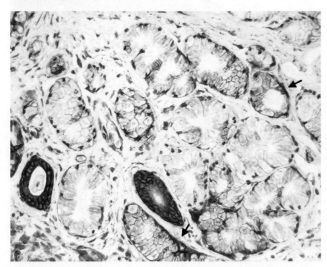

Figure 1.18.5   Cowper glands lined by HMWCK-positive basal cells (*arrows*).

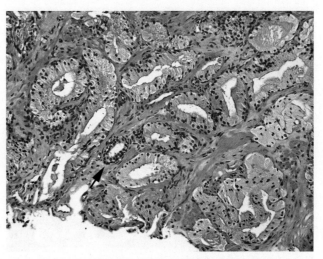

Figure 1.18.6   Foamy gland carcinoma infiltrating in prostate stroma around the benign gland (*arrow*).

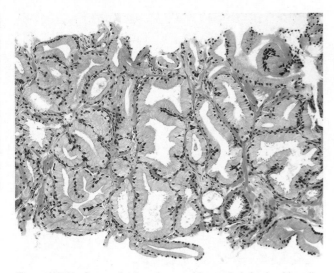

Figure 1.18.7 Foamy gland carcinoma with crowded glands with well-formed open lumina.

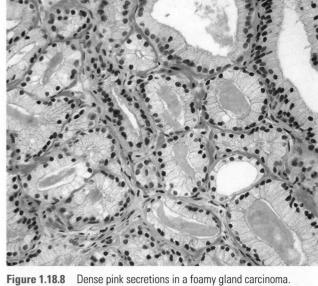

Figure 1.18.8 Dense pink secretions in a foamy gland carcinoma.

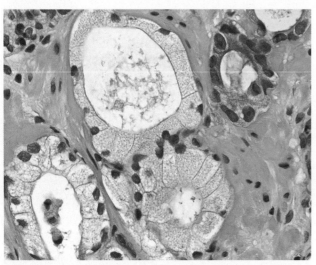

Figure 1.18.9 Foamy gland carcinoma with cuboidal to columnar bland nuclei. More atypical nuclei are seen in adjacent nonfoamy gland carcinoma (*upper right*).

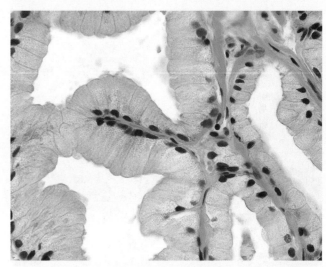

Figure 1.18.10 Foamy gland carcinoma with bland nuclei and columnar cells with abundant xanthomatous-appearing cytoplasm.

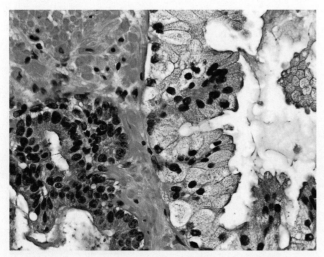

Figure 1.18.11 Foamy gland carcinoma (*right*) with bland nuclei compared to usual prostate cancer with greater cytologic atypia (*left*).

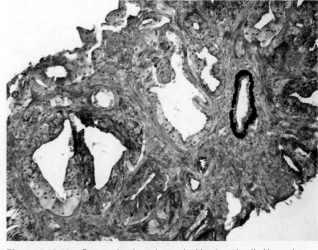

Figure 1.18.12 Foamy gland carcinoma lacking basal cells (*brown*) and positive for AMACR (*red*). An entrapped benign gland surrounded by basal cells is present (same case as Fig. 1.18.6).

	Adenosis	Prostatic Adenocarcinoma
Age	Adults, more commonly on TURP or radical prostatectomy compared to needle biopsy. Diffuse adenosis of the peripheral zone (DAPZ) predilection for men in their 40s–50s	Typically 50 to elderly, although not rare in 40s
Location	Transition > peripheral zone. DAPZ: Predominantly the peripheral zone	Peripheral > transition zone
Symptoms	Asymptomatic	Typically asymptomatic. Advanced disease with urinary obstructive symptoms and/or hematuria or from distant metastases
Signs	None	Serum PSA levels variably elevated
Etiology	No known risk factors	Cases mimicking adenosis consist of individual glands of Gleason pattern 3
Histology	1. Lobular collection of glands, easier to appreciate on TURP or radical prostatectomy compared to needle biopsy *(Figs. 1.19.1–1.19.3)*. Can be minimal infiltration at periphery 2. Typically small but can extensively involve the entire core or large percentage of a TURP specimen. DAPZ involves multiple cores 3. Glands can be as crowded as cancer with back-to-back glands *(Figs. 1.19.2–1.19.4)* 4. Small glands share features with admixed larger more benign-appearing glands *(Fig. 1.19.4)* 5. Scattered poorly formed glands and single cells can be seen due to tangential sectioning *(Fig. 1.19.5)* 6. Pale–clear cytoplasm 7. Indistinct or small- or medium-sized nucleoli 8. Blue mucinous secretions rare 9. Corpora amylacea common *(Fig. 1.19.6)* 10. Intraluminal crystalloids common *(Fig. 1.19.7)* 11. Can be admixed with basal cell hyperplasia or clear cell cribriform hyperplasia	1. Haphazard growth pattern, easier to appreciate on TURP or radical prostatectomy compared to needle biopsy *(Fig. 1.19.9)*. Some cases may appear lobular, mimicking adenosis *(Figs. 1.19.10–1.19.12)* 2. Range in size from focal to extensive 3. Glands often crowded, yet not a differentiating feature from adenosis 4. Small glands differ from adjacent benign glands in terms of nuclear, cytoplasmic, or luminal features *(Fig. 1.19.11)* 5. Scattered poorly formed glands and single cells can be seen due to tangential sectioning of Gleason pattern 3 6. Occasionally amphophilic cytoplasm 7. Range of size of nucleoli with occasionally large nucleoli 8. Blue mucinous secretions common 9. Corpora amylacea rare 10. Intraluminal crystalloids common 11. Typically not admixed with benign mimickers of carcinoma

	Adenosis	**Prostatic Adenocarcinoma**
Special Studies	• HMWCK and p63 positive, yet typically only a few glands per nodule having immunoreactive basal cells. Positive glands typically show patchy basal cell staining of one to two basal cells per glands *(Fig. 1.19.8)* • AMACR positive in 10%–25% of cases	• Carcinomas are negative for HMWCK and p63 with uncommon exceptions (see Sections 1.46 and 1.47) *(Fig. 1.19.12)* • AMACR positive in 80% of carcinomas on biopsy
Treatment	None	Grade and stage dependent
Prognosis	Also known as atypical adenomatous hyperplasia (AAH), which is not a preferred term since not associated with an increased risk of subsequent adenocarcinoma. DAPZ has an increased risk of prostate adenocarcinoma on subsequent rebiopsy	Cases mimicking adenosis typically Gleason scores 6

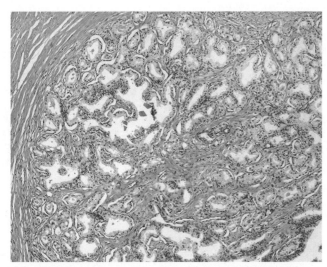

Figure 1.19.1   Lobular focus of adenosis. Glands lack interspersed large bundles of smooth muscle.

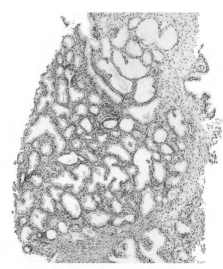

Figure 1.19.2   Adenosis on needle where a lobular pattern can still be appreciated.

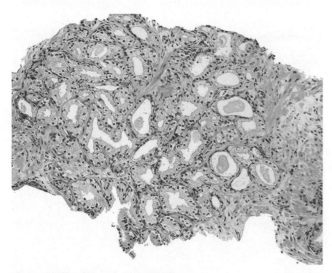

Figure 1.19.3   Adenosis on needle biopsy.

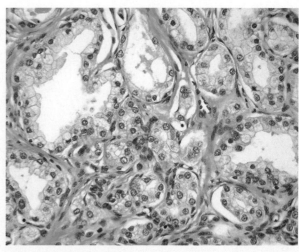

Figure 1.19.4   Same case as Figure 1.19.1 with small crowded glands sharing cytoplasmic and nuclear features with more benign-appearing glands (*left*).

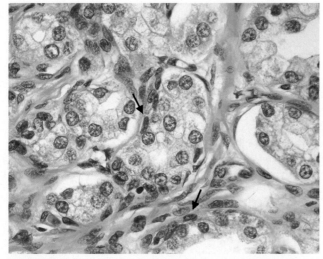

Figure 1.19.5   Same case as Figure 1.19.1 with some glands with a visible basal cell layer (*arrows*). Some of the glands are tangentially sectioned (*left*).

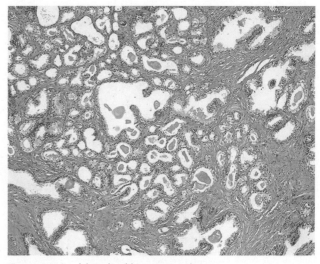

Figure 1.19.6   Adenosis with corpora amylacea.

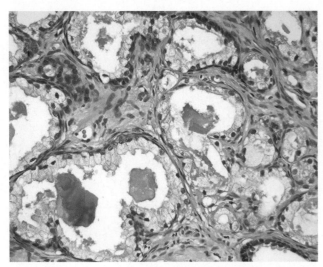

Figure 1.19.7   Same case as Figure 1.19.1 with crystalloids.

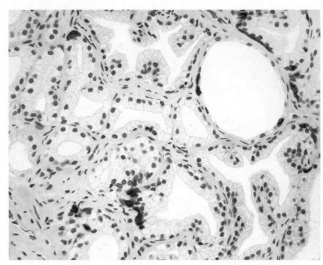

Figure 1.19.8   Same case as Figure 1.19.1 with adenosis showing some glands with HMWCK patchy, positive basal cells and other glands negative. Negative glands have the same morphology as positive glands.

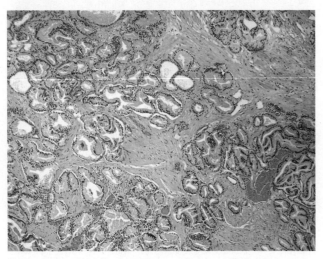

Figure 1.19.9   Irregular growth pattern of cancer with glands interspersed between large bundles of smooth muscle.

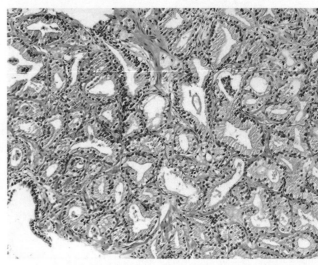

Figure 1.19.10   Adenocarcinoma mimicking adenosis on needle biopsy.

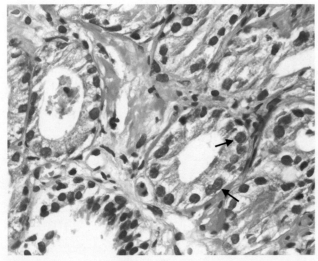

Figure 1.19.11   Same case as Figure 1.19.10 with adenocarcinoma showing prominent nucleoli (*arrows*) compared to benign gland (*lower left*).

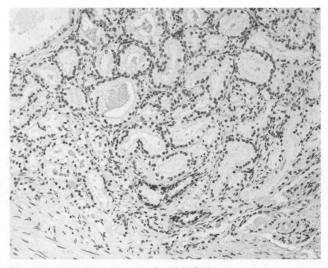

Figure 1.19.12   Negative stains for HMWCK (same case as Figs. 1.19.10 and 1.19.11). Note entrapped benign glands (*bottom*) with circumferential staining.

	Sclerosing Adenosis	High-Grade Prostatic Adenocarcinoma
Age	Typically adults, more commonly on TURP or radical prostatectomy. Rare on needle biopsy	Typically 50 to elderly, although not rare in 40s
Location	Transition zone	Peripheral > transition zone
Symptoms	Asymptomatic	Typically asymptomatic. Advanced disease with urinary obstructive symptoms and/or hematuria or from distant metastases
Signs	None	Serum PSA levels variably elevated
Etiology	No known risk factors	See Section 1.6
Histology	1. Mixture of well-formed glands, single epithelial cells, and cellular spindle cells *(Figs. 1.20.1–1.20.3)* 2. Usually focal, although uncommonly can be extensive 3. Relatively circumscribed with minimal infiltration at its perimeter 4. Glandular component composed of cells with pale to clear cytoplasm and relatively benign-appearing nuclei *(Figs. 1.20.4 and 1.20.5)* 5. Hyaline sheath of collagen surrounds some of the glands *(Figs. 1.20.4, 1.20.5, and 1.20.7)* 6. Individual cells may have very prominent nucleoli 7. Associated dense, spindle cell component *(Figs. 1.20.1, 1.20.4, and 1.20.6)*	1. Lesions mimicking sclerosing adenosis would typically be graded as Gleason score 3 + 5 = 8 *(Fig. 1.20.10)* 2. Range in size from focal to extensive 3. Irregularly infiltrative 4. Gleason pattern 3 may have cells with amphophilic cytoplasm and prominent nucleoli 5. Absence of periglandular collagenous sheath 6. Individual cancer cells can be identical to single cells in sclerosing adenosis 7. Usually, no apparent stromal response or at most a hypocellular fibrotic reaction
Special Studies	• HMWCK and p63 positive around some of the glands *(Fig. 1.20.8)* • Positive for muscle-specific actin and S100 protein consistent with myoepithelial cell differentiation in some of the spindle cells and basal cell *(Fig. 1.20.9)* • Spindle cell component keratin positive, consistent with myoepithelial cell differentiation	• Absence of HMWCK and p63 • Muscle-specific actin negative • Stroma surrounding cancer glands that are keratin negative
Treatment	None	Stage dependent
Prognosis	Benign with no risk of subsequent carcinoma	Variably aggressive depending on stage. Gleason score 8 treated by radical prostatectomy approximately 60% cure rate

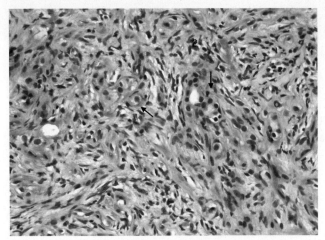

Figure 1.20.1 Sclerosing adenosis with scattered glands and single epithelial cells (*arrows*) with cellular stroma background.

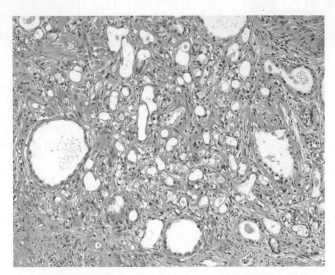

Figure 1.20.2 Limited focus of sclerosing adenosis on TURP.

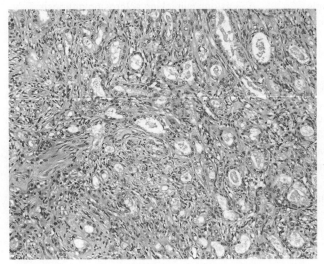

Figure 1.20.3 Sclerosing adenosis consisting of well-formed glands (*right*) and poorly formed glands (*left*) with cellular spindle cells in background.

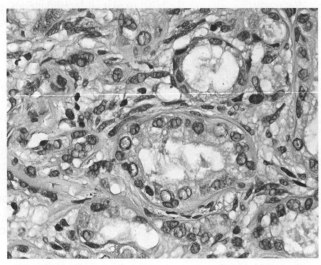

Figure 1.20.4 Higher magnification of Figure 1.20.2 showing a gland surrounded by hyaline rim of connective tissue. Background of cellular spindle cells.

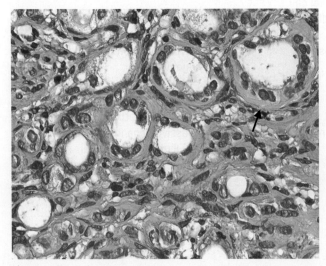

Figure 1.20.5 Higher magnification of Figure 1.20.3 with atrophic glands having hyaline rim (*arrow*).

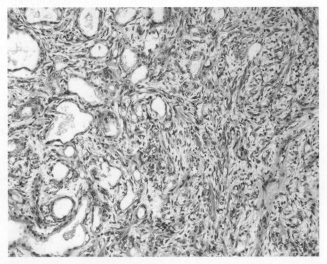

Figure 1.20.6 Sclerosing adenosis.

1.20 Sclerosing Adenosis vs. High-Grade Prostatic Adenocarcinoma   **61**

1 PROSTATE

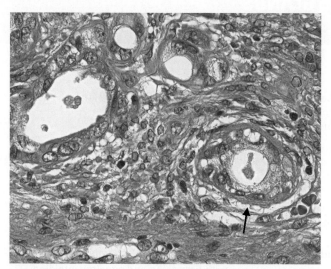

Figure 1.20.7   Higher magnification of Figure 1.20.6 with a gland having hyaline rim of connective tissue (*arrow*). Glands have nuclei with prominent nucleoli.

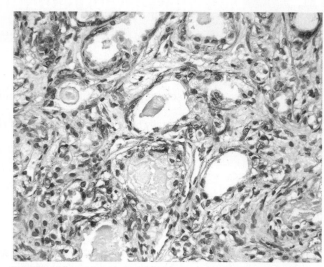

Figure 1.20.8   Same case of Figures 1.20.6 and 1.20.7 with HMWCK positivity of basal cells.

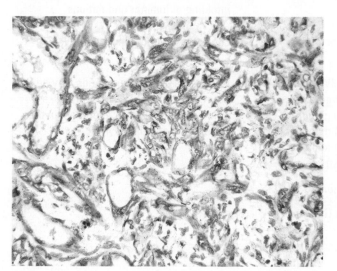

Figure 1.20.9   Same case as Figures 1.20.6–1.20.8 with S100 protein showing myoepithelial cell differentiation in basal and some spindle cells.

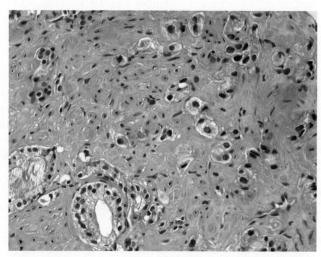

Figure 1.20.10   Adenocarcinoma, Gleason score 5 + 3 = 8 lacking cellular background stroma and hyaline rim of connective tissue around glands.

	Pseudohyperplastic Prostate Adenocarcinoma	Crowded Benign Prostate Glands
Age	Typically 50 to elderly, although not rare in 40s	Typically adults
Location	Peripheral > transition zone	Peripheral = transition zone
Symptoms	Typically asymptomatic	Asymptomatic
Signs	Serum PSA levels variably elevated	None
Etiology	See Section 1.6	No known risk factors. Commonly seen
Histology	1. Crowded focus of larger glands with branching and papillary infolding *(Figs. 1.21.1–1.21.5)* 2. Crowded large glands with abundant cytoplasm and a sharp, straight, luminal border *(Figs. 1.21.6–1.21.9)* 3. Typically requires prominent nucleoli for diagnosis *(Figs. 1.21.5 and 1.21.6)*	1. Crowded variably sized glands often with branching and papillary infolding *(Fig. 1.21.10)* 2. Large benign glands with abundant cytoplasm typically have papillary infolding or luminar undulations *(Fig. 1.21.10)* 3. Lack of prominent nucleoli *(Fig. 1.21.11)*
Special Studies	• Diagnosis verified with absent HMWCK/p63 in many cytologically atypical glands *(Figs. 1.21.3, 1.21.7, and 1.21.9)*. A few glands absent for HMWCK or p63 are not diagnostic of carcinoma, as HGPIN can have same histology and immunohistochemistry	• Although a few benign glands may be entirely absent for HMWCK or p63, a patchy basal cell layer is present in the setting of more glands *(Fig. 1.21.12)*
Treatment	Same as usual prostate adenocarcinoma	None
Prognosis	Equivalent to usual adenocarcinoma Gleason score 3 + 3 = 6	Benign

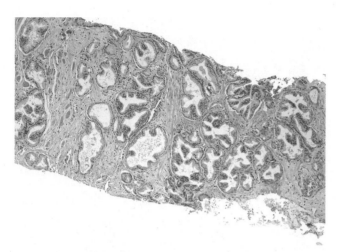

Figure 1.21.1   Pseudohyperplastic carcinoma with large crowded glands with papillary infolding.

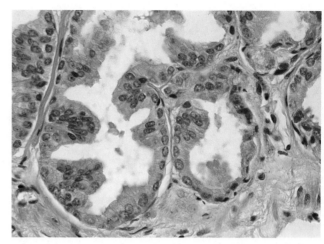

Figure 1.21.2   Same case as Figure 1.21.1 with numerous prominent nucleoli.

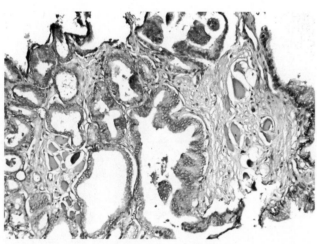

Figure 1.21.3   Same case as Figures 1.21.1 and 1.21.2 with absence of a basal cell layer. Note benign gland with basal cells (*right*).

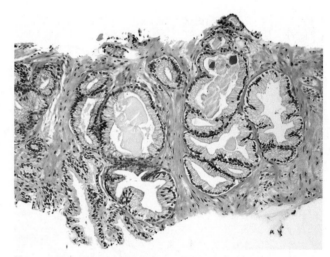

Figure 1.21.4   Pseudohyperplastic carcinoma with crowded glands with papillary infolding.

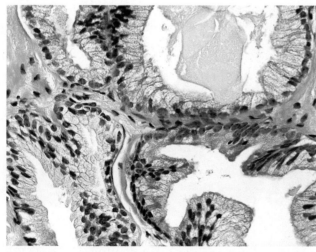

Figure 1.21.5   Same case as Figure 1.21.4 with numerous prominent nucleoli in cancer glands (*right*) compared to benign gland (*lower left*). Stains showed an absence of basal cells.

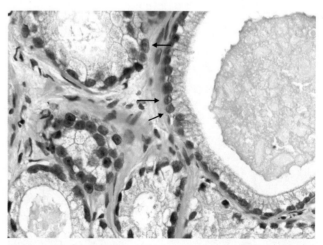

Figure 1.21.6   Pseudohyperplastic carcinoma with large glands with straight luminal borders and abundant cytoplasm and prominent nucleoli (*arrows*).

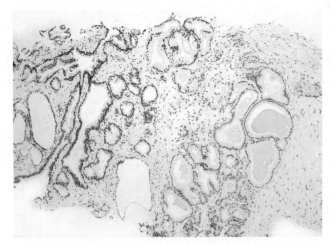

Figure 1.21.7   Same case as Figure 1.21.6 with absence of a basal cell layer in large glands with straight luminal border (*right*). Less crowded benign glands without atypia have a basal cell layer (*left*).

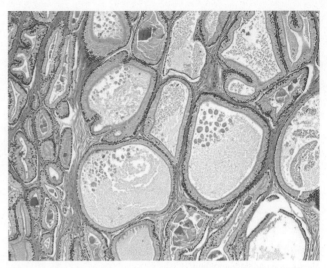

Figure 1.21.8   Pseudohyperplastic carcinoma with large glands with straight luminal borders and abundant cytoplasm.

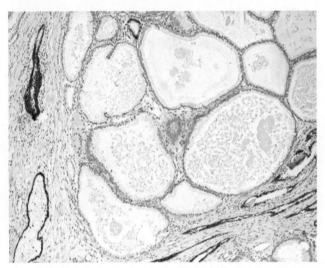

Figure 1.21.9   Same case as Figure 1.21.8 with absence of a basal cell layer in large glands with straight luminal border.

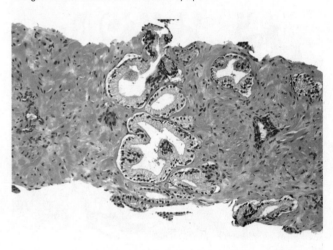

Figure 1.21.10   Benign crowded cluster of larger glands with papillary infolding.

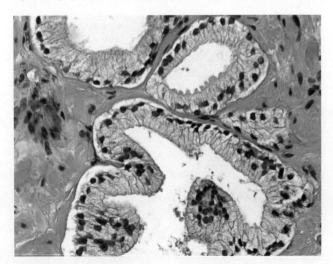

Figure 1.21.11   Same case as Figure 1.21.10 with totally benign cytology.

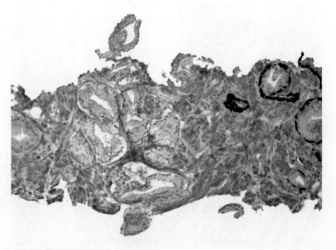

Figure 1.21.12   Same case as Figures 1.21.10 and 1.21.11 with absence of a basal cell layer. As the focus on H&E is totally benign, negative staining for basal cells in a small focus of glands is still consistent with a benign diagnosis.

	Benign Prostate Glands with Perineural Indentation	Prostate Adenocarcinoma with Perineural Invasion
Age	Typically adults, equally common on TURP, radical prostatectomy, and needle biopsy	Typically 50 to elderly, although not rare in 40s
Location	Peripheral > transition zone	Peripheral > transition zone
Symptoms	Asymptomatic	Typically asymptomatic. Advanced disease with urinary obstructive symptoms and/or hematuria or from distant metastases
Signs	None	Serum PSA levels variably elevated
Etiology	Unknown	Initially thought to be pathway of least resistance. Currently, related to complex interactions between nerves and carcinoma. Present in 20% of needle biopsies of the prostate showing adenocarcinoma
Histology	1. Glands typically have benign cytology without prominent nucleoli *(Fig. 1.22.1)* 2. Architecturally larger glands typically with papillary infolding *(Fig. 1.22.2)* 3. Glands only partially encircle *(Figs. 1.22.1 and 1.22.2)* 4. May show intraneural growth *(Fig. 1.22.3)* 5. Perineural indentation may be present *(Fig. 1.22.4)*	1. Vast majority of cases have malignant features such as visible nucleoli, nuclear enlargement, nuclear hyperchromasia, amphophilic cytoplasm, or blue luminal mucin *(Figs. 1.22.6–1.22.8)* 2. Small glands with straight luminal border 3. Glands in some cases circumferentially surround the nerve. Even if benign cytology, if totally surrounding a nerve, then diagnostic of carcinoma *(Fig. 1.22.9)* 4. Intraneural growth rare *(Fig. 1.22.7)* 5. Perineural indentation may be present
Special Studies	• Basal cell stains typically positive *(Fig. 1.22.5)* • AMACR negative • S100 not needed to highlight nerve	• Basal cell stains typically negative • AMACR positive • In rare equivocal cases, S100 protein immunohistochemistry can be performed to verify the presence of a nerve *(Fig. 1.22.10)*
Treatment	None	Can affect the type of radiotherapy regimen used. Less affect on treatment by radical prostatectomy. Should not exclude a patient from active surveillance
Prognosis	No prognostic significance	Perineural invasion associated with an increased risk of extraprostatic extension

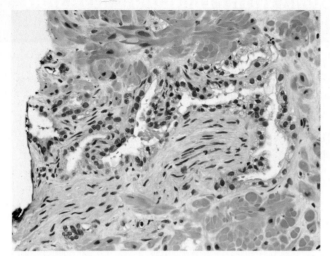

Figure 1.22.1 Benign gland with bland cytology partially wrapping around a nerve.

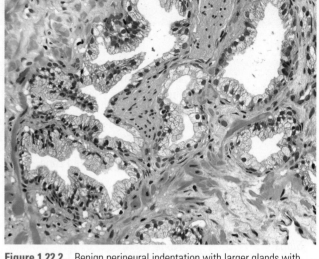

Figure 1.22.2 Benign perineural indentation with larger glands with papillary infolding surrounding a nerve.

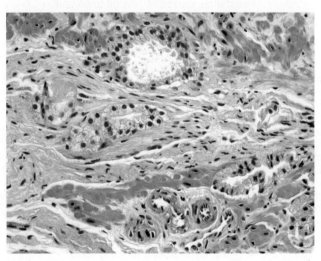

Figure 1.22.3 Benign intraneural prostate gland with benign cytology.

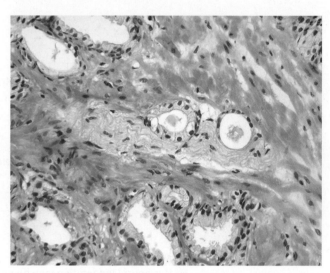

Figure 1.22.4 Partially atrophic benign gland indenting a nerve.

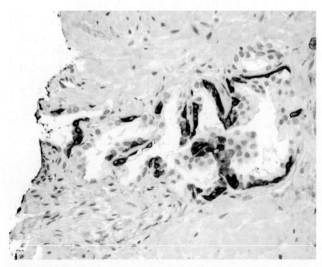

Figure 1.22.5 Same case as Figure 1.22.1 with a patchy basal cell layer shown by HMWCK.

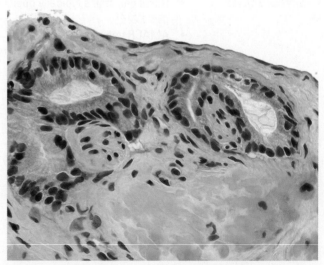

Figure 1.22.6 Adenocarcinoma with small glands with amphophilic cytoplasm and luminal blue mucin partially encircling a nerve.

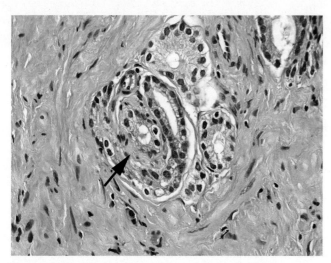

Figure 1.22.7   Adenocarcinoma with prominent nucleoli both surrounding and within a nerve (*arrow*).

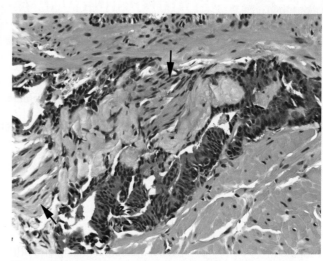

Figure 1.22.8   Adenocarcinoma with amphophilic cytoplasm partially surrounding a nerve (*arrows*). Also present is less cellular collagen of mucinous fibroplasia (collagenous micronodule).

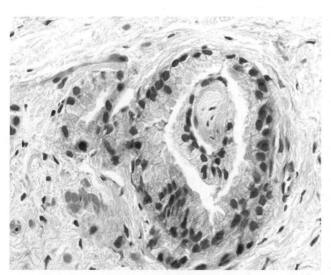

Figure 1.22.9   Adenocarcinoma totally surrounding a nerve. In some cases, there is a gland within a gland formation with the nerve in the center superficially resembling a benign gland with papillary infolding.

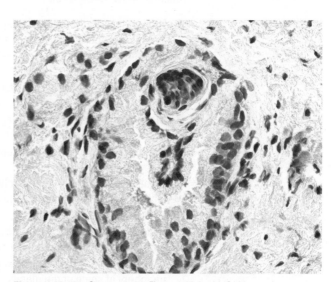

Figure 1.22.10   Same case as Figure 1.22.9 with S100 protein highlighting nerve.

	Clear Cell Cribriform Hyperplasia	Cribriform Prostatic Carcinoma
Age	Typically 50 to elderly, although not rare in 40s	Typically 50 to elderly, although not rare in 40s
Location	Transition zone	Peripheral > transition zone
Symptoms	Asymptomatic	Typically asymptomatic. Advanced disease with urinary obstructive symptoms and/or hematuria or from distant metastases
Signs	None. Incidental finding on TURP and less commonly on needle biopsy	Serum PSA levels variably elevated
Etiology	Unknown if variant of usual hyperplasia or distinct entity. Uncommon	One of the common patterns of Gleason pattern 4
Histology	1. Numerous cribriform glands separated by a modest amount of stroma in a pattern of nodular hyperplasia or diffusely infiltrative (Figs. 1.23.1–1.23.4) 2. Gland contour typically rounded (Figs. 1.23.1–1.23.4) 3. Glands same size or slightly larger than normal benign glands (Figs. 1.23.1–1.23.4) 4. Lightly eosinophilic to more clear cytoplasm (Figs. 1.23.5–1.23.8) 5. Small, bland secretory cell nuclei with inconspicuous or small nucleoli (Figs. 1.23.5–1.23.8) 6. A strikingly prominent basal cell layer, consisting of a row or small cluster of cells with scant cytoplasm is seen at the periphery of some of the glands. The basal cell layer may be incomplete or not visible around some glands. Basal cell nuclei may have prominent nucleoli (Figs. 1.23.5–1.23.8)	1. Cribriform glands that may appear crowded or infiltrative between benign glands (Fig. 1.23.10) 2. Gland contour may be rounded or irregular 3. Gland size variable from size of normal benign glands to much larger 4. Variable cytoplasm from pale, lightly eosinophilic to amphophilic (Fig. 1.23.10) 5. Typically enlarged nuclei with prominent nucleoli (Fig. 1.23.10) 6. Absent basal cell layer although on occasion compressed cancer cells at the periphery may mimic a basal cell layer
Special Studies	• Basal cell stains patchy positive around some of the glands (Fig. 1.23.9). Some glands are negative • AMACR negative	• Basal cell stains typically negative although positive basal cell labeling may be see around some of the glands, representing intraductal spread of carcinoma • AMACR typically positive
Treatment	None	Age and stage dependent
Prognosis	Totally benign without increased risk of carcinoma	All cribriform carcinoma without necrosis represents Gleason pattern 4 with a relatively poor prognosis. The likelihood of being cured after diagnosed with Gleason score 4 + 4 = 8 on biopsy and subsequently treated by radical prostatectomy is approximately 63%. Cribriform carcinoma with necrosis is assigned Gleason pattern 5

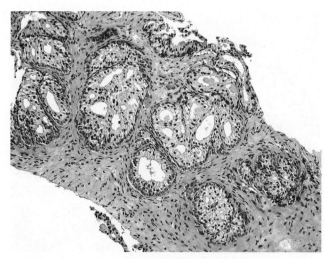

Figure 1.23.1 Clear cell cribriform hyperplasia with numerous cribriform glands on needle biopsy.

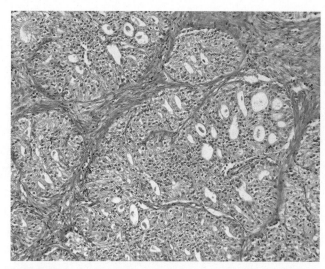

Figure 1.23.2 Back-to-back cribriform glands in clear cell cribriform hyperplasia.

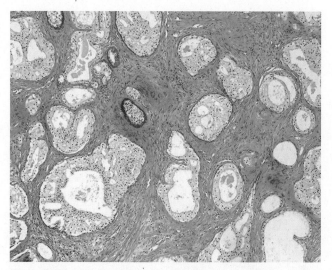

Figure 1.23.3 Cribriform glands of clear cell cribriform hyperplasia with pale cytoplasm.

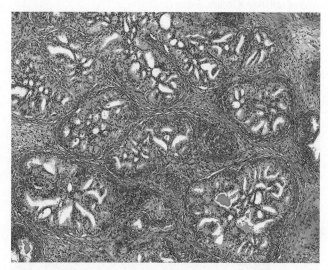

Figure 1.23.4 Clear cell cribriform hyperplasia with multiple cribriform glands.

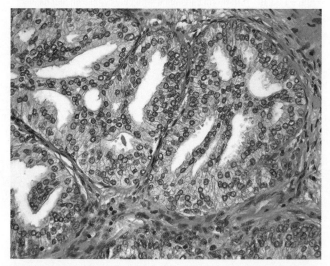

Figure 1.23.5 Higher magnification of Figure 1.23.4 with back-to-back cribriform glands with bland cytology and lightly eosinophilic cytoplasm. A basal cell layer is not evident.

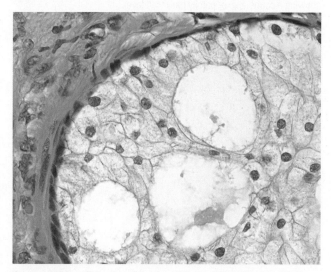

Figure 1.23.6 Higher magnification of Figure 1.23.3 showing cribriform gland with clear cytoplasm and an obvious basal cell layer.

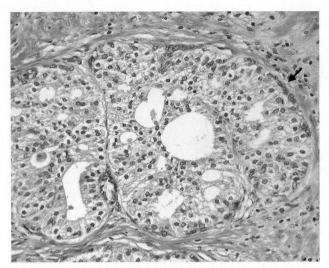

Figure 1.23.7   Higher magnification of Figure 1.23.2 with back-to-back cribriform glands with bland cytology and lightly eosinophilic cytoplasm. A basal cell layer is focally evident (*arrow*).

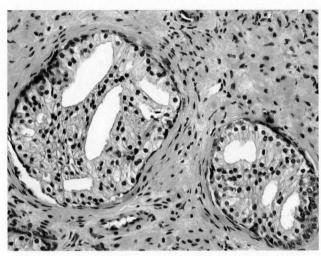

Figure 1.23.8   Higher magnification of Figure 1.23.1 showing cribriform glands with lightly eosinophilic cytoplasm and an obvious basal cell layer.

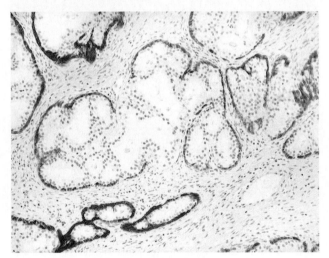

Figure 1.23.9   HMWCK staining of clear cell cribriform hyperplasia showing a continuous or patchy basal cell layer.

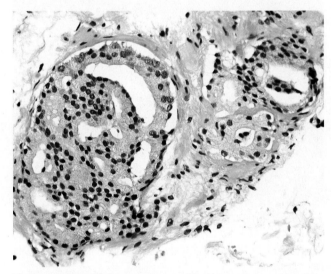

Figure 1.23.10   Cribriform carcinoma with pale cytoplasm and focally prominent nucleoli (*arrow*).

	Clear Cell Cribriform Hyperplasia	Cribriform High-Grade Prostatic Intraepithelial Neoplasia (HGPIN)
Age	Typically 50 to elderly, although not rare in 40s	Typically 50 to elderly, although not rare in 40s
Location	Transition zone	Peripheral > transition zone
Symptoms	Asymptomatic	Asymptomatic
Signs	None. Incidental finding on TURP and less commonly on needle biopsy	None. Incidental finding on needle biopsy and less commonly on TURP
Etiology	Considered by some to be a cribriform variant of BPH	An uncommon variant of PIN compared to flat, tufted, and micropapillary variants
Histology	1. Numerous cribriform glands separated by a modest amount of stroma in a pattern of nodular hyperplasia or diffusely infiltrative *(Fig. 1.24.1)* 2. Gland contour typically rounded *(Figs. 1.24.1 and 1.24.2)* 3. Glands same size or slightly larger than normal benign glands *(Figs. 1.24.1 and 1.24.2)* 4. Pale lightly eosinophilic cytoplasm *(Figs. 1.24.3 and 1.24.4)* 5. Small bland nuclei with inconspicuous or small nucleoli *(Fig. 1.24.4)* 6. A strikingly prominent basal cell layer, consisting of a row or small cluster of cells with scant cytoplasm is seen at the periphery of some of the glands. The basal cell layer may be incomplete or not visible around some glands. Basal cell nuclei may have prominent nucleoli	1. Cribriform glands separated by a modest amount of stroma, typically not in a nodular pattern *(Figs. 1.24.4 and 1.24.5)* 2. Gland contour typically rounded *(Figs. 1.24.4 and 1.24.5)* 3. Glands same size or slightly larger than normal benign glands 4. Variable cytoplasm, typically eosinophilic to amphophilic *(Figs. 1.24.6–1.24.8)* 5. HGPIN nuclei toward the periphery have enlarged nuclei with prominent nucleoli. HGPIN nuclei toward the center of the gland may appear more bland without visible nucleoli *(Figs. 1.24.7 and 1.24.8)* 6. A basal cell layer is typically unapparent, consisting of a row or small cluster of cells with scant cytoplasm is seen at the periphery of some of the glands. The basal cell layer may be incomplete or not visible around some glands. Basal cell nuclei may have prominent nucleoli
Special Studies	• Basal cell stains patchy positive around some of the glands. Some glands are negative • AMACR negative	• Basal cell stains patchy positive around some of the glands. Some glands are negative • AMACR typically positive
Treatment	None	None
Prognosis	Totally benign without increased risk of carcinoma	There are scant data on the risk of subsequent carcinoma following the diagnosis of cribriform HGPIN. Reasonable to recommend repeat biopsy within 6 mo

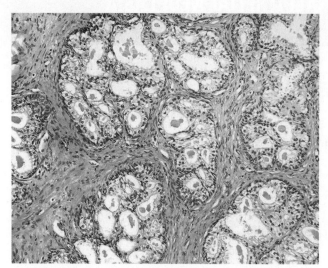

Figure 1.24.1 Clear cell cribriform hyperplasia with numerous cribriform glands.

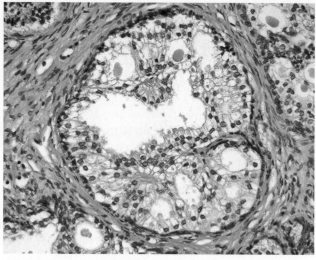

Figure 1.24.2 Clear cell cribriform hyperplasia showing cribriform gland with clear cytoplasm and an obvious basal cell layer.

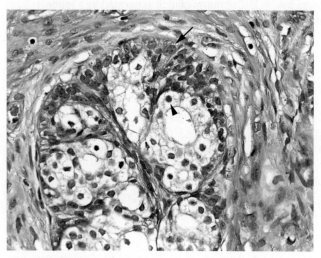

Figure 1.24.3 Clear cell cribriform hyperplasia with pale cytoplasm. Multilayered basal cells (*arrow*) with scant cytoplasm show prominent nucleoli. Secretory cells with pale cytoplasm lack cytologic atypia (*arrowhead*).

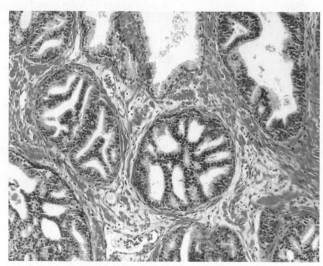

Figure 1.24.4 Cribriform PIN with cribriform glands approximately the same size as adjacent benign glands (*top*) separated by stroma.

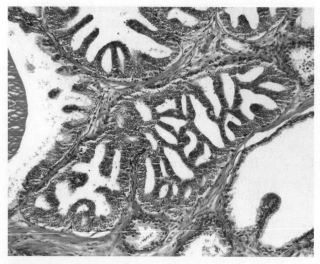

Figure 1.24.5 Cribriform PIN with surrounding micropapillary PIN.

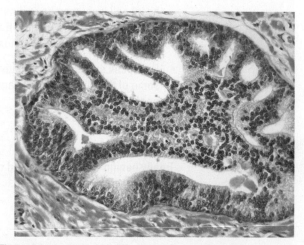

Figure 1.24.6 Higher magnification of Figure 1.24.4 showing a cribriform gland with eosinophilic cytoplasm and no obvious basal cell layer. Prominent nucleoli are seen in the PIN nuclei at the perimeter of the gland, with more bland nuclei toward the center.

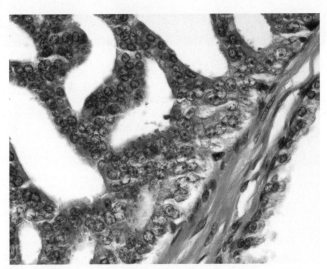

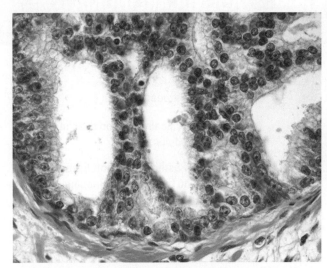

Figure 1.24.7   Higher magnification of Figure 1.24.5 showing cribriform gland with eosinophilic cytoplasm and no obvious basal cell layer. Prominent nucleoli are seen in the PIN nuclei at the perimeter of the gland, with more bland nuclei toward the center.

Figure 1.24.8   Cribriform PIN with gradual maturation of nuclei from periphery with prominent nucleoli to center without visible nucleoli.

	Paraganglia	Poorly Differentiated Prostatic Adenocarcinoma
Age	Typically seen on specimens from adults	Typically 50 to elderly, although not rare in 40s
Location	Posterolateral soft tissue exterior to the prostate. Uncommonly, in the lateral prostatic stroma or in the bladder neck smooth muscle	Peripheral > transition zone
Symptoms	Asymptomatic	Typically asymptomatic. Advanced disease with urinary obstructive symptoms and/or hematuria or from distant metastases
Signs	None. Incidental finding on TURP or needle biopsy	Serum PSA levels variably elevated
Etiology	Normal structure identified in 8% of radical prostatectomy specimens. Less commonly seen on needle biopsy and TURP	Gleason score 10 carcinoma is not frequently seen, but there is a tendency for pathologists to undergrade Gleason pattern 5
Histology	1. Typically small solid cluster of cells (Fig. 1.25.1), yet occasionally larger (Figs. 1.25.2 and 1.25.3) 2. Cells are not present in the prostate, but either in thick muscles of bladder neck or in periprostatic soft tissue (Figs. 1.25.1 and 1.25.2). 3. Usually, cytoplasm deeply amphophilic and granular, although uncommonly pale–clear (Figs. 1.25.4–1.25.7) 4. Thin vascular network apparent (Figs. 1.25.3–1.25.7) 5. Small bland nuclei with inconspicuous or small nucleoli with occasional more pleomorphic nuclei with degenerative atypia 6. May be intimately related to nerves and ganglia	1. Typically Gleason score 10 adenocarcinoma is extensive on TURP and needle biopsy, although uncommon cases exist with small foci of high-grade cancer (Fig. 1.25.8) 2. Although Gleason score 10 adenocarcinoma may show extraprostatic extension on biopsy, most of the tumor will be intraprostatic. 3. Lacks prominent thin vascular network (Fig. 1.25.8) 4. Variable cytoplasm from pale lightly eosinophilic to amphophilic (Fig. 1.25.8) 5. Typically enlarged nuclei with prominent nucleoli 6. May show perineural invasion
Special Studies	• Negative immunoreactivity for PSA, PSAP, and keratins • Diffusely positive for neuroendocrine markers • S100 protein labels sustentacular cells	• Best keratins that label high-grade prostate adenocarcinoma are CAM5.2 and AE1/AE3. PSA and PSAP may be negative in Gleason score 10 adenocarcinoma. More sensitive prostate-specific markers are p501S (prostein) and NKX3.1 • Although neuroendocrine markers may be focally positive in prostate carcinoma, they are typically not diffusely positive • S100 negative

	Paraganglia	**Poorly Differentiated Prostatic Adenocarcinoma**
Treatment	None	Age and stage dependent. Often not a candidate for radical prostatectomy
Prognosis	Totally benign normal anatomical finding	The likelihood of being cured after diagnosed with Gleason score 9–10 on biopsy and subsequently treated by radical prostatectomy is approximately 34%. However, this is a better prognosis than for all patients with Gleason score 9–10, as these men have less advanced disease based on digital rectal examination, serum PSA levels, extent of cancer on biopsy, and imaging studies, enabling them to be candidates for an attempt at curative surgery

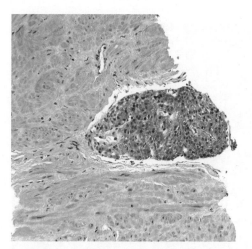

Figure 1.25.1 Small focus of paraganglia in muscle bundles on prostate needle biopsy.

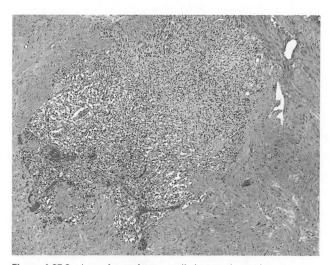

Figure 1.25.2 Large focus of paraganglia in smooth muscle.

1 PROSTATE

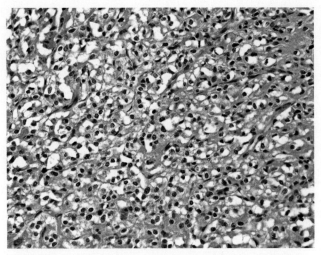

Figure 1.25.3   Higher magnification of Figure 1.25.2 with cells having amphophilic cytoplasm and thin capillaries with distributed throughout the lesion.

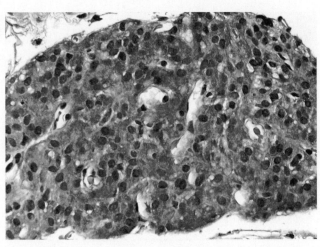

Figure 1.25.4   Higher magnification of Figure 1.25.1 with cells having deeply amphophilic cytoplasm. Note thin capillaries with erythrocytes distributed throughout the lesion.

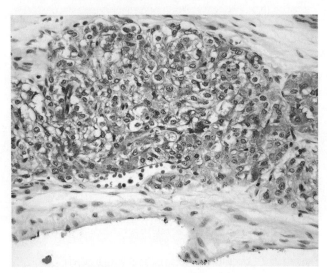

Figure 1.25.5   Paraganglia with scattered thin vessels.

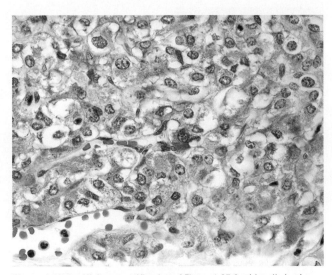

Figure 1.25.6   Higher magnification of Figure 1.25.3 with cells having amphophilic cytoplasm separated by thin capillaries.

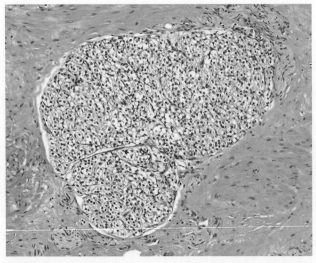

Figure 1.25.7   Paraganglia with pale cells separated by thin capillaries.

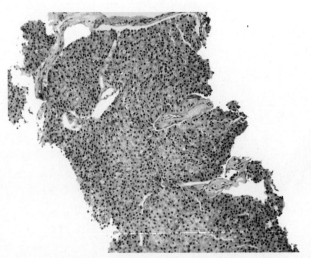

Figure 1.25.8   Extensive adenocarcinoma of the prostate Gleason score 5 + 5 = 10 with amphophilic cytoplasm. Sheets of tumor lack network of fine capillaries.

	Distorted Colon	Prostatic Adenocarcinoma
Age	Typically seen on specimens from adults	Typically 50 to elderly, although not rare in 40s
Location	Only seen on transrectal needle biopsy	Peripheral > transition zone
Symptoms	Asymptomatic	Typically asymptomatic. Advanced disease with urinary obstructive symptoms and/or hematuria or from distant metastases
Signs	None. Incidental finding on needle biopsy	Serum PSA levels variably elevated
Etiology	Small fragments of colon are not uncommonly seen on transrectal needle biopsy	Same as usual adenocarcinoma of the prostate (see Section 1.6)
Histology	1. If distorted, can consist of crowded glands *(Fig. 1.26.1)* 2. Fragment of tissue with colon is detached *(Fig. 1.26.2)* 3. Fragment contains loose lamina propria with chronic inflammation and sometimes identifiable muscularis propria *(Figs. 1.26.1–1.26.3)* 4. Cells may have prominent nucleoli, mitotic activity, and rarely show adenomatous change *(Figs. 1.26.4 and 1.26.5)* 5. Colonic cells typically have goblet cells *(Figs. 1.26.6–1.26.8)*, yet occasionally absent in distorted glands *(Figs. 1.26.5–1.26.8)* 6. Intraluminal and extracellular blue-tinged mucinous secretions may be seen *(Fig. 1.26.7)*	1. Adenocarcinoma mimicking a distorted colon would be Gleason score 3 + 3 = 6 and could consist of crowded glands 2. Uncommon for the only Gleason score 3 + 3 = 6 adenocarcinoma in a specimen to be a small detached fragment. Typically seen in cribriform Gleason score 4 + 4 = 8 *(Fig. 1.26.10)* 3. Lacks lamina propria, thick muscle bundles of muscularis propria, and associated inflammation usually lacking 4. Cells may have prominent nucleoli and mitotic activity 5. Goblet cells are not a feature of adenocarcinoma 6. Intraluminal and extracellular blue-tinged mucinous secretions may be seen
Special Studies	• HMWCK and p63 are negative, and AMACR is positive *(Fig. 1.26.9)* • Negative immunoreactivity for PSA, PSAP, and other prostate-specific markers	• HMWCK and p63 are negative, and AMACR is positive • Gland-forming adenocarcinomas are typically positive for PSA, PSAP, and other prostate-specific markers
Treatment	None	Age and stage dependent
Prognosis	Totally benign normal anatomical finding	Adenocarcinomas potentially confused with distorted colonic mucosa are Gleason score 3 + 3 = 6 with an excellent prognosis

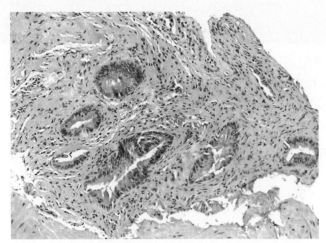

Figure 1.26.1 Colon fragment on prostate needle biopsy with crowded glands. Glands are associated with cellular stroma consistent with lamina propria.

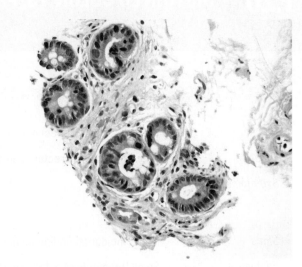

Figure 1.26.2 Detached colon fragment on prostate needle biopsy.

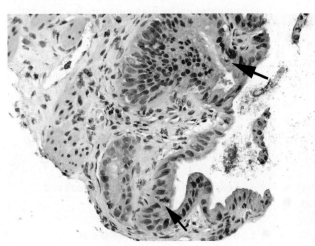

Figure 1.26.3 Distorted colon fragment with mitoses (*arrows*) and associated cellular stromal consistent with the lamina propria. The cells lack obvious goblet cells.

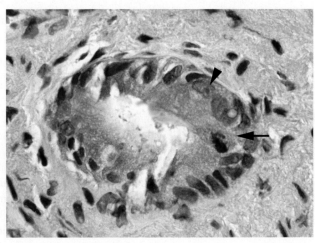

Figure 1.26.4 Higher magnification of Figure 1.26.1 with the colonic gland with the mitotic figure (*arrow*) and occasional prominent nucleoli (*arrowhead*).

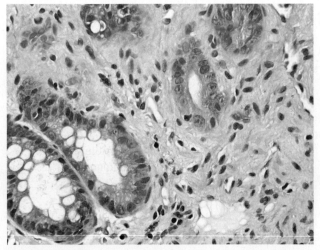

Figure 1.26.5 Higher magnification of Figure 1.26.2 with colonic glands showing prominent nucleoli. Glands in lower left have numerous goblet cells.

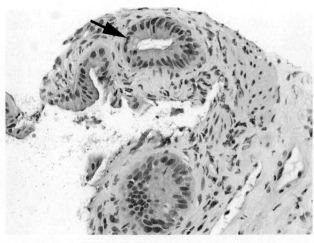

Figure 1.26.6 Colonic glands on prostate biopsy with rare goblet cells (*arrow*).

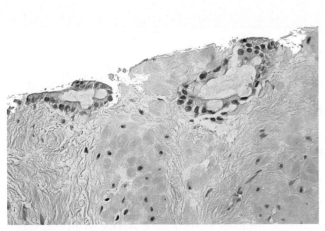

Figure 1.26.7 Colonic glands on prostate biopsy with goblet cells and intraluminal blue mucin.

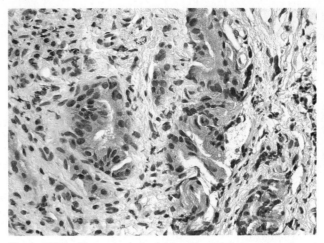

Figure 1.26.8 Distorted colonic glands without obvious goblet cells, yet having the lamina propria.

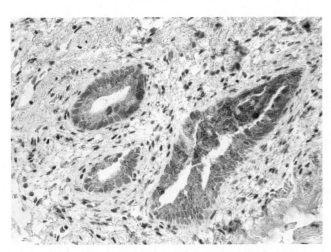

Figure 1.26.9 Same case as Figure 1.26.8 negative for HMWCK and p63 and positive for AMACR.

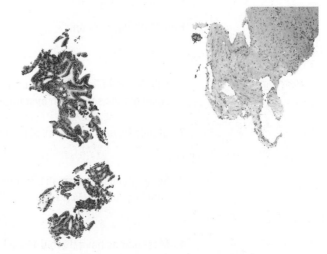

Figure 1.26.10 Small detached fragments of cribriform Gleason score 4 + 4 = 8 adenocarcinoma on needle biopsy.

	Mesonephric Hyperplasia	Prostatic Adenocarcinoma
Age	Typically 50 to elderly, although not rare in 40s	Typically 50 to elderly, although not rare in 40s
Location	Two sites: (1) anterior fibromuscular stroma and (2) toward the base posterior and posterolaterally either within or exterior to the prostate and around the seminal vesicle	Peripheral > transition zone
Symptoms	Asymptomatic	Typically asymptomatic. Advanced disease with urinary obstructive symptoms and/or hematuria or from distant metastases
Signs	None. Incidental finding on TURP and in radical prostatectomy	Serum PSA levels variably elevated
Etiology	Rare Wolffian remnants	Adenocarcinomas potentially confused with mesonephric hyperplasia are Gleason score 3 + 3 = 6
Histology	1. Lobular or infiltrative proliferation of small glands some with cyst formation (Figs. 1.27.1 and 1.27.2) 2. Glands have markedly atrophic cytoplasm (Figs. 1.27.3–1.27.5) 3. Some glands have small intraluminal papillary tufting (Figs. 1.27.6 and 1.27.7) 4. Most glands have thyroid-like deeply eosinophilic "watery" secretions (Fig. 1.27.7) 5. Glands lack cytologic atypia (Figs. 1.27.3–1.27.5)	1. Infiltrative growth pattern of small glands 2. Uncommon to be atrophic, but atrophic adenocarcinomas of the prostate exist (Fig. 1.27.8) 3. Adenocarcinomas of the prostate in general rarely have papillary projections, yet this finding is absent in atrophic adenocarcinomas (Figs. 1.27.9 and 1.27.10) 4. Glands may have dense amorphous not thyroid-like intraluminal pink secretions 5. Glands typically have cytologic atypia (Fig. 1.27.8)
Special Studies	• HMWCK diffusely positive in one-half of cases with remaining cases focally positive. Stains for p63 negative or only focally positive • AMACR positive in about one-half of cases • Prostate-specific markers negative • All cases diffusely positive for PAX8	• HMWCK and p63 negative • AMACR positive • Gland-forming adenocarcinomas typically positive for PSA, PSAP, and other prostate-specific markers • PAX8 negative
Treatment	None	Age and stage dependent
Prognosis	Totally benign without increased risk of carcinoma	The likelihood of being cured after diagnosed with Gleason score 6 on biopsy and subsequently treated by radical prostatectomy is approximately 95%

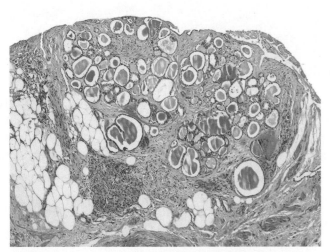

Figure 1.27.1 Mesonephric hyperplasia with lobular proliferation of glands with eosinophilic secretions in periprostatic adipose tissue.

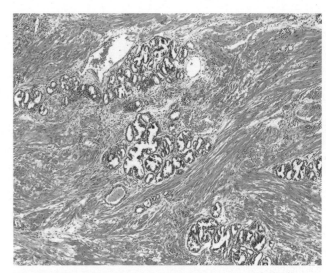

Figure 1.27.2 Infiltrative pattern of mesonephric hyperplasia in prostatic stroma.

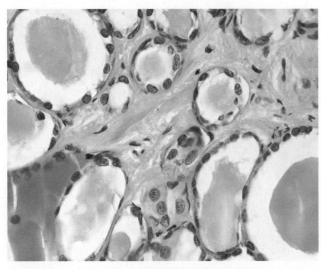

Figure 1.27.3 Same case as Figure 1.27.1 with atrophic tubules with no nuclear atypia containing eosinophilic secretions.

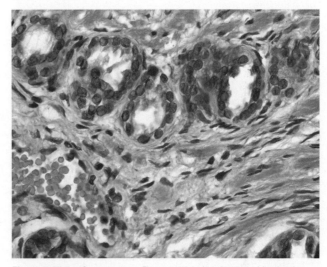

Figure 1.27.4 Same case as Figure 1.27.2 showing atrophic glands with bland cytology.

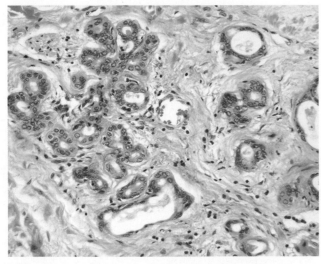

Figure 1.27.5 Mesonephric hyperplasia with atrophic glands.

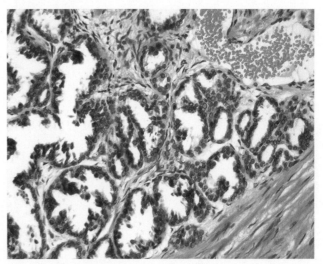

Figure 1.27.6 Same case as Figure 1.27.2 showing glands with papillary infolding.

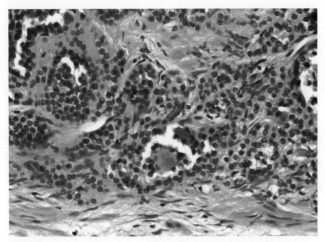

Figure 1.27.7   Mesonephric hyperplasia with papillary tufts and calcification.

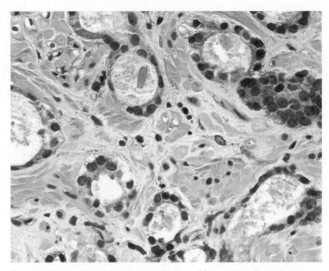

Figure 1.27.8   Atrophic adenocarcinoma with occasional prominent nucleoli.

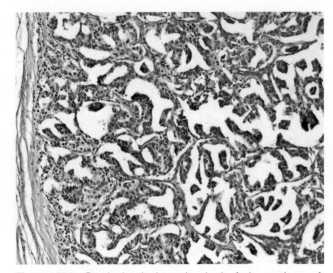

Figure 1.27.9   Rare back-to-back complex glands of adenocarcinoma of the prostate with micropapillary projections.

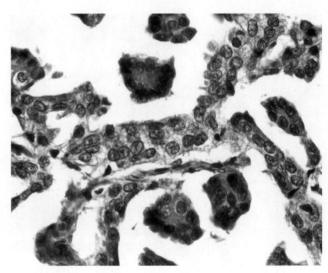

Figure 1.27.10   Same case as Figure 1.27.9 with micropapillary features.

	Nephrogenic Adenoma	Prostatic Adenocarcinoma
Age	Any age. When on prostate biopsy same age distribution as adenocarcinoma	Typically 50 to elderly, although not rare in 40s
Location	Transition > peripheral zone (12% arise in the urethra). Rare on needle biopsy	Peripheral > transition zone
Symptoms	Typically asymptomatic	Typically asymptomatic
Signs	None	Serum PSA levels variably elevated
Etiology	Setting of prior injury with implantation of shed renal tubular cells	Same as usual adenocarcinoma of the prostate (see Section 1.6)
Histology	1. Small tubules, lined by low columnar to cuboidal epithelial cells with eosinophilic cytoplasm. May have prominent nucleoli *(Figs. 1.28.1–1.28.3)* 2. Vascular-like structures with attenuated epithelium, with or without hobnail nuclei *(Figs. 1.28.1, 1.28.2, and 1.28.4)*. May show reactive and degenerative atypia 3. Papillary fronds lined by bland cuboidal epithelium *(Fig. 1.28.5)* 4. Small tubules lined by one or two cells with crescentic nuclei mimicking signet ring cells *(Fig. 1.28.6)* 5. Small tubules with atrophic cytoplasm and dense eosinophilic secretions resembling thyroid follicles *(Fig. 1.28.7)* 6. Thickened hyaline sheath around some of the tubules *(Fig. 1.28.8)* 7. Mitoses absent 8. Typically associated with acute and chronic inflammation *(Fig. 1.28.4)* 9. May be seen infiltrating muscle bundle of suburethral prostate tissue but not infiltrate between benign prostate glands *(Fig. 1.28.7)*	1. Adenocarcinoma usually not as atrophic as nephrogenic adenoma, but atrophic variants exist (see Section 1.10) *(Figs. 1.28.10 and 1.28.11)* 2. No analogous vascular-like structures in prostate cancer 3. Papillary architecture only in ductal adenocarcinoma (see Section 1.37) when lined by variably atypical pseudostratified columnar epithelium 4. No analogous signet-ring cell–like structures in prostate cancer 5. No analogous thyroid-like follicular structures in prostate cancer 6. Lack hyaline rim of collagen around cancerous glands 7. Mitotic figures uncommon; if present virtually rules out nephrogenic adenoma 8. Uncommon to have associated inflammation (see Section 1.8) 9. Similar infiltrative appearance to nephrogenic adenoma, although may also see atypical glands infiltrating between benign prostate glands *(Fig. 1.28.12)*

	Nephrogenic Adenoma	Prostatic Adenocarcinoma
Special studies	• HMWCK and p63 positive in about 50% of cases, yet not in a basal cell distribution. Pancytokeratin positive • AMACR strongly and diffusely positive in 60% of cases *(Fig. 1.28.9)* • PSA and PSAP may be weakly positive *(Fig. 1.28.9)* • PAX2 and PAX8 positive	• HMWCK and p63 negative. Pancytokeratin positive • AMACR often positive • Gland-forming adenocarcinomas typically strongly positive for PSA and PSAP • PAX2 and PAX8 negative
Treatment	None	Stage and grade dependent
Prognosis	Entirely benign although can "recur" following biopsy	Adenocarcinomas potentially confused with nephrogenic adenoma are Gleason score 3 + 3 = 6 with an excellent prognosis

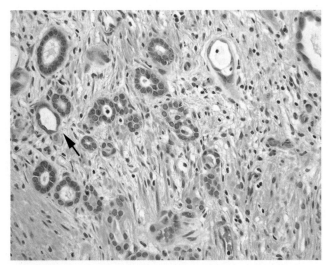

Figure 1.28.1   Nephrogenic adenoma composed of small atrophic tubules. Some tubules are lined by flattened epithelium where the structure resembles a vessel (*arrow*).

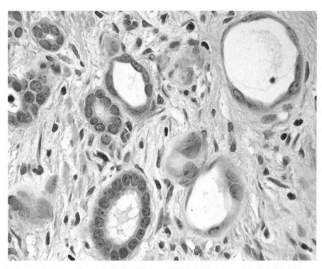

Figure 1.28.2   Same case as Figure 1.28.1 with some tubules having prominent nucleoli. Some tubules resemble vessels lined by attenuated epithelium.

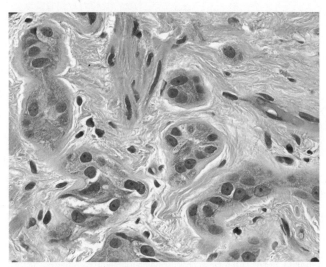

Figure 1.28.3   Nephrogenic adenoma with cords of cells with some having large nucleoli. Note hyaline rim of connective tissue around most of the glands.

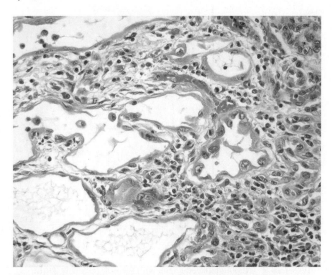

Figure 1.28.4   Nephrogenic adenoma composed of tubules lined by flattened epithelium, some with a reactive hobnail appearance, resembling vessels. Surrounding stroma is inflamed.

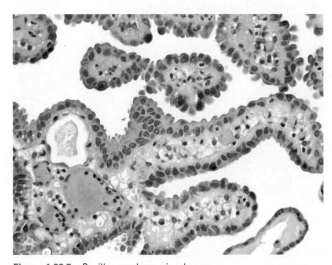

Figure 1.28.5   Papillary nephrogenic adenoma.

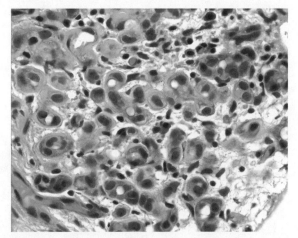

Figure 1.28.6   Nephrogenic adenoma with small tubules surrounded by hyaline rim of connective tissue. Some tubules cut in a section where only one nucleus visible resembling a signet ring cell. Glands contain blue mucinous secretions.

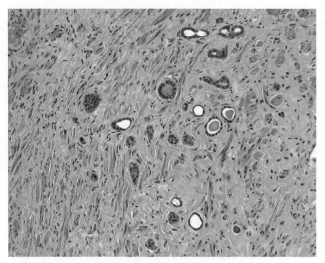

Figure 1.28.7   Atrophic glands of nephrogenic adenoma in smooth muscle. Tubules have thyroid-like secretions.

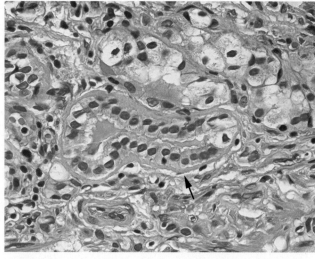

Figure 1.28.8   Nephrogenic adenoma surrounded by thickened rim of collagen (*arrow*).

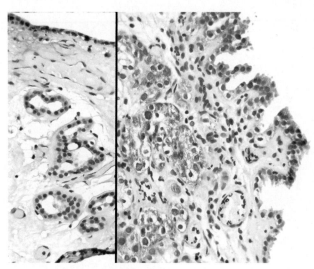

Figure 1.28.9   Nephrogenic adenoma with AMACR positivity (**right**) and weak PSA staining (**left**).

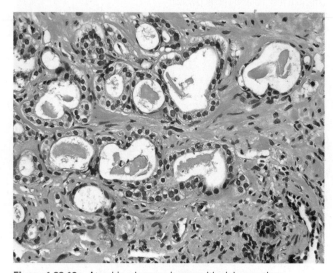

Figure 1.28.10   Atrophic adenocarcinoma with pink secretions.

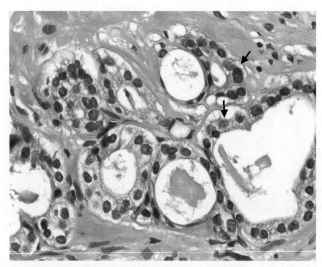

Figure 1.28.11   Higher magnification of Figure 1.28.10 showing occasional nucleoli.

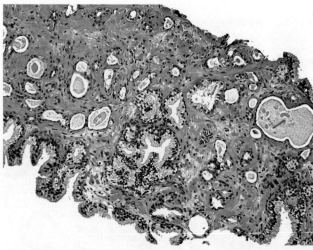

Figure 1.28.12   Atrophic adenocarcinoma infiltrating between benign prostate glands.

	Verumontanum Gland Hyperplasia (VMGH)	Adenocarcinoma
Age	Any age, although when seen on prostate biopsy same age distribution as adenocarcinoma	Typically 50 to elderly, although not rare in 40s
Location	Transition > peripheral zone. Rare on needle biopsy	Peripheral > transition zone
Symptoms	Asymptomatic	Typically asymptomatic. Advanced disease with urinary obstructive symptoms and/or hematuria or from distant metastases
Signs	No signs or symptoms	Serum PSA levels variably elevated
Etiology	A variant of normal histology	Same as usual adenocarcinoma of the prostate (see Section 1.6)
Histology	1. Proliferation of small crowded glands resembling adenosis of the prostate (see Section 1.18) *(Figs. 1.29.1–1.29.4)* 2. Merges in with overlying urothelium where the prostatic ducts empty into the prostatic urethra 3. Lobular noninfiltrative appearance *(Fig. 1.29.1)* 4. May have papillary fronds lined by bland cuboidal epithelium *(Fig. 1.29.5)* 5. Lacks any cytologic atypia 6. Characteristic red-orange and occasional purple-gray concretions and corpora amylacea *(Figs. 1.29.2–1.29.5)*	1. May also consist of crowded glands 2. Uncommon for prostate cancer to be situated immediately beneath the urethra 3. Typically has an infiltrative appearance 4. Papillary architecture only seen in prostatic ductal adenocarcinoma (see Section 1.37) when lined by variably atypical pseudostratified columnar epithelium 5. Variable cytologic atypia, although typically some nuclei with prominent nucleoli *(Fig. 1.29.6)* 6. Uncommonly has corpora amylacea and when present eosinophilic *(Fig. 1.29.6)*
Special studies	• Stains for HMWCK and p63 positive in all cases in a basal cell distribution • AMACR typically negative • PSA and PSAP positive	• Stains for HMWCK and p63 negative • AMACR often positive • Gland-forming adenocarcinomas typically strongly positive for PSA and PSAP
Treatment	None	Stage and grade dependent
Prognosis	Entirely benign	Adenocarcinomas potentially confused with VMGH are Gleason score 3 + 3 = 6 with an excellent prognosis

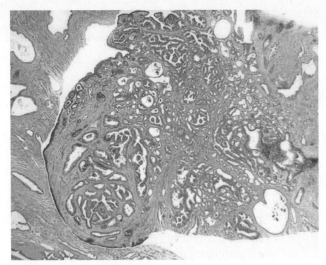

Figure 1.29.1 Crowded lobular proliferation of glands at the verumontanum.

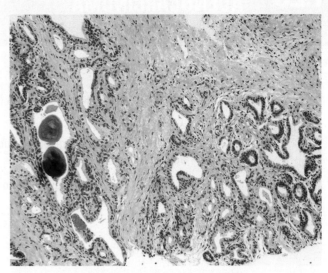

Figure 1.29.2 Higher magnification of verumontanum gland hyperplasia with crowded benign glands. Corpora amylacea have rust color.

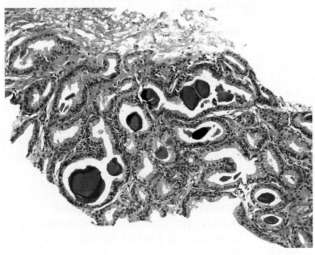

Figure 1.29.3 Verumontanum gland hyperplasia with crowded benign-appearing glands containing red-orange and gray corpora amylacea.

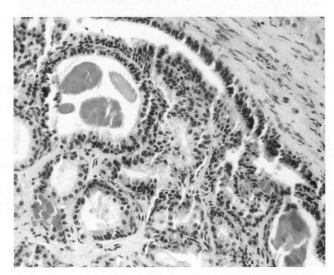

Figure 1.29.4 Verumontanum gland hyperplasia with crowded benign glands containing red-orange corpora amylacea.

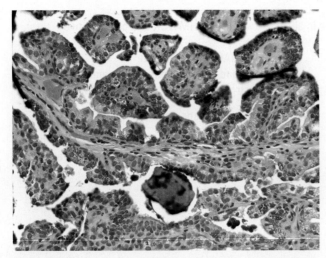

Figure 1.29.5 Verumontanum gland hyperplasia with papillary fronds. Note rust color corpora amylacea (*bottom*).

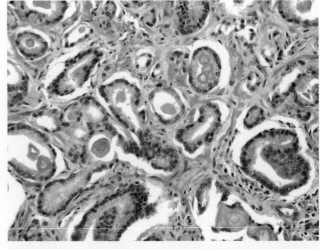

Figure 1.29.6 Adenocarcinoma with cytologic atypia and typical red corpora amylacea.

	Central Zone Glands	High-Grade Prostatic Intraepithelial Neoplasia (HGPIN)
Age	Any age	Typically 50 to elderly, although not rare in 40s
Location	Located at the base of the prostate around the ejaculatory duct but can extend to mid gland	Peripheral > transition zone
Symptoms	Asymptomatic	Asymptomatic incidentally discovered on biopsy
Signs	Does not elevate serum PSA levels	By itself not elevate serum PSA
Etiology	A variant of normal histology that can be prominent in a small percent of cases	Unknown
Histology	1. Medium to large glands that are of the size of normal prostatic acini (*Figs. 1.30.1 and 1.30.2*) 2. Stands out at low magnification as being darker than normal glands (*Figs. 1.30.1 and 1.30.2*) 3. May have papillary infolding, cribriform formation, and Roman bridges (*Figs. 1.30.3–1.30.5*) 4. Lined by tall pseudostratified epithelium with eosinophilic cytoplasm (*Fig. 1.30.6*) 5. Lacks prominent nucleoli (*Figs. 1.30.3, 1.30.5, and 1.30.6*) 6. Some of the nuclei in cribriform and Roman bridges stream parallel to the bridges (*Fig. 1.30.5*) 7. A prominent basal cell layer surrounds some of the glands, seen even at low magnification (*Figs. 1.30.4 and 1.30.6*)	1. Medium to large glands that are of the size of normal prostatic acini (*Figs. 1.30.7–1.30.9*) 2. Stands out at low magnification as being darker than normal glands (*Figs. 1.30.7 and 1.30.9*) 3. May have papillary infolding, cribriform formation, and Roman bridges (*Figs. 1.30.9 and 1.30.10*) 4. Lined by tall pseudostratified epithelium with amphophilic cytoplasm (*Fig. 1.30.7*) 5. Some nuclei with prominent nucleoli, especially toward the periphery of the gland (*Figs. 1.30.7–1.30.10*) 6. Nuclei in cribriform and Roman bridges are round and lack streaming in relation to the bridges (*Fig. 1.30.10*) 7. A basal cell layer indistinct on H&E stain
Special studies	• A patchy basal cell layer seen with HMWCK and p63 • AMACR negative	• A patchy or continuous basal cell layer seen with HMWCK and p63 with occasional glands negative • Variably AMACR positive
Treatment	None	None
Prognosis	Entirely benign	See Section 1.31

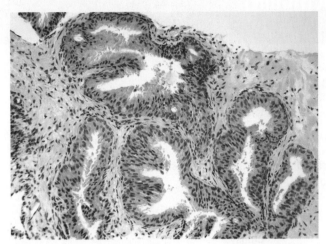

Figure 1.30.1   Central zone composed of normal-sized glands with a darker appearance at low magnification.

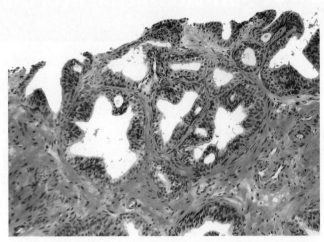

Figure 1.30.2   Normal-sized glands of central zone with Roman bridges.

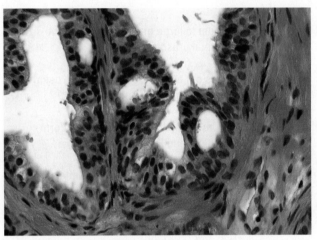

Figure 1.30.3   Same case as Figure 1.30.2 with Roman bridge formation. Cells lack prominent nucleoli.

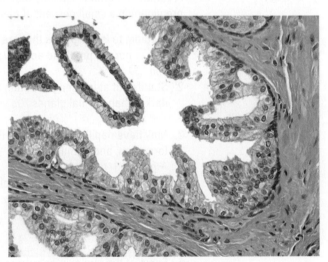

Figure 1.30.4   Central zone with Roman bridge formation, an obvious basal cell layer, and bland cytology.

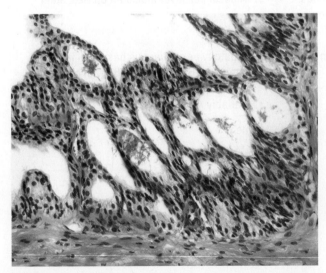

Figure 1.30.5   Cribriform formation in the central zone gland. Note lack of cytologic atypia. Nuclei stream parallel to the bridges.

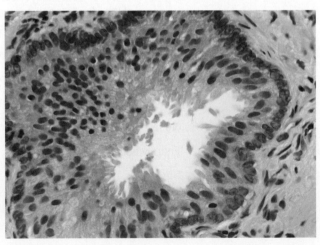

Figure 1.30.6   Higher magnification of Figure 1.30.1. Pseudostratified columnar cells with eosinophilic cytoplasm. A prominent basal cell layer is seen.

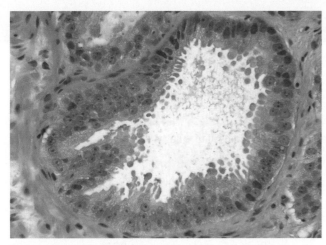

Figure 1.30.7   Normal-sized gland with flat, high-grade PIN with numerous prominent nucleoli.

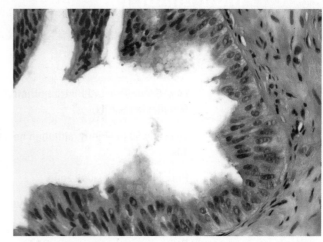

Figure 1.30.8   Slightly tufted high-grade PIN with prominent nucleoli at the periphery of the gland.

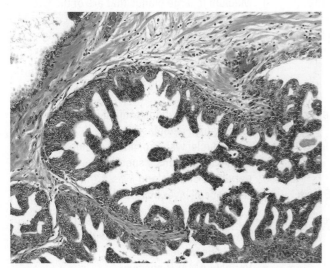

Figure 1.30.9   Large gland of high-grade PIN with cribriform and Roman bridge formation.

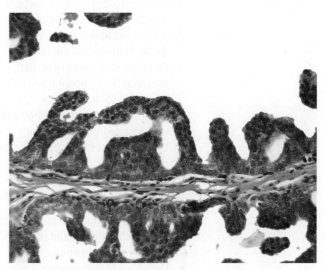

Figure 1.30.10   Higher magnification of Figure 1.30.9 with nucleoli visible in cells toward the basement membrane. Cells within Roman bridges lack orientation (i.e., do not stream parallel to the bridge).

	Low-Grade Prostatic Intraepithelial Neoplasia (LGPIN)	High-Grade Prostatic Intraepithelial Neoplasia (HGPIN)
Age	Typically 50 to elderly, although not rare in 40s	Typically 50 to elderly, although not rare in 40s
Location	Peripheral > transition zone	Peripheral > transition zone
Symptoms	Asymptomatic incidentally discovered on biopsy	Asymptomatic incidentally discovered on biopsy
Signs	By itself not elevate serum PSA	By itself not elevate serum PSA
Etiology	Unknown	Unknown
Histology	1. Medium to large glands that are of the size of normal prostatic acini 2. Stands out at low magnification as being darker than normal glands 3. Usually tufted but may be flat, micropapillary infolding with rare cribriform formation *(Figs. 1.31.1–1.31.6)* 4. Lined by tall pseudostratified epithelium with amphophilic cytoplasm 5. Lacks prominent nucleoli with 20× lens *(Figs. 1.31.1–1.31.6)* 6. A basal cell layer indistinct on H&E stain	1. Medium to large glands that are of the size of normal prostatic acini 2. Stands out at low magnification as being darker than normal glands 3. May have flat, tufted, micropapillary, and cribriform formation *(Figs. 1.31.7–1.31.12)* 4. Lined by tall pseudostratified epithelium with amphophilic cytoplasm 5. Some nuclei with prominent nucleoli seen with 20× lens, especially toward the periphery of the gland *(Figs. 1.31.7–1.31.12)* 6. A basal cell layer indistinct on H&E stain
Special studies	• Usually a continuous basal cell layer seen with HMWCK and p63 with occasional glands negative • Variably AMACR positive	• A patchy or continuous basal cell layer seen with HMWCK and p63 with occasional glands negative • Variably AMACR positive
Treatment	None	None
Prognosis	No increased risk of cancer on repeat biopsy, so typically should not even be mentioned in pathology reports	No increased risk of cancer on repeat biopsy done within 1 y of initial diagnosis of HGPIN if found on one core (unifocal). Little data on the long-term risk so may be reasonable to do repeat biopsy 2–3 y later. If more than one core with HGPIN (multifocal), risk of cancer on repeat biopsy is 40% warranting repeat biopsy within 6 mo of initial biopsy

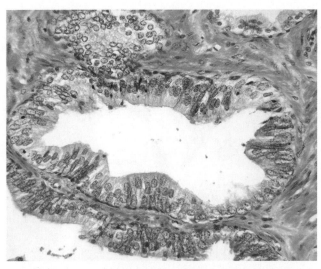

Figure 1.31.1   Flat low-grade PIN with crowded piled up enlarged nuclei lacking prominent nucleoli.

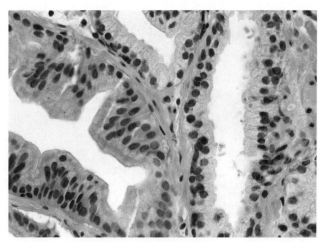

Figure 1.31.2   Tufted low-grade PIN (*left*) with enlarged hyperchromatic nuclei lacking prominent nucleoli compared to benign glands (*right*).

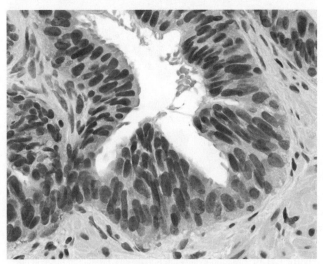

Figure 1.31.3   Tufted low-grade PIN.

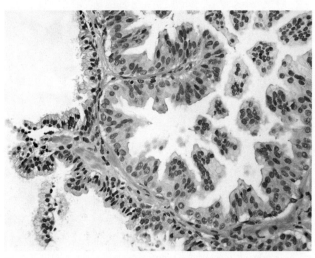

Figure 1.31.4   Low-grade micropapillary PIN with enlarged nuclei (*right*) compared to the benign gland (*left*).

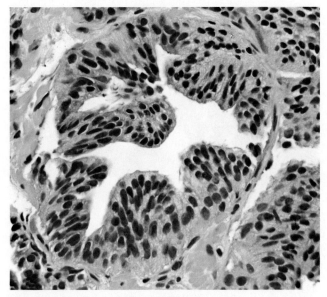

Figure 1.31.5   Micropapillary low-grade PIN.

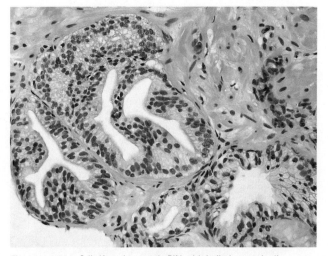

Figure 1.31.6   Cribriform low-grade PIN with indistinct nucleoli.

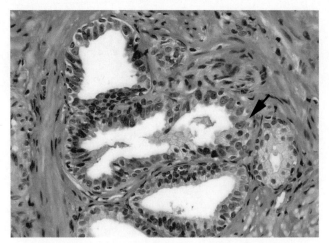

Figure 1.31.7   Flat high-grade PIN with focal prominent nucleoli.

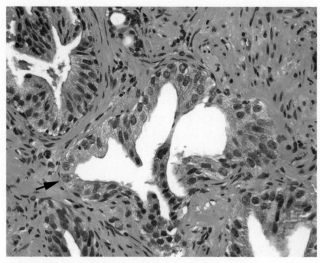

Figure 1.31.8   Tufted high-grade PIN.

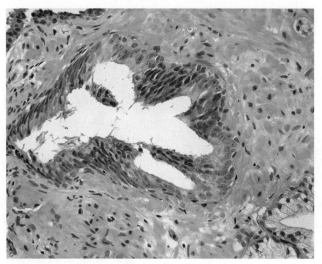

Figure 1.31.9   Tufted high-grade PIN.

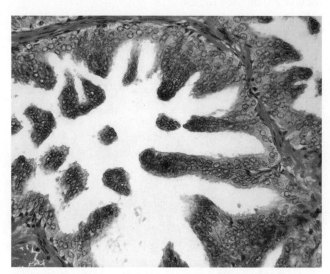

Figure 1.31.10   Micropapillary high-grade PIN. Prominent nucleoli are visible toward the periphery of the gland. More benign nuclei are seen toward the center.

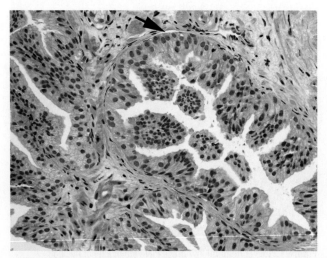

Figure 1.31.11   Micropapillary high-grade PIN. Focal prominent nucleoli are seen (*arrow*).

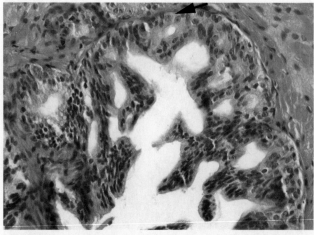

Figure 1.31.12   Cribriform high-grade PIN with prominent nucleoli toward the periphery of the gland (*arrow*). More benign-appearing nuclei are present toward the center.

	PINATYP	HGPIN with Adjacent Carcinoma
Age	Typically 50 to elderly, although not rare in 40s	Typically 50 to elderly, although not rare in 40s
Location	Peripheral > transition zone	Peripheral > transition zone
Symptoms	Asymptomatic incidentally discovered on biopsy	Asymptomatic incidentally discovered on biopsy
Signs	By itself not elevate serum PSA	If substantial cancer volume may elevate serum PSA
Etiology	HGPIN with either out pouching or tangential sections off of HGPIN or HGPIN with adjacent carcinoma	See Section 1.6
Histology	1. Small glands adjacent to HGPIN having identical atypical cytology *(Figs. 1.32.1–1.32.8)* 2. Typically only a few small atypical glands in close proximity to HGPIN 3. More numerous small atypical glands may be seen if extensive HGPIN 4. A basal cell layer indistinct on H&E stain	1. Small glands adjacent to HGPIN having identical atypical cytology 2. Glands trail away from HGPIN *(Figs. 1.32.9–1.32.12)* 3. More numerous small atypical glands even if focal HGPIN 4. A basal cell layer indistinct on H&E stain
Special studies	• A patchy basal cell layer seen with HMWCK and p63 in some of the small atypical glands without a cluster of negative glands *(Figs. 1.32.1–1.32.8)* • HGPIN surrounded by a patchy basal cell layer in area of adjacent small glands • Variably AMACR positive	• Absent basal cell layer seen with HMWCK and p63 in adjacent small glands. Still diagnosable as cancer if few patchy small glands next to HGPIN as long as cluster of negative glands trailing away from HGPIN *(Figs. 1.32.9–1.32.12)* • HGPIN may be surrounded by an intact basal cell layer in area of adjacent small glands *(Figs. 1.32.11 and 1.32.12)* • Variably AMACR positive
Treatment	None	None
Prognosis	Risk of cancer on repeat biopsy is 40% warranting repeat biopsy within 6 mo of initial biopsy	Typically cancer in this differential diagnosis is Gleason score 3 + 3 = 6 with excellent prognosis

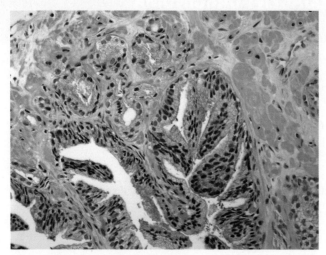

Figure 1.32.1 High-grade PIN (*bottom*) with adjacent small glands that could represent adjacent carcinoma or outpouching off of high-grade PIN.

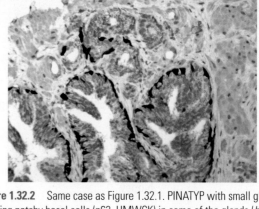

Figure 1.32.2 Same case as Figure 1.32.1. PINATYP with small glands showing patchy basal cells (p63, HMWCK) in some of the glands (*brown*). Although there are a few glands without visible basal cells, they are insufficient in number to diagnose carcinoma. The adjacent larger PIN gland demonstrates a patchy basal cell layer with both HGPIN- and AMACR-positive small glands (*red*).

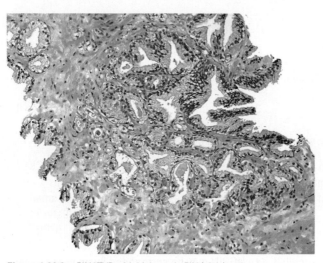

Figure 1.32.3 PINATYP with high-grade PIN (*right*) and numerous adjacent small glands that could represent adjacent carcinoma or outpouching off of high-grade PIN.

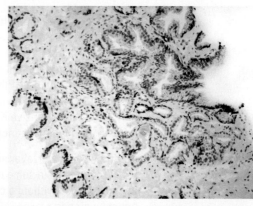

Figure 1.32.4 Same case as Figure 1.32.3. PIN4 cocktail showing HGPIN with budding off of small glands, some showing patchy brown-labeled basal cells (p63, HMWCK). Although there are a few glands without visible basal cells, they are insufficient in number to diagnose carcinoma. The adjacent larger PIN gland demonstrates a patchy basal cell layer with both HGPIN- and AMACR-positive (*red*) small glands.

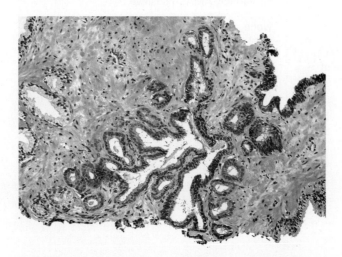

Figure 1.32.5 PINATYP with high-grade PIN (*center*) and numerous adjacent small glands that could represent adjacent carcinoma or outpouching off of high-grade PIN.

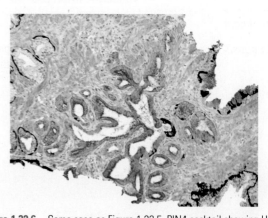

Figure 1.32.6 Same case as Figure 1.32.5. PIN4 cocktail showing HGPIN and a few small glands both showing patchy brown-labeled basal cells (p63, HMWCK). Although there are a few small glands without visible basal cells, they are insufficient in number and too close to the PIN gland to diagnose carcinoma. Larger PIN and AMACR-positive (*red*) small glands.

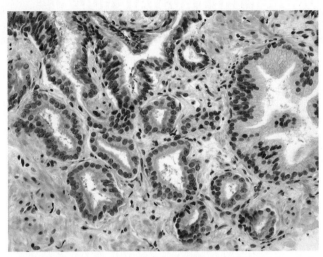

Figure 1.32.7 PINATYP with part of a high-grade PIN gland (*upper left*) and adjacent small glands suspicious for infiltrating carcinoma but could be outpouching off of high-grade PIN.

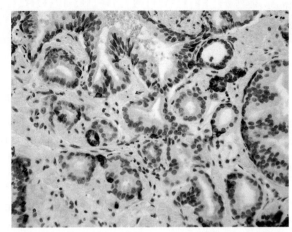

Figure 1.32.8 Same case as Figure 1.32.7. Many of the small glands adjacent to HGPIN show patchy brown-labeled basal cells (HMWCK). Although there are a few small glands without visible basal cells, they are insufficient in number to diagnose carcinoma.

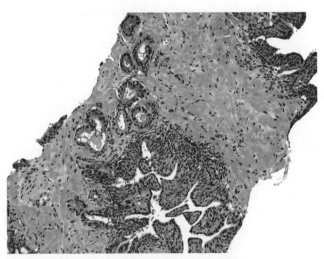

Figure 1.32.9 High-grade PIN gland (*lower left*) surrounded by several small atypical glands suspicious for carcinoma.

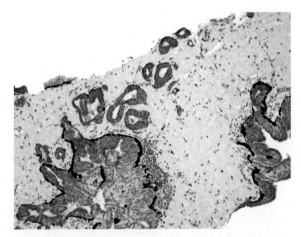

Figure 1.32.10 Same case as Figure 1.32.9 with small glands trailing away from HGPN negative for basal cell markers (*brown*) and positive for AMACR (*red*). There are enough small glands that are far enough away from the HGPIN to be diagnostic of carcinoma.

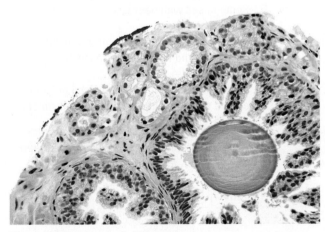

Figure 1.32.11 High-grade PIN gland containing corpora amylacea surrounded by several small atypical glands suspicious for carcinoma.

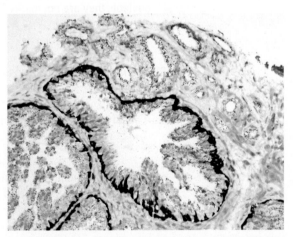

Figure 1.32.12 Same case as Figure 1.32.11 with small glands all negative for basal cell markers (*brown*) and positive for AMACR (*red*). The high-grade PIN has an intact basal cell layer, such that the atypical small glands cannot be attributed as outpouching off the PIN gland and are diagnostic of carcinoma.

	High-Grade Prostatic Intraepithelial Neoplasia (HGPIN)	Intraductal Adenocarcinoma of the Prostate (IDC-P)
Age	Typically 50 to elderly, although not rare in 40s	Typically 50 to elderly, although not rare in 40s
Location	Peripheral > transition zone	Peripheral > transition zone
Symptoms	Asymptomatic incidentally discovered on biopsy	Asymptomatic incidentally discovered on biopsy
Signs	By itself not elevate serum PSA	By itself not elevate serum PSA, although typically associated with high-grade cancer and elevated serum PSA levels. DRE may be abnormal if associated infiltrating carcinoma
Etiology	Unknown	Typically, represents intraductal spread of carcinoma within preexisting ducts and acini. In the absence of infiltrating carcinoma, it is distinct from HGPIN and represents a late event in prostate cancer evolution
Histology	1. Medium to large glands that are of the size of normal prostatic acini 2. Stands out at low magnification as being darker than normal glands 3. May have flat, tufted, micropapillary, and cribriform formation 4. Cribriform glands have loose fenestrations with >70% of the area of the gland containing lumina *(Fig. 1.33.1)* 5. Lacks solid nests of cells 6. Although nuclei enlarged with prominent nucleoli, they are not markedly anaplastic 7. Necrosis absent 8. Cribriform pattern involves the entire gland 9. A basal cell layer indistinct on H&E stain	1. Medium to large glands, the latter representing normal prostatic acini expanded in size 2. Stands out at low magnification as being darker than normal glands 3. May have flat, tufted, micropapillary, cribriform, and solid nest formation 4. Cribriform glands with dense cribriform structures with >70% of the area of the gland containing epithelial bridges *(Figs. 1.33.2–1.33.6)* 5. Some cases with solid nests of cells *(Figs. 1.33.7 and 1.33.8)* 6. Some cases with marked nuclear pleomorphism with 6× size, the size of normal nuclei *(Figs. 1.33.9 and 1.33.10)* 7. Some cases with necrosis *(Figs. 1.33.11 and 1.33.12)* 8. In some cases, cribriform pattern focally involves gland with abrupt transition to normal gland 9. A basal cell layer in some involved glands can be seen, and in other glands, indistinct on H&E stain
Special studies	• A patchy or continuous basal cell layer seen with HMWCK and p63 with occasional glands negative • Variably AMACR positive	• A patchy or continuous basal cell layer seen with HMWCK and p63 *(Figs. 1.33.6, 1.33.8, 1.33.10, and 1.33.12)* • Variably AMACR positive

	High-Grade Prostatic Intraepithelial Neoplasia (HGPIN)	Intraductal Adenocarcinoma of the Prostate (IDC-P)
Treatment	None	Recommend treating patients with IDC-P on biopsy with definitive therapy even in the absence of documented infiltrating cancer
Prognosis	See Section 1.31	Frequently associated with high-grade cancer at radical prostatectomy or advanced disease where surgery is not an option

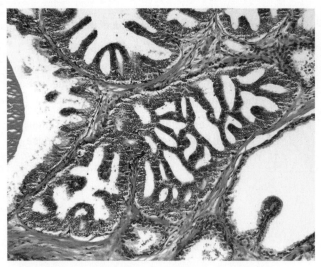

Figure 1.33.1 Cribriform high-grade PIN with open fenestrations occupying >70% of the area of the gland (i.e., loose cribriform).

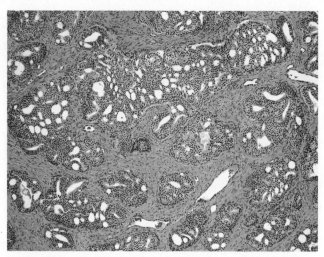

Figure 1.33.2 Cribriform lesion borderline between cribriform high-grade PIN and intraductal carcinoma (IDC-P).

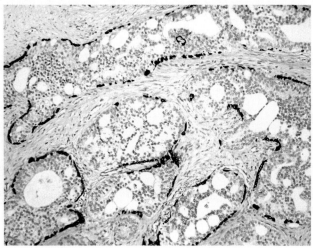

Figure 1.33.3 High molecular weight cytokeratin outlines glands seen in Figure 1.33.2.

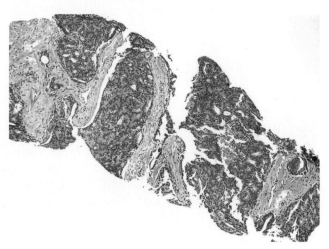

Figure 1.33.4 IDC-P with cribriform glands where the lumina occupy <30% of the luminal space (i.e., dense cribriform).

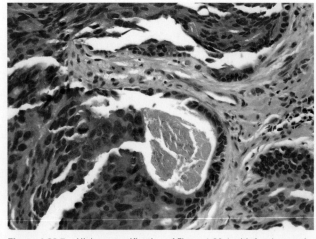

Figure 1.33.5 Higher magnification of Figure 1.33.4 with focal necrosis.

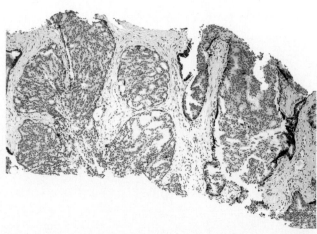

Figure 1.33.6 High molecular weight cytokeratin outlines glands seen in Figures 1.33.4 and 1.33.5.

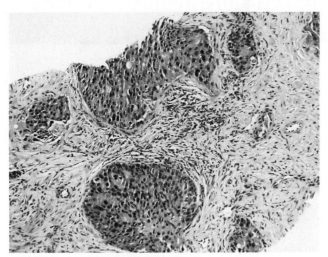

Figure 1.33.7   IDC-P with solid nests of cells.

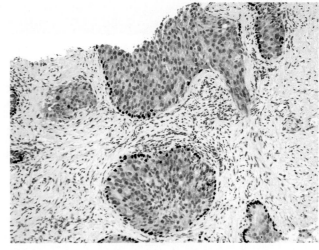

Figure 1.33.8   p63 outline glands seen in Figure 1.33.7.

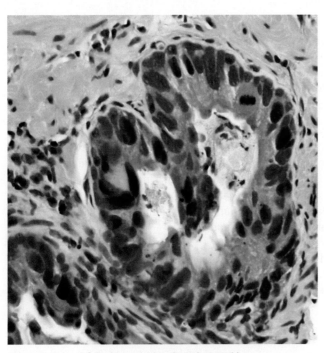

Figure 1.33.9   IDC-P with marked nuclear pleomorphism.

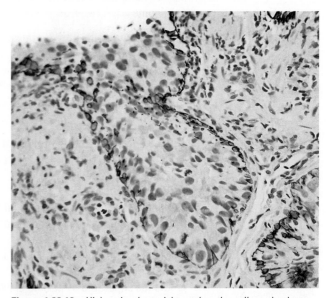

Figure 1.33.10   High molecular weight cytokeratin outlines gland seen in Figure 1.33.9.

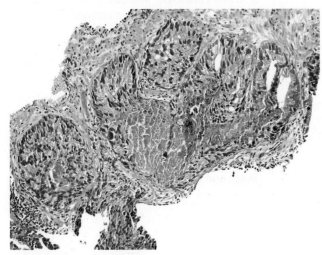

Figure 1.33.11   IDC-P with necrosis.

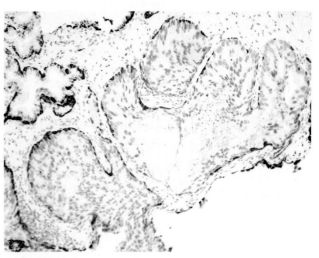

Figure 1.33.12   High molecular weight cytokeratin outlines gland seen in Figure 1.33.11.

	Intraductal Adenocarcinoma of the Prostate (IDC-P)	Infiltrating High-Grade Prostate Adenocarcinoma
Age	Typically 50 to elderly, although not rare in 40s	Typically 50 to elderly, although not rare in 40s
Location	Peripheral > transition zone	Peripheral > transition zone
Symptoms	Asymptomatic incidentally discovered on biopsy	Variable depending if advanced disease
Signs	By itself does not elevate serum PSA, although typically associated with high-grade cancer and elevated serum PSA levels. DRE may be abnormal if associated infiltrating carcinoma	Serum PSA levels variably elevated
Etiology	Typically, represents intraductal spread of carcinoma within preexisting ducts and acini. In the absence of infiltrating carcinoma, it is a distinct lesion from high-grade PIN and represents a late event in prostate cancer evolution	See Section 1.6
Histology	1. Medium to large cribriform glands, the latter representing normal prostatic acini expanded in size 2. Conforms to the shape of normal glands with rounded edges and occasional branching *(Figs. 1.34.1–1.34.3)* 3. May have "dense" cribriform glands or solid nests *(Figs. 1.34.4–1.34.7)* 4. Glands separated by stroma similar to normal glands *(Fig. 1.34.1)* 5. Some cases with marked nuclear pleomorphism with 6× size, the size of normal nuclei 6. Some cases with necrosis 7. Some glands partially involved with abrupt interface with normal gland 8. A basal cell layer in some involved glands can be seen, and in other glands, indistinct on H&E stain *(Fig. 1.34.2)*	1. Small to medium to large to very large glands, the latter larger than could be expected even in normal expanded acini *(Fig. 1.34.8)* 2. Glands with irregular edges, without branching *(Fig. 1.34.9)* 3. May have cribriform glands, solid nests, or single cells 4. Some cases with back-to-back glands inconsistent with IDC-P *(Fig. 1.34.10)* 5. Some cases with marked nuclear pleomorphism with 6× size, the size of normal nuclei 6. Some cases with necrosis 7. No partial glandular involvement 8. A basal cell layer indistinct on H&E stain
Special studies	• A patchy or continuous basal cell layer seen with HMWCK and p63 • Variably AMACR positive	• Some glands with a negative basal cell layer seen with HMWCK and p63 *(Figs. 1.34.11 and 1.34.12)* • Variably AMACR positive
Treatment	See Section 1.33	Stage and extent on biopsy dependent

	Intraductal Adenocarcinoma of the Prostate (IDC-P)	Infiltrating High-Grade Prostate Adenocarcinoma
Prognosis	See Section 1.33	As difference in prognosis and treatment for IDC-P and high-grade prostate adenocarcinoma is typically not different, typically not necessary to do stains to differentiate between the two entities. IDC-P and infiltrating adenocarcinoma should be combined when recording the extent of carcinoma

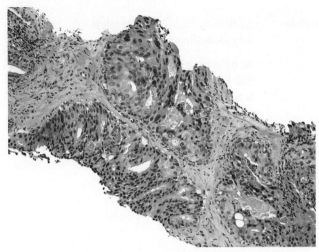

Figure 1.34.1   IDC-P with dense cribriform glands with >70% epithelium relative to lumens. Glands are of the size, contour, and spatial arrangement of normal glands.

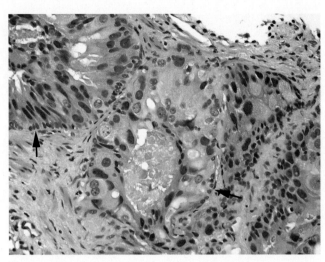

Figure 1.34.2   Same case as Figure 1.34.1 with a visible basal cell layer (*arrows*) on H&E stain.

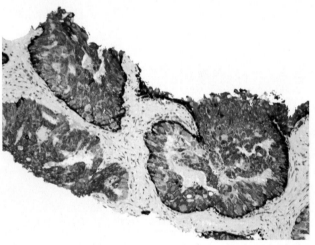

Figure 1.34.3   Same case as Figures 1.34.1 and 1.34.2 with a variably intact basal cell layer on PIN4 stain.

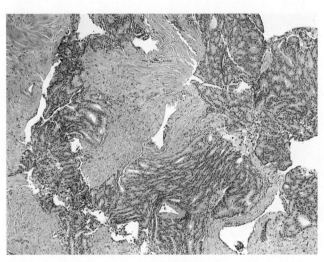

Figure 1.34.4   IDC-P with dense cribriform glands mimicking infiltrative Gleason score 4 + 4 = 8 adenocarcinoma.

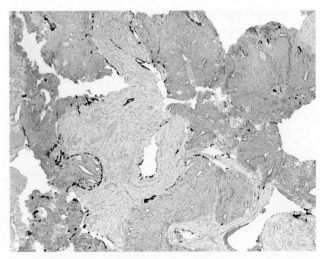

Figure 1.34.5   Same case as Figure 1.34.4 with triple stain showing a patchy intact basal cell layer.

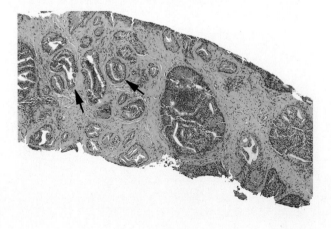

Figure 1.34.6   Small glands of Gleason score 3 + 3 = 6 with adjacent cribriform glands. Some of the cribriform glands are small and more consistent with infiltrating Gleason pattern cancer (*arrows*). Other cribriform glands are larger and could on the H&E stain represent either IDC-P or infiltrating carcinoma.

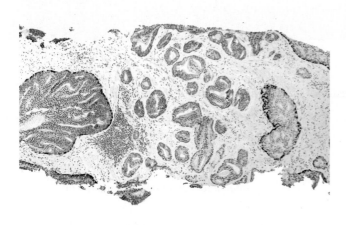

Figure 1.34.7 Triple stain with Gleason score 3 + 4 = 7 carcinoma (*center*) lacking basal cells and adjacent IDC-P surrounded by basal cells.

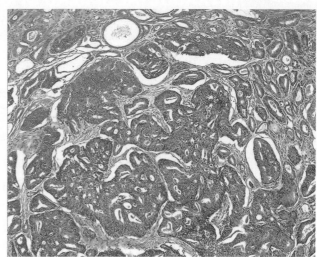

Figure 1.34.8 Infiltrating cribriform carcinoma admixed with small glands of Gleason score 6 cancer. The cribriform glands are too large and irregular to represent IDC-P.

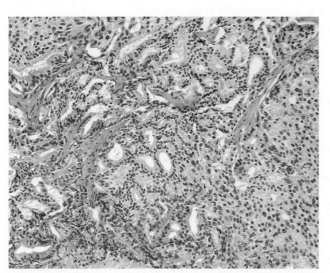

Figure 1.34.9 Irregular infiltrating cribriform glands of Gleason pattern 4.

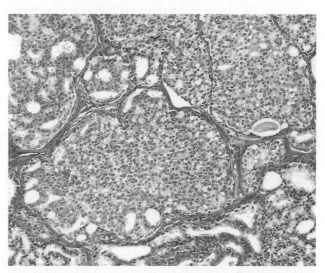

Figure 1.34.10 Back-to-back cribriform glands of Gleason pattern 4.

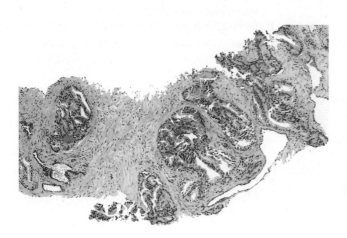

Figure 1.34.11 Dense cribriform glands with a differential diagnosis of IDC-P and infiltrating carcinoma.

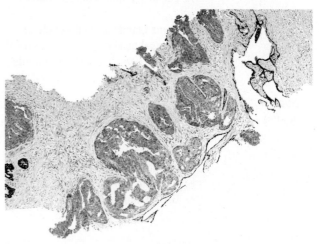

Figure 1.34.12 Same case as Figure 1.34.11 stained with HMWCK/p6/AMACR lacking negative basal cells in the cribriform glands, consistent with infiltrating carcinoma. The diagnosis of carcinoma in this case can only be made after stains for basal cells confirm their absence.

	Intraductal Adenocarcinoma of the Prostate (IDC-P)	Intraductal Spread of Urothelial Carcinoma (UC)
Age	Typically 50 to elderly, although not rare in 40s	Typically 50 to elderly, although not rare in 40s
Location	Peripheral > transition zone	Transition > peripheral zone
Symptoms	Asymptomatic incidentally discovered on biopsy	Asymptomatic incidentally discovered on biopsy
Signs	Typically associated with high-grade cancer and elevated serum PSA levels. DRE may be abnormal if associated infiltrating carcinoma	PSA may be elevated and DRE abnormal
Etiology	Typically, represents intraductal spread of carcinoma within preexisting ducts and acini. In the absence of infiltrating carcinoma, it is a distinct lesion from high-grade PIN and represents a late event in prostate cancer evolution	Represents spread of CIS from the bladder to the prostatic urethra and then down into prostatic ducts and acini
Histology	1. Normal or slightly expanded glands compared to normal 2. Stands out at low magnification as being darker than normal glands 3. May have flat, tufted, micropapillary, cribriform, or solid formation *(Figs. 1.35.1–1.35.7)* 4. Some cases with marked nuclear pleomorphism with 6× size, the size of normal nuclei 5. Some cases with necrosis *(Figs. 1.35.1 and 1.35.2)* 6. Some cases with subtle attempt at cribriform gland formation with rosette-like structures *(Figs. 1.35.4 and 1.35.5)* 7. Lacks squamous differentiation 8. Some glands partially involved 9. A basal cell layer in some involved glands can be seen, and in other glands, indistinct on H&E stain	1. Normal or slightly expanded glands compared to normal 2. Stands out at low magnification as being darker than normal glands 3. Typically solid nests filling up acini *(Figs. 1.35.7–1.35.12)* 4. Typically marked nuclear pleomorphism with 6× size, the size of normal nuclei 5. Some cases with necrosis *(Fig. 1.35.8)* 6. Lacks rosette-like structures 7. May have squamous differentiation with eosinophilic cytoplasm *(Fig. 1.35.9)* 8. Some glands partially involved *(Fig. 1.35.8)* 9. A basal cell layer in some involved glands can be seen, and in other glands, indistinct on H&E stain
Special studies	• A patchy or continuous basal cell layer seen with HMWCK and p63 *(Figs. 1.35.3 and 1.35.5)* • Variably AMACR positive • Prostate markers positive • GATA3 negative	• A patchy or continuous basal cell layer seen with HMWCK and p63 (one-third of cases) *(Fig. 1.35.10)* with HMWCK and/or p63 staining of tumor cells (two-third of cases) *(Fig. 1.35.11)* • Variably AMACR positive • Prostate markers negative • Malignant cells GATA3 positive *(Fig. 1.35.12)*

	Intraductal Adenocarcinoma of the Prostate (IDC-P)	Intraductal Spread of Urothelial Carcinoma (UC)
Treatment	Recommend treating patients with IDC-P on biopsy with definitive therapy even in the absence of documented infiltrating cancer	If intraductal UC on TURP, typically treated with radical cystoprostatectomy as BCG not effective in this setting
Prognosis	Frequently associated with high-grade cancer at radical prostatectomy or advanced disease where surgery is not an option	Intraductal UC on biopsy usually associated with infiltrating UC elsewhere in the prostate and poor prognosis. If only intraductal spread of UC at cystectomy, prognosis depends on the stage of the cancer in the bladder

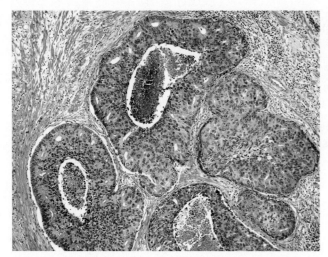

Figure 1.35.1 IDC-P with cribriform glands and necrosis. A patchy basal cell layer labeled with p63 and HMWCK (not shown).

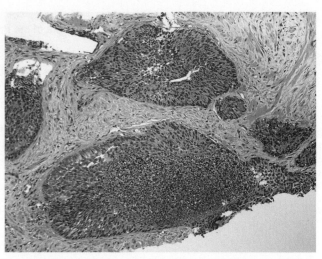

Figure 1.35.2 IDC-P with solid nests and central necrosis. Would need immunohistochemistry to differentiate from urothelial carcinoma. Other stains verified prostatic origin.

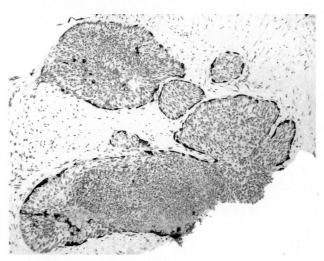

Figure 1.35.3 High molecular weight cytokeratin stain of Figure 1.35.1 showing intraductal growth. Could still represent either IDC-P or urothelial carcinoma, as one-third of urothelial carcinomas are negative for HMWCK.

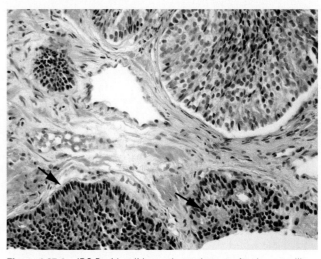

Figure 1.35.4 IDC-P with solid growth, yet there are focal rosette-like structures (*arrows*) indicating rudimentary cribriform gland formation.

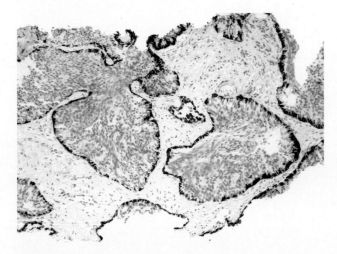

Figure 1.35.5 Same case as Figure 1.35.4 showing an intact basal cell layer labeled with HMWCK and p63.

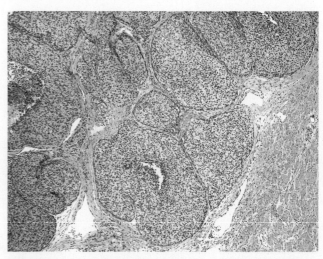

Figure 1.35.6 Expanded prostatic ducts and acini filled with urothelial carcinoma in a patient with CIS.

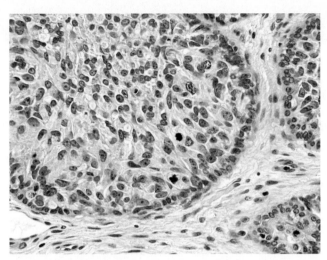

Figure 1.35.7   Same case as Figure 1.35.6 showing a preserved basal cell layer. On H&E, this could represent either urothelial carcinoma or IDC-P.

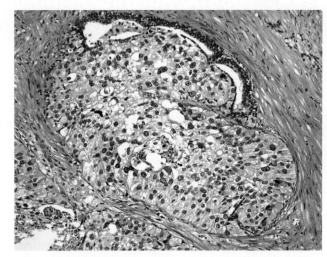

Figure 1.35.8   Intraductal spread of urothelial carcinoma with partial involvement and focal necrosis.

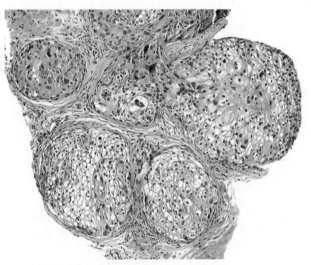

Figure 1.35.9   Intraductal spread of urothelial carcinoma with squamous differentiation.

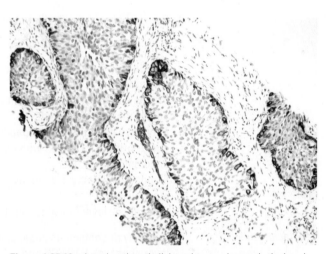

Figure 1.35.10   Intraductal urothelial carcinoma where only the basal cells label with HMWCK. Cannot be used to differentiate from IDC-P.

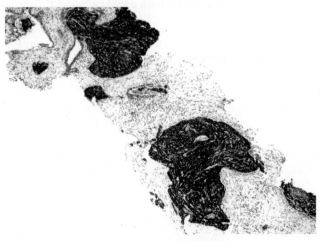

Figure 1.35.11   Intraductal urothelial carcinoma where tumor cells also label with HMWCK, in contrast to what is seen with IDC-P.

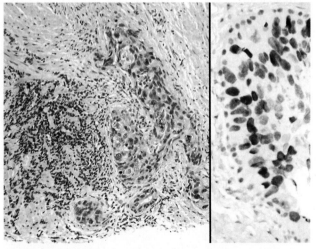

Figure 1.35.12   Intraductal urothelial carcinoma (**left**) labeled with GATA3 (**right**). GATA3 also more faintly labels prostatic basal cells but would be negative in the tumor cells of IDC-P.

	Prostatic Intraepithelial Neoplasia (PIN)	**PIN-Like Ductal Adenocarcinoma**
Age	Typically 50 to elderly, although not rare in 40s	Typically 50 to elderly, although not rare in 40s
Location	Peripheral > transition zone	Peripheral > transition zone
Symptoms	Asymptomatic incidentally discovered on biopsy	Asymptomatic incidentally discovered on biopsy
Signs	By itself not elevate serum PSA	Variably elevated serum PSA levels
Etiology	Unknown	Unknown. Variant of ductal adenocarcinoma
Histology	1. Medium to large glands that are of the size of normal prostatic acini *(Fig. 1.36.1)* 2. Rare to have cystically dilated glands 3. Glands may be crowded or spaced apart similar to benign glands 4. Stands out at low magnification as being darker than normal glands 5. May have flat, tufted, micropapillary, and cribriform formation with flat PIN uncommon *(Fig. 1.36.2)* 6. Elongated nuclei with some prominent nucleoli *(Fig. 1.36.2)* 7. A basal cell layer indistinct on H&E stain	1. Some medium to large glands that are of the size of normal prostatic acini *(Figs. 1.36.3–1.36.5)* 2. Some glands cystically dilated manifested by strips of epithelium along the edge of the tissue *(Figs. 1.36.3–1.36.10)* 3. Glands may be crowded or spaced apart similar to benign glands *(Figs. 1.36.3 and 1.36.11)* 4. Stands out at low magnification as being darker than normal glands 5. May have flat, tufted, and micropapillary formation with preponderance of flat lining *(Figs. 1.36.3 and 1.36.4)* 6. Elongated nuclei that typically lack prominent nucleoli *(Figs. 1.36.4 and 1.36.7)* 7. A basal cell layer indistinct on H&E stain
Special studies	• A patchy or continuous basal cell layer seen with HMWCK and p63 with occasional glands negative • Variably AMACR positive	• All glands negative for basal cell markers *(Figs. 1.36.8, 1.36.10, and 1.36.12)* • Variably AMACR positive *(Figs. 1.36.5, 1.36.8, and 1.36.12)*
Treatment	None	Same as usual prostate adenocarcinoma
Prognosis	No increased risk of cancer on repeat biopsy done within 1 y of initial diagnosis of HGPIN if found on one core (unifocal). No data on the long-term risk, so may be reasonable to do repeat biopsy 2–3 y later. If more than 1 core with HGPIN (multifocal), risk of cancer on repeat biopsy is 40% warranting repeat biopsy within 6 mo of initial biopsy	This variant of ductal adenocarcinoma, prognosis is equivalent to acinar Gleason score 3 + 3 = 6 adenocarcinoma

1.36 Prostatic Intraepithelial Neoplasia (PIN) vs. PIN-Like Ductal Adenocarcinoma   **111**

1 PROSTATE

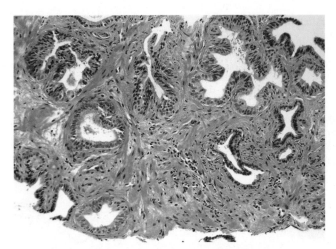

Figure 1.36.1   High-grade PIN with both flat and tufted pattern.

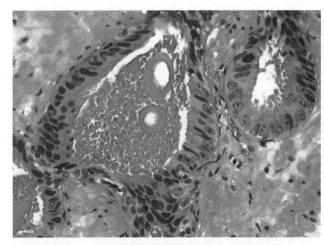

Figure 1.36.2   Flat high-grade PIN with prominent nucleoli.

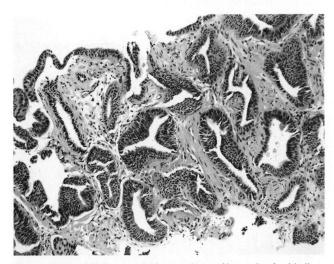

Figure 1.36.3   PIN-like ductal adenocarcinoma. Note strip of epithelium (*top*) that runs along length of core.

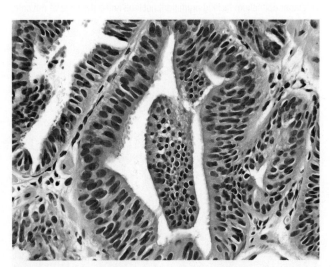

Figure 1.36.4   Same case as Figure 1.36.3. Despite appearance of extensive high-grade PIN at low magnification, the nuclei lack prominent nucleoli.

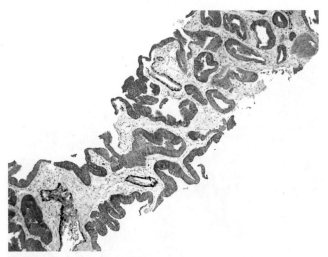

Figure 1.36.5   Same case as Figures 1.36.3 and 1.36.4 with triple stain showing positive AMACR (*red*) and lack of basal cells (*brown*) in all the PIN-like glands.

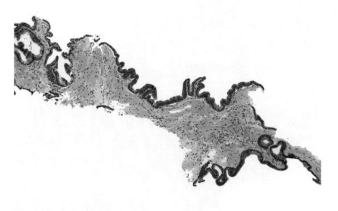

Figure 1.36.6   PIN-like ductal adenocarcinoma with strip of epitheliums that run along the bottom and top lengths of the core.

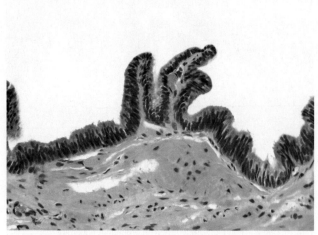

Figure 1.36.7   Same case as Figure 1.36.6 with pseudostratified columnar epithelium lacking prominent nucleoli lining the edge of the core.

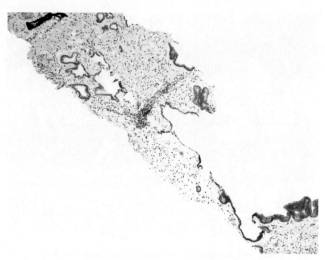

Figure 1.36.8   Same case as Figures 1.36.6 and 1.36.7, negative for basal cells (*brown*) and focally positive for AMACR (*red*).

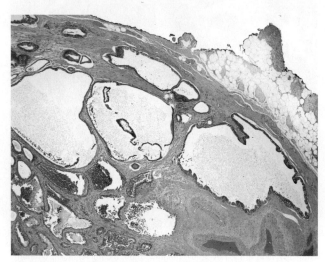

Figure 1.36.9   Radical prostatectomy with cystic glands of PIN-like ductal adenocarcinoma.

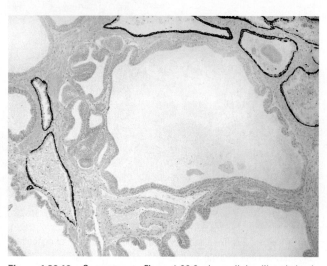

Figure 1.36.10   Same case as Figure 1.36.9 where all the dilated glands lined by columnar epithelium are negative for HMWCK.

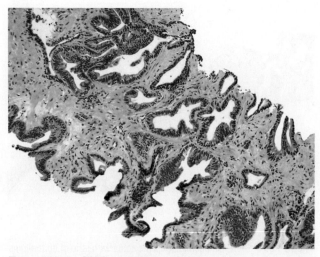

Figure 1.36.11   PIN-like ductal adenocarcinoma with somewhat more crowded glands than typical high-grade PIN.

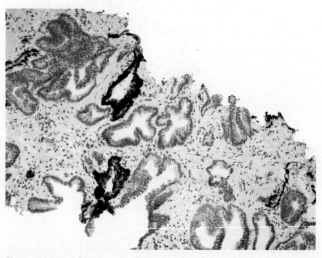

Figure 1.36.12   Same case as Figure 1.36.11 with triple stain showing positive AMACR (*red*) and lack of basal cells (*brown*) in all the PIN-like glands.

	Prostatic Urethral Polyp	Prostatic Ductal Adenocarcinoma
Age	From adolescence to elderly	Typically 50 to elderly, although not rare in 40s
Location	Arises from prostatic urethra. Typically on TURP. Rarely on needle biopsy	Most arise from verumontanum in prostatic urethra and underlying periurethral prostatic ducts but also can arise in smaller peripheral prostatic ducts and acini
Symptoms	Gross or microscopic hematuria, hematospermia, dysuria, and frequency	If urethral, gross or microscopic hematuria, hematospermia, dysuria, and frequency. If peripheral, asymptomatic incidentally discovered on biopsy
Signs	Does not elevate serum PSA levels	Variably elevated serum PSA levels. Less elevation than comparably sized acinar carcinomas
Etiology	Unknown	Unknown. Variant of prostate adenocarcinoma
Histology	1. Low-power polypoid growth lacking fronds or broad papillae (*Figs. 1.37.1 and 1.37.2*). Uncommon cases with occasional true papillary fronds (*Figs. 1.37.3 and 1.37.4*) 2. Surface lining by either low cuboidal benign prostate cells or benign urothelium (*Figs. 1.37.1–1.37.5*) 3. Suburethral or intrapapillae glands composed of crowded benign prostate glands (*Figs. 1.37.1, 1.37.2, and 1.37.5*) 4. A basal cell layer indistinct on H&E stain	1. Low-power thin papillary growth with fibrovascular cores (*Figs. 1.37.6–1.37.10*) 2. Surface lining by cells with pseudostratified columnar nuclei with variable cytologic atypia (*Figs. 1.37.8 and 1.37.10*) 3. Suburethral glands may be cribriform lined by cells with pseudostratified columnar nuclei. Papillary fronds contain central fibrovascular cores lined by columnar epithelium without any glands 4. A basal cell layer indistinct on H&E stain
Special studies	• Glands positive labeling for basal cell markers • AMACR negative	• When arising in large ducts, some involved may be positive for basal cell markers. Other areas may be negative • Variably AMACR positive
Treatment	None	Same as usual prostate adenocarcinoma
Prognosis	Entirely benign	Papillary and cribriform ductal adenocarcinoma's prognosis is equivalent to acinar Gleason score 4 + 4 = 8 adenocarcinoma

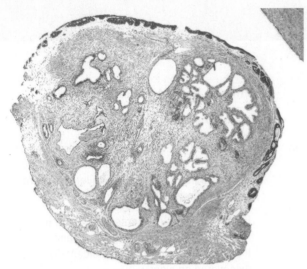

Figure 1.37.1   Rounded polypoid prostatic urethral polyp lined by urothelium.

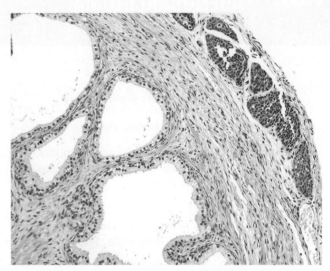

Figure 1.37.2   Same case as Figure 1.37.1 with denuded surface and underlying von Brunn nests and center of polyp with benign prostate glands.

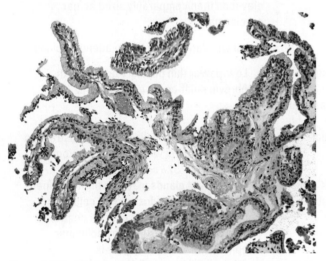

Figure 1.37.3   Prostatic urethral polyp lined by prostatic epithelium with occasional papillary fronds.

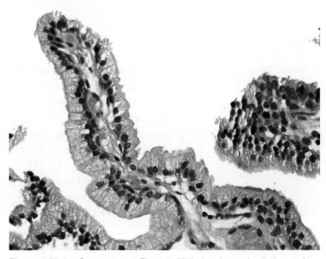

Figure 1.37.4   Same case as Figure 1.37.3 showing a simple layer of round nuclei without atypia.

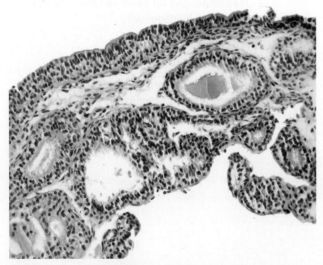

Figure 1.37.5   Prostatic urethral polyp with urothelial lining and underlying benign prostate glands.

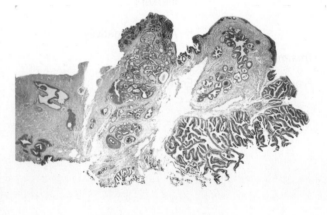

Figure 1.37.6   Prostatic duct adenocarcinoma arising from large ducts entering into the verumontanum.

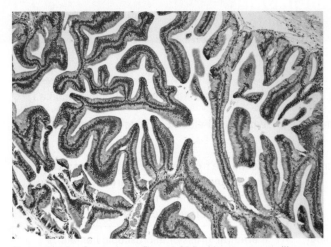

Figure 1.37.7 Same case as Figure 1.37.6 with numerous papillary fronds.

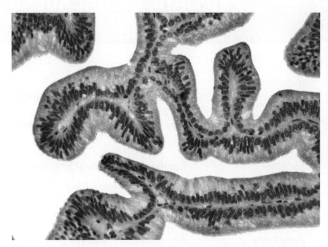

Figure 1.37.8 Same case as Figures 1.37.6 and 1.37.7 with papillary fronds lined by pseudostratified columnar cells with relatively bland nuclei.

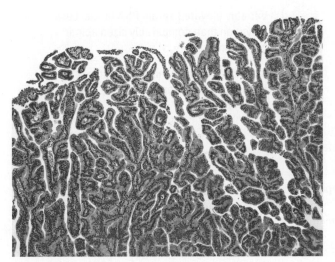

Figure 1.37.9 Numerous papillary fronds of prostatic duct adenocarcinoma.

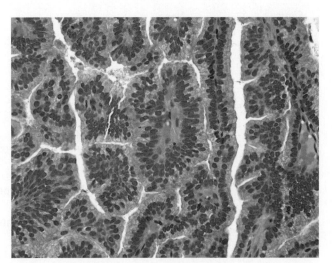

Figure 1.37.10 Same case as Figure 1.37.9 with papillary fronds lined by pseudostratified columnar cells with some nuclei having visible nucleoli.

	Hyperplastic Benign Prostate Glands	Papillary Prostatic Ductal Adenocarcinoma
Age	Any age, although typically sampled in adults	Typically 50-elderly, although not rare in 40s
Location	Can be the peripheral or transition zone	Most arise from verumontanum in prostatic urethra and underlying periurethral prostatic ducts but also can arise in smaller peripheral prostatic ducts and acini
Symptoms	Asymptomatic. Variant of normal histology	If urethral, gross or microscopic hematuria, hematospermia, dysuria, and frequency. If peripheral, asymptomatic incidentally discovered on biopsy
Signs	None	Variably elevated serum PSA levels. Less elevation than comparably sized acinar carcinomas
Incidence	Uncommon	If pure, <1%, and if mixed with acinar adenocarcinoma, approximately 5% of prostate carcinomas
Etiology	A variant of normal histology. Not necessarily indication of benign prostatic hyperplasia	
Histology	1. Dilated glands with occasional papillary fronds *(Figs. 1.38.1–1.38.6)* 2. Surface lining by low cuboidal benign prostate cells 3. Cytologically bland nuclei *(Figs. 1.38.2, 1.38.3, 1.38.5, and 1.38.6)* 4. A basal cell layer indistinct on H&E stain	1. Thin papillary growth with fibrovascular cores *(Figs. 1.38.7–1.38.10)* 2. Surface lining by cells with pseudostratified columnar nuclei *(Figs. 1.38.8–1.38.10)* 3. Variable cytologic atypia with some cases having nuclear enlargement with prominent nucleoli *(Figs. 1.38.8–1.38.10)* 4. A basal cell layer indistinct on H&E stain
Special studies	• Glands positive for basal cell markers • AMACR negative	• When arising in large ducts, some involved may be positive for basal cell markers. Other areas may be negative • Variably AMACR positive
Treatment	None	Same as usual prostate adenocarcinoma
Prognosis	Entirely benign	Papillary and cribriform ductal adenocarcinoma's prognosis is equivalent to acinar Gleason score 4 + 4 = 8 adenocarcinoma

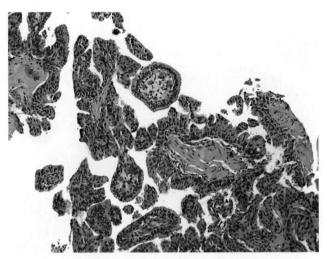

Figure 1.38.1   Hyperplastic benign glands with papillary fronds.

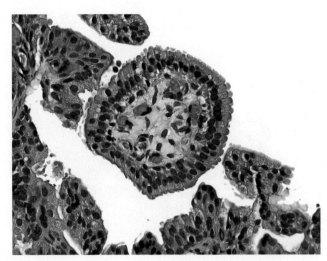

Figure 1.38.2   Same case as Figure 1.38.1 with epithelium lining papillary fronds composed of nonstratified round benign nuclei.

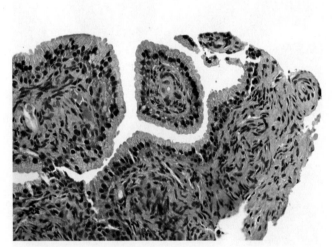

Figure 1.38.3   Hyperplastic benign glands with papillary fronds lined by nonstratified round benign nuclei.

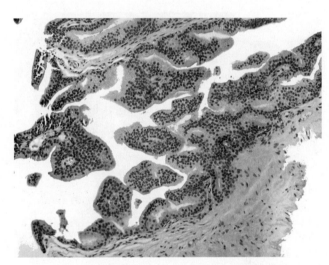

Figure 1.38.4   Hyperplastic benign glands with papillary fronds.

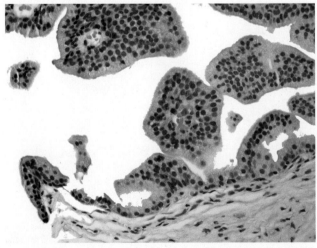

Figure 1.38.5   Same case as Figure 1.38.4 with epithelium lining papillary fronds composed of round benign nuclei.

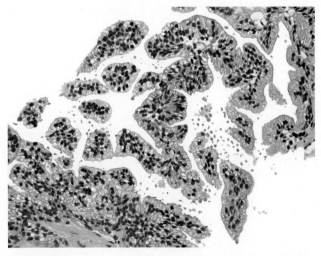

Figure 1.38.6   Hyperplastic benign glands with papillary fronds lined by round benign nuclei.

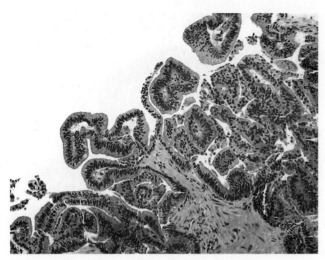

Figure 1.38.7   Papillary prostatic duct adenocarcinoma.

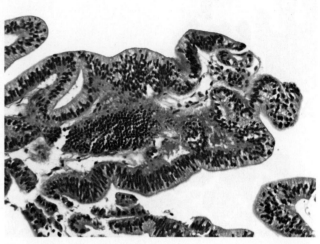

Figure 1.38.8   Same case as Figure 1.38.7 with papillary fronds lined by bland pseudostratified columnar cells.

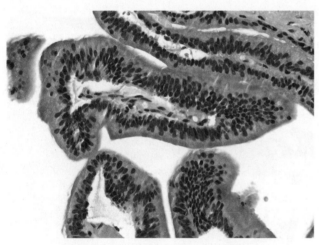

Figure 1.38.9   Papillary prostatic duct adenocarcinoma lined by bland pseudostratified columnar cells.

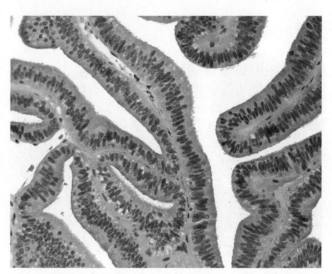

Figure 1.38.10   Papillary prostatic duct adenocarcinoma lined by pseudostratified columnar cells with some visible nucleoli.

	Prostatic Ductal Adenocarcinoma	Prostatic Acinar Adenocarcinoma
Age	Typically 50-elderly, although not rare in 40s	Typically 50-elderly, although not rare in 40s
Location	Most arise from verumontanum in prostatic urethra and underlying periurethral prostatic ducts found on TURP but also can arise in smaller peripheral prostatic ducts and acini found on needle biopsy	85%–90% arise in the peripheral zone and detected on needle biopsy, yet remaining arise in the transition zone and can be found either on needle biopsy or on TURP
Symptoms	If urethral, gross or microscopic hematuria, hematospermia, dysuria, and frequency. If peripheral, asymptomatic incidentally discovered on biopsy	Typically asymptomatic. Advanced disease with urinary obstructive symptoms and/or hematuria or from distant metastases
Signs	Variably elevated serum PSA levels. Less elevation than comparably sized acinar carcinomas	Variably elevated serum PSA levels
Etiology	Unknown. Variant of prostatic adenocarcinoma	See Section 1.6
Histology	1. Cribriform, papillary, PIN-like 2. Glands or papillary fronds lined by cells with pseudostratified columnar nuclei *(Figs. 1.39.1–1.39.7)*, which is the hallmark of ductal adenocarcinoma 3. Variable cytologic atypia with some cases having nuclear enlargement with prominent nucleoli 4. Cribriform glands tend to have slit-like spaces *(Figs. 1.39.1, 1.39.3, and 1.39.7)* 5. Cytoplasm typically amphophilic yet rarely lightly eosinophilic 6. PIN-like pattern consists of markedly dilated glands (see Section 1.37) 7. A basal cell layer indistinct on H&E stain	1. Cribriform, small glands, individual cells, solid nests 2. Cells are cuboidal *(Figs. 1.39.5–1.39.10)*, which is the key to defining acinar differentiation 3. Variable cytologic atypia with some cases having nuclear enlargement with prominent nucleoli 4. Cribriform glands tend to have punched out round lumina, although not required to define acinar adenocarcinoma *(Figs. 1.39.7 and 1.39.8)* 5. Cytoplasm variable ranging from lightly eosinophilic to amphophilic 6. Pseudohyperplastic variant can have markedly dilated glands (see Section 1.21) 7. A basal cell layer indistinct on H&E stain
Special studies	• When arising in large ducts, some involved may be positive for basal cell markers. Other areas may be negative • Variably AMACR positive	• With very rare exception, negative for basal cell markers. May be associated with intraductal spread with positive basal cells (see Section 1.35) • Variably AMACR positive
Treatment	Same as usual prostate adenocarcinoma	Stage and grade dependent

	Prostatic Ductal Adenocarcinoma	Prostatic Acinar Adenocarcinoma
Prognosis	Papillary and cribriform ductal adenocarcinoma's prognosis is equivalent to acinar Gleason score 4 + 4 = 8 adenocarcinoma	Individual well-formed glands are Gleason pattern 3 with excellent prognosis and no potential for metastases. Cribriform, poorly formed, and fused glands are Gleason pattern 4 with capacity for metastatic spread; increasing risk of progression from 3 + 4 = 7 to 4 + 3 = 7 to 4 + 4 = 8. Single cells, solid nests, and cribriform glands with central necrosis are Gleason pattern 5 with typically a poor prognosis

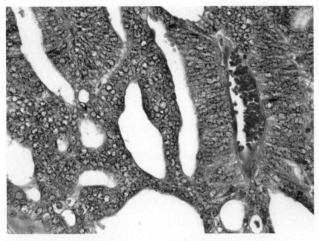

Figure 1.39.1   Ductal adenocarcinoma with slit-like spaces lined by pseudostratified columnar cells.

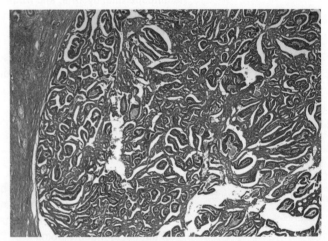

Figure 1.39.2   Large nodule of papillary and cribriform ductal adenocarcinoma surrounded by acinar adenocarcinoma (*left*).

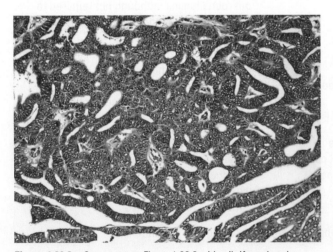

Figure 1.39.3   Same case as Figure 1.39.2 with cribriform ductal adenocarcinoma.

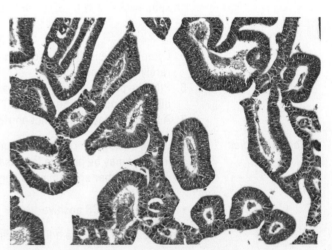

Figure 1.39.4   Same case as Figures 1.39.2 and 1.39.3 with papillary ductal adenocarcinoma.

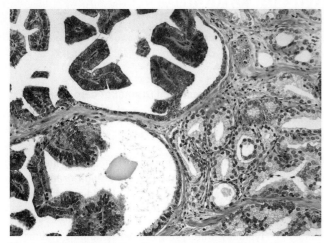

Figure 1.39.5 Same case as Figures 1.39.2–1.39.4 with papillary ductal adenocarcinoma (*left*) and acinar adenocarcinoma (*right*).

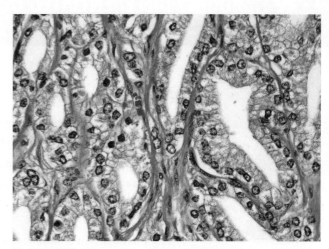

Figure 1.39.6 Same case as Figures 1.39.2–1.39.5 with acinar adenocarcinoma composed of cuboidal epithelium lacking pseudostratification.

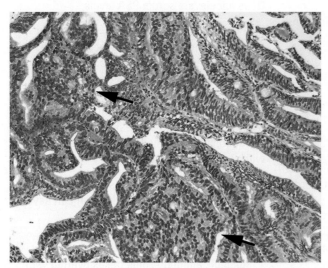

Figure 1.39.7 Mixed cribriform ductal adenocarcinoma with slit-like spaces lined by pseudostratified columnar cells and acinar (*arrows*) adenocarcinoma with rounded lumens and cuboidal epithelium.

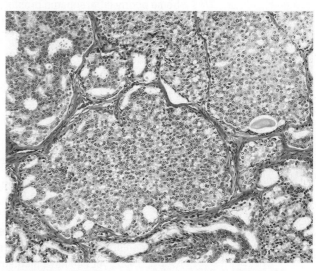

Figure 1.39.8 Cribriform acinar adenocarcinoma with cuboidal epithelium and rounded lumens.

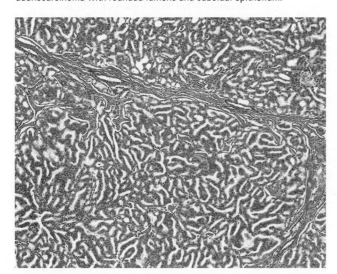

Figure 1.39.9 Cribriform acinar adenocarcinoma with more elongated lumens than usual.

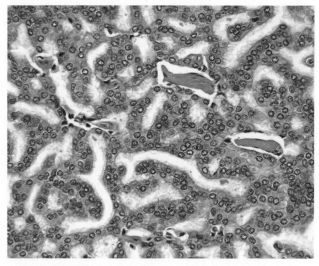

Figure 1.39.10 Same case as Figure 1.39.9 with rounded nuclei, diagnostic of acinar differentiation.

	Poorly Differentiated Prostatic Adenocarcinoma	Poorly Differentiated Urothelial Carcinoma
Age	Typically 50 to elderly, although not rare in 40s	Typically 50 to elderly, although not rare in 40s
Location	85%–90% arise in the peripheral zone (PZ), yet can invade the transition zone (TZ) from PZ and can be found either on needle biopsy or on TURP	Most commonly seen on TUR of bladder neck where clinically could be either high-grade prostate adenocarcinoma or bladder urothelial carcinoma
Symptoms	Typically asymptomatic. Advanced disease with urinary obstructive symptoms and/or hematuria or from distant metastases	Typically urinary obstructive symptoms and/or hematuria
Signs	Some poorly differentiated prostate carcinomas lack significant PSA production	Does not elevate serum PSA levels
Etiology	See Section 1.6	Numerous environmental risk factors. Most common is history of smoking, accounting for 60% and 30% of all urothelial carcinomas in males and females, respectively. Other risk factors include exposure to various chemicals (especially aromatic amines), heredity, infection, prior radiation, prior chemotherapy with cyclophosphamide, and diet
Histology	1. Cribriform glands, large solid nests, cords of cells 2. Nuclei more uniform with centrally located prominent eosinophilic nucleoli *(Fig. 1.40.1)*, yet can have pleomorphic giant cell features *(Fig. 1.40.2)* 3. Tumor can have a pseudopapillary appearance due to tumor necrosis or as a result of an artifact *(Figs. 1.40.3–1.40.5)* 4. May have subtle rudimentary cribriform formation with rosette-like formation *(Figs. 1.40.6 and 1.40.7)* 5. Mitotic figures are typically not frequent 6. Necrosis uncommon 7. Stromal inflammation uncommon 8. Squamous differentiation rare and typically seen with prior hormonal therapy	1. Typically variably sized nests *(Fig. 1.40.9)*. Lacks cribriform glands, although can have glandular differentiation 2. Cytologically, tends to show greater nuclear pleomorphism, variably prominent nucleoli, although some cases overlap with prostate cancer with more uniform cytology *(Figs. 1.40.10 and 1.40.11)* 3. True papillary fronds may be present 4. Lacks rosette-like formation 5. Increased mitotic activity not uncommon 6. Necrosis not uncommon 7. Stromal inflammation common *(Fig. 1.40.10)* 8. Squamous differentiation seen in 14% of cases

	Poorly Differentiated Prostatic Adenocarcinoma	**Poorly Differentiated Urothelial Carcinoma**
Special studies	• Occasionally can aberrantly express HMWCK in a nonbasal cell distribution; less commonly seen with p63 • GATA3, thrombomodulin, uroplakin negative • Variably and focally positive for prostate markers (PSA, PSMA, P501S, NKX3.1) *(Figs. 1.40.3 and 1.40.5)*. Small percent negative for PSA such that other prostate markers should be done before assuming PSA-negative cancer is urothelial carcinoma. Critical to have strong positive control of benign prostate tissue since prostate carcinoma shows lower expression *(Fig. 1.40.8)* • Variably AMACR positive	• Approximately two-thirds of cases positive for HMWCK or p63 • Most sensitive and specific marker is GATA3 with fewer cases positive for thrombomodulin *(Fig. 1.40.12)*. Uroplakin is not that sensitive in high-grade urothelial carcinomas • Negative for prostate markers • Variably AMACR positive
Treatment	Critical to recognize as prostatic in origin since advanced high-grade prostatic adenocarcinoma treated with antiandrogen therapy	Important to diagnose correctly as urothelial carcinoma since effective chemotherapy tailored to urothelial carcinoma exists
Prognosis	Some patients respond well for many years before developing hormone-resistant cancer	Urothelial carcinoma directly invading the prostate is stage T4 with a poor prognosis

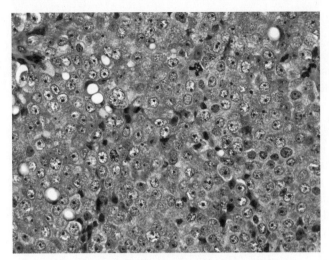

Figure 1.40.1 Gleason score 5 + 5 = 10 prostatic adenocarcinoma. Despite prominent nucleoli and atypical mitotic figure, nuclei are relatively uniform in terms of size and shape.

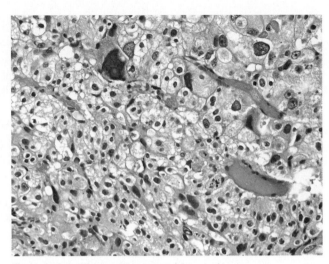

Figure 1.40.2 Pleomorphic prostate adenocarcinoma.

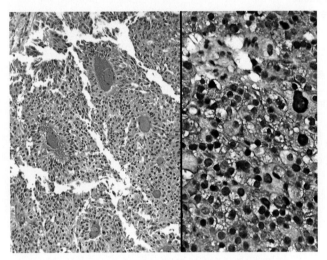

Figure 1.40.3 Same case as Figure 1.40.2 with pseudopapillary formation due to artifactual tumor falling apart (*left*) and NKX3.1 positivity (*right*).

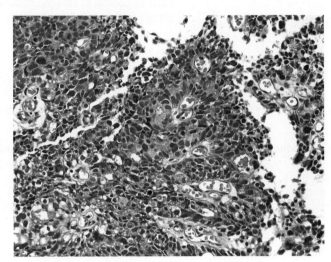

Figure 1.40.4 Pleomorphic adenocarcinoma of the prostate with pseudopapillary formation.

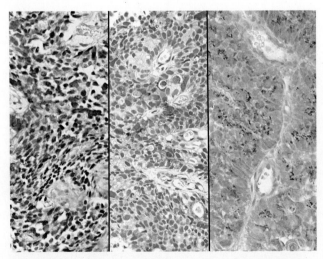

Figure 1.40.5 Same case as Figure 1.40.4 with positivity for NKX3.1 (*left*), PSA (*middle*), and P501S (*right*).

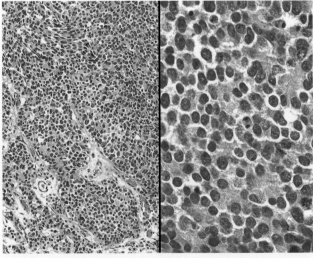

Figure 1.40.6 Poorly differentiated prostate adenocarcinoma (*left*) with higher magnification (*right*) showing rosette-like formation.

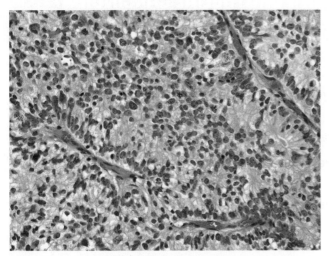

Figure 1.40.7   Poorly differentiated prostate adenocarcinoma rosette-like formation. The presence of thin capillaries could be mistaken for papillary urothelial carcinoma.

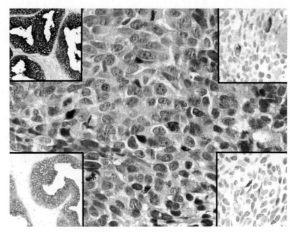

Figure 1.40.8   High-grade prostate adenocarcinoma (**center**). **Lower left inset** is benign prostate tissue PSA control from referring institution, which shows weak staining. Prostate cancer stained at the referring institution was negative (**lower right inset**). **Upper left inset** is benign prostate tissue PSA control from Hopkins, which shows strong staining. Prostate cancer stained at Hopkins showed focal positive staining (**upper right inset**).

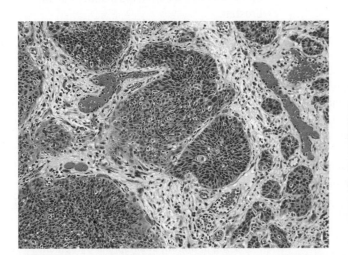

Figure 1.40.9   Variably sized irregular nests of infiltrating urothelial carcinoma.

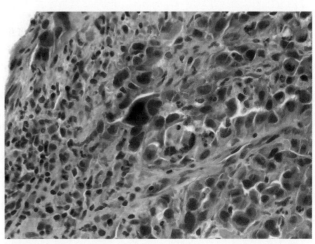

Figure 1.40.10   Infiltrating urothelial carcinoma with pleomorphic nuclei and associated inflammation.

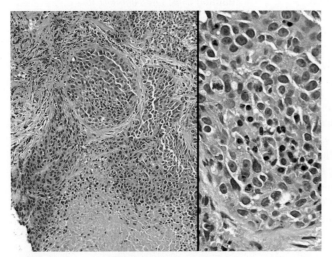

Figure 1.40.11   Nests of infiltrating urothelial carcinoma with necrosis (**left**) and relatively uniform nuclei with prominent nucleoli, mimicking prostate adenocarcinoma (**right**).

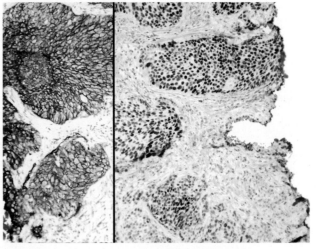

Figure 1.40.12   Same case as Figure 1.40.11 with positive thrombomodulin (**left**) and GATA3 (**right**).

	Prostatic Intraductal Urothelial Carcinoma	**Intraductal and Infiltrating Urothelial Carcinoma**
Age	Typically 50 to elderly, although not rare in 40s	Typically 50 to elderly, although not rare in 40s
Location	Most commonly seen on TUR of bladder neck but can be seen on needle biopsy	Most commonly seen on TUR of bladder neck but can be seen on needle biopsy
Symptoms	Typically urinary obstructive symptoms and/or hematuria	Typically urinary obstructive symptoms and/or hematuria
Signs	Does not elevate serum PSA levels	Does not elevate serum PSA levels
Etiology	Spread from CIS of the bladder to prostatic urethra and then down to prostatic ducts and acini	Invasion from intraductal urothelial carcinoma within the prostate as opposed to direct extension of an invasive urothelial carcinoma directly from the bladder into the prostate
Histology	1. Urothelial carcinoma involving nests that are in general the same size as normal prostatic acini *(Figs. 1.41.1 and 1.41.2)*. In some cases, ducts are expanded with intraductal urothelial carcinoma showing central necrosis *(Figs. 1.41.3 and 1.41.4)* 2. Nests may be numerous, crowded, and complex *(Figs. 1.41.5 and 1.41.6)* 3. Lacks carcinoma manifesting as individual cells and small nests with retraction artifact 4. Paradoxical differentiation absent 5. Typically stroma surrounding nests lacks inflammation and desmoplastic reaction, although occasionally may be present *(Fig. 1.41.4)* 6. A basal cell layer can in some cases be visualized around nests of carcinoma *(Fig. 1.41.2)*, and in some glands, only partial involvement is seen *(Figs. 1.41.7 and 1.41.8)*	1. An intraductal component is urothelial carcinoma involving nests that are in general the same size as normal prostatic acini 2. Intraductal urothelial carcinoma nests may be numerous, crowded, and complex 3. Carcinoma invades as individual cells and small nests sometimes with retraction artifact *(Figs. 1.41.9 and 1.41.10)* 4. Some infiltrating tumor may show paradoxical differentiation with cells having abundant eosinophilic cytoplasm 5. Typically stroma surrounding nests exhibits an inflammation and desmoplastic reaction *(Figs. 1.41.9 and 1.41.10)* 6. A basal cell layer is absent
Special studies	• In difficult cases, pancytokeratin or CK7 can help document the absence of individual infiltrating tumor cells • In one-third of cases, HMWCK outlines basal cells of preexisting prostatic acini and are negative in the tumor (remaining two-thirds of cases also labels tumor) helping to identify the nest as not being invasive carcinoma	• In difficult cases, pancytokeratin or CK7 can help document individual infiltrating tumor cells • In one-third of cases, HMWCK outlines basal cells of preexisting prostatic acini and are negative in the tumor helping to identify small irregular nests without basal cell as being invasive carcinoma

	Prostatic Intraductal Urothelial Carcinoma	**Intraductal and Infiltrating Urothelial Carcinoma**
Treatment	In TURP specimens, the presence of intraductal urothelial carcinoma typically leads to cystoprostatectomy as intravesicle BCG is not effective to treat intraprostatic disease	Typically treated with cystoprostatectomy
Prognosis	In cystoprostatectomy specimens, intraductal urothelial carcinoma has no prognostic significance. Prognosis is dependent on tumor stage in bladder	The presence of infiltrating urothelial carcinoma is associated with a worse prognosis yet not equivalent to pT4, which is direct extension of a muscle invasive bladder urothelial carcinoma into the prostatic stroma. When there is prostatic intraductal and associated infiltrating urothelial carcinoma, it is staged as pT2 urethral carcinoma. The prognosis is also dependent on the stage of carcinoma within the bladder

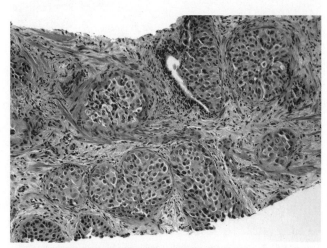

Figure 1.41.1   Intraductal urothelial carcinoma on needle biopsy. The involved glands are of the size and distribution of normal prostate glands.

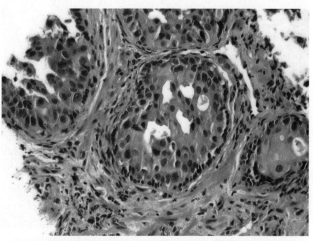

Figure 1.41.2   Same case as Figure 1.41.1 showing a preserved basal cell layer.

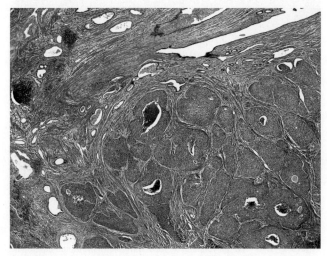

Figure 1.41.3   Expanded nests of intraductal urothelial carcinoma.

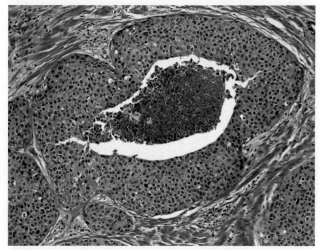

Figure 1.41.4   Same case as Figure 1.41.3 showing intraductal urothelial carcinoma with central necrosis. The surrounding tissue lacks a stromal reaction.

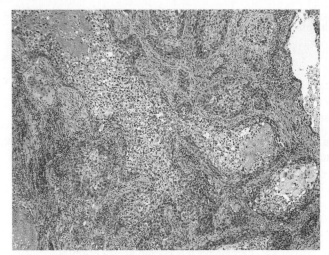

Figure 1.41.5   Complex intraductal urothelial carcinoma. Ducts maintain their branching morphology. Surrounding stroma is inflamed but not desmoplastic.

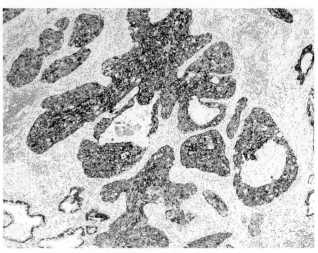

Figure 1.41.6   Same case as Figure 1.41.5 with pancytokeratin highlighting normal ductal contours and absence of infiltrating small nests and individual cells.

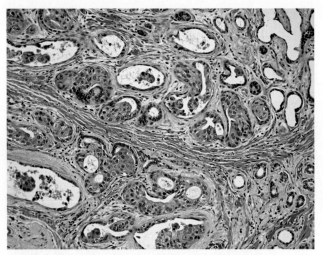

Figure 1.41.7   Intraductal urothelial carcinoma involving small atrophic prostate glands.

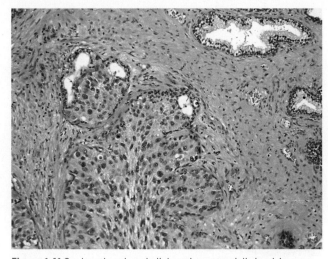

Figure 1.41.8   Intraductal urothelial carcinoma partially involving prostate glands.

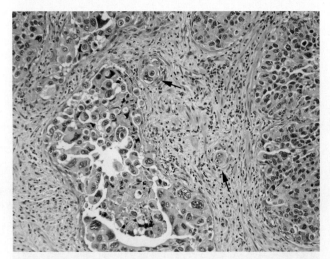

Figure 1.41.9   Larger rounded nests of intraductal urothelial carcinoma with small nests of infiltrating urothelial carcinoma (*arrows*). Stroma is inflamed and shows desplasia.

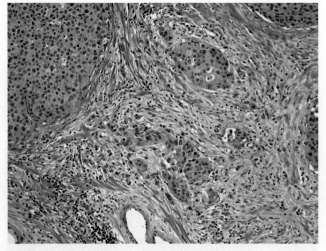

Figure 1.41.10   Larger rounded nests of intraductal urothelial carcinoma (*top*) with small irregular nests of infiltrating urothelial carcinoma in a desmoplastic stroma.

	Prostatic Infarct	Infiltrating Urothelial Carcinoma
Age	Typically 50 to elderly	Typically 50 to elderly, although not rare in 40s
Location	Most commonly seen on TURPs done for BPH but can occasionally be seen on needle biopsy	Most commonly seen on TUR of bladder. Occasionally on needle biopsy of the prostate
Symptoms	Typically urinary obstructive symptoms and/or hematuria	Typically urinary obstructive symptoms and/or hematuria
Signs	Can markedly elevate serum PSA levels	Does not elevate serum PSA levels
Etiology	Typically associated with large size of BPH. Also associated with generalized severe atherosclerosis	See Section 1.40
Histology	1. On TURP, can appear as lobular lesion *(Figs. 1.42.1 and 1.42.2)* 2. On TURP, zonation with center of the infarct having acute coagulative necrosis and recent hemorrhage with adjacent reactive epithelial nests. Progressing away from infarct, more mature squamous metaplasia with fibrosis. Zonation not as easily identified on biopsy *(Figs. 1.42.3 and 1.42.4)* 3. Reactive urothelium may be pleomorphic with irregular nuclei and prominent nucleoli *(Figs. 1.42.4–1.42.8)* 4. Increased mitotic activity not uncommon *(Figs. 1.42.4, 1.42.6 and 1.42.8)* 5. Necrosis common in center of nests often with neutrophils and acellular debris *(Fig. 1.42.9)* 6. Stromal recent hemorrhage or hemosiderin common *(Figs. 1.42.7 and 1.42.8)*	1. Irregular low-magnification appearance without lobularity 2. Lacks zonation with atypical urothelium usually consistently throughout the lesion 3. Neoplastic urothelium may be pleomorphic with irregular nuclei and prominent nucleoli 4. Increased mitotic activity not uncommon 5. Necrosis not common and typically lacks neutrophils and central debris 6. Stromal recent hemorrhage or hemosiderin uncommon *(Fig. 1.42.10)*
Special studies	• Not helpful in this differential	• Not helpful in this differential
Treatment	None	Typically would be treated with chemotherapy
Prognosis	Entirely benign	Infiltrating urothelial carcinoma on prostate needle biopsy is pT4 disease with a poor prognosis

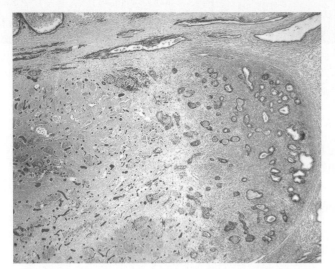

Figure 1.42.1 Lobular appearance of recent prostatic infarct (*left*).

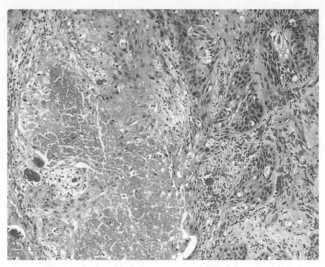

Figure 1.42.2 Same case as Figure 1.42.1 with reactive urothelial metaplasia (*right*) adjacent to infarct (*left*).

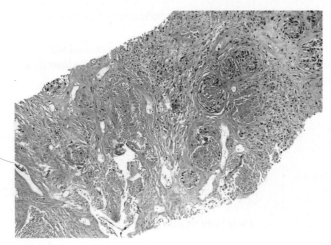

Figure 1.42.3 Infarct on needle biopsy with necrosis (*left*) and reactive urothelial metaplasia (*upper right*).

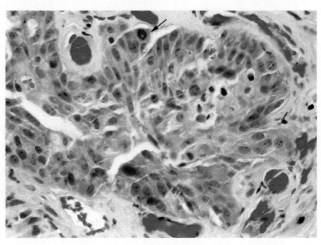

Figure 1.42.4 Same case as Figure 1.42.3 with reactive urothelial metaplasia with moderate pleomorphism and mitotic figure (*arrow*).

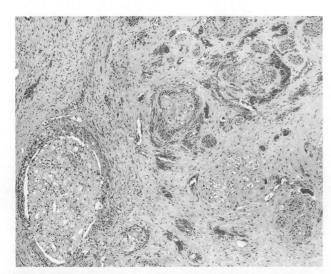

Figure 1.42.5 Infarct with reactive urothelial and squamous metaplasia with stromal hemorrhage.

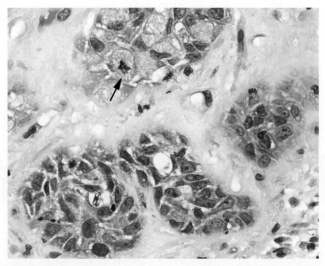

Figure 1.42.6 Same case as Figure 1.42.5 with cytologic atypia and mitotic figure (*arrow*).

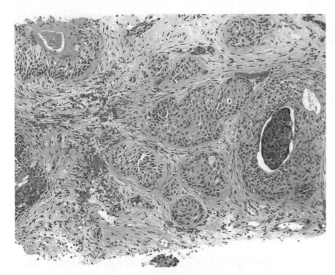

Figure 1.42.7 Infarct with reactive urothelial nests with central necrosis. Stromal hemorrhage is prominent.

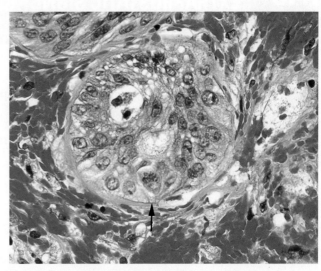

Figure 1.42.8 Same case as Figure 1.42.7 with cytologic atypia and mitotic figure (*arrow*) and surrounding stromal hemorrhage.

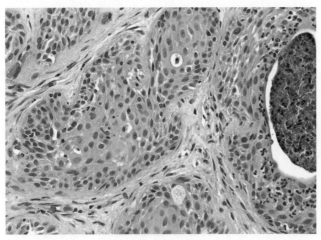

Figure 1.42.9 Same case as Figures 1.42.7 and 1.42.8 showing reactive urothelial nests with central collection of neutrophils (*right*).

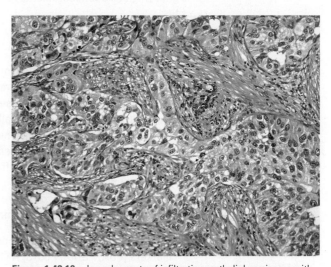

Figure 1.42.10 Irregular nests of infiltrating urothelial carcinoma with surrounding stroma lacking changes seen with prostatic infarct.

	Signet-Ring Cell–Like High-grade Prostate Adenocarcinoma	Extraprostatic Signet-Ring Cell Carcinoma
Age	Typically 50 to elderly, although not rare in 40s	Typically 50 to elderly, although not rare in 40s
Location	Not localized to a specific area	If extension from the rectum, predominantly involves posterior prostate
Symptoms	Typically asymptomatic	Typically asymptomatic
Signs	Variably elevated serum PSA levels	Typically not elevated PSA levels
Etiology	All grades of prostate adenocarcinoma can have empty cytoplasmic vacuoles. With Gleason pattern 5 cancer, can resemble signet-ring cell adenocarcinomas from other sites	Most common signet-ring cell adenocarcinoma to invade the prostate is from the rectum
Histology	1. Individual cells or cords of cells (*Figs. 1.43.1 and 1.43.2*) 2. If there are also glands, typical of usual prostate cancer with minimal pleomorphism and rarely necrosis 3. Nuclei are eccentric with centrally located prominent eosinophilic nucleoli. However, nucleoli not always visible 4. Mitotic figures are typically not frequent 5. Clear cytoplasmic vacuoles (*Figs. 1.43.1 and 1.43.2*) 6. Stromal inflammation is uncommon	1. Individual cells or cords of cells (*Figs. 1.43.3–1.43.6*) 2. If there are glands, typical of colon cancer with prominent pleomorphism and often necrosis 3. Nuclei are eccentric with centrally located prominent eosinophilic nucleoli. However, nucleoli not always visible 4. Mitotic figures are typically not frequent 5. Cytoplasmic vacuoles have a bluish tinge (*Figs. 1.43.4 and 1.43.5*) 6. Stromal inflammation is common
Special studies	• Variably and focally positive for prostate markers (PSA, PSMA, P501S, NKX3.1) • Variably AMACR positive • CDX2 can be uncommonly positive • Nuclear beta-catenin negative • Mucin stains negative	• Negative for prostate markers (PSA, PSMA, P501S, NKX3.1) • Variably AMACR positive • CDX2 commonly positive (*Fig. 1.43.6*) • Nuclear beta-catenin can be positive • Mucin stains positive (*Fig. 1.43.6*)
Treatment	Same as usual prostate adenocarcinoma	Critical to recognize as nonprostatic in origin since treatment tailored to the specific primary
Prognosis	Critical to recognize as prostatic in origin since advanced high-grade prostatic adenocarcinoma treated with antiandrogen therapy	Dismal since stage T4, regardless of the primary

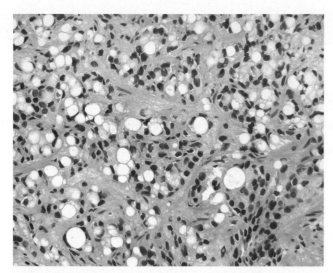

Figure 1.43.1 Signet-ring cell–like adenocarcinoma with individual cells having clear cytoplasmic vacuoles and eccentric nuclei.

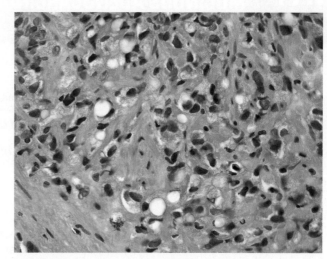

Figure 1.43.2 Prostate with scattered signet-ring cell–like adenocarcinoma cells (*left*).

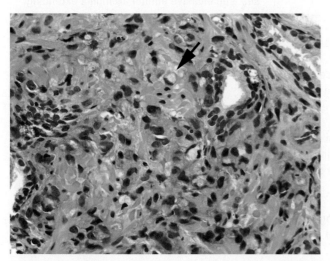

Figure 1.43.3 Signet-ring cell adenocarcinoma of the rectum invading the prostate. True signet ring cells have lightly blue-tinged cytoplasm (*arrow*).

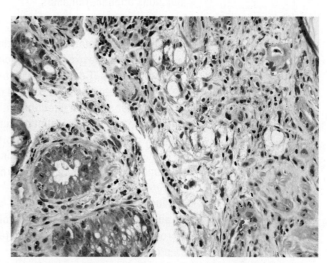

Figure 1.43.4 Same case as Figure 1.43.3 with primary signet-ring cell adenocarcinoma of the rectum.

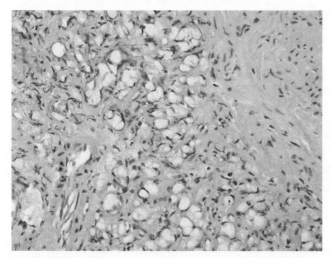

Figure 1.43.5 Signet-ring cell adenocarcinoma of the gastrointestinal tract invading prostate stroma. Cells lack clear empty cytoplasmic vacuoles of prostatic signet-ring cell–like adenocarcinoma.

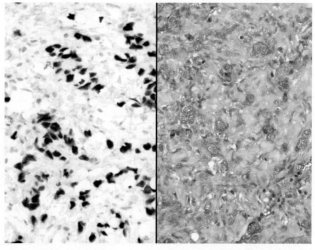

Figure 1.43.6 Same case as Figure 1.43.5 with diffuse CDX2 (**left**) and mucicarmine (**right**) staining.

	Mucinous Prostatic Adenocarcinoma	Urethral Mucinous Adenocarcinoma
Age	Typically 50 to elderly, although not rare in 40s	Typically 50 to elderly, although not rare in 40s
Location	Most are located in the peripheral zone, detected on needle biopsy	Arises from prostatic urethra without bladder involvement
Symptoms	Typically asymptomatic	Typically hematuria and occasionally mucusuria
Signs	Variably elevated serum PSA levels, no different than usual prostate cancer	PSA levels typically not elevated
Etiology	All grades of prostate adenocarcinoma can be mucinous. 0.2% of prostate cancers are mucinous adenocarcinomas	Glandular metaplasia of the prostatic urethra that progresses to dysplasia, carcinoma *in situ*, and invasive adenocarcinoma extending into the prostate
Histology	1. "Mucinous prostatic adenocarcinoma" requires >25% extracellular mucin. Diagnosed as "Carcinoma with focal mucinous features" if <25% or if on biopsy, as in latter situation need the entire prostate to assess percent mucin 2. Most common pattern is cribriform glands floating in mucin, less common individual round glands, least common cords of cells *(Figs. 1.44.1–1.44.3)* 3. Nuclei are typical of prostate adenocarcinoma with bland cytology, round nuclei with centrally located prominent nucleoli 4. Mitotic figures are typically not frequent 5. Can have signet-ring cell–like features with clear cytoplasmic vacuoles 6. Surface of urethra is uninvolved and lined by normal urothelium	1. Lakes of extracellular mucin *(Figs. 1.44.4 and 1.44.5)* 2. Mucin lined by tall columnar epithelium with scattered goblet cells *(Fig. 1.44.6)*. Lacks glands floating within mucin 3. Nuclei are variably atypical from relatively bland to overtly pleomorphic *(Fig. 1.44.7)* 4. Mitotic figures are not uncommon 5. Can have true signet ring cells with cytoplasm having bluish tinge on H&E *(Fig. 1.44.8)* 6. Surface of urethra is lined by either flat epithelium or villous adenoma, both with variably atypical glandular epithelium *(Figs. 1.44.9 and 1.44.10)*
Special studies	• Variably and focally positive for prostate markers (PSA, PSMA, P501S, NKX3.1). Small percent of high-grade prostate adenocarcinomas negative for PSA such that other prostate markers should be done before assuming PSA-negative cancer is not prostate carcinoma • HMWCK negative • CDX2 can be uncommonly positive • Nuclear beta-catenin negative • Intraluminal mucin stains are positive, yet no mucin-positive signet ring cells	• Negative for prostate markers (PSA, PSMA, P501S, NKX3.1) • Variably positive for HMWCK • CDX2 more commonly positive • Nuclear beta-catenin can be positive • Mucin stains are positive intraluminally, within goblet cells, and in signet ring cells if present

	Mucinous Prostatic Adenocarcinoma	**Urethral Mucinous Adenocarcinoma**
Treatment	Same as usual prostate adenocarcinoma	Radical prostatectomy
Prognosis	Mucinous adenocarcinoma at radical prostatectomy has a favorable prognosis, where grade is based on the underlying architectural pattern. Same metastatic pattern as usual prostate adenocarcinoma	Aggressive with approximately 50% dead of disease at an average of about 4 y from presentation. Metastases typically to the lung and liver and not to bone

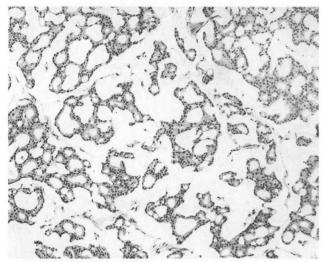

Figure 1.44.1 Mucinous adenocarcinoma of the prostate with cribriform glands floating in mucin.

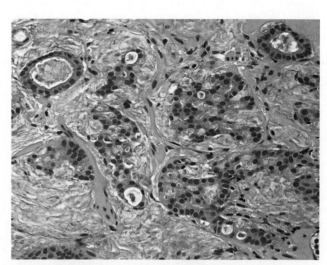

Figure 1.44.2 Mucinous adenocarcinoma of the prostate with cribriform and simple round glands floating in mucin.

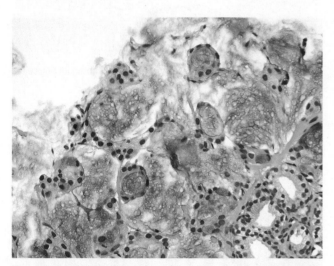

Figure 1.44.3 Mucinous adenocarcinoma of the prostate with simple round glands floating in mucin.

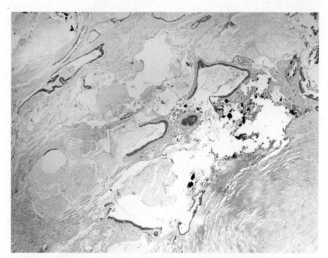

Figure 1.44.4 Prostatic urethral adenocarcinoma with lakes of mucin lined by epithelium.

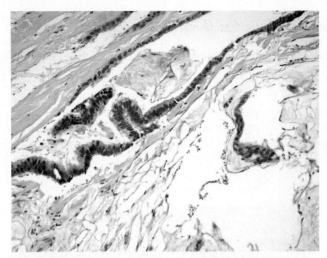

Figure 1.44.5   Same case as Figure 44.4 with strips of atypical glandular epithelium lining mucin.

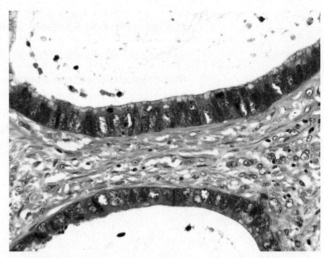

Figure 1.44.6   Prostatic urethral adenocarcinoma with lakes of mucin lined by atypical columnar epithelium.

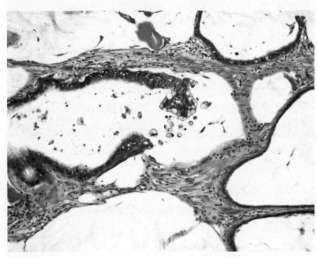

Figure 1.44.7   Prostatic urethral adenocarcinoma with lakes of mucin lined by epithelium, some composed of goblet cells.

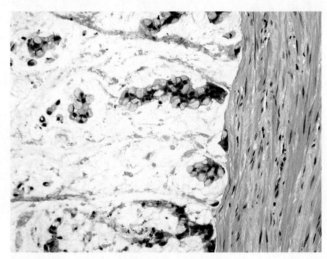

Figure 1.44.8   Prostatic urethral adenocarcinoma with signet ring cells floating in mucin.

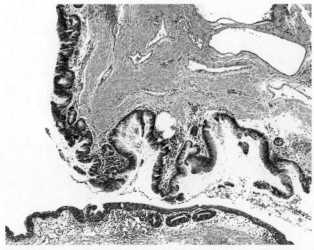

Figure 1.44.9   Same case as Figures 1.44.6–1.44.8 with prostatic urethra lined by intestinal metaplasia.

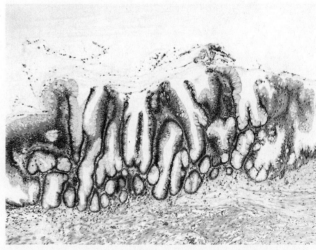

Figure 1.44.10   Same case as Figures 1.44.6–1.44.9 with prostatic urethra lined by intestinal metaplasia with numerous goblet cells.

	p63-Positive Prostate Adenocarcinoma	Basal Cell Carcinoma
Age	Typically 50 to elderly, although not rare in 40s	Typically 50 to elderly, although not rare in 40s
Location	Most are peripheral zone carcinomas detected on needle biopsy, although some are in the transition zone	Most are located within the transition zone and seen on TURP, yet can also uncommonly be detected on needle biopsy
Symptoms	Typically asymptomatic. Advanced disease with urinary obstructive symptoms and/or hematuria or from distant metastases	Usually present with urinary obstructive symptoms
Signs	Variably elevated serum PSA levels, no different than usual prostate cancer	Does not elevate serum PSA levels
Etiology	Unknown	Unknown. Not thought to arise from basal cell hyperplasia, with possible rare exceptions
Histology	1. Typically forms individual glands but can also form cords (Figs. 1.45.1 and 1.45.2) 2. Usually atrophic cytoplasm, although can have more abundant cytoplasm 3. Usually has distinctive morphology with multilayered streaming nuclei and lack prominent pleomorphism (Figs. 1.45.3 and 1.45.4), and in other cases, identical to usual atrophic prostate cancer with a single cell layer (Figs. 1.45.5 and 1.45.6) 4. Mitotic figures are typically not frequent 5. Widely infiltrative in between benign prostate glands 6. Some cases distinctive morphology admixed with usual prostate adenocarcinoma (Figs. 1.45.7 and 1.45.8)	1. Variable architecture: (a) large solid basaloid nests; (b) adenoid cystic; (c) anastomosing variably sized nests with central tubules; (d) individual glands. Only the latter resembles p63-positive prostate carcinoma (Fig. 1.45.10) 2. Atrophic cytoplasm (Figs. 1.45.11 and 1.45.12) 3. Multilayered ranging from subtle 2 cell thickness to solid nests (Figs. 1.45.10–1.45.12) 4. Mitotic figures are typically not frequent in the pattern composed of individual glands 5. Widely infiltrative in between benign prostate glands 6. Not admixed with usual prostate adenocarcinoma
Special studies	• Intense diffuse positivity for p63 in all tumor cells, without a flattened positive basal cell layer and a negative secretory cell layer seen in benign glands • Negative reactivity for HMWCK (Fig. 1.45.9) • Positive for prostate markers (PSA, PSMA, P501S, NKX3.1)	• Positive for p63 in multilayered cells, with some centrally located cells negative • HMWCK positive in the same distribution as p63-positive cells (Figs. 1.45.10 and 1.45.12) • Negative for prostate markers (PSA, PSMA, P501S, NKX3.1)
Treatment	Same as usual prostate adenocarcinoma	Radical prostatectomy for younger men and radical TURP for the elderly

	p63-Positive Prostate Adenocarcinoma	Basal Cell Carcinoma
Prognosis	Little is known about the prognosis and whether different than usual Gleason score 6 adenocarcinoma. Can coexist with other foci of prostate cancer that do not express p63	The variant of basal cell carcinoma composed of individual glands resembling p63-positive prostate carcinoma can locally infiltrate out of the prostate into periprostatic adipose tissue or bladder neck. It does not typically metastasize to distant sites

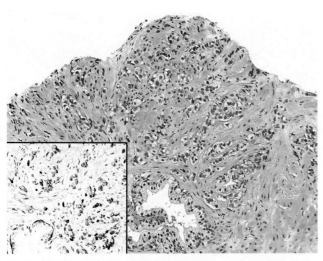

Figure 1.45.1   p63-positive prostate adenocarcinoma with cords of cells. **Inset** shows carcinoma labeled with p63 only compared to benign prostate glands (**lower left**) labeled with p63 and HMWCK.

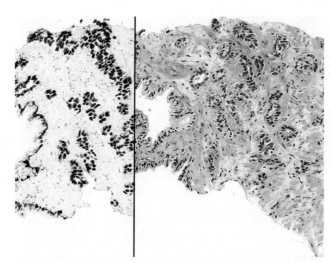

Figure 1.45.2   p63-positive prostate adenocarcinoma with multilayered glands with atrophic cytoplasm (**right panel**). Carcinoma labels with p63 only (**left panel**) compared to benign prostate glands (**far left**) labeled with p63 and HMWCK.

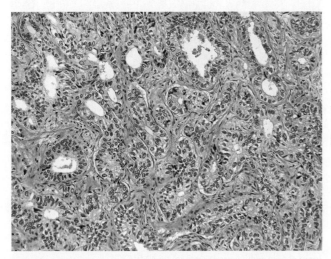

Figure 1.45.3   Distinctive morphology of p63-positive prostate adenocarcinoma with multilayered glands with slightly spindled nuclei and atrophic cytoplasm.

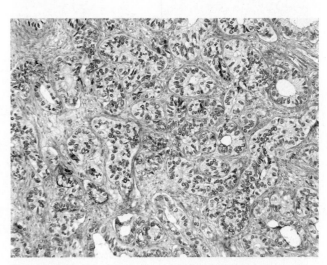

Figure 1.45.4   Same case as Figure 1.45.3 with PIN4 cocktail showing only p63 staining of nuclei and absent cytoplasmic HMWCK labeling.

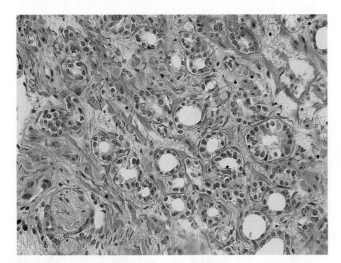

Figure 1.45.5   p63-positive adenocarcinoma resembling usual atrophic prostate cancer with perineural invasion (*lower left*).

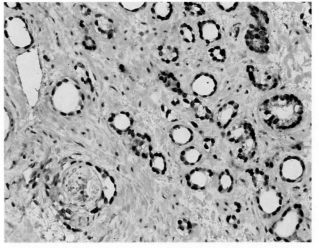

Figure 1.45.6   Same case as Figure 1.45.5 with PIN4 cocktail showing only p63 staining of nuclei and absent cytoplasmic HMWCK labeling.

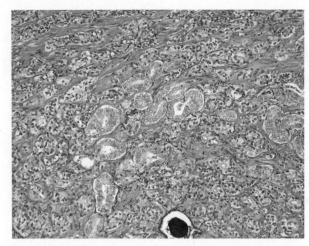

Figure 1.45.7   Mixture of usual prostate adenocarcinoma (*center*) with abundant cytoplasm and a single cell layer admixed with p63-positive prostate cancer with multilayering.

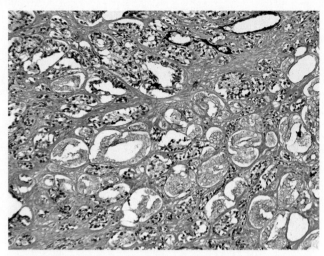

Figure 1.45.8   Same case as Figure 1.45.7 with PIN4 cocktail. Usual prostate adenocarcinoma lacks positivity for HMWCK and p63, whereas distinctive multilayered prostate glands are positive for p63.

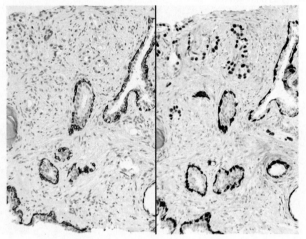

Figure 1.45.9   Adenocarcinoma labeled with HMWCK only (**left**) showing absence of staining in small glands of carcinoma. Same carcinoma labeled with HMWCK/p63 cocktail (**right**) demonstrating p63-positive prostate carcinoma glands labeling nuclei only (**top**) compared to surrounding benign glands with both nuclear and cytoplasmic positivity for p63 and HMWCK, respectively.

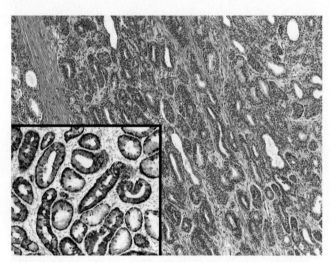

Figure 1.45.10   Basal cell carcinoma with single multilayered glands. **Inset** shows multilayered positivity for HMWCK.

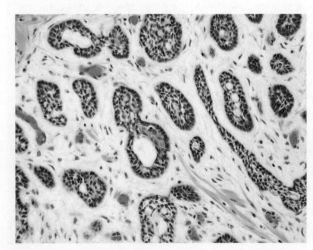

Figure 1.45.11   Basal cell carcinoma with multilayered glands with atrophic cytoplasm and solid nests.

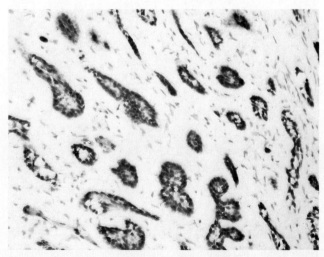

Figure 1.45.12   Same case as Figure 1.45.11 positive for p63 and HMWCK.

	Small Cell Carcinoma	High-Grade Prostatic Adenocarcinoma
Age	Typically 50 to elderly, although not rare in 40s	Typically 50 to elderly, although not rare in 40s
Location	May be seen on biopsy or TURP	May be seen on biopsy or TURP
Symptoms	Predilection to spread to unusual sites such as soft tissue and brain. Bone metastases typically lytic	Most common metastatic sites: Osteoblastic bone lesions; pelvic and para-aortic lymph nodes; lung and liver although typically small deposits
Signs	At diagnosis, 70% pure small cell carcinoma with remaining mixed with acinar adenocarcinoma. Serum PSA level may be elevated yet decrease with the onset of the small cell component	Variably elevated serum PSA levels
Etiology	14%–35% have a history of prostate cancer with progression to high-grade neuroendocrine differentiation	See Section 1.6
Histology	1. Sheets and less frequently cords of cells without glandular differentiation unless mixed with usual prostate adenocarcinoma (*Figs. 1.46.1–1.46.5*) 2. Tumor appears very blue at low power (*Figs. 1.46.1 and 1.46.2*) 3. Very high nuclear to cytoplasmic (N/C) ratio (*Fig. 1.46.6*) 4. Nuclei tend to mold against each other (*Fig. 1.46.6*) 5. Nuclei vary from lacking to small visible nucleoli (*Figs. 1.46.6 and 1.46.7*) 6. Mitotic figures and/or apoptotic bodies numerous (*Figs. 1.46.6 and 1.46.7*) 7. Sheets of geographic necrosis not uncommon (*Fig. 1.46.8*)	1. Cribriform glands, large solid nests, cords of cells 2. At low power, tumor has a lighter more eosinophilic appearance (*Fig. 1.46.2*) 3. More cytoplasm results in lower N/C ratio (*Fig. 1.46.11*) 4. No nuclear molding 5. Prominent nucleoli are typical (*Fig. 1.46.11*) 6. Variable mitotic figures, yet less than small cell carcinoma (*Fig. 1.46.11*) 7. Focal necrosis can be seen in solid nests of Gleason pattern 5 (*Fig. 1.46.12*)
Special studies	• 18% positive for PSA, 29% for p501S (prostein), yet focally • 88% positive for at least one neuroendocrine marker (*Figs. 1.46.9 and 1.46.10*) • TTF-1 positive in 50% of cases (*Figs. 1.46.9 and 1.46.10*) • Ki-67 positive in >70% of cells	• >90% positive for prostate markers (PSA, P501S, NKX3.1), yet often focally • Can have focal neuroendocrine differentiation • TTF-1 negative • Ki-67 positive in <50% of cells
Treatment	Treated with same chemotherapy as small cell carcinoma of the lung, possibly also with antiandrogen therapy if mixed with usual adenocarcinoma	Advanced high-grade prostatic adenocarcinoma treated with antiandrogen therapy
Prognosis	Tumors initially respond to chemotherapy but relapse within a year and almost all are dead within 1–2 y. A few case reports of cures with chemotherapy. >90% present with stage T3 or T4 disease	Some patients respond well for many years before developing hormone-resistant cancer

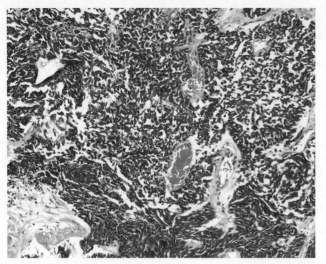

Figure 1.46.1   Small cell carcinoma at low magnification composed of sheets of "blue cells."

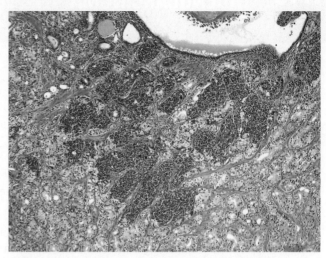

Figure 1.46.2   Mixed small cell carcinoma, which is "blue" at a low magnification, and paler usual prostate adenocarcinoma.

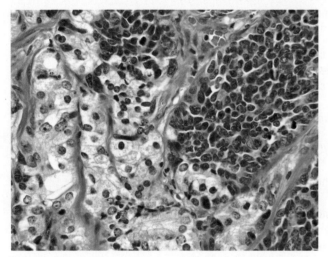

Figure 1.46.3   Same case as Figure 1.46.2 with small cell carcinoma (*right*) and usual prostate adenocarcinoma (*left*).

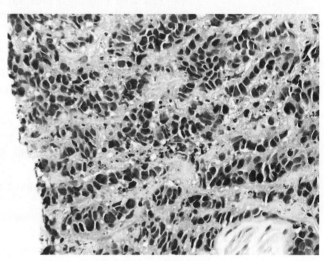

Figure 1.46.4   Cords of small cell carcinoma.

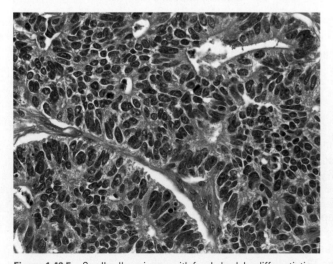

Figure 1.46.5   Small cell carcinoma with focal glandular differentiation.

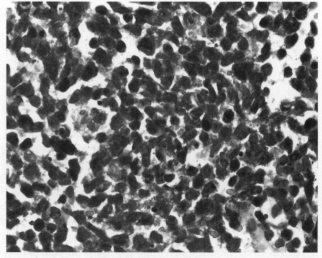

Figure 1.46.6   Typical cytology of small cell carcinoma. Numerous apoptotic bodies are present.

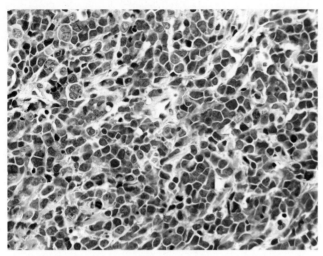

Figure 1.46.7 Occasional small cell carcinomas can have visible nucleoli, yet still have scant cytoplasm, nuclear molding, and frequent mitotic figures and apoptotic bodies.

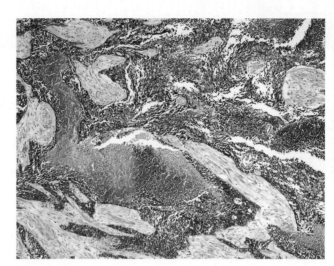

Figure 1.46.8 Small cell carcinoma with sheets of cancer with large areas of necrosis.

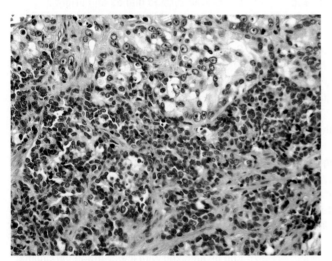

Figure 1.46.9 Mixed small cell carcinoma (*bottom*) and usual prostate adenocarcinoma (*top*).

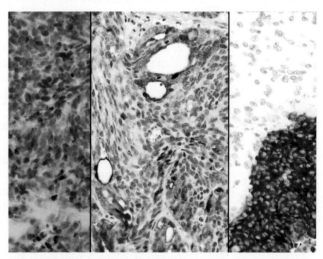

Figure 1.46.10 Same case as Figure 1.46.9. Small cell carcinoma with TTF-1 (**left**) and synaptophysin (**right**) positivity. Adenocarcinoma component is PSA (**center**) positive, whereas small cell carcinoma is PSA negative.

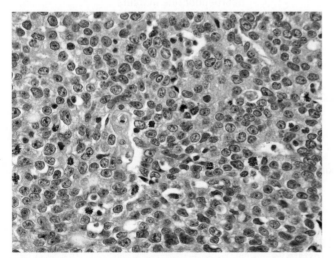

Figure 1.46.11 Prostatic adenocarcinoma with sheets of cells composed of cells with abundant cytoplasm and nuclei with prominent nucleoli. Numerous mitotic figures are present.

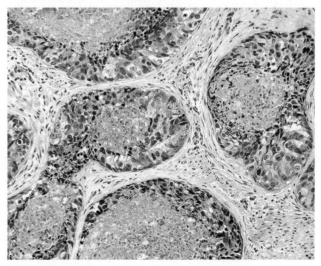

Figure 1.46.12 Gleason pattern 5 adenocarcinoma with nests of tumor with comedonecrosis.

	Adenocarcinoma with Paneth Cell–Like Change	High-Grade Prostatic Adenocarcinoma
Age	Typically 50 to elderly, although not rare in 40s	Typically 50 to elderly, although not rare in 40s
Location	Most detected in the peripheral zone (PZ)	85%–90% arise in (PZ), yet can arise in or involve the transition zone (TZ)
Symptoms	Typically asymptomatic	Variably symptomatic
Signs	Variably elevated serum PSA levels, no different than usual prostate cancer	Variably elevated serum PSA levels
Etiology	Unknown. Corresponds to numerous neurosecretory granules	See Section 1.6
Histology	1. Some cases with well-formed glands and bright coarse eosinophilic cytoplasmic granules 2. Some cases with small nests and cords of cells mimicking high-grade carcinoma with cytoplasm having abundant to sparse eosinophilic granules or amphophilic *(Figs. 1.47.1–1.47.10)* 3. Nuclei are small, very uniform, without prominent nucleoli *(Fig. 1.47.2)* 4. Combined architecture and cytology resembles carcinoid tumor *(Fig. 1.47.3)* 5. Mitotic figures are typically absent 6. Infiltrative in between benign prostate glands but tends to be relatively small focus 7. Can be admixed with usual acinar adenocarcinoma of varying grades	1. Lacks well-formed glands and bright coarse eosinophilic cytoplasmic granules *(Figs. 1.47.11 and 1.47.12)* 2. Cribriform glands, large solid nests, cords of cells lacking granules 3. Nuclei enlarged, typically with prominent nucleoli 4. High-grade acinar adenocarcinoma does not resemble carcinoid tumor 5. Mitotic figures frequent 6. Infiltrative and typically extensive although small foci may be seen on needle biopsy and less likely on TURP 7. Can be admixed with lower-grade carcinoma
Special studies	• Strong diffuse immunoreactivity for neuroendocrine markers (CD56, synaptophysin, chromogranin) *(Fig. 1.47.9)* • Can be negative for prostate markers (PSA, PSMA, P501S, NKX3.1) • Negative for basal cell markers (p63, HMWCK) • Ki-67 very low *(Fig. 1.47.10)*	• May show focal immunoreactivity for neuroendocrine markers • >90% of high-grade carcinomas positive for prostate markers (PSA, PSMA, P501S, NKX3.1). Occasionally focally but can be more diffuse • Negative for basal cell markers (p63, HMWCK). • Ki-67 higher than cases with Paneth cell–like neuroendocrine change
Treatment	Same as usual prostate adenocarcinoma, Gleason score 3 + 3 = 6	Stage and biopsy extent dependent
Prognosis	If Gleason scored, would be pattern 5 due to lack of gland formation. However, should not be assigned a Gleason score as typically can coexists Gleason score 3 + 3 = 6 prostate cancer and overall has a favorable prognosis	Associated with a poor prognosis, which is stage dependent

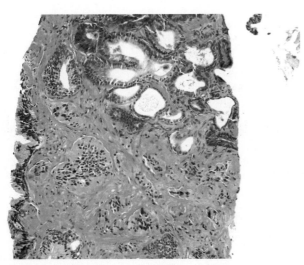

Figure 1.47.1 Adenocarcinoma with Paneth cell–like change. Areas of tumor are composed of well-formed gland with eosinophilic granules (*top*) and others nests of cells (*bottom*).

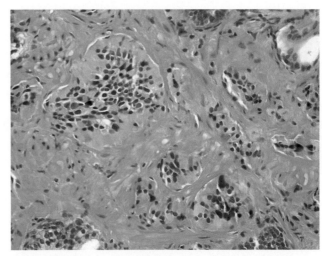

Figure 1.47.2 Same case as Figure 1.47.1 composed of nests of cells with abundant amphophilic cytoplasm and bland nuclei.

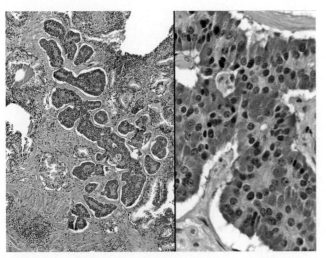

Figure 1.47.3 Adenocarcinoma with Paneth cell–like change resembling carcinoid tumor (**left**). Higher magnification shows uniform nuclei with cytoplasmic eosinophilic granules.

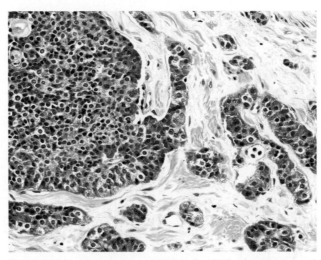

Figure 1.47.4 Adenocarcinoma with Paneth cell–like change composed of variably sized nests of bland cells with numerous cytoplasmic eosinophilic granules.

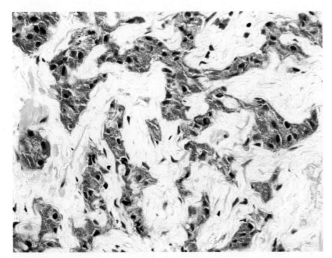

Figure 1.47.5 Adenocarcinoma with Paneth cell–like change composed of cords of bland cells with numerous cytoplasmic eosinophilic granules, mimicking high-grade prostate cancer.

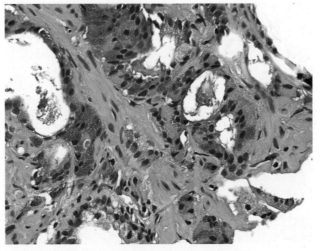

Figure 1.47.6 Adenocarcinoma with Paneth cell–like change composed of glands with some cells displaying cytoplasmic eosinophilic granules and others dense amphophilic cytoplasm.

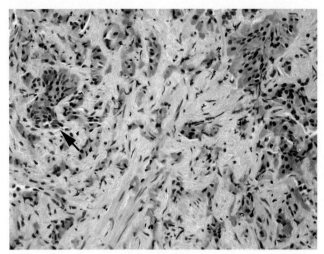

Figure 1.47.7   Adenocarcinoma with Paneth cell–like change composed of nests and cords with focal cells displaying cytoplasmic eosinophilic granules (*arrow*) and others dense amphophilic cytoplasm.

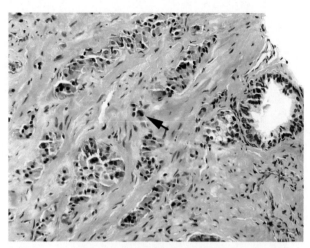

Figure 1.47.8   Adenocarcinoma with Paneth cell–like change composed of nests and cords with rare cells displaying cytoplasmic eosinophilic granules (*arrow*) and others dense amphophilic cytoplasm.

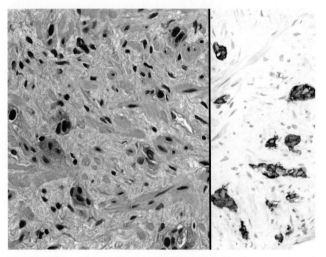

Figure 1.47.9   Adenocarcinoma with Paneth cell–like change composed of small nests of cells with bland cytology and dense amphophilic cytoplasm (**left**) and diffuse synaptophysin positivity (**right**).

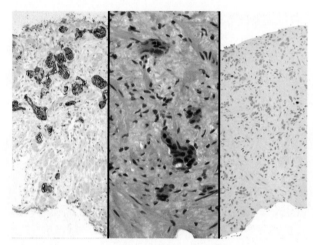

Figure 1.47.10   Adenocarcinoma with Paneth cell–like change composed of small nests of cells with bland cytology and dense amphophilic cytoplasm (**center**), diffuse synaptophysin positivity (**left**), and low Ki-67 rate (**right**).

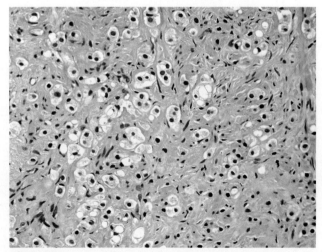

Figure 1.47.11   Gleason score 5 + 5 = 10 adenocarcinoma with nests and single cells lacking the dense amphophilic cytoplasm of adenocarcinoma with Paneth cell–like change.

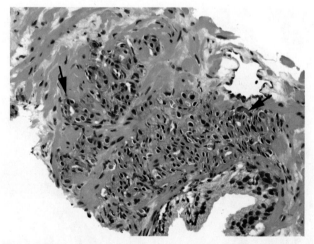

Figure 1.47.12   Gleason score 5 + 3 = 8 adenocarcinoma with nests and occasional glands (*arrows*). Cells are not as uniform, lacking the resemblance to carcinoid tumor, compared to adenocarcinoma with Paneth cell–like change.

	Sarcomatoid Carcinoma (Carcinosarcoma)	Sarcoma
Age	Typically 50 to elderly, although not rare in 40s	Typically 50 to elderly, although not rare in 40s
Location	Mostly detected on TURP but can be seen on needle biopsy as well	Can be found either on needle biopsy or on TURP
Symptoms	Symptomatic. Advanced disease with symptoms from urinary obstruction, hematuria, or from distant metastases	Symptomatic. Advanced disease with symptoms from urinary obstruction, hematuria, or from distant metastases
Signs	Typically not elevated serum PSA levels	Does not elevate serum PSA levels
Etiology	Two-thirds of cases with prior history, typically 5–10 y in the past, of usual adenocarcinoma of the prostate. Often but not necessary there is a prior treatment with irradiation	Usually no prior history of prostate adenocarcinoma or irradiation
Histology	1. Adenocarcinoma component can be acinar, ductal, squamous, small cell *(Figs. 1.48.1–1.48.3)* 2. Mesenchymal component can be pleomorphic giant cells, nonspecific malignant spindle cells, chondrosarcoma, osteogenic sarcoma, rhabdomyosarcoma *(Figs. 1.48.1–1.48.7)*	1. Lacks an adenocarcinoma component 2. Most common sarcoma in adults is leiomyosarcoma composed of sweeping intersecting fascicles *(Fig. 1.48.8)*. Even poorly differentiated leiomyosarcomas, maintain their fascicular pattern in areas
Special studies	• May express focal actin and desmin in sarcomatoid areas • In spindle cell component, keratin (especially, HMWCK) is focally positive. However, in limited material, keratin may be negative. In epithelial component, best marker is CAM5.2. If epithelial component is adenocarcinoma will be HMWCK negative • p63 is another sensitive marker for epithelial differentiation in the spindle cell component	• Expresses actin and desmin • One quarter of case express cytokeratin • No data on p63 in prostate leiomyosarcomas, although p63 is with rare exception negative in leiomyosarcomas in general
Treatment	Radical prostatectomy if early stage. Optimal treatment for metastatic disease not known	Optimal treatment requires a multimodal approach
Prognosis	Poor outcome with an actuarial risk of death of 20% within the first year and frequent widespread metastases to bone, the liver, and the lung	Poor outcome, with multiple recurrences. Majority (50%–75%) die from disease within 2–5 y with metastatic spread most commonly to the lungs, often several years following initial diagnosis. Better prognosis for men who present without distant metastases and those who are able to undergo complete surgical resection with microscopically negative margins

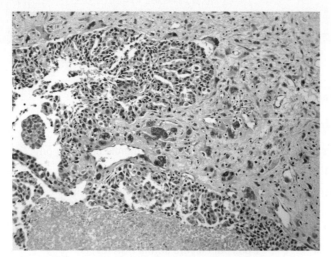

Figure 1.48.1 Sarcomatoid carcinoma with epithelial component of cribriform acinar adenocarcinoma and mesenchymal component consisting of nonspecific pleomorphic spindle cells.

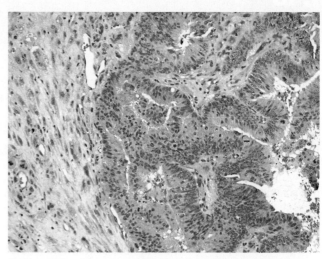

Figure 1.48.2 Sarcomatoid carcinoma with epithelial component of ductal adenocarcinoma and mesenchymal component consisting of nonspecific malignant spindle cells.

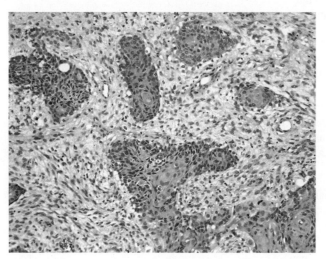

Figure 1.48.3 Sarcomatoid carcinoma with epithelial component of squamous cell carcinoma and mesenchymal component consisting of hypercellular spindle cells.

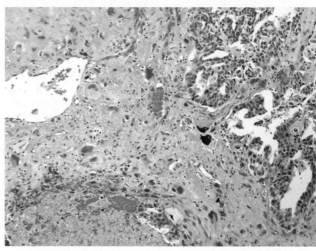

Figure 1.48.4 Sarcomatoid carcinoma with epithelial component of acinar adenocarcinoma and mesenchymal component consisting of nonspecific pleomorphic giant and spindle cells.

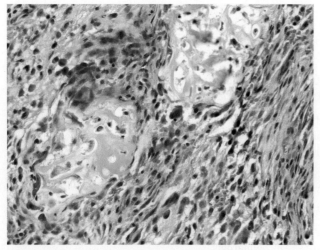

Figure 1.48.5 Sarcomatoid carcinoma (epithelial component not shown) with mesenchymal component consisting of osteogenic sarcoma and cellular malignant spindle cells.

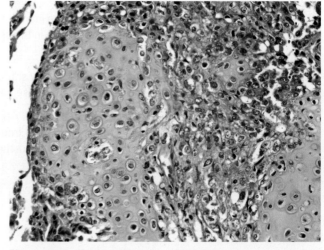

Figure 1.48.6 Sarcomatoid carcinoma (epithelial component not shown) with mesenchymal component consisting of chondrosarcoma and cellular malignant spindle cells.

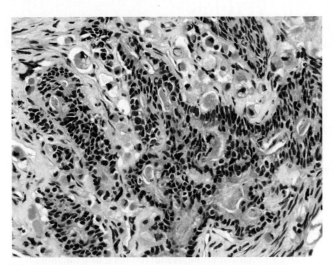

Figure 1.48.7 Sarcomatoid carcinoma with epithelial component of acinar adenocarcinoma and mesenchymal component consisting of rhabdomyosarcoma.

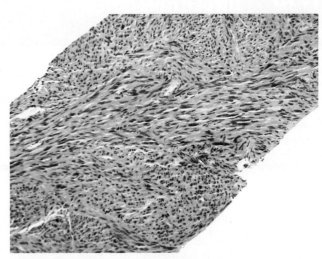

Figure 1.48.8 Leiomyosarcoma of the prostate consisting of uniform long fascicles cut in both longitudinal and cross-section with marked increase in cellularity and occasional hyperchromatic nuclei.

	Stromal Nodule of Hyperplasia	Stromal Tumor of Uncertain Malignant Potential (STUMP)
Age	Typically 50 to elderly	Typically 50 to elderly, although not rare in 40s
Location	Transition zone lesion, yet can be found either on needle biopsy or on TURP	Peripheral or transition zone lesion and can be found either on needle biopsy or on TURP
Symptoms	May be incidental finding or patients may be symptomatic with lower urinary tract obstruction	Most commonly present with lower urinary tract obstruction, followed by an abnormal digital rectal examination, hematuria, hematospermia, rectal fullness, or a palpable rectal mass
Signs	Does not elevate serum PSA levels	Does not elevate serum PSA levels
Etiology	Component of BPH	Unknown
Histology	1. May be pure spindle cell nodule or mixed glandular–stromal nodule 2. Normocellular or slightly hypercellular stroma without atypia 3. BPH stroma is not as cellular as second pattern of STUMP and lacks eosinophilic cytoplasm 4. Can have extensive stromal nodular hyperplasia with cellular stroma mimicking the third pattern of STUMP. In contrast to STUMP, BPH myxoid stroma has nodularity and numerous thick-walled arterioles *(Figs. 1.49.1–1.49.3)* 5. Rarely, BPH can have small fibroadenomatoid foci mimicking the fourth pattern of STUMP. Lesions are small and incidentally found without complex glandular proliferations *(Figs. 1.49.4–1.49.7)*	1. May be pure spindle cell nodule or mixed glandular–stromal nodule with several patterns that can be pure or mixed in a given case 2. Most common pattern with slightly hypercellular or normocellular stroma with scattered atypical, but degenerative-appearing cell glands. Glands can be crowded with basal cell hyperplasia, adenosis, cribriform hyperplasia, squamous and urothelial metaplasia. Does not mimic BPH 3. Second pattern with hypercellular stroma consisting of bland fusiform stromal cells with eosinophilic cytoplasm admixed with benign glands *(Figs. 1.49.8 and 1.49.9)* 4. Third pattern with myxoid stroma containing bland stromal cells and often lacking admixed glands in sheets of stroma without nodularity *(Fig. 1.49.10)*. Lacks thick-walled arterioles 5. Fourth pattern is phyllodes with leaf-like hypocellular fibrous stroma covered by benign-appearing prostatic epithelium *(Figs. 1.49.11 and 1.49.12)*. Can have associated complex glandular proliferations of basal cell hyperplasia, adenosis, cribriform hyperplasia, squamous and urothelial metaplasia
Special studies	• Positive for CD34, smooth muscle actin, desmin, and progesterone receptor-2	• Not helpful in this differential. Same as nonneoplastic prostatic stroma
Treatment	Same as for usual BPH	Usually, radical prostatectomy for relatively young men and surveillance for elderly

	Stromal Nodule of Hyperplasia	**Stromal Tumor of Uncertain Malignant Potential (STUMP)**
Prognosis	If removed by TURP, BPH does not recur for many years if at all. No association with malignancy	STUMPS may recur within a few months or years after TURP only. STUMPs have been associated with stromal sarcoma on concurrent biopsy material or have demonstrated stromal sarcoma on repeat biopsy, suggesting a malignant progression in at least some cases. If a STUMP is entirely resected and there is no sarcomatous component, then the lesion is entirely cured

1 PROSTATE

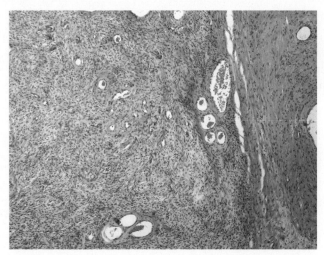

Figure 1.49.1 BPH stromal nodule (*left*) with numerous thick-walled arterioles.

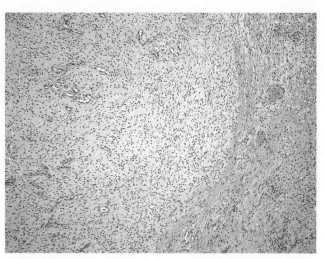

Figure 1.49.2 Myxoid BPH stromal nodule with numerous thick-walled arterioles.

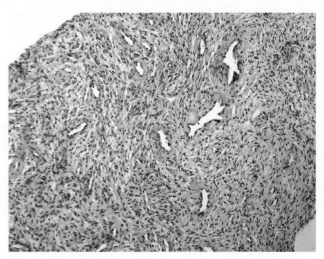

Figure 1.49.3 BPH stromal nodule on needle biopsy with numerous thick-walled arterioles.

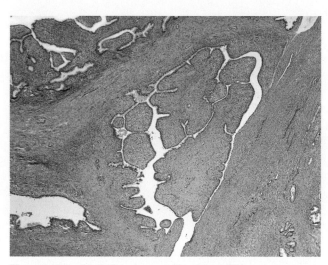

Figure 1.49.4 Small fibroadenomatoid nodule of BPH.

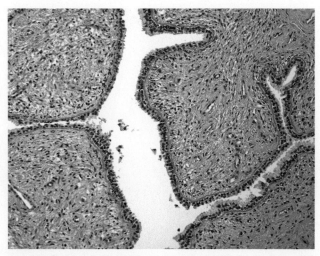

Figure 1.49.5 Higher magnification of Figure 1.49.4.

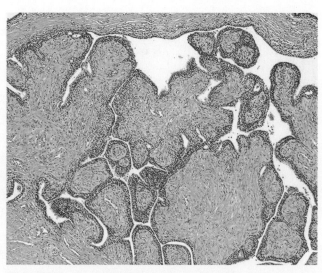

Figure 1.49.6 Small fibroadenomatoid nodule of BPH.

1.49 Stromal Nodule of Hyperplasia vs. Stromal Tumor of Uncertain Malignant Potential (STUMP)   **153**

1   PROSTATE

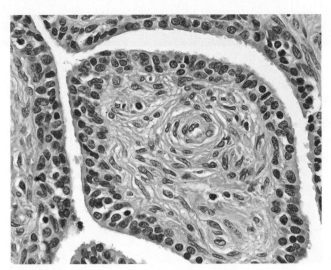

Figure 1.49.7   Higher magnification of Figure 1.49.6.

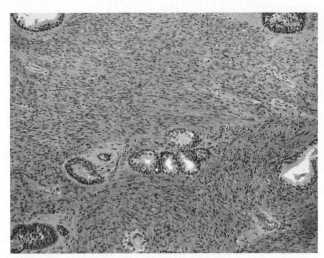

Figure 1.49.8   STUMP with markedly hypercellular stroma composed of cells with eosinophilic cytoplasm.

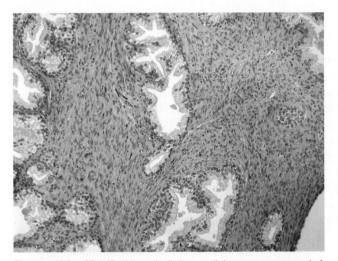

Figure 1.49.9   STUMP with markedly hypercellular stroma composed of cells with eosinophilic cytoplasm.

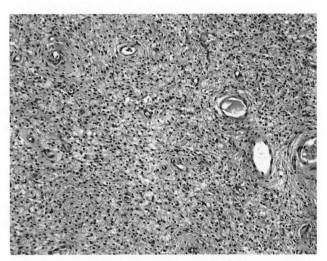

Figure 1.49.10   Myxoid STUMP. This lesion consisted of a 70 g TURP with sheets of hypercellular myxoid stroma without nodularity.

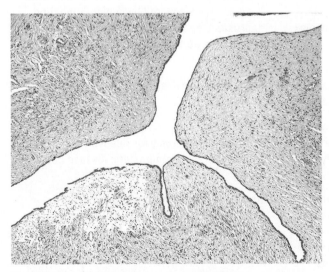

Figure 1.49.11   Benign phyllodes pattern of STUMP.

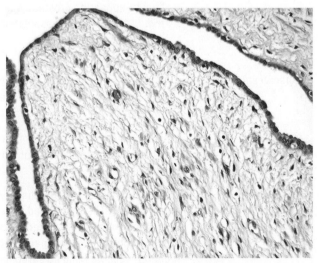

Figure 1.49.12   Same case as Figure 1.49.11 with hypocellular fibrous tissue. Lesion was a large mass that rapidly recurred following TURP.

	Stromal Tumor of Uncertain Malignant Potential (STUMP)	Stromal Sarcoma
Age	Between the ages of 27 and 83 y, with a median age of 58 y, and a peak incidence in the sixth and seventh decades	Somewhat younger than patients with STUMPS with approximately half of all reported cases of stromal sarcoma occurring before the age of 50 y
Location	Peripheral or transition zone lesion	Peripheral or transition zone lesion
Symptoms	Usually lower urinary tract obstruction, followed by an abnormal digital rectal examination, hematuria, hematospermia, rectal fullness, or a palpable rectal mass	Same as STUMP
Signs	Does not elevate serum PSA levels	Does not elevate serum PSA levels
Etiology	Unknown	Unknown. In some cases, progression from STUMP
Histology	1. Most common pattern slightly hypercellular or normocellular stroma with scattered atypical, but degenerative-appearing stromal cells (Figs. 1.50.1–1.50.4). Lacks atypical mitotic figures. Glands can be crowded with basal cell hyperplasia, adenosis, cribriform hyperplasia, squamous and urothelial metaplasia (Fig. 1.50.4) 2. Myxoid stroma with bland stromal cells and often lacking admixed glands in sheets of stroma without nodularity 3. Phyllodes pattern with leaf-like hypocellular fibrous stroma covered by benign-appearing prostatic epithelium (Fig. 1.50.5). Can have associated complex glandular proliferations	1. Can resemble STUMP with scattered atypical, but degenerative-appearing stromal cells. However, intervening stroma is too hypercellular for STUMP. Can have atypical mitotic figures (Fig. 1.50.6). Similar glands to STUMP 2. Can be epithelioid or spindled with marked hypercellularity and increased mitotic activity but rare to have myxoid features (Figs. 1.50.7–1.50.9). Other patterns are storiform, epithelioid, fibrosarcomatous, or patternless 3. Malignant phyllodes pattern with hypercellular mitotically active stroma with some atypia covered by benign-appearing prostatic epithelium (Figs. 1.50.10–1.50.12). Can have associated complex glandular proliferations
Special studies	• Most cases positive for CD34, smooth muscle actin, desmin, and progesterone receptor	• Not helpful in this differential. Same as STUMP
Treatment	Usually, radical prostatectomy for relatively young men and surveillance for elderly	Radical prostatectomy for relatively young men. Optimal therapy for metastatic disease not known
Prognosis	May recur within a few months or years after TURP. Can be associated with stromal sarcoma on concurrent material or on repeat biopsy, suggesting a malignant progression. If entirely resected and no sarcomatous component, then entirely cured	Stromal sarcomas can extend out of the prostate and metastasize to distant sites, such as bone, lung, abdomen, and retroperitoneum

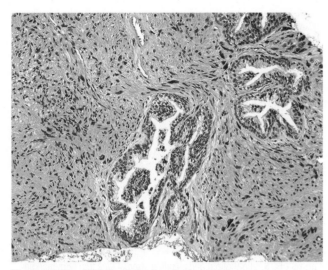

Figure 1.50.1 STUMP with benign glands with intervening hypercellular stroma containing atypical cells.

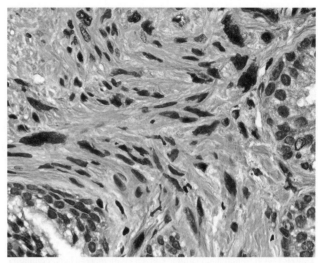

Figure 1.50.2 Same case as Figure 1.50.1 with enlarged pleomorphic nuclei with a degenerative appearance. Nuclei lack well-defined chromatin and lack mitotic activity.

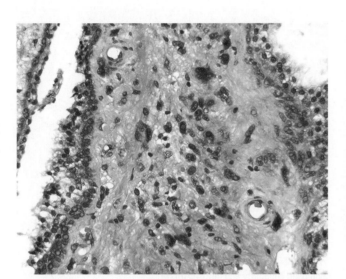

Figure 1.50.3 STUMP with benign glands with intervening hypercellular stroma containing atypical but degenerative-appearing nuclei.

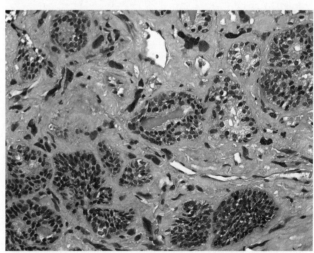

Figure 1.50.4 STUMP with benign glands showing basal cell hyperplasia with intervening normocellular stroma containing atypical but degenerative-appearing nuclei.

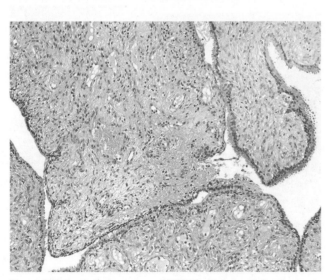

Figure 1.50.5 Phyllodes pattern of STUMP with hypocellular stroma.

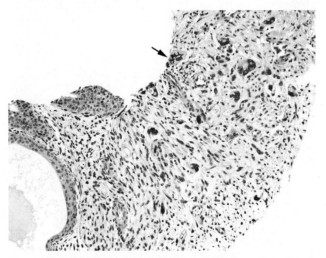

Figure 1.50.6 Stromal sarcoma with hypercellular stroma and atypical nuclei, including one with an atypical mitotic figure (*arrow*).

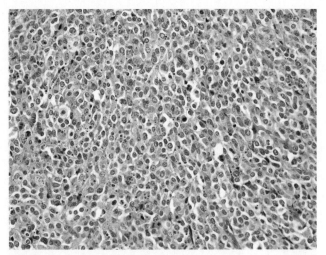

Figure 1.50.7 Epithelioid stromal sarcoma with marked hypercellularity and numerous apoptotic bodies.

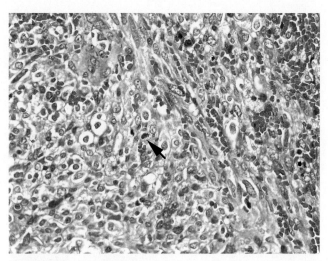

Figure 1.50.8 Epithelioid and spindled stromal sarcoma with marked hypercellularity and mitotic activity (*arrow*).

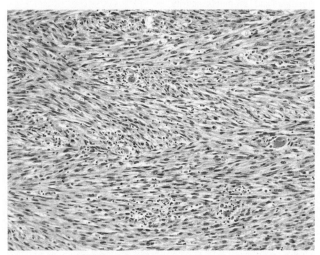

Figure 1.50.9 Spindled stromal sarcoma with marked hypercellularity and mitotic activity. If other more specific sarcomas (i.e., neural, smooth muscle, etc.) are excluded, then consistent with stromal sarcoma.

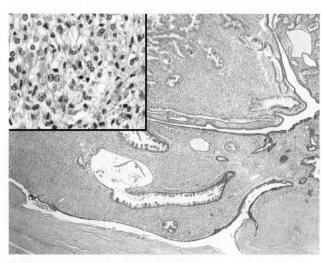

Figure 1.50.10 Malignant phyllodes pattern of stromal sarcoma with increased cellularity and mitoses (**inset**).

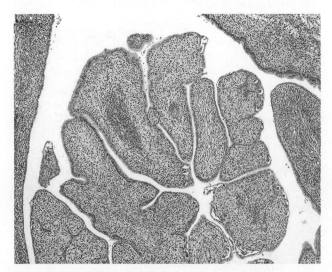

Figure 1.50.11 Malignant phyllodes pattern of stromal sarcoma.

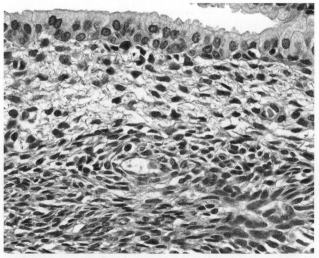

Figure 1.50.12 Same case as Figure 1.50.11 with marked increase in stromal cellularity.

	"Prostatic" Gastrointestinal Stromal Tumor (GIST)	Mimickers of "Prostatic" GIST
Age	Typically from 40s to 50s	Lesions in the differential diagnosis of GIST include solitary fibrous tumor (SFT), schwannoma, leiomyosarcoma, or stromal sarcoma and occur typically in adults, yet wide age range including patients in their 20s
Location	Posterior of the prostate. Most cases of "prostatic" GISTs are sampled on prostatic needle biopsy, although rarely on transurethral resection	Lesions, other than schwannoma, are peripheral or transition zone lesions and can be found either on needle biopsy or on TURP
Symptoms	Most commonly present with lower urinary tract obstruction, followed by an abnormal digital rectal examination, rectal fullness, or a palpable rectal mass	Most commonly present with lower urinary tract obstruction, followed by an abnormal digital rectal examination, hematuria, hematospermia, rectal fullness, or a palpable rectal mass
Signs	Does not elevate serum PSA levels	Does not elevate serum PSA levels
Etiology	Typically large masses (1.0 cm to over 8.0 cm) arising from GISTs of the rectum or perirectal space that compress but do not invade the prostate. Exceptionally, malignant GISTs may also invade the prostate. No convincing case of a true intraprostatic GIST	Schwannoma typically periprostatic and sampled on needle biopsy
Histology	1. Fascicular or palisading growth pattern and perinuclear vacuoles with a lack of collagen deposition between tumor cells (Figs. 1.51.1 and 1.51.2). Lesion is very cellular with elongated nuclei, yet lacks pleomorphism (Fig. 1.51.3) 2. As GISTs are extraprostatic, needle biopsies containing GIST typically lack prostate glands (Fig. 1.51.4)	1. Fascicular or palisading growth pattern and perinuclear vacuoles along with a lack of collagen deposition differentiate from stromal sarcoma and SFT (Figs. 1.51.6–1.51.8). Stromal sarcomas usually more pleomorphic. Could mimic cellular schwannoma or leiomyosarcoma 2. May be associated with prostate glands if arise in prostate gland
Special studies	• CD117/c-kit is uniformly expressed in all cases, and CD34 is positive in almost all cases studied (Fig. 1.51.5) • S100, desmin, and smooth muscle actin negative	• CD117/c-kit is negative in all mimickers. CD34 is positive in SFT and stromal sarcoma and variably in schwannoma • S100 positive in schwannoma; strong diffuse desmin diagnostic of leiomyosarcoma
Treatment	c-Kit tyrosine kinase inhibitor imatinib (Gleevec)	Typically surgical resection with no role for tyrosine kinase inhibitor therapy

	"Prostatic" Gastrointestinal Stromal Tumor (GIST)	Mimickers of "Prostatic" GIST
Prognosis	A subset of patients treated with Gleevec shown reduction in tumor size. Tumors with malignant potential show elevated mitotic rates of >5 per 50 HPF, cytologically malignant features (high cellularity and overlapping nuclei), or necrosis	Schwannoma is benign. Prognosis in SFT depends if malignant features present, yet usually a benign clinical course. Stromal sarcomas can extend out of the prostate and metastasize to distant sites, such as bone, lung, abdomen, and retroperitoneum. Majority (50%–75%) of patients with prostatic leiomyosarcomas die from disease within 2–5 y with metastatic spread most commonly to the lungs, often several years following initial diagnosis

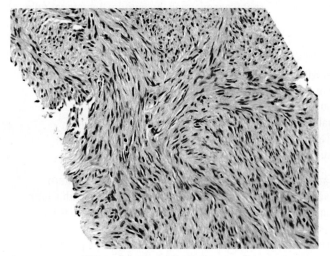

Figure 1.51.1   GIST on prostate needle biopsy.

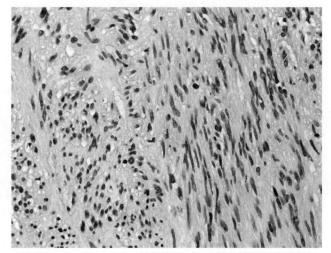

Figure 1.51.2   GIST on prostate needle biopsy with elongated nuclei and occasional perinuclear vacuoles (*left*).

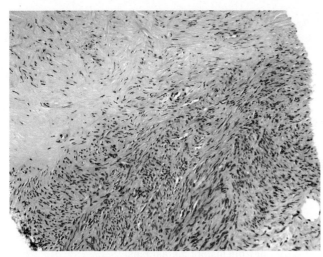

Figure 1.51.3 GIST on prostate needle biopsy with fibrosis yet lack of collagen between lesional cells.

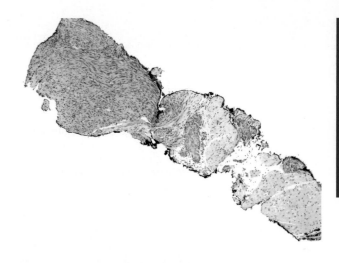

Figure 1.51.4 GIST on prostate needle biopsy with no involvement of prostate tissue.

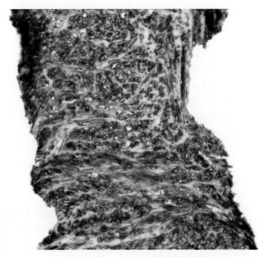

Figure 1.51.5 GIST on prostate needle biopsy with diffuse strong CD117 positivity.

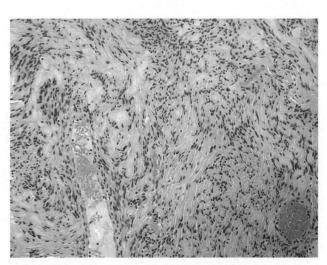

Figure 1.51.6 Solitary fibrous tumor (SFT) on TURP with bands of collagen between spindle cells.

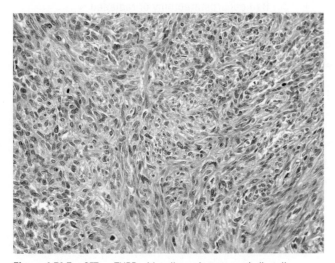

Figure 1.51.7 SFT on TURP with collagen between spindle cells.

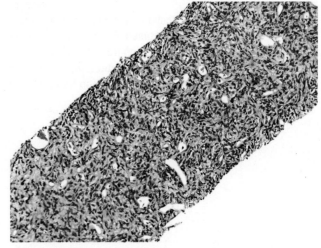

Figure 1.51.8 SFT on prostate needle biopsy with hemangiopericytomatous pattern.

	Gleason Pattern 3	Gleason Pattern 4
Age	Typically 50 to elderly, although not rare in 40s	Typically 50 to elderly, although not rare in 40s
Location	85%–90% arise in the peripheral zone and detected on needle biopsy, yet remaining arise in the transition zone and can be found either on needle biopsy or on TURP	85%–90% arise in the peripheral zone and detected on needle biopsy, yet remaining arise in the transition zone and can be found either on needle biopsy or on TURP
Symptoms	Typically asymptomatic. Advanced disease with urinary obstructive symptoms and/or hematuria or from distant metastases	Typically asymptomatic. Advanced disease with urinary obstructive symptoms and/or hematuria or from distant metastases
Signs	Variably elevated serum PSA levels	Variably elevated serum PSA levels
Etiology	See Section 1.6	See Section 1.6
Histology	1. Individual small glands, yet can be crowded back to back *(Figs. 1.52.1 and 1.52.2)* 2. A few poorly formed glands due to tangential sectioning *(Fig. 1.52.3)* 3. Lack of cribriform glands and lack of glomerulations. May see telescoping of glands mimicking glomerulations *(Fig. 1.52.4)* 4. Glands with perineural invasion or mucinous fibroplasia appear more complex *(Figs. 1.52.5 and 1.52.6)* 5. Typically lack of detached carcinoma glands on needle biopsy 6. Variable cytologic atypia	1. Fused glands *(Fig. 1.52.7)* 2. Cluster of poorly formed glands with enough glands that cannot be attributed to a tangential section off of Gleason pattern 3 glands *(Figs. 1.52.8 and 1.52.9)* 3. Cribriform glands or glands with glomerulations *(Figs. 1.52.10–1.52.12)* 4. Perineural or mucinous fibroplasia with cribriform glands 5. Detached cribriform glands on needle biopsy due to lack of stroma in large cribriform glands 6. Variable cytologic atypia including some cases with bland cytology
Special studies	Not helpful in this differential	Not helpful in this differential
Treatment	Radical prostatectomy or radiation	Radical prostatectomy or radiation
Prognosis	Excellent prognosis with no potential for metastases. Biopsy Gleason score 6: 94.6% progression free after radical prostatectomy. Radical prostatectomy Gleason score 6: 96.6% progression free after radical prostatectomy	Capacity for metastatic spread; increasing risk of progression from 3 + 4 = 7 to 4 + 3 = 7 to 4 + 4 = 8. Biopsy Gleason score 3 + 4 = 7: 82.7% progression free after radical prostatectomy. Radical prostatectomy Gleason score 3 + 4 = 7: 88.1% progression free after radical prostatectomy. Biopsy Gleason score 4 + 3 = 7: 65.1% progression free after radical prostatectomy. Radical prostatectomy Gleason score 4 + 3 = 7: 69.7% progression free after radical prostatectomy. Biopsy Gleason score 4 + 4 = 8: 63.1% progression free after radical prostatectomy. Radical prostatectomy Gleason score 4 + 4 = 8: 63.7% progression free after radical prostatectomy

1.52 Gleason Pattern 3 vs. Gleason Pattern 4   **161**

1   PROSTATE

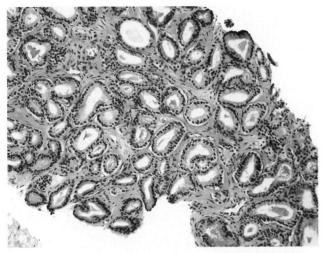

Figure 1.52.1   Gleason score 3 + 3 = 6 with individual well-formed glands.

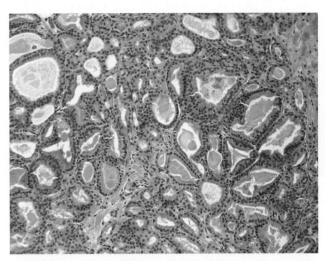

Figure 1.52.2   Gleason score 3 + 3 = 6 with crowded but still individual well-formed glands.

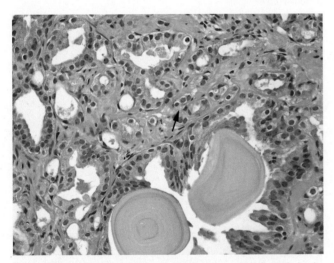

Figure 1.52.3   Gleason score 3 + 3 = 6 with a few poorly formed glands (*arrow*) that most likely represent tangential sections off of adjacent well-formed glands.

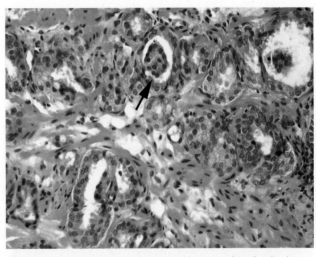

Figure 1.52.4   Gleason score 3 + 3 = 6 with telescoping of a gland (*arrow*). The gland lacks the cribriform structure of glomerulation.

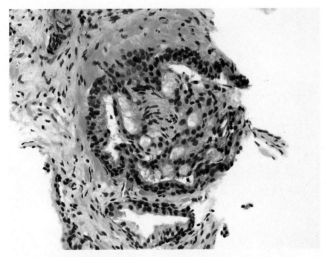

Figure 1.52.5   Gleason score 3 + 3 = 6 with perineural invasion. There is an absence of well-formed cribriform glands required for the diagnosis of Gleason pattern 4.

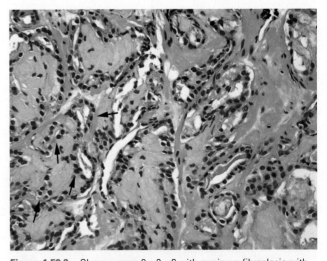

Figure 1.52.6   Gleason score 3 + 3 = 6 with mucinous fibroplasia with individual glands (*arrows*) distorted by ingrowth of fibrous tissue. There is an absence of well-formed cribriform glands required for the diagnosis of Gleason pattern 4.

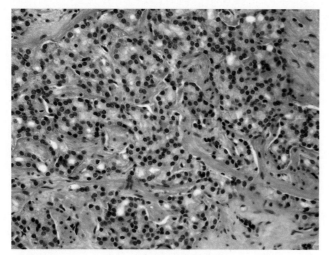

Figure 1.52.7   Fused glands of Gleason score 4 + 4 = 8.

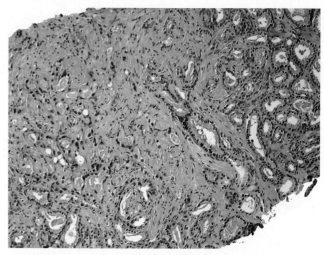

Figure 1.52.8   Gleason score 3 + 4 = 7 with poorly formed glands of Gleason pattern 4 (*left*) compared to well-formed glands of Gleason pattern 3 (*upper right*).

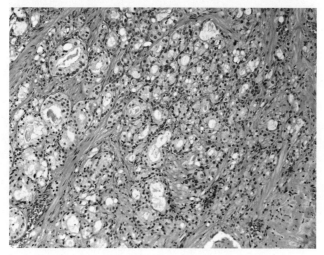

Figure 1.52.9   Gleason score 3 + 4 = 7 with poorly formed glands of Gleason pattern 4 (*upper right*) compared to well-formed glands of Gleason pattern 3 (*lower left*).

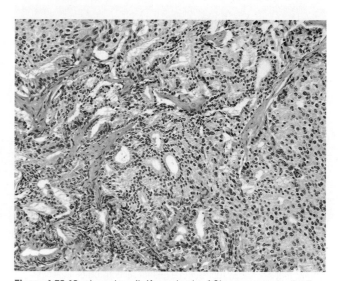

Figure 1.52.10   Irregular cribriform glands of Gleason score 4 + 4 = 8.

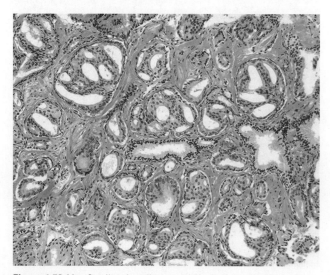

Figure 1.52.11   Small and medium rounded cribriform glands of Gleason score 4 + 4 = 8.

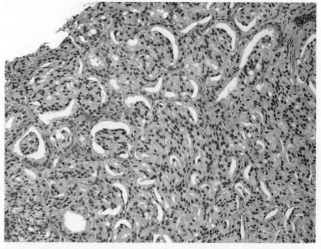

Figure 1.52.12   Gleason score 4 + 4 = 8 with irregular cribriform glands and glomerulations, which are cribriform glands protruding into a dilated gland, attached on only one side mimicking a glomerulus.

	Gleason Pattern 4	**Gleason Pattern 5**
Age	Typically 50 to elderly, although not rare in 40s	Typically 50 to elderly, although not rare in 40s
Location	85%–90% arise in the peripheral zone and detected on needle biopsy, yet remaining arise in the transition zone and can be found either on needle biopsy or on TURP	85%–90% arise in the peripheral zone and detected on needle biopsy, yet remaining arise in the transition zone and can be found either on needle biopsy or on TURP
Symptoms	Typically asymptomatic. Advanced disease with urinary obstructive symptoms and/or hematuria or from distant metastases	Typically asymptomatic. Advanced disease with urinary obstructive symptoms and/or hematuria or from distant metastases
Signs	Variably elevated serum PSA levels	Variably elevated serum PSA levels
Etiology	See Section 1.6	See Section 1.6
Histology	1. Fused glands 2. Poorly formed glands *(Figs. 1.53.1 and 1.53.2)* 3. Cribriform glands *(Figs. 1.53.3 and 1.53.4)* 4. Lacks necrosis 5. Variable cytologic atypia including some cases with bland cytology	1. Cords of cells *(Fig. 1.53.5)* 2. Single cells *(Fig. 1.53.6)* 3. Very ill-defined fused or cribriform glands to solid sheets *(Figs. 1.53.7–1.53.10)* 4. Nests and gland with central necrosis *(Figs. 1.53.11 and 1.53.12)* 5. Variable cytologic atypia including some cases with bland cytology
Special studies	Not helpful in this differential	Not helpful in this differential
Treatment	Radical prostatectomy or radiation	Radical prostatectomy for limited disease on biopsy. Otherwise, neoadjuvant hormone therapy followed by external beam and interstitial radiotherapy
Prognosis	Capacity for metastatic spread; increasing risk of progression from 3 + 4 = 7 to 4 + 3 = 7 to 4 + 4 = 8. Biopsy Gleason score 3 + 4 = 7: 82.7% progression free after radical prostatectomy. Radical prostatectomy Gleason score 3 + 4 = 7: 88.1% progression free after radical prostatectomy. Biopsy Gleason score 4 + 3 = 7: 65.1% progression free after radical prostatectomy. Radical prostatectomy Gleason score 4 + 3 = 7: 69.7% progression free after radical prostatectomy. Biopsy Gleason score 4 + 4 = 8: 63.1% progression free after radical prostatectomy. Radical prostatectomy Gleason score 4 + 4 = 8: 63.7% progression free after radical prostatectomy	High risk of metastatic spread. Biopsy Gleason score 9–10: 34.5% progression free after radical prostatectomy. Radical prostatectomy Gleason score 9–10: 34.5% progression free after radical prostatectomy

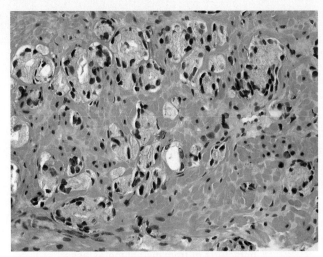

Figure 1.53.1 Gleason score 4 + 4 = 8 with poorly formed glands with occasional single cells that could represent a tangential section off a poorly formed gland.

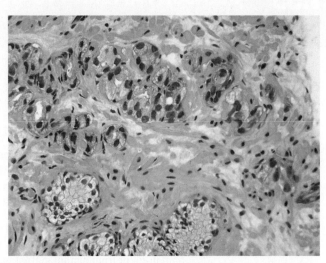

Figure 1.53.2 Gleason score 4 + 3 = 7 with poorly formed glands with occasional single cells that could represent a tangential section off a poorly formed gland.

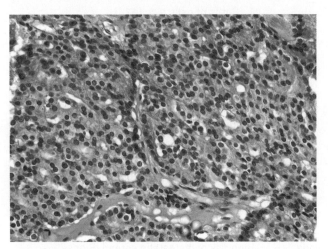

Figure 1.53.3 Cribriform Gleason score 4 + 4 = 8 with well-developed although small lumens.

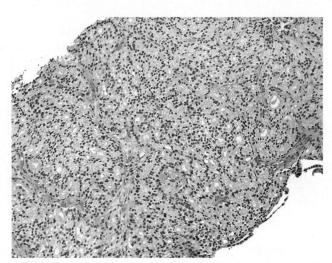

Figure 1.53.4 Cribriform Gleason score 4 + 4 = 8 with well-developed although small lumens.

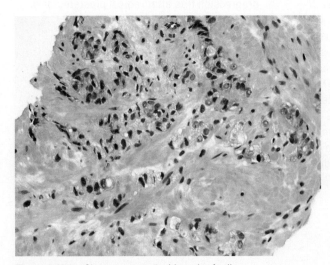

Figure 1.53.5 Gleason pattern 5 with cords of cells.

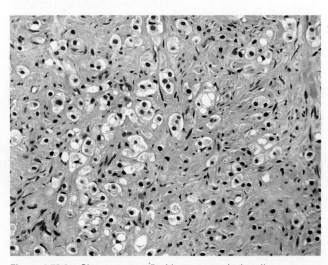

Figure 1.53.6 Gleason pattern 5 with numerous single cells.

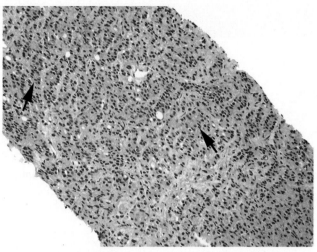

Figure 1.53.7   Gleason pattern 5 with such barely perceptible glands (*arrows*) and mostly no gland formation.

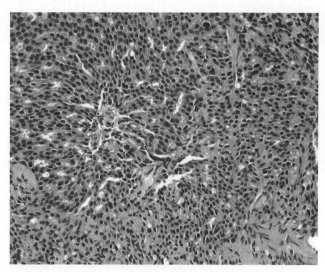

Figure 1.53.8   Gleason pattern 4 (*top*) with cribriform gland merging with solid sheets with barely developed lumens (*bottom*) of Gleason pattern 5.

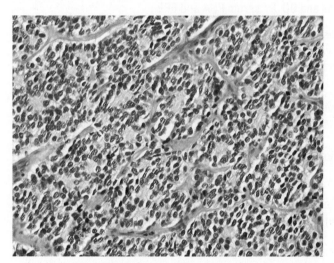

Figure 1.53.9   Gleason pattern 5 with lack of true cribriform glands and merely rosettes of cytoplasm as an attempt at rudimentary cribriform gland formation.

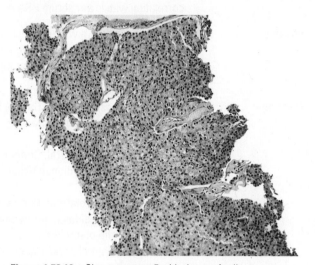

Figure 1.53.10   Gleason pattern 5 with sheets of cells.

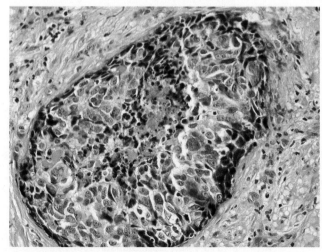

Figure 1.53.11   Gleason pattern 5 with solid nests of cancer with central necrosis.

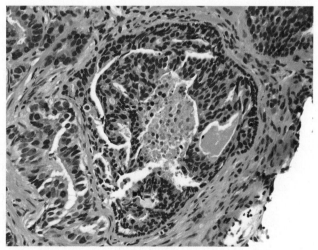

Figure 1.53.12   Gleason pattern 5 with cribriform gland with central necrosis.

	Organ-confined at Radical Prostatectomy	Extraprostatic Extension (EPE) at Radical Prostatectomy
Age	Typically 50 to elderly, although not rare in 40s	Typically 50 to elderly, although not rare in 40s
Location	85% of cancers predominantly in the peripheral zone with remaining predominantly in the transition zone	85% of cancers predominantly in the peripheral zone with remaining predominantly in the transition zone with location of EPE paralleling tumor location
Symptoms	Asymptomatic	Asymptomatic
Signs	Variably elevated serum PSA levels. Can be organ-confined with relatively high serum PSA levels, although in general, there is a correlation with lower serum PSA levels and OC	Variably elevated serum PSA levels. Can have EPE with relatively low serum PSA level, although in general, there is a correlation with serum PSA and EPE
Etiology	Despite the lack of a well-defined prostatic capsule, the edge of the prostate provides a barrier against spread of tumor into the periprostatic soft tissue	Posterior and posterolaterally, tumor tends to spread out of the prostate via perineural invasion. Anteriorly via direct spread through the stroma
Histology	1. Posterior/posterolateral: Cancer within condensed smooth muscle (Figs. 1.54.1 and 1.54.2) 2. Posterior/posterolateral: Cancer not in or at same plane as adipose tissue 3. Posterior/posterolateral: Cancer can extend on both sides of large blood vessels at edge of the gland (Fig. 1.54.3) 4. Posterior/posterolateral: Cancer does not protrude beyond contour of normal prostate 5. Anterior: Cancer does not extend into adipose tissue 6. At apex, if cancer is present in skeletal muscle, yet not at the inked margin, the convention is to call it organ confined as the boundaries of the prostate are vague in this region and patients do well with this finding (Fig. 1.54.4)	1. Posterior/posterolateral: Cancer beyond condensed smooth muscle (Figs. 1.54.5–1.54.8) 2. Posterior/posterolateral: Cancer in or at same plane as adipose tissue (Figs. 1.54.9 and 1.54.10) 3. Posterior/posterolateral: Cancer extends beyond large blood vessels at edge of the gland 4. Posterior/posterolateral: Cancer protrudes beyond contour of normal prostate 5. Anterior: Cancer extends into adipose tissue (Fig. 1.54.11) 6. At apex, if cancer at inked margin in region of skeletal muscle, then cannot tell if tumor is organ confined or EPE since the boundaries of the prostate are vague in this region. Tumor is reported as pT2+ or pT2x, meaning that the status of EPE is unknown (Fig. 1.54.12)
Special studies	Not helpful in this differential	Not helpful in this differential
Treatment	Not applicable	Not applicable
Prognosis	Radical prostatectomy Gleason score 6: 98% 5-y biochemical-free recurrence (BCR). Gleason score 3 + 4 = 7: 89% 5-y BCR. Gleason score 4 + 3 = 7: 5-y 76% BCR. Gleason score 4 + 4 = 8: 74% 5-y BCR. Gleason score 9–10: 5-y 69% BCR	Nonfocal EPE with no seminal vesicle invasion or lymph node metastases. Radical prostatectomy Gleason score 6: 84% 5-y biochemical-free recurrence (BCR). Gleason score 3 + 4 = 7: 70% 5-y BCR. Gleason score 4 + 3 = 7: 5-y 42% BCR. Gleason score 4 + 4 = 8: 42% 5-y BCR. Gleason score 9–10: 5-y 27% BCR

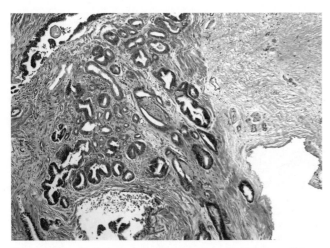

Figure 1.54.1 Posterior organ-confined carcinoma with tumor within condensed smooth muscle.

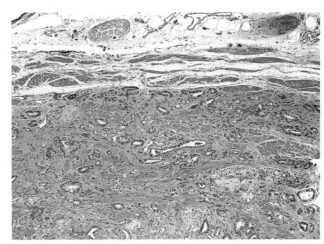

Figure 1.54.2 Posterior organ-confined carcinoma with tumor within condensed smooth muscle.

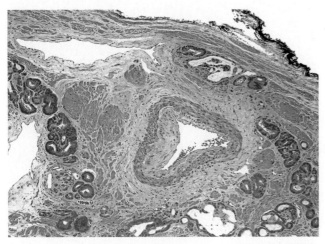

Figure 1.54.3 Posterior organ-confined carcinoma with tumor on both sides of large blood vessel mimicking EPE.

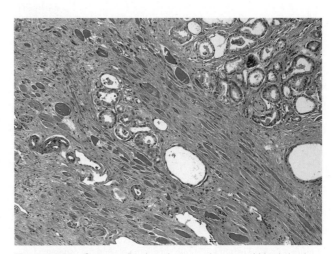

Figure 1.54.4 Organ-confined carcinoma at the apex within skeletal muscle not at the margin.

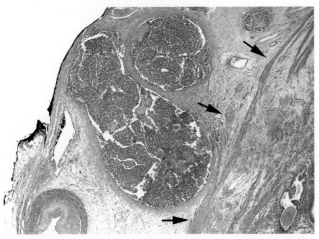

Figure 1.54.5 Posterior nonfocal EPE with large nests of carcinoma beyond the condensed smooth muscle (*arrows*) of the prostate.

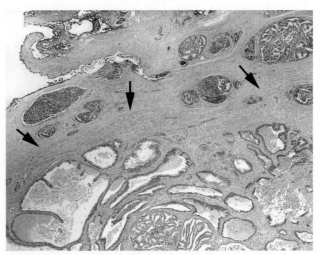

Figure 1.54.6 Posterior nonfocal EPE with large nests of carcinoma beyond the condensed smooth muscle (*arrows*) of the prostate.

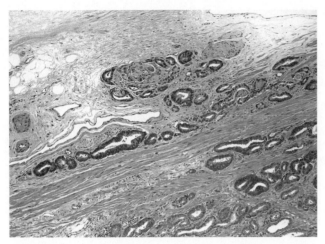

Figure 1.54.7   Posterior focal EPE with limited carcinoma just beyond the condensed smooth muscle of the prostate.

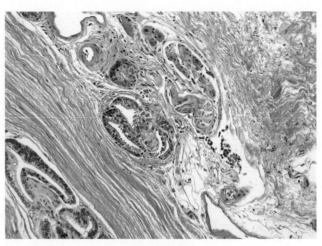

Figure 1.54.8   Posterior focal EPE with limited carcinoma just beyond the condensed smooth muscle of the prostate.

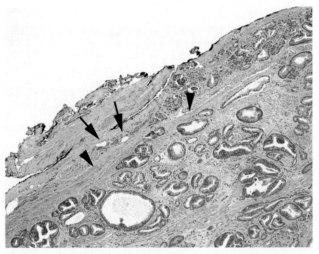

Figure 1.54.9   Posterior EPE with carcinoma beyond the condensed smooth muscle of the prostate (*arrowheads*) and beyond the level of adipose tissue (*arrows*).

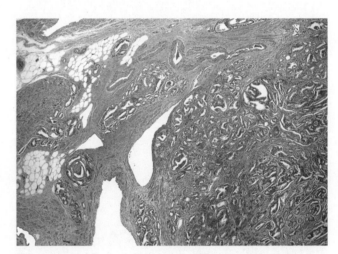

Figure 1.54.10   Posterolateral nonfocal EPE with carcinoma infiltrating adipose tissue.

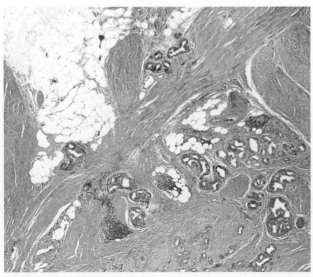

Figure 1.54.11   Anterior nonfocal EPE with tumor infiltrating adipose tissue.

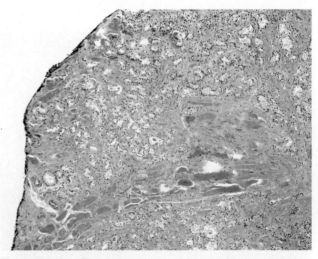

Figure 1.54.12   pT2+ cancer at the apex where carcinoma extends to the inked margin in an area within skeletal muscle where the boundary of the prostate is ambiguous.

	Pelvic Lymph Nodes with Reaction to Hip Replacement	Metastatic Prostatic Adenocarcinoma in Lymph Nodes
Age	Typically 50 to elderly	Typically 50 to elderly
Location	Ipsilateral pelvic lymph nodes on the same side as prosthetic hip replacement	Pelvic lymph nodes
Symptoms	Asymptomatic relative to the hip replacement. Clinical history must be elicited from clinician	Typically nodal metastases asymptomatic
Signs	Variably elevated serum PSA levels	Serum PSA levels tend to be higher than cases without nodal metastases, yet exceptions occur
Etiology	Histiocytic reaction to microscopic particles, such as titanium or cobalt–chromium and methyl methacrylate that constantly shed off from hip prosthesis as a result of wear and tear	Metastases from Gleason score 7 or higher adenocarcinoma. Metastases tend to be ipsilateral to the dominant tumor nodule. Uncommonly, men may have received neoadjuvant antiandrogen therapy if there is a delay between diagnosis and treatment, giving rise to cancer with hormonal therapy affect
Histology	1. Nodule within node composed of cells with dense eosinophilic cytoplasm *(Fig. 1.55.1)* 2. No glandular differentiation 3. Nuclei with at most small nucleoli 4. Scattered small black irregular particles overlying eosinophilic cells (titanium or cobalt–chromium) *(Fig. 1.55.2)* 5. Scattered small refractile polarizable irregular particles overlying eosinophilic cells (polyethylene) *(Fig. 1.55.3)*	1. Nodule within node composed of cells with cytoplasm ranging from lightly pale eosinophilic to dense eosinophilic to amphophilic *(Fig. 1.55.4)* 2. Even in high-grade adenocarcinoma, often a hint of glandular differentiation *(Fig. 1.55.5)*. With prior hormonal therapy, glandular cells become loosely cohesive, resulting in cleft-like spaces containing detached tumor cells 3. Typically enlarged nuclei with prominent nucleoli. In setting of prior hormone therapy, cells have pyknotic nuclei where cells resembling lymphocytes or histiocytes depending on the extent of cytoplasm *(Fig. 1.55.6)* 4. Lack of black particles overlying tumor cells 5. Lack of refractile polarizable particles overlying tumor cells
Special studies	• Eosinophilic cells positive for histiocytic markers, such as CD68 • Eosinophilic cells negative for prostate markers (PSA, P501S, NKX3.1) and negative for epithelial markers (CAM5.2, AE1/AE3)	• Tumor cells negative for histiocytic markers, such as CD68 • Tumor cells variably and often only focally positive for prostate markers (PSA, P501S, NKX3.1) and more diffusely positive for epithelial markers (CAM5.2, AE1/AE3)

	Pelvic Lymph Nodes with Reaction to Hip Replacement	**Metastatic Prostatic Adenocarcinoma in Lymph Nodes**
Treatment	None for the node involvement	Antiandrogen therapy
Prognosis	Dependent on the grade, stage, and margins of tumor in radical prostatectomy specimen	Ultimately, all men with pelvic lymph node metastases will die of prostate cancer if live long enough. For men undergoing radical prostatectomy with positive pelvic lymph nodes, approximately 50% are dead of cancer at around 10 y

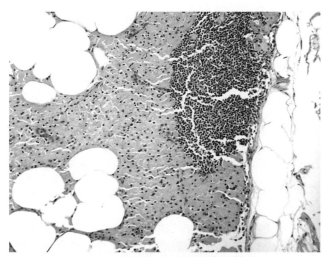

Figure 1.55.1 Large dense pink histiocytes in pelvic lymph node reacting to hip replacement material.

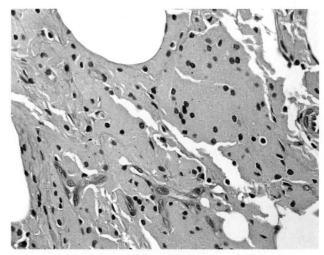

Figure 1.55.2 Same case as Figure 1.55.1 with numerous scattered small black foreign particles within cytoplasm.

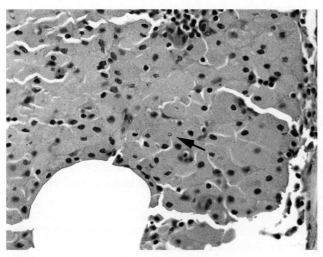

Figure 1.55.3 Same case as Figure 1.55.1 with small refractile polarizable irregular particles (*arrow*).

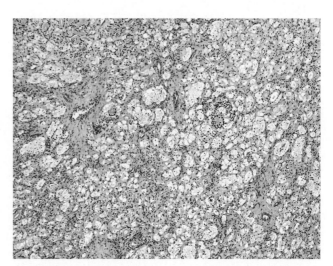

Figure 1.55.4 Metastatic prostate adenocarcinoma to a pelvic lymph node with hormone therapy affect. Cytoplasm tends to be paler than the dense cytoplasm seen in reaction to hip replacement.

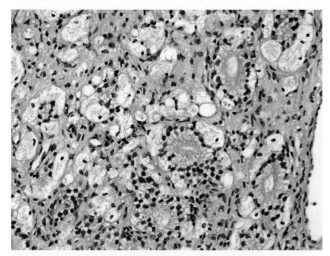

Figure 1.55.5 Same case as Figure 1.55.4 with many cells resembling histiocytes, yet focal glandular differentiation seen.

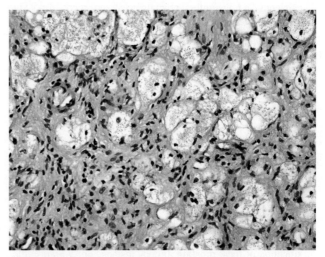

Figure 1.55.6 Same case as Figures 1.55.4 and 1.55.5 with treated carcinoma having pyknotic nuclei and abundant pale cytoplasm.

SUGGESTED READINGS

1.1–1.6

Chu PG, Huang Q, Weiss LM. Incidental and concurrent malignant lymphomas discovered at the time of prostatectomy and prostate biopsy: a study of 29 cases. *Am J Surg Pathol.* 2005;29:693–699.

Eisenberger CF, Walsh PC, Eisenberger MA, et al. Incidental non-Hodgkin's lymphoma in patients with localized prostate cancer. *Urology.* 1999;53:175–179.

Epstein JI, Hutchins GM. Granulomatous prostatitis: distinction among allergic, nonspecific, and post-transurethral resection lesions. *Hum Pathol.* 1984;15:818–825.

Gorelick JI, Senterfit LB, Vaughan ED, Jr. Quantitative bacterial tissue cultures from 209 prostatectomy specimens: findings and implications. *J Urol.* 1988;139:57–60.

Kohnen PW, Drach GW. Patterns of inflammation in prostatic hyperplasia: a histologic and bacteriologic study. *J Urol.* 1979; 121:755–760.

Moser PL, Brunner A, Horninger W, et al. Correlation between inflammatory cells (T and B lymphocytes, macrophages) in prostate biopsies and elevated PSA levels in a PSA screening population. *Urology.* 2002;59:68–72.

Okada K, Kojima M, Naya Y, et al. Correlation of histological inflammation in needle biopsy specimens with serum prostate-specific antigen levels in men with negative biopsy for prostate cancer. *Urology.* 2000;55:892–898.

Oppenheimer JR, Kahane H, Epstein JI. Granulomatous prostatitis on needle biopsy. *Arch Pathol Lab Med.* 1997;121:724–729.

Stillwell TJ, Engen DE, Farrow GM. The clinical spectrum of granulomatous prostatitis: a report of 200 cases. *J Urol.* 1987;138:320–323.

Weir EG, Epstein JI. Incidental small lymphocytic lymphoma/chronic lymphocytic leukemia in pelvic lymph nodes excised at radical prostatectomy. *Arch Pathol Lab Med.* 2003;127:567–572.

1.7

Alguacil-Garcia A. Artifactual changes mimicking signet ring cell carcinoma in transurethral prostatectomy specimens. *Am J Surg Pathol.* 1986;10:795–800.

Ro JY, el-Naggar A, Ayala AG, et al. Signet-ring-cell carcinoma of the prostate. electron-microscopic and immunohistochemical studies of eight cases. *Am J Surg Pathol.* 1988;12:453–460.

1.10–1.11

Adley BP, Yang XJ. Alpha-methylacyl coenzyme A racemase immunoreactivity in partial atrophy of the prostate. *Am J Clin Pathol.* 2006;126:849–855.

Billis A, Meirelles L, Freitas LL. Mergence of partial and complete atrophy in prostate needle biopsies: a morphologic and immunohistochemical study. *Virchows Arch.* 2010;456:689–694.

De Marzo AM, Platz EA, Epstein JI, et al. A working group classification of focal prostate atrophy lesions. *Am J Surg Pathol.* 2006;30:1281–1291.

Farinola MA, Epstein JI. Utility of immunohistochemistry for alpha-methylacyl-CoA racemase in distinguishing atrophic prostate cancer from benign atrophy. *Hum Pathol.* 2004;35: 1272–1278.

Humphrey PA. Atrophy of the prostate on needle biopsy and false-positive diagnosis of malignancy. *J Urol.* 2011;186:2065–2066.

Oppenheimer JR, Wills ML, Epstein JI. Partial atrophy in prostate needle cores: another diagnostic pitfall for the surgical pathologist. *Am J Surg Pathol.* 1998;22:440–445.

Przybycin CG, Kunju LP, Wu AJ, et al. Partial atrophy in prostate needle biopsies: a detailed analysis of its morphology, immunophenotype, and cellular kinetics. *Am J Surg Pathol.* 2008;32: 58–64.

Wang W, Sun X, Epstein JI. Partial atrophy on prostate needle biopsy cores: a morphologic and immunohistochemical study. *Am J Surg Pathol.* 2008;32:851–857.

1.13

Bostwick DG, Egbert BM, Fajardo LF. Radiation injury of the normal and neoplastic prostate. *Am J Surg Pathol.* 1982;6:541–551.

Brawer MK, Nagle RB, Pitts W, et al. Keratin immunoreactivity as an aid to the diagnosis of persistent adenocarcinoma in irradiated human prostates. *Cancer.* 1989;63:454–460.

Crook J, Malone S, Perry G, et al. Postradiotherapy prostate biopsies: what do they really mean? Results for 498 patients. *Int J Rad Onc Biol Phys.* 2000;48:355–367.

Magi-Galluzzi C, Sanderson H, Epstein JI. Atypia in nonneoplastic prostate glands after radiotherapy for prostate cancer: duration of atypia and relation to type of radiotherapy. *Am J Surg Pathol.* 2003;27:206–212.

Yang XJ, Laven B, Tretiakova M, et al. Detection of alpha-methylacyl-coenzyme A racemase in postradiation prostatic adenocarcinoma. *Urology.* 2003;62:282–286.

1.14

Armas OA, Aprikian AG, Melamed J, et al. Clinical and pathobiological effects of neoadjuvant total androgen ablation therapy on clinically localized prostatic adenocarcinoma. *Am J Surg Pathol.* 1994;18:979–991.

Chuang AY, Epstein JI. Xanthoma of the prostate: a mimicker of high-grade prostate adenocarcinoma. *Am J Surg Pathol.* 2007;31:1225–1230.

Murphy WM, Soloway MS, Barrows GH. Pathologic changes associated with androgen deprivation therapy for prostate cancer. *Cancer.* 1991;68:821–828.

Smith DM, Murphy WM. Histologic changes in prostate carcinomas treated with leuprolide (luteinizing hormone-releasing hormone effect). Distinction from poor tumor differentiation. *Cancer.* 1994;73:1472–1477.

Tetu B, Srigley JR, Boivin JC, et al. Effect of combination endocrine therapy (LHRH agonist and flutamide) on normal prostate and prostatic adenocarcinoma. A histopathologic and immunohistochemical study. *Am J Surg Pathol.* 1991;15:111–120.

Vailancourt L, Ttu B, Fradet Y, et al. Effect of neoadjuvant endocrine therapy (combined androgen blockade) on normal prostate and prostatic carcinoma. A randomized study. *Am J Surg Pathol.* 1996;20:86–93.

1.15–1.17

Ali TZ, Epstein JI. Basal cell carcinoma of the prostate: a clinicopathologic study of 29 cases. *Am J Surg Pathol.* 2007; 31:697–705.

Epstein JI, Armas OA. Atypical basal cell hyperplasia of the prostate. *Am J Surg Pathol.* 1992;16:1205–1214.

Hosler GA, Epstein JI. Basal cell hyperplasia: an unusual diagnostic dilemma on prostate needle biopsies. *Hum Pathol.* 2005;36:480–485.

Iczkowski KA, Ferguson KL, Grier DD, et al. Adenoid cystic/basal cell carcinoma of the prostate: clinicopathologic findings in 19 cases. *Am J Surg Pathol.* 2003;27:1523–1529.

McKenney JK, Amin MB, Srigley JR, et al. Basal cell proliferations of the prostate other than usual basal cell hyperplasia: a clinicopathologic study of 23 cases, including four carcinomas, with a proposed classification. *Am J Surg Pathol* 2004;28:1289–1298.

Rioux-Leclercq NC, Epstein JI. Unusual morphologic patterns of basal cell hyperplasia of the prostate. *Am J Surg Pathol.* 2002;26:237–243.

Yang XJ, McEntee M, Epstein JI. Distinction of basaloid carcinoma of the prostate from benign basal cell lesions by using immunohistochemistry for bcl-2 and ki-67. *Hum Pathol.* 1998;29:1447–1450.

Yang XJ, Tretiakova MS, Sengupta E, et al. Florid basal cell hyperplasia of the prostate: a histological, ultrastructural, and immunohistochemical analysis. *Hum Pathol.* 2003;34:462–470.

1.18

Cina SJ, Silberman MA, Kahane H, et al. Diagnosis of Cowper's glands on prostate needle biopsy. *Am J Surg Pathol.* 1997;21:550–555.

Nelson RS, Epstein JI. Prostatic carcinoma with abundant xanthomatous cytoplasm. foamy gland carcinoma. *Am J Surg Pathol.* 1996;20:419–426.

Saboorian MH, Huffman H, Ashfaq R, et al. Distinguishing Cowper's glands from neoplastic and pseudoneoplastic lesions of prostate: immunohistochemical and ultrastructural studies. *Am J Surg Pathol.* 1997;21:1069–1074.

1.19

Gaudin PB, Epstein JI. Adenosis of the prostate. histologic features in needle biopsy specimens. *Am J Surg Pathol.* 1995;19: 737–747.

Gaudin PB, Epstein JI. Adenosis of the prostate. Histologic features in transurethral resection specimens. *Am J Surg Pathol.* 1994;18:863–870.

Lotan TL, Epstein JI. Diffuse adenosis of the peripheral zone in prostate needle biopsy and prostatectomy specimens. *Am J Surg Pathol.* 2008;32:1360–1366.

1.20

Grignon DJ, Ro JY, Srigley JR, et al. Sclerosing adenosis of the prostate gland. A lesion showing myoepithelial differentiation. *Am J Surg Pathol.* 1992;16:383–391.

Luque RJ, Lopez-Beltran A, Perez-Seoane C, et al. Sclerosing adenosis of the prostate. Histologic features in needle biopsy specimens. *Arch Pathol Lab Med.* 2003;127:e14–e16.

Sakamoto N, Tsuneyoshi M, Enjoji M. Sclerosing adenosis of the prostate. Histopathologic and immunohistochemical analysis. *Am J Surg Pathol.* 1991;15:660–667.

1.21

Humphrey PA, Kaleem Z, Swanson PE, et al. Pseudohyperplastic prostatic adenocarcinoma. *Am J Surg Pathol.* 1998;22: 1239–1246.

Levi AW, Epstein JI. Pseudohyperplastic prostatic adenocarcinoma on needle biopsy and simple prostatectomy. *Am J Surg Pathol.* 2000;24:1039–1046.

Yaskiv O, Cao D, Humphrey PA. Microcystic adenocarcinoma of the prostate: a variant of pseudohyperplastic and atrophic patterns. *Am J Surg Pathol.* 2010;34:556–561.

1.22

Ali TZ, Epstein JI. Perineural involvement by benign prostatic glands on needle biopsy. *Am J Surg Pathol.* 2005;29:1159–1163.

Baisden BL, Kahane H, Epstein JI. Perineural invasion, mucinous fibroplasia, and glomerulations: diagnostic features of limited cancer on prostate needle biopsy. *Am J Surg Pathol.* 1999;23:918–924.

Carstens PH. Perineural glands in normal and hyperplastic prostates. *J Urol.* 1980;123:686–688.

1.23–1.24

Ayala AG, Srigley JR, Ro JY, et al. Clear cell cribriform hyperplasia of prostate. Report of 10 cases. *Am J Surg Pathol.* 1986;10:665–671.

1.25

Kawabata K. Paraganglion of the prostate in a needle biopsy: a potential diagnostic pitfall. *Arch Pathol Lab Med.* 1997;121: 515–516.

Ostrowski ML, Wheeler TM. Paraganglia of the prostate. Location, frequency, and differentiation from prostatic adenocarcinoma. *Am J Surg Pathol.* 1994;18:412–420.

1.26

Schowinsky JT, Epstein JI. Distorted rectal tissue on prostate needle biopsy: a mimicker of prostate cancer. *Am J Surg Pathol.* 2006;30:866–870.

1.27

Bostwick DG, Qian J, Ma J, et al. Mesonephric remnants of the prostate: incidence and histologic spectrum. *Mod Pathol.* 2003;16:630–635.

Chen YB, Fine SW, Epstein JI. Mesonephric remnant hyperplasia involving prostate and periprostatic tissue: findings at radical prostatectomy. *Am J Surg Pathol.* 2011;35:1054–1061.

Gikas PW, Del Buono EA, Epstein JI. Florid hyperplasia of mesonephric remnants involving prostate and periprostatic tissue. Possible confusion with adenocarcinoma. *Am J Surg Pathol.* 1993;17:454–460.

1.28

Chuang AY, Epstein JI. Xanthoma of the prostate: a mimicker of high-grade prostate adenocarcinoma. *Am J Surg Pathol.* 2007;31:1225–1230.

Sebo TJ, Bostwick DG, Farrow GM, et al. Prostatic xanthoma: a mimic of prostatic adenocarcinoma. *Hum Pathol.* 1994;25:386–389.

1.29

Allan CH, Epstein JI. Nephrogenic adenoma of the prostatic urethra: a mimicker of prostate adenocarcinoma. *Am J Surg Pathol.* 2001;25:802–808.

Gupta A, Wang HL, Policarpio-Nicolas ML, et al. Expression of alpha-methylacyl-coenzyme A racemase in nephrogenic adenoma. *Am J Surg Pathol.* 2004;28:1224–1229.

Mazal PR, Schaufler R, Altenhuber-Muller R, et al. Derivation of nephrogenic adenomas from renal tubular cells in kidney-transplant recipients. *N Engl J Med.* 2002;347:653–659.

Skinnider BF, Oliva E, Young RH, et al. Expression of alpha-methylacyl-CoA racemase (P504S) in nephrogenic adenoma: a significant immunohistochemical pitfall compounding the differential diagnosis with prostatic adenocarcinoma. *Am J Surg Pathol.* 2004;28: 701–705.

Tong GX, Melamed J, Mansukhani M, et al. PAX2: a reliable marker for nephrogenic adenoma. *Mod Pathol.* 2006;19:356–363.

1.30

Gaudin PB, Wheeler TM, Epstein JI. Verumontanum mucosal gland hyperplasia in prostatic needle biopsy specimens. A mimic of low grade prostatic adenocarcinoma. *Am J Clin Pathol.* 1995;104:620–626.

Gagucas RJ, Brown RW, Wheeler TM. Verumontanum mucosal gland hyperplasia. *Am J Surg Pathol.* 1995;19:30–36.

1.31

Srodon M, Epstein JI. Central zone histology of the prostate: a mimicker of high-grade prostatic intraepithelial neoplasia. *Hum Pathol.* 2002;33:518–523.

1.32–1.33

Bostwick DG, Amin MB, Dundore P, et al. Architectural patterns of high-grade prostatic intraepithelial neoplasia. *Hum Pathol.* 1993;24:298–310.

Epstein JI, Grignon DJ, Humphrey PA, et al. Interobserver reproducibility in the diagnosis of prostatic intraepithelial neoplasia. *Am J Surg Pathol.* 1995;19:873–886.

Kronz JD, Allan CH, Shaikh AA, et al. Predicting cancer following a diagnosis of high-grade prostatic intraepithelial neoplasia on needle biopsy: data on men with more than one follow-up biopsy. *Am J Surg Pathol.* 2001;25:1079–1085.

Kronz JD, Shaikh AA, Epstein JI. High-grade prostatic intraepithelial neoplasia with adjacent small atypical glands on prostate biopsy. *Hum Pathol.* 2001;32:389–395.

Lefkowitz GK, Sidhu GS, Torre P, et al. Is repeat prostate biopsy for high-grade prostatic intraepithelial neoplasia necessary after routine 12-core sampling? *Urology.* 2001;58:999–1003.

McNeal JE, Bostwick DG. Intraductal dysplasia: a premalignant lesion of the prostate. *Hum Pathol.* 1986;17:64–71.

Merrimen JL, Jones G, Srigley JR. Is high grade prostatic intraepithelial neoplasia still a risk factor for adenocarcinoma in the era of extended biopsy sampling? *Pathology.* 2010;42:325–329.

Merrimen JL, Jones G, Walker D, et al. Multifocal high grade prostatic intraepithelial neoplasia is a significant risk factor for prostatic adenocarcinoma. *J Urol.* 2009;182:485–490; discussion 490.

1.34–1.36

Cohen RJ, McNeal JE, Baillie T. Patterns of differentiation and proliferation in intraductal carcinoma of the prostate: significance for cancer progression. *Prostate.* 2000;43:11–19.

Guo CC, Epstein JI. Intraductal carcinoma of the prostate on needle biopsy: histologic features and clinical significance. *Mod Pathol.* 2006;19:1528–1535.

Henry PC, Evans AJ. Intraductal carcinoma of the prostate: a distinct histopathological entity with important prognostic implications. *J Clin Pathol.* 2009;62:579–583.

Robinson B, Magi-Galluzzi C, Zhou M. Intraductal carcinoma of the prostate. *Arch Pathol Lab Med.* 2012;136:418–425.

Robinson BD, Epstein JI. Intraductal carcinoma of the prostate without invasive carcinoma on needle biopsy: emphasis on radical prostatectomy findings. *J Urol.* 2010;184:1328–1333.

Shah RB, Zhou M. Atypical cribriform lesions of the prostate: clinical significance, differential diagnosis and current concept of intraductal carcinoma of the prostate. *Adv Anat Pathol.* 2012;19:270–278.

Van der Kwast T, Al Daoud N, Collette L, et al. Biopsy diagnosis of intraductal carcinoma is prognostic in intermediate and high risk prostate cancer patients treated by radiotherapy. *Eur J Cancer.* 2012;48:1318–1325.

1.37

Tavora F, Epstein JI. High-grade prostatic intraepithelial neoplasia-like ductal adenocarcinoma of the prostate: a clinicopathologic study of 28 cases. *Am J Surg Pathol.* 2008;32:1060–1067.

Hameed O, Humphrey PA. Stratified epithelium in prostatic adenocarcinoma: a mimic of high-grade prostatic intraepithelial neoplasia. *Mod Pathol.* 2006;19:899–906.

1.38–1.40

Bostwick DG, Kindrachuk RW, Rouse RV. Prostatic adenocarcinoma with endometrioid features. Clinical, pathologic, and ultrastructural findings. *Am J Surg Pathol.* 1985;9:595–609.

Brinker DA, Potter SR, Epstein JI. Ductal adenocarcinoma of the prostate diagnosed on needle biopsy: correlation with clinical and radical prostatectomy findings and progression. *Am J Surg Pathol.* 1999;23:1471–1479.

Butterick JD, Schnitzer B, Abell MR. Ectopic prostatic tissue in urethra: a clinocopathological entity and a significant cause of hematuria. *J Urol.* 1971;105:97–104.

Craig JR, Hart WR. Benign polyps with prostatic-type epithelium of the urethra. *Am J Clin Pathol.* 1975;63:343–347.

Epstein JI, Woodruff JM. Adenocarcinoma of the prostate with endometrioid features. A light microscopic and immunohistochemical study of ten cases. *Cancer.* 1986;57:111–119.

Herawi M, Epstein JI. Immunohistochemical antibody cocktail staining (p63/HMWCK/AMACR) of ductal adenocarcinoma and Gleason pattern 4 cribriform and noncribriform acinar adenocarcinomas of the prostate. *Am J Surg Pathol.* 2007;31:889–894.

1.41–1.43

Chuang AY, DeMarzo AM, Veltri RW, et al. Immunohistochemical differentiation of high-grade prostate carcinoma from urothelial carcinoma. *Am J Surg Pathol.* 2007;31:1246–1255.

Esheba GE, Longacre TA, Atkins KA, et al. Expression of the urothelial differentiation markers GATA3 and placental S100 (S100P) in female genital tract transitional cell proliferations. *Am J Surg Pathol.* 2009;33:347–353.

Esrig D, Freeman JA, Elmajian DA, et al. Transitional cell carcinoma involving the prostate with a proposed staging classification for stromal invasion. *J Urol.* 1996;156:1071–1076.

Genega EM, Hutchinson B, Reuter VE, et al. Immunophenotype of high-grade prostatic adenocarcinoma and urothelial carcinoma. *Mod Pathol.* 2000;13:1186–1191.

Higgins JP, Kaygusuz G, Wang L, et al. Placental S100 (S100P) and GATA3: markers for transitional epithelium and urothelial carcinoma discovered by complementary DNA microarray. *Am J Surg Pathol.* 2007;31:673–680.

Milord RA, Kahane H, Epstein JI. Infarct of the prostate gland: experience on needle biopsy specimens. *Am J Surg Pathol.* 2000;24:1378–1384.

Mostofi FK, Morse WH. Epithelial metaplasia in "prostatic infarction". *AMA Arch Pathol.* 1951;51:340–345.

Oliai BR, Kahane H, Epstein JI. A clinicopathologic analysis of urothelial carcinomas diagnosed on prostate needle biopsy. *Am J Surg Pathol.* 2001;25:794–801.

Ordonez NG. Thrombomodulin expression in transitional cell carcinoma. *Am J Clin Pathol.* 1998;110:385–390.

Parker DC, Folpe AL, Bell J, et al. Potential utility of uroplakin III, thrombomodulin, high molecular weight cytokeratin, and cytokeratin 20 in noninvasive, invasive, and metastatic urothelial (transitional cell) carcinomas. *Am J Surg Pathol.* 2003;27:1–10.

Schellhammer PF, Bean MA, Whitmore WF, Jr. Prostatic involvement by transitional cell carcinoma: pathogenesis, patterns and prognosis. *J Urol.* 1977;118:399–403.

Shen SS, Lerner SP, Muezzinoglu B, et al. Prostatic involvement by transitional cell carcinoma in patients with bladder cancer and its prognostic significance. *Hum Pathol.* 2006;37:726–734.

Varma M, Morgan M, Amin MB, et al. High molecular weight cytokeratin antibody (clone 34betaE12): a sensitive marker for differentiation of high-grade invasive urothelial carcinoma from prostate cancer. *Histopathology.* 2003;42:167–172.

1.44

Osunkoya AO, Netto GJ, Epstein JI. Colorectal adenocarcinoma involving the prostate: report of 9 cases. *Hum Pathol.* 2007;38:1836–1841.

Owens CL, Epstein JI, Netto GJ. Distinguishing prostatic from colorectal adenocarcinoma on biopsy samples: the role of morphology and immunohistochemistry. *Arch Pathol Lab Med.* 2007;131:599–603.

Ro JY, el-Naggar A, Ayala AG, et al. Signet-ring-cell carcinoma of the prostate. Electron-microscopic and immunohistochemical studies of eight cases. *Am J Surg Pathol.* 1988;12:453–460.

1.45

Epstein JI, Lieberman PH. Mucinous adenocarcinoma of the prostate gland. *Am J Surg Pathol.* 1985;9:299–308.

Lane BR, Magi-Galluzzi C, Reuther AM, et al. Mucinous adenocarcinoma of the prostate does not confer poor prognosis. *Urology.* 2006;68:825–830.

Osunkoya AO, Epstein JI. Primary mucin-producing urothelial-type adenocarcinoma of prostate: report of 15 cases. *Am J Surg Pathol.* 2007;31:1323–1329.

Osunkoya AO, Nielsen ME, Epstein JI. Prognosis of mucinous adenocarcinoma of the prostate treated by radical prostatectomy: A study of 47 cases. *Am J Surg Pathol.* 2008;32:468–472.

Ro JY, Grignon DJ, Ayala AG, et al. Mucinous adenocarcinoma of the prostate: histochemical and immunohistochemical studies. *Hum Pathol.* 1990;21:593–600.

Tran KP, Epstein JI. Mucinous adenocarcinoma of urinary bladder type arising from the prostatic urethra. Distinction from mucinous adenocarcinoma of the prostate. *Am J Surg Pathol.* 1996;20:1346–1350.

1.46

Ali TZ, Epstein JI. Basal cell carcinoma of the prostate: a clinicopathologic study of 29 cases. *Am J Surg Pathol.* 2007;31: 697–705.

Osunkoya AO, Hansel DE, Sun X, et al. Aberrant diffuse expression of p63 in adenocarcinoma of the prostate on needle biopsy and radical prostatectomy: report of 21 cases. *Am J Surg Pathol.* 2008;32:461–467.

1.47

Ro JY, Tetu B, Ayala AG, et al. Small cell carcinoma of the prostate. II. Immunohistochemical and electron microscopic studies of 18 cases. *Cancer.* 1987;59:977–982.

Tetu B, Ro JY, Ayala AG, et al. Small cell carcinoma of the prostate. Part I. A clinicopathologic study of 20 cases. *Cancer.* 1987;59:1803–1809.

Yao JL, Madeb R, Bourne P, et al. Small cell carcinoma of the prostate: an immunohistochemical study. *Am J Surg Pathol.* 2006;30:705–712.

Wang W, Epstein JI. Small cell carcinoma of the prostate. A morphologic and immunohistochemical study of 95 cases. *Am J Surg Pathol.* 2008;32:65–71.

1.48

Tamas EF, Epstein JI. Prognostic significance of paneth cell-like neuroendocrine differentiation in adenocarcinoma of the prostate. *Am J Surg Pathol.* 2006;30:980–985.

1.49

Dundore PA, Cheville JC, Nascimento AG, et al. Carcinosarcoma of the prostate. Report of 21 cases. *Cancer.* 1995;76:1035–1042.

Hansel DE, Epstein JI. Sarcomatoid carcinoma of the prostate: a study of 42 cases. *Am J Surg Pathol.* 2006;30:1316–1321.

1.50–1.51

Bostwick DG, Hossain D, Qian J, et al. Phyllodes tumor of the prostate: long-term follow-up study of 23 cases. *J Urol.* 2004;172:894–899.

Gaudin PB, Rosai J, Epstein JI. Sarcomas and related proliferative lesions of specialized prostatic stroma: a clinicopathologic study of 22 cases. *Am J Surg Pathol.* 1998;22:148–162.

Herawi M, Epstein JI. Specialized stromal tumors of the prostate: a clinicopathologic study of 50 cases. *Am J Surg Pathol.* 2006;30:694–704.

Herawi M, Epstein JI. Solitary fibrous tumor on needle biopsy and transurethral resection of the prostate: a clinicopathologic study of 13 cases. *Am J Surg Pathol.* 2007;31:870–876.

Nagar M, Epstein JI. Epithelial proliferations in prostatic stromal tumors of uncertain malignant potential (STUMP). *Am J Surg Pathol.* 2011;35:898–903.

1.52

Hansel DE, Herawi M, Montgomery E, et al. Spindle cell lesions of the adult prostate. *Mod Pathol.* 2007;20:148–158.

Herawi M, Montgomery EA, Epstein JI. Gastrointestinal stromal tumors (GISTs) on prostate needle biopsy: a clinicopathologic study of 8 cases. *Am J Surg Pathol.* 2006;30:1389–1395.

1.53–1.54

Epstein JI. *The Gleason Grading System: A Complete Guide for Pathologists and Clinicians.* Philadelphia, PA: Lippincott Williams & Wilkins; 2013.

1.55

Magi-Galluzzi C, Evans AJ, Delahunt B, et al.; ISUP Prostate Cancer Group. International society of urological pathology (ISUP) consensus conference on handling and staging of radical prostatectomy specimens. working group 3: Extraprostatic extension, lymphovascular invasion and locally advanced disease. *Mod Pathol.* 2011;24:26–38.

Evans AJ, Henry PC, Van der Kwast TH, et al. Interobserver variability between expert urologic pathologists for extraprostatic extension and surgical margin status in radical prostatectomy specimens. *Am J Surg Pathol.* 2008;32:1503–1512.

1.56

Albores-Saavedra J, Vuitch F, Delgado R, et al. Sinus histiocytosis of pelvic lymph nodes after hip replacement. A histiocytic proliferation induced by cobalt-chromium and titanium. *Am J Surg Pathol.* 1994;18:83–90.

Bjornsson BL, Truong LD, Cartwright J Jr, et al. Pelvic lymph node histiocytosis mimicking metastatic prostatic adenocarcinoma: association with hip prostheses. *J Urol.* 1995;154: 470–473.

2

Kidney

	Wilms Tumor (WT)	Clear Cell Sarcoma
Age	Peak 2–5 y. 90% by 6 y	Rare < 6 months old. Most occur in 2nd and 3rd year of life
Location	Renal cortex or medulla. Typically unifocal. Bilateral (5%) and multifocal (7%), typically in syndromic forms	Renal medulla. Always unifocal, no bilateral occurrence
Symptoms	Pain, hematuria, or hypertension	Due to large abdominal mass. In advanced cases, symptoms resulting from associated widespread bone and brain metastasis
Signs	Abdominal mass. Rarely, acquired von Willebrand factor; renin or erythropoietin is secreted leading to coagulopathy or polycythemia	Large abdominal mass (up to 11 cm) on imaging. More frequently cystic
Etiology	Unknown in majority of cases. Association with dysmorphic syndromes such as WAGR (WT, aniridia, and genital anomalies) and Denys-Drash (pseudohermaphroditism, glomerulopathy, and WT)	Unknown. No risk association with any of the dysmorphic syndromes associated with WT
Gross and Histology	1. Variable size. Sharply defined, rounded, multinodular mass. Can see botryoid intrapelvic growth, involvement of the renal vein, and precursor nephrogenic rests (NRs) 2. Triphasic histology (blastemal, stromal, and epithelial), although monophasic or biphasic examples are not infrequent *(Figs. 2.1.1 and 2.1.2)*. Blastemal predominant can be confused with clear cell sarcoma 3. Blastemal component with a typical "small blue cell" appearance with primitive cells displaying molded round-oval nuclei with coarse chromatin and a high N/C ratio 4. Frequent mitotic figures including atypical forms *(Fig. 2.1.3)*. 5. Blastemal with diffuse or nested patterns, the latter serpentine or nodular *(Fig. 2.1.4)* 6. Epithelial component includes tubule and glomeruloid structures. Mucinous or squamous differentiation can be seen 7. The stromal component encompasses myxoid, myofibroblastic, smooth and skeletal muscle, lipid, cartilage, osseous, and neuroglial elements	1. Generally larger in size. Irregular mass with mucoid homogenous cut surface. Lack botryoid intrapelvic growth, involvement of the renal vein, or precursor NRs 2. Monomorphous nests and cords of spindle-to-epithelioid cells loosely set in an extracellular myxoid material. May have intracytoplasmic vacuoles with mucopolysaccharides *(Figs. 2.1.5 and 2.1.6)* 3. Nuclei are monotonous with dispersed "empty" chromatin pattern lacking the molding and overlapping pattern seen in WT *(Fig. 2.1.7)* 4. Mitotic activity is deceptively low. 5. Nests separated by arborizing fibrovascular septa ranging from a thin chicken-wire network to thickened sheaths of fibroblastic cells encircling capillaries. Epithelioid variant may have condensation of nested cells with "cohesive" ribbons, tubular, or rosette-like patterns around the vascular network *(Figs. 2.1.8 and 2.1.9)* 6. Subtle infiltrative peripheral border of clear cell sarcoma of the kidney (CCSK) can entrap native tubules that may undergo "embryonal" metaplastic change mimicking a biphasic tumor *(Fig. 2.1.10)* 7. Spindle cell variant lacks heterologous elements. Other variants include sclerosing hyalinized, cystic, pericytomatous, and pleomorphic patterns

	Wilms Tumor (WT)	**Clear Cell Sarcoma**
Special studies	• WT1 positive in the blastemal and epithelial component but not in stromal elements • Epithelial component keratin AE1/AE3 positive. Stromal component expresses typical markers according to the line of differentiation	• Lacks immunoexpression of WT1 • Negative for keratins AE1/AE3 and CAM5.2
Treatment	Stage dependent. Nephrectomy with chemotherapy with or without radiotherapy. Diffuse anaplasia dictates a more aggressive treatment regimen	Nephrectomy with chemotherapy
Prognosis	Overall survival >90%. Negative prognostic factors include older age, higher stage, and unfavorable histology (anaplasia) with markedly enlarged hyperchromatic nuclei seen on 10× objective and abnormal mitotic figures	First metastases may present over a decade posttreatment. Stage I more favorable outcome. Stage II and III cases account for over 70% of patients with 75% 6-y survival

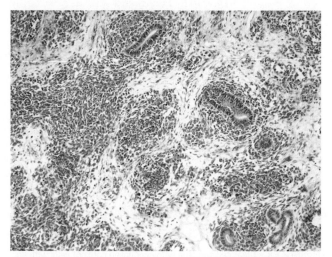

Figure 2.1.1   Wilms tumor displaying triphasic histology (blastemal, stromal, and epithelial).

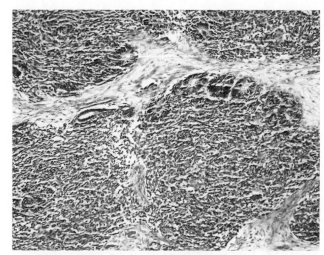

Figure 2.1.2   Wilms tumor with mostly blastemic and focal tubular differentiation at the periphery of the blastema.

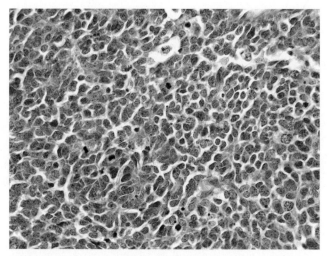

Figure 2.1.3   Wilms tumor with a high nuclear-to-cytoplasmic ratio, coarse chromatin, and numerous mitotic figures.

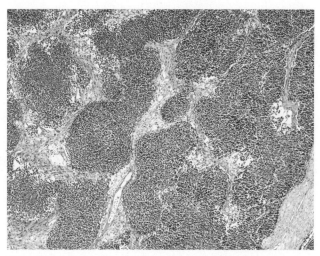

Figure 2.1.4   Wilms tumor with serpentine growth pattern.

2 KIDNEY

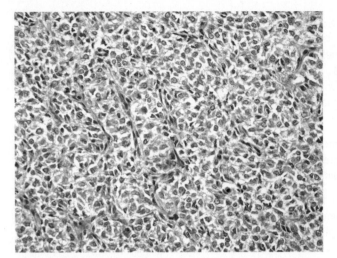

Figure 2.1.5 Classic clear cell sarcoma with nests separated by evenly dispersed small vascular channels.

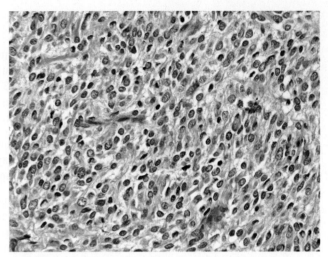

Figure 2.1.6 Clear cell sarcoma with nests separated by small thin-walled vessels.

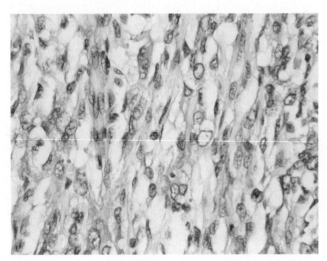

Figure 2.1.7 Clear cell sarcoma with open nuclei and uncommon mitotic figures.

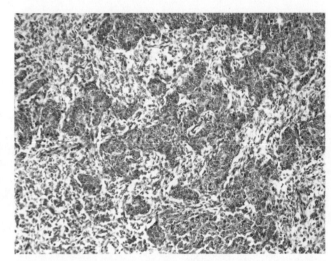

Figure 2.1.8 Clear cell sarcoma with condensed cords of cells with an epithelioid appearance that can mimic Wilms tumor.

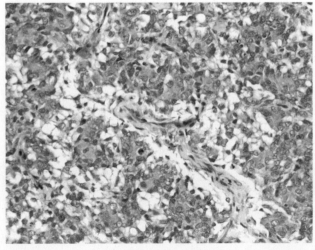

Figure 2.1.9 Clear cell sarcoma with condensed tumor cells in myxoid stroma separated by fine vascular network.

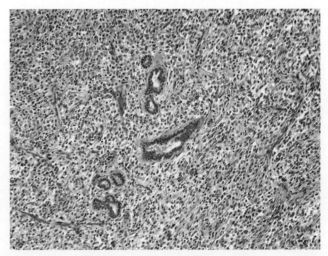

Figure 2.1.10 Clear cell sarcoma with entrapped tubules.

	Wilms Tumor	Metanephric Adenoma
Age	Peak 2–5 y with 90% by 6 y. Adult Wilms tumor usually in 20s–30s but can rarely occur as late as the seventh decade	Usually adults but may occur as early as the first decade of life
Location	Renal cortex or medulla; unifocal in 90% of cases. Bilateral and multifocal in 5% and 7% of cases, respectively, typically in syndromic forms	Renal cortex. Well circumscribed. Very rarely multifocal and no bilateral occurrence
Symptoms	Pain, hematuria, or hypertension	Nonspecific. Pain, hematuria. Polycythemia in 12% of patients
Signs	See Section 2.1	Abdominal mass, incidentally detected on imaging
Etiology	See Section 2.1	Unknown. No association with dysmorphic syndromes associated with WT
Gross and Histology	1. Variable size. Sharply defined rounded multinodular mass. Can see botryoid intrapelvic growth, involvement of the renal vein, and precursor nephrogenic rests (NRs) 2. Has a "blue" appearance at scanning magnification due to cell's scant cytoplasm 3. Typically displays triphasic histology (blastemal, stromal, and epithelial) although monophasic or biphasic examples are not infrequent. Epithelial WT most likely to be confused with metanephric adenoma 4. Attempts to recapitulate epithelial nephrogenesis with tubules and glomeruloid structures 5. High N/C ratio. Molded round-oval nuclei with coarse chromatin and a high N/C ratio *(Figs. 2.2.1 and 2.2.2)*. Focally, can have tubules lined by similar bland cells seen in metanephric adenoma. Some cases with nuclear anaplasia (see Section 2.3) 6. Frequent mitotic figures 7. Can have prominent calcifications and cystic change 8. Stromal component encompasses myxoid, myofibroblastic, smooth and skeletal muscle, lipid, cartilage, osseous, and neuroglial elements	1. Variable in size (< 1–20 cm). Well-circumscribed mass with a solid cut surface. Occasional hemorrhage, calcification, and cystic 2. Has a "blue" appearance at scanning magnification due to cell's scant cytoplasm *(Fig. 2.2.3)* 3. Lacks a triphasic appearance. Epithelial component and solid areas could mimic blastemal areas *(Figs. 2.2.4 and 2.2.5)* 4. Composed of tubules, glomeruloid, and aborted papillary structures. Most cases are tubular but uncommonly mostly papillary *(Fig. 2.2.6)* 5. High N/C ratio. Small bland round-to-oval nuclei that may overlap and contain grooves. Nucleoli are not discernible 6. Mitotic figures are rare 7. Can have prominent calcifications and cystic change *(Fig. 2.2.7)* 8. Stromal component is often myxoid and lacks heterologous components *(Fig. 2.2.8)*
Special studies	Epithelial component positive for keratins AE1/AE3 and CAM5.2 and WT1	Not helpful in this differential as identical to WT

	Wilms Tumor	**Metanephric Adenoma**
Treatment	Stage dependent. Nephrectomy with chemotherapy with or without radiotherapy. Anaplastic Wilms tumor treated with a more aggressive treatment regimen	Partial nephrectomy
Prognosis	Overall survival exceeding 90%. (see Section 2.1)	Benign

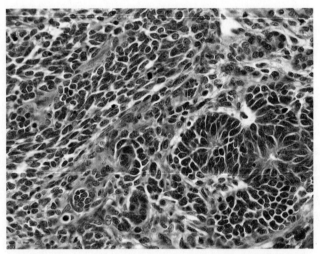

Figure 2.2.1   Wilms tumor with tubules and blastema. The blastema has a high mitotic rate. The tubules are lined by overlapping nuclei with a high N/C ratio.

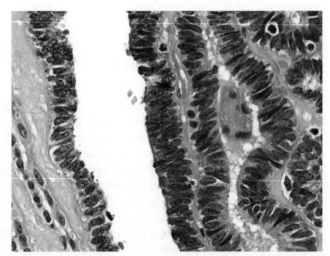

Figure 2.2.2   Wilms tumor with tubules having atypical elongated nuclei with an overlapping and high N/C ratio.

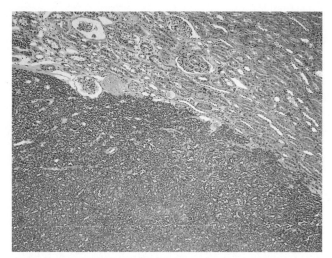

Figure 2.2.3   Metanephric adenoma showing well-circumscribed border and "blue," low-power appearance.

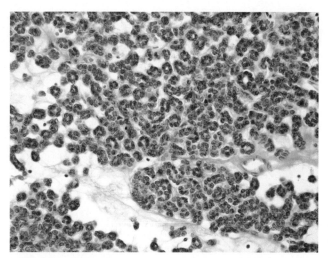

Figure 2.2.4   Metanephric adenoma composed of small tubules in a myxoid background.

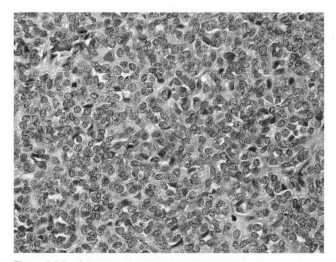

Figure 2.2.5   Solid area of metanephric adenoma that is composed of uniform small nuclei without mitoses.

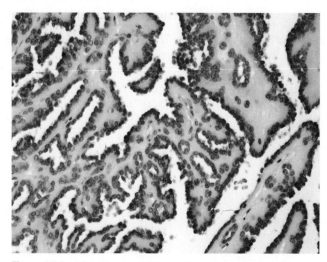

Figure 2.2.6   Metanephric adenoma with papillary morphology.

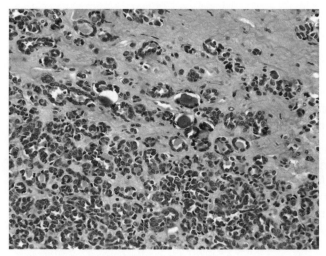

Figure 2.2.7   Metanephric adenoma with calcifications.

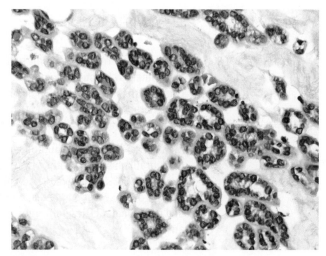

Figure 2.2.8   Metanephric adenoma with myxoid stroma.

	Wilms Tumor (WT) of Favorable Histology	Wilms Tumor of Unfavorable Histology (Anaplastic WT)
Age	Peak 2–5 y. 90% by 6 y	Never in 1st year of life. Rare in 2nd year with subsequent increase in incidence. 10% of WT after 5 y of age anaplastic WT
Location	See Section 2.1	Same as WT with favorable histology
Symptoms	See Section 2.1	Same as WT with favorable histology
Signs	See Section 2.1	Same as WT with favorable histology
Etiology	Unknown in majority of cases. A risk association with several dysmorphic syndromes (see Section 2.1). p53 mutations not present in WT with favorable histology	"Anaplastic nuclear change," the hallmark of unfavorable histology, correlates with p53 mutation
Gross and Histology	1. Typically displays triphasic histology (blastemal, stromal, and epithelial), although monophasic or biphasic examples are not infrequent 2. Lacks "anaplastic nuclear change" *(Figs. 2.3.1 and 2.3.2)*	1. Other than "anaplastic nuclear change," remaining histologic features do not differ than those of WT with favorable histology 2. "Anaplastic nuclear change" is the hallmark of unfavorable histology, defined by (a) markedly enlarged hyperchromatic nuclei seen on 10× objective *(Figs. 2.3.3 and 2.3.4)*; and (b) polyploidy/multipolar mitotic figures *(Fig. 2.3.5)*. Can be segregated into focal anaplasia (FA) and diffuse anaplasia (DA). FA has "anaplastic nuclear change" in discrete 1 or more foci while background tumor cells show no nuclear unrest (features approaching but not satisfying nuclear criteria of anaplasia). DA is defined by diffuse presence of "anaplastic nuclear change" or nuclear unrest in WT with focal nuclear anaplasia
Special studies	• Lacks p53 expression	• p53 immunoaccumulation in areas of nuclear anaplasia *(Fig. 2.3.6)*
Treatment	Stage dependent. Nephrectomy with chemotherapy (dactinomycin, cyclophosphamide, doxorubicin) with or without radiotherapy. The presence of LOH 1p and 16q dictates a more aggressive treatment regimen	Nephrectomy with chemotherapy (dactinomycin, cyclophosphamide, doxorubicin) with or without radiotherapy depending on stage, FA vs. DA, and LOH of chromosomal loci 1p and 16q
Prognosis	Majority have favorable outcome and are of favorable histology with overall survival exceeding 90%. Negative prognostic factors include older age at diagnosis, higher stage, and presence of LOH of chromosomal loci 1p and 16q	Anaplasia thought to be an indicator of resistance to chemotherapy rather than an inherent marker of WT aggressiveness. Stage I WT with only FA has a favorable prognosis. Higher stage, presence of DA, and LOH of chromosomal loci 1p and 16q are negative prognosticators and require a more aggressive treatment regimen

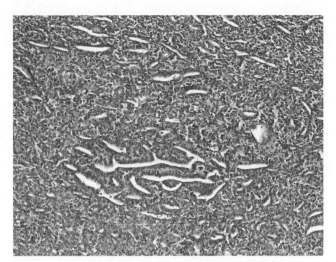

Figure 2.3.1   Wilms tumor with favorable histology. Nuclear pleomorphism is lacking even at a low magnification.

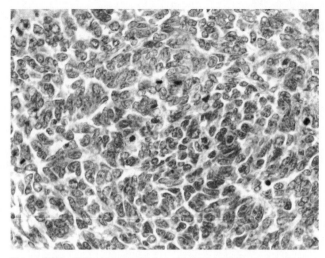

Figure 2.3.2   Wilms tumor with favorable histology. Abnormal mitotic figures are not found. Nuclear pleomorphism is lacking.

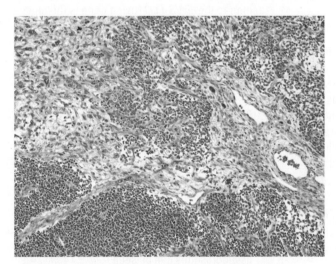

Figure 2.3.3   Wilms tumor with unfavorable histology. "Anaplastic nuclear change" is the hallmark of unfavorable histology; markedly enlarged hyperchromatic nuclei seen on 10× objective.

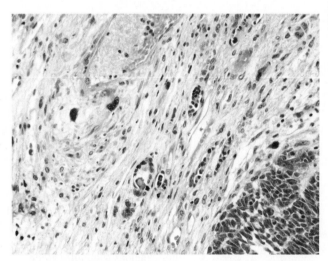

Figure 2.3.4   Wilms tumor with unfavorable histology with markedly enlarged hyperchromatic nuclei (*upper left*) compared to favorable histology in *lower right*.

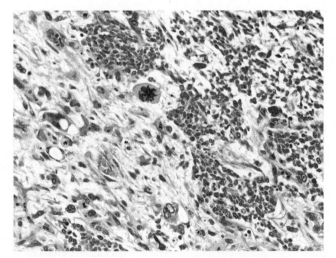

Figure 2.3.5   Wilms tumor with unfavorable histology. Polyploidy/multipolar mitotic figures.

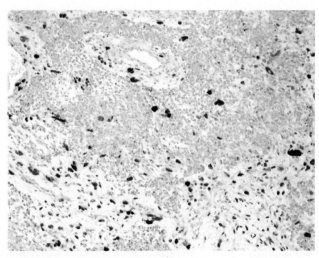

Figure 2.3.6   Wilms tumor with unfavorable histology. p53 positivity in areas of anaplastic nuclear change.

2   KIDNEY

	Wilms Tumor (WT)	Primitive Neuroectodermal Tumor (PNET)
Age	Peak incidence 2–5 y. 90% by 6 y	Adolescent and young adult, average age 23–27 y, but ranges from first to eighth decades
Location	Renal cortex or medulla. Typically unifocal. Bilateral (5%) and multifocal (7%), typically in syndromic forms	Not specific. Large mass replacing the entire kidney
Symptoms	Pain, hematuria, or hypertension	Pain, hematuria. Abdominal mass in 25% of cases. Constitutional symptoms (fever, weight loss)
Signs	See Section 2.1	Abdominal mass, detectable on imaging
Etiology	See Section 2.1	Chromosomal translocation t(11;22)(q24;q12) leading to the *EWS-FLI1* fusion gene is the most frequent underlying genetic alteration
Gross and Histology	1. Variable size. Sharply defined rounded multinodular mass. Can see botryoid intrapelvic growth, involvement of the renal vein, and precursor nephrogenic rests (NRs) 2. Differential diagnosis with PNET limited to WT of monophasic blastemal patterns. Blastema has typical "small blue cell" appearance with primitive cells having molded round-oval nuclei with coarse chromatin and a high N/C ratio *(Fig. 2.4.1)* 3. Frequent mitotic figures including atypical forms 4. Lacks Homer-Wright rosette and perivascular pseudorosettes 5. Diffuse or nested patterns, the latter can be serpentine or nodular	1. Size ranges from 4 to 22 cm (average 12.5 cm). Lobulated cut surface with areas of hemorrhage and necrosis 2. Small blue cell morphology with monotonous polygonal cells with thin rim of cleared cytoplasm. Nuclei are less hyperchromatic than those of WT blastemal cells and more evenly spaced *(Figs. 2.4.2 and 2.4.3)*. Micronucleoli can be encountered 3. Frequent mitotic activity 4. Homer-Wright rosette and perivascular pseudorosettes can be seen *(Figs. 2.4.4 and 2.4.5)* 5. Serpentine or nodular patterns not seen
Special studies	• WT1 positive in blastemal and epithelial components but not in stromal elements • CD99 in a minority of WT, yet not diffuse strong crisp membranous staining • Blastemal component is negative for AE1/AE3, CAM 5.2 • Negative for FLI 1 • Negative for synaptophysin and chromogranin • Lacks *EWS-FLI1* fusion	• WT1 is negative • CD99 positivity in a diffuse distinct crisp membranous pattern *(Fig. 2.4.6)* • AE1/AE3 and CAM5.2 positivity in a minority (20%) • FLI 1 nuclear immunoexpression • Rare positivity for synaptophysin and chromogranin • FISH or RT-PCR detection of t(11;22)(q24;q12) leading to the *EWS-FLI1* fusion gene
Treatment	Stage dependent. Nephrectomy with chemotherapy (dactinomycin, cyclophosphamide, doxorubicin) with or without radiotherapy	Stage dependent. Nephrectomy with an aggressive multidrug chemotherapy regimen
Prognosis	Overall survival >90%. Negative prognostic factors (see Chapters 1 and 3)	Stage dependent. Overall aggressive behavior

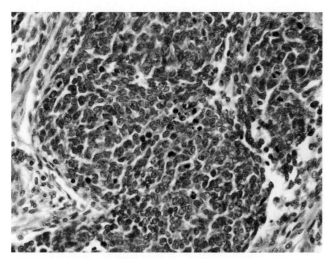

Figure 2.4.1   Wilms tumor with blastema showing hyperchromatic overlapping nuclei.

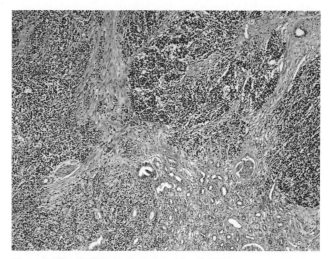

Figure 2.4.2   PNET/Ewing tumor involving the kidney.

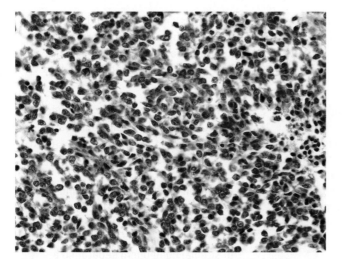

Figure 2.4.3   Same case as Figure 2.4.2 with monotonous polygonal cells with thin rim of cleared cytoplasm. Less hyperchromatic nuclei than WT blastemal cells and more evenly spaced.

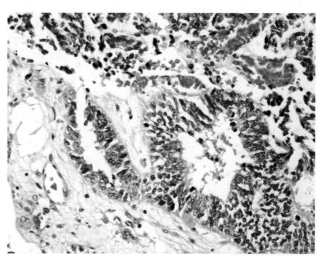

Figure 2.4.4   Renal PNET/Ewing tumors arranged in Homer-Wright rosettes.

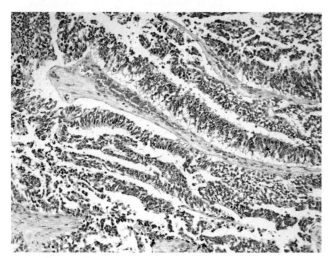

Figure 2.4.5   Same case as Figure 2.4.4 with perivascular pseudorosettes.

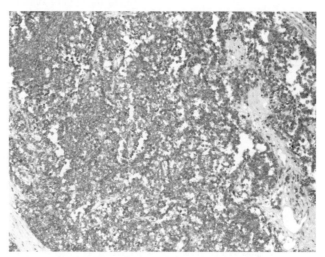

Figure 2.4.6   Same case as Figures 2.4.4 and 2.4.5 with diffuse membranous CD99 positivity.

	Wilms Tumor (WT)	Nephrogenic Rest (NR)
Age	Peak incidence 2–5 y. 90% by 6 y	Same age as WT. 1% incidence in infant autopsy series and 4% incidence in dysplastic kidneys
Location	Renal cortex or medulla. Unifocal in 90% of cases. Occasionally bilateral (5%) and multifocal (7%), typically in syndromic forms	Renal cortex or medulla. Perilobar rests (PLNR) are more likely unifocal compared to intralobar rests (ILNR). Bilateral and multifocal (nephroblastomatosis) are typically found in syndromic forms
Symptoms	See Section 2.1	None specific to NR
Signs	See Section 2.1	None specific to NR
Etiology	Unknown in majority of cases. A risk association with several dysmorphic syndromes (see Section 2.1)	Precursor lesions for WT found in up to 25% of nephrectomies performed for unilateral WT and up to 80% of bilateral WT *(Fig. 2.5.2)*. Same etiology as WT (see Section 2.1)
Gross and Histology	1. Variable size. Sharply defined rounded multinodular mass. Can see botryoid intrapelvic growth, involvement of the renal vein, and precursor NRs 2. Often triphasic histology (blastemal, stromal, and epithelial) although monophasic or biphasic examples are not infrequent 3. Blastemal and epithelial component with primitive cells displaying molded round-oval nuclei with coarse chromatin and a high N/C ratio 4. Frequent mitotic figures including atypical forms 5. Blastema with serpentine or nodular appearance *(Fig. 2.5.1)*	1. Smaller lesions, many only microscopic. PLNR peripheral sharply demarcated nodules. ILNR randomly interspersed in renal cortex and medulla with irregular borders 2. PLNR composed of blastemal and tubular embryonal structures with little stromal component *(Figs. 2.5.3 and 2.5.4)*. ILNR composed predominantly of stromal component separating a lesser amount of blastemal and tubular elements *(Figs. 2.5.5 and 2.5.6)* 3. Blastemal component identical to WT. "Sclerosing/involuting" NR composed of tubules lined by a single layer of basophilic epithelium encased by collagenous stroma. "Hyperplastic" NR has diffuse or focal proliferation without distorting the original contour of the NR 4. Mitotic figures present with a lower mitotic rate in sclerosing/involuting NR 5. Lacks serpentine or nodular pattern
Special studies	WT1 positivity in the blastemal and epithelial component but not in stromal elements. Epithelial component also expresses AE1/AE3 and CAM 5.2	Same as WT

	Wilms Tumor (WT)	**Nephrogenic Rest (NR)**
Treatment	Stage dependent (see Section 2.1)	Usually in nephrectomies done for WT, the latter dictating therapy. With diffuse hyperplastic nephroblastomatosis, chemotherapy reduces the precursor burden in an attempt to decrease the risk of development of WT and preserve function followed by close imaging surveillance
Prognosis	See Section 2.1	Marker for metachronous or synchronous multifocal WT in both the kidneys. Diffuse hyperplastic nephroblastomatosis increases the risk of anaplastic WT

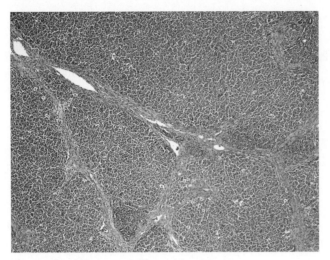

Figure 2.5.1   Wilms tumor with a nodular pattern.

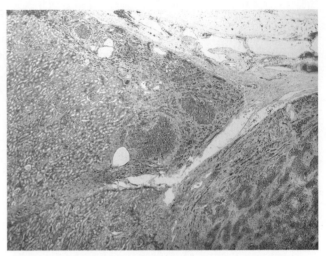

Figure 2.5.2   Nephrogenic rest (*center and upper left*) adjacent to serpentine pattern of Wilms tumor (*lower right*).

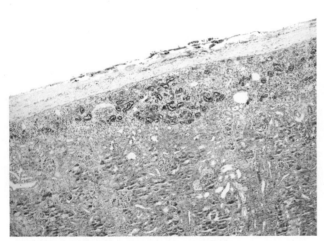

Figure 2.5.3   Perilobar sclerosing nephrogenic rest.

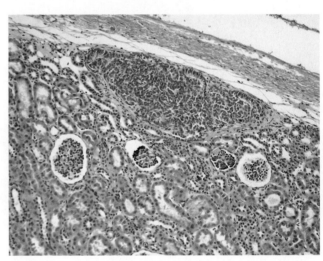

Figure 2.5.4   Perilobar nephrogenic rest. (Courtesy of Dr. Peter Argani.)

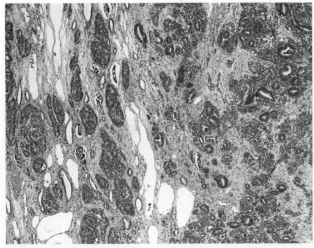

Figure 2.5.5   Intralobar rest admixed with normal kidney (*left*) adjacent to solid Wilms tumor (*right*). (Courtesy of Dr. Peter Argani.)

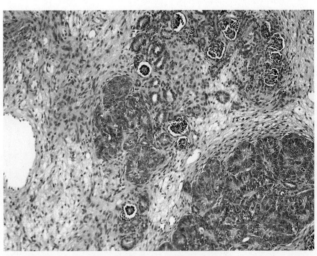

Figure 2.5.6   Same case as Figure 2.5.5 with intralobar rest and associated stroma admixed with a normal kidney.

	Rhabdoid Tumor of the Kidney	Renal Tumors with Rhabdoid Features
Age	Peak age at diagnosis 1 y. 80% by 2 y, never over 5 y	Depends on the underlying tumor
Location	Renal cortex or medulla. Unifocal	Depends on the underlying tumor
Symptoms	Hematuria and symptoms related to wide metastatic disease	Depends on the underlying tumor
Signs	Abdominal mass, detectable on imaging. Posterior fossa brain mass with PNET-like morphology in 15% of patients	Depends on the underlying tumor
Etiology	Unknown. Biallelic inactivation of the tumor suppressor gene *hSNF5/INI1* on long arm of chromosome 22 is frequently detected. Germ line *hSNF5/INI1* mutation in patients with rhabdoid tumor of the kidney and PNET-like tumors in the brain	Rhabdoid cells can be seen in WT, rhabdomyosarcoma, leiomyosarcoma, mesoblastic nephroma, medullary carcinoma, collecting duct carcinoma, and urothelial carcinoma, metastatic melanoma, metastatic hepatocellular carcinoma
Gross and Histology	1. Large unencapsulated irregular mass with extensive necrosis and hemorrhage 2. Discohesive sheets of undifferentiated polygonal large-sized cells with abundant cytoplasm and eccentric nuclei ("rhabdoid") *(Fig. 2.6.1)*. Typically, large nuclei with vesicular chromatin and large cherry-red nucleoli *(Figs. 2.6.2 and 2.6.3)*. Cord-like, pseudoglandular, alveolar, and peritheliomatous spindle cell patterns can be seen. Stroma is occasionally hyalinized and myxoid/chondroid. Striations and "tadpole" cells of rhabdomyosarcoma not seen. Extensive vascular invasion and infiltration of surrounding tissue are common	1. Gross depends on the underlying neoplasm 2. Lack of true myogenic differentiation helps differentiates rhabdoid tumor from WT with heterologous stroma and primary rhabdomyosarcoma *(Figs. 2.6.4 and 2.6.5)*. Rhabdoid tumor with large vesicular nuclei with cherry-red nucleoli, association with cranial midline mass, disseminated metastatic disease helps rule out mesoblastic nephroma. Older age, sickle cell trait (medullary carcinoma), and tubular features (collecting duct carcinoma) help rule out rhabdoid tumor of the kidney (Fig. 2.6.6)

	Rhabdoid Tumor of the Kidney	Renal Tumors with Rhabdoid Features
Special studies	• Nuclear loss of *hSNF5/INI1* expression. Immunoexpression is complicated by nonspecific entrapment of antibodies in the cytoplasmic hyaline inclusion of intermediate filaments. The latter should be remembered when myoglobin, desmin, and actin staining is encountered. Nuclear staining for myogenin is not present. Cytokeratins, EMA, and vimentin positivity is seen	• Lack of true myogenic differentiation immunohistochemically helps rule out WT with heterologous stroma and primary rhabdomyosarcoma. Loss of INI1 nuclear expression, positive AE1/AE3, and EMA helps rule out mesoblastic nephroma. Lack of S100, HMB-45, Melan A, miTF, and SOX2 helps rule out metastatic melanoma. HEP-PAR1 and canalicular CD10 and polyclonal CEA help establish diagnosis of secondary involvement of the kidney by hepatocellular carcinoma. Differential with collecting duct carcinoma and medullary carcinoma cannot be made based on IHC given the similar profile including loss of INI1 expression
Treatment	Nephrectomy with chemotherapy	Depends on the underlying tumor
Prognosis	Dismal, 80% of patients die of disease by 2 y from diagnosis	Depends on the underlying tumor

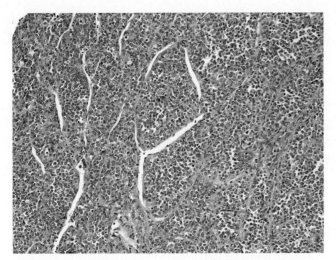

Figure 2.6.1   Rhabdoid tumor of the kidney with discohesive sheets of undifferentiated tumor.

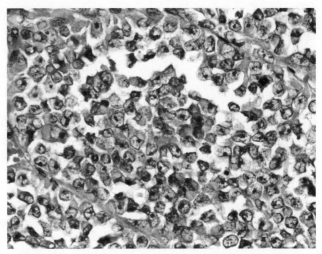

Figure 2.6.2   Same case as Figure 2.6.1 with polygonal, large-sized cells with abundant cytoplasm and eccentric nuclei containing prominent nucleoli.

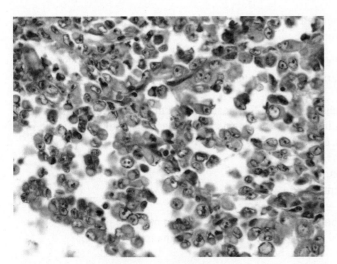

Figure 2.6.3   Rhabdoid tumor of the kidney.

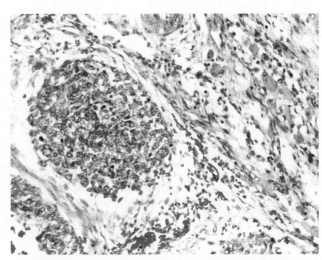

Figure 2.6.4   Wilms tumor with blastema and rhabdoid cells.

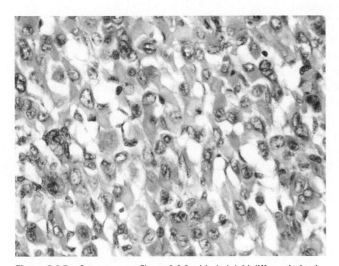

Figure 2.6.5   Same case as Figure 2.6.3 with rhabdoid differentiation in stromal component.

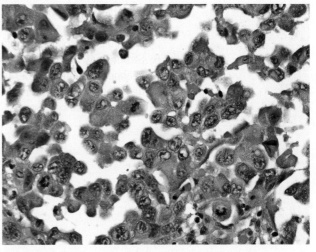

Figure 2.6.6   Medullary carcinoma of the kidney with rhabdoid features.

	Mesoblastic Nephroma	Clear Cell Sarcoma
Age	Can be seen as young as newborns (congenital). Median age at diagnosis is 2 mo. 90% of cases occur in first year	Rare before 6 mo of age. Most cases occur in 2nd and 3rd year of life with mean age at diagnosis at 36 mo
Location	Unifocal, centered in hilar region	Renal medulla. Always unifocal, no bilateral occurrence
Symptoms	Abdominal mass. Polyhydramnios, premature delivery	In advanced cases, symptoms related to associated widespread bone and brain metastasis
Signs	Abdominal mass detected *in utero* during fetal ultrasound. Hypercalcemia due to prostaglandin E production	Large abdominal mass (up to 11 cm), detectable on imaging
Etiology	Unknown. Occasional cases associated with Beckwith-Wiedemann syndrome	Unknown
Gross and Histology	1. 0.8- to 14-cm well-demarcated solid mass. Necrosis, hemorrhage, and cystic change 2. Classic and cellular types: Fascicles of monomorphous spindle fibroblastic- and myofibroblastic-type cells. Classic mesoblastic nephroma reminiscent of infantile fibromatosis. Cellular mesoblastic nephroma same entity as infantile renal fibrosarcoma 3. Bands of spindle cells extend beyond gross mass into hilar extrarenal and parenchymal tissue *(Fig. 2.7.1)* 4. Bland vesicular nuclei *(Fig. 2.7.2)*. Coarse granular nuclear chromatin pattern and moderate pleomorphism in cellular mesoblastic nephroma *(Fig. 2.7.3)* 5. Variable mitotic activity; usually higher in cellular mesoblastic nephroma 6. Stroma may contain nodules of hyaline cartilage and extramedullary hematopoiesis but not rhabdomyogenic or heterologous elements *(Fig. 2.7.4)*	1. Irregular mass with mucoid homogenous cut surface 2. Classic pattern display monomorphous nests and cords of spindle to epithelioid cells 3. Spindle cells do not typically extend beyond gross mass 4. Nuclei are monotonous with dispersed "empty" chromatin pattern *(Fig. 2.7.5)* 5. Mitotic activity is deceptively low 6. Loose myxoid stroma with an extracellular myxoid material that may falsely appears intracytoplasmic. Arborizing fibrovascular septa (chicken-wire network) *(Fig. 2.7.6)*. No heterologous component

	Mesoblastic Nephroma	Clear Cell Sarcoma
Special studies	• May show scattered positive cells in stroma for desmin and muscle-specific actin • Negative for keratins (AE1/AE3 and CAM5.2), EMA, S100, CD99, and WT1 • The t(12;15) *ETV6-NTRK3* fusion gene in cellular mesoblastic nephroma/infantile fibrosarcoma	• Negative for desmin and muscle-specific actin • Negative for keratins (AE1/AE3 and CAM5.2), EMA, S100, CD99, and WT1 • Lacks the t(12;15) *ETV6-NTRK3* fusion gene
Treatment	Nephrectomy	Nephrectomy with chemotherapy (doxorubicin)
Prognosis	Overall, good prognosis with low incidence of metastasis. Stage and age dependent. Recurrence/metastasis more likely in patients older than 6 mo who tend to present with the cellular type of mesoblastic nephroma	Stage dependent. 6-y survival 75% with doxorubicin. First metastases may present over a decade posttreatment

2 KIDNEY

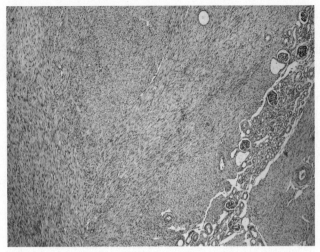

Figure 2.7.1   Mesoblastic nephroma extending into surrounding the kidney.

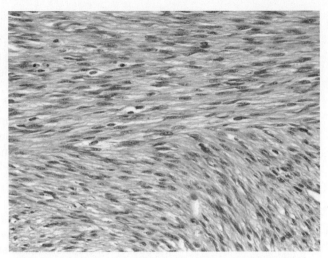

Figure 2.7.2   Same case as Figure 2.7.1 with monomorphous spindle fibroblastic- and myofibroblastic-type cells.

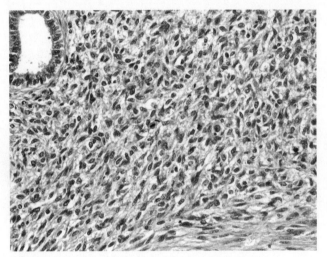

Figure 2.7.3   Cellular mesoblastic nephroma with moderate pleomorphism, greater cellularity, and increased mitotic activity.

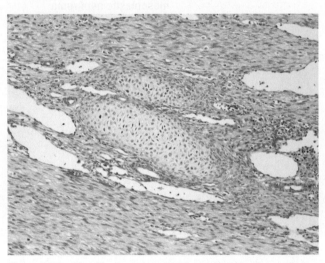

Figure 2.7.4   Mesoblastic nephroma with nodules of hyaline cartilage.

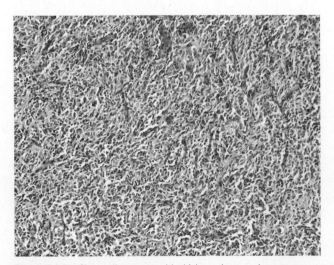

Figure 2.7.5   Clear cell sarcoma with chicken-wire vascular pattern.

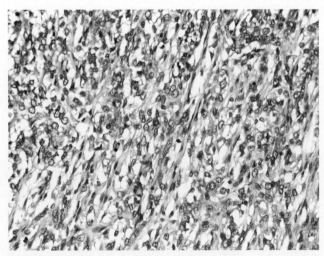

Figure 2.7.6   Same case as Figure 2.7.5 with monomorphous spindle to epithelioid cells loosely set in extracellular myxoid material.

	Atypical Renal Cyst	Cystic Renal Cell Carcinoma
Age	Adults	Adults
Location	Predominantly cortical. Often multifocal	Cortical. Almost always unifocal
Symptoms	Typically asymptomatic	Pain, hematuria, or in current times typically asymptomatic
Signs	Usually incidental on imaging study	Usually incidental on imaging study
Etiology	Unknown. *vHL* gene mutation in renal cyst precursors of RCC does not imply malignant potential. Also be seen with end-stage renal disease and acquired cystic kidney disease with or without carcinoma	An intrinsic component of either papillary or clear cell renal cell carcinoma. Can also result from necrosis, which does not enter into this differential diagnosis
Histology	1. Variable-sized typically unilocular or less commonly multilocular cysts lined by piled up flattened to cuboidal eosinophilic to clear cells *(Figs. 2.8.1 and 2.8.2)*. Nuclei are cytologically bland. Lacks solid clusters/aggregates or nodules of clear cells within the wall of the cyst. Cyst with a single cell layer lined by clear cells not diagnosed as atypical cyst but rather simple cyst with clear cell lining *(Fig. 2.8.3)* 2. Unilocular cyst focally lined by short, simple papillary structures or tufts without cytologic atypia *(Figs. 2.8.4–2.8.6)*	1. Either multilocular or unilocular cyst with some septae containing small aggregates of polygonal epithelial cells with typical features of clear cell renal cell carcinoma. Typically, Fuhrman grade 1 or 2 2. Papillary renal cell carcinoma has much more complex papillary growth characterized by multiple papillary fronds within a cystic space *(Figs. 2.8.7 and 2.8.8)*. Fuhrman grade can vary
Special studies	• Immunohistochemical stains not helpful in this differential diagnosis	• Immunohistochemical stains not helpful in this differential diagnosis
Treatment	Excision	Partial or total nephrectomy
Prognosis	Benign	Varies according to the grade and stage. Often cystic renal cell carcinoma has a better prognosis than solid lesion

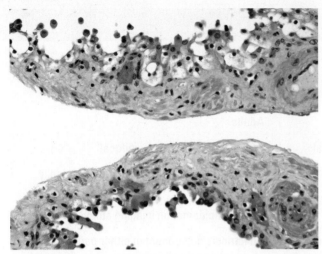

Figure 2.8.1 Atypical cyst with piled up clear cells but lacking clear cells within the wall of the septae.

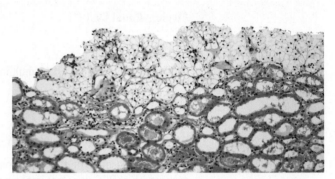

Figure 2.8.2 Atypical cyst piled up clear cells with abortive papillae.

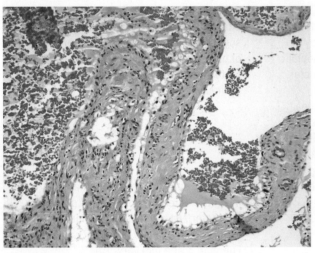

Figure 2.8.3 Simple cyst lined by a single layer of clear cells.

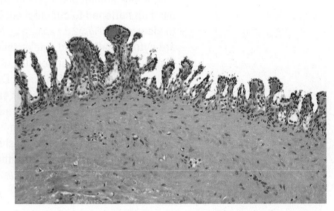

Figure 2.8.4 Atypical cyst with papillary projections lined by cuboidal epithelium with clear cytoplasm.

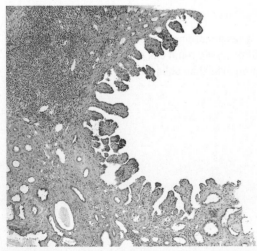

Figure 2.8.5 Unilocular cyst with short papillary projections into the cyst. This lesion is incapable of metastatic behavior and should not be designated as carcinoma.

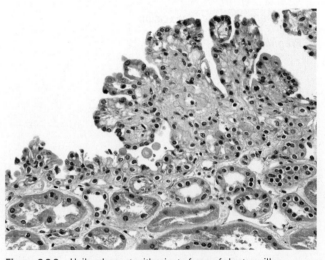

Figure 2.8.6 Unilocular cyst with minute focus of short papillary projections lined by bland cuboidal cells. This lesion is incapable of metastatic behavior and should not be designated as carcinoma.

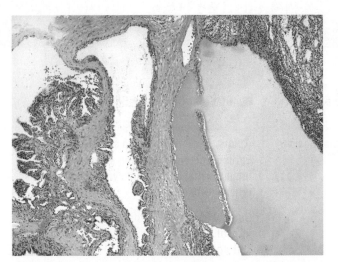

Figure 2.8.7   Cystic papillary RCC with complex papillary nodule (*left*) and nodule of tubules lined by clear cells (*upper right*).

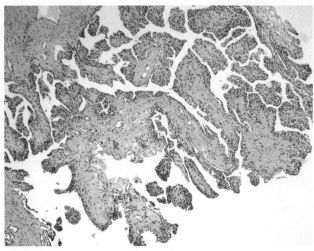

Figure 2.8.8   Cystic papillary RCC.

	Multicystic Renal Cell Neoplasm of Low Malignant Potential	Cystic Clear Cell Renal Cell Carcinoma
Age	Peak sixth decade, mean age at diagnosis 54.3 y (30–80 y)	Adults, peak incidence in sixth decade. Earlier incidence (starting second decade) in familial renal carcinoma syndromes such as vHL syndrome
Location	Almost always unifocal	Usually unifocal. Multifocal and bilateral in <5% of cases, mainly in familial syndromic setting
Symptoms	Pain, hematuria yet most often asymptomatic	Currently, incidentally detected during abdominal and pelvic imaging
Signs	Abdominal mass, many incidentally detectable on imaging studies	Pain, hematuria, flank mass are the classic triad of presentation
Etiology	Unknown. *vHL* gene mutation documented in up to 25% of cases	Somatic *vHL* gene inactivation in two-third of sporadic cases. Inherited germ line *vHL* mutation (3p25-26) in vHL syndrome
Gross and Histology	1. Grossly, multilocular cystic gross appearance, encapsulated, mean size 4.9 cm (1–14 cm) 2. Cysts have smooth lining filled with straw-colored fluid 3. Solid component limited to small-sized nonexpansile yellow-gray areas within septa 4. No necrosis 5. Variable-sized cysts lined by flattened to cuboidal clear cells. Occasional septa contain small aggregates of epithelial cells typical of clear cell RCC (*Figs. 2.9.1–2.9.4*) 6. Optically clear cytoplasm, distinct cell border, and round to ovoid nuclei 7. Fuhrman grade 1 or 2 8. Tumor is organ confined and does not invade vessels	1. Solid and cystic mass with distinct pushing borders. Mean size 7 cm (wide size range) 2. Cysts have smooth lining filled with straw-colored fluid 3. Cystic spaces surrounded by nodular solid areas, typically golden to yellow in color 4. Associated necrosis and hemorrhage are relatively common in larger masses. Calcifications are encountered 5. Variable-sized cysts lined by cuboidal clear cells. Septae and wall of cysts contain sheets of cells with expansile solid appearance (*Figs. 2.9.5–2.9.10*) 6. Cytoplasm ranges from optically clear to granular eosinophilic 7. Nuclear and nucleolar size varies according to tumor 8. Extrarenal extension uncommon in cystic clear cell RCC
Special studies	Not helpful in this differential as identical to cystic clear cell RCC	PAX8, CAIX, RCC, CD10, vimentin, AE1/AE3, positive
Treatment	Excision, partial or total nephrectomy	Partial or radical nephrectomy for localized disease. Targeted therapy is increasingly used for metastatic disease including VEGF receptors, tyrosine kinase receptors, and mTOR inhibitors

	Multicystic Renal Cell Neoplasm of Low Malignant Potential	Cystic Clear Cell Renal Cell Carcinoma
Prognosis	Surgical removal is curative. Cases with >95% cyst formation and rare nonexpansile low-grade clear cell nests in the septae never been shown to exhibit malignant behavior. We diagnose these lesions as "multicystic renal cell neoplasm of low malignant potential" rather than benign given the lack of long-term follow-up data. Also avoids labeling patients as having "carcinoma," which has psychosocial and financial implications. Others use "multicystic renal cell carcinoma" for these lesions. In cases with >20% solid areas, uniformly accepted as cystic carcinomas. Unclear of the malignant potential of 5%–20% solid areas, but the current convention is to diagnose "RCC with cystic change" with a comment that their prognosis is favorable	Primarily stage, grade, and clinical performance status dependent

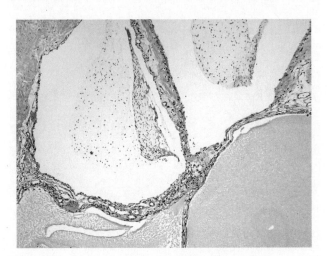

Figure 2.9.1 Multicystic renal cell neoplasm of low malignant potential (LMP) showing variable-sized cysts lined by cuboidal clear cells.

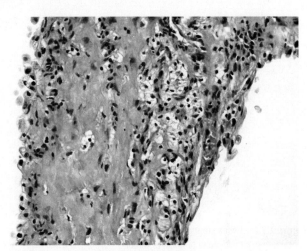

Figure 2.9.2 Same case as Figure 2.9.1 with septae containing rare small nonexpansile aggregates of cells with clear cytoplasm and round-to-ovoid nuclei.

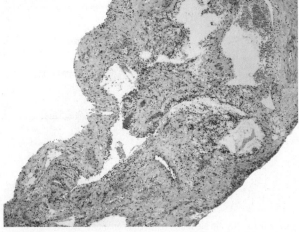

Figure 2.9.3 Multicystic renal cell neoplasm of low malignant potential (LMP) without obvious carcinoma at low magnification.

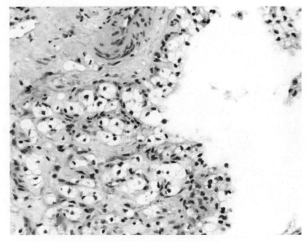

Figure 2.9.4 Same case as Figure 2.9.3 with cytologically benign nonexpansile clear cells within septae.

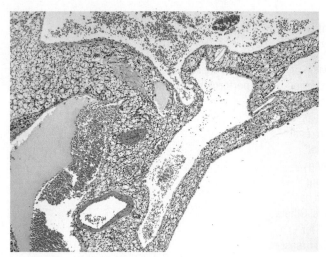

Figure 2.9.5   Cystic clear cell renal cell carcinoma showing variable-sized cysts lined by cuboidal clear cells. Septa contain expansile solid tumor.

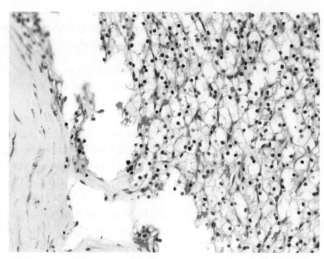

Figure 2.9.6   Same case as Figure 2.9.5 with solid nests of clear cells.

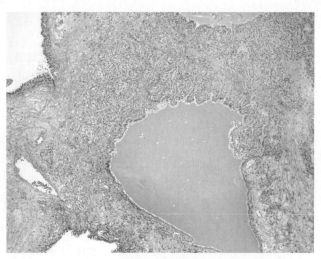

Figure 2.9.7   Cystic clear cell renal cell carcinoma with septae containing expansile solid of nests of tumor.

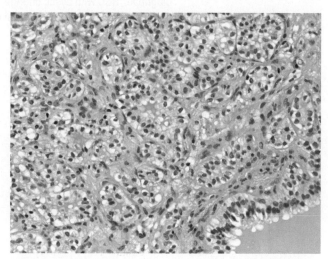

Figure 2.9.8   Same case as Figure 2.9.7 with low-grade renal cell carcinoma within septae.

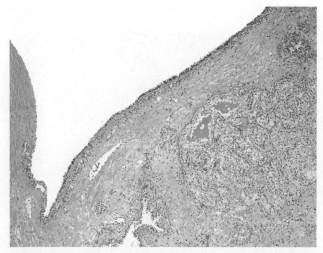

Figure 2.9.9   Cystic clear cell renal cell carcinoma with nodule of carcinoma within wall.

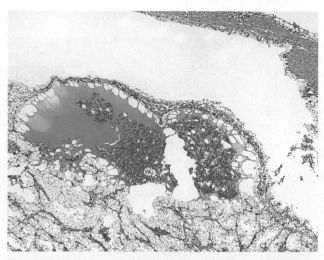

Figure 2.9.10   Cystic clear cell renal cell carcinoma with nodule of carcinoma within wall.

	Solid Papillary Renal Cell Carcinoma	Metanephric Adenoma
Age	Adults, peak incidence in fifth to sixth decades. Earlier incidence (starting second decade) in hereditary renal carcinoma syndromes	Usually adult but may occur as early as the first decade of life
Location	Usually unifocal. Multifocal and bilateral in hereditary papillary RCC	Renal cortex. Almost always unifocal
Symptoms	Currently, incidentally detected during abdominal and pelvic imaging	Usually asymptomatic
Signs	Pain, hematuria, flank mass are the classic triad of presentation	Pain, hematuria. Polycythemia in 12% of patients. Incidentally detected on imaging
Etiology	Trisomy 7, 17, and loss of chromosome Y. Inherited germ line c-met mutation (7q31) is responsible for hereditary papillary RCC syndrome	Unknown
Gross and Histology	1. Grossly encapsulated with distinct pushing borders. Variable size; by definition >0.5 cm. Cystic change, necrosis, and hemorrhage are relatively common in larger masses. Calcifications are encountered 2. Light eosinophilic low-power appearance imparted by a low N/C ratio *(Figs. 2.10.1 and 2.10.2)* 3. Composed of stubby glomeruloid papillary structures admixed with tubular proliferation lined by polygonal epithelial cells with moderate amount of granular/foamy eosinophilic cytoplasm *(Figs. 2.10.3 and 2.10.4)* 4. Foamy histiocytes in fibrovascular cores. Hemosiderin deposition in histiocytes and neoplastic epithelium may be seen 5. Psammomatous calcifications are frequently present 6. Solid papillary RCC are usually of the type 1 papillary RCC morphology with generally low Fuhrman grades (1–2). Higher-grade examples, however, display conspicuous to prominent nucleoli (Fuhrman grades 3–4) 7. Mitotic figures can be seen in higher-grade lesions 8. Extrarenal extension including invasion of the renal sinus and renal vein branches may occur in locally advanced papillary RCC	1. Variable in size (<1–20 cm). Well-circumscribed solid mass. Occasional hemorrhage, calcification, and cystic 2. Low-power "blue/basophilic" appearance due to scant neoplastic cell cytoplasm (high N/C ratio) *(Fig. 2.10.5)* 3. Composed of tightly packed tubules admixed with glomeruloid to aborted papillary structure lined by bland cells *(Figs. 2.10.6–2.10.9)* 4. Occasionally, foamy histiocytes within fibrovascular cores 5. Calcifications can be present 6. Nuclei are small round to oval, may overlap, and contain grooves. Nucleoli not discernible 7. Mitotic figures rare 8. No extrarenal extension

	Solid Papillary Renal Cell Carcinoma	Metanephric Adenoma
Special studies	CK7 positive and WT1 negative	Negative CK7 and positive WT1 *(Fig. 2.10.10)*
Treatment	Partial or radical nephrectomy	Partial nephrectomy
Prognosis	Primarily stage, grade, and clinical performance status dependent	Surgical resection is curative

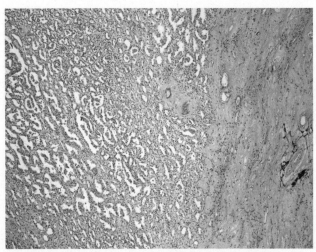

Figure 2.10.1   Solid papillary renal cell carcinoma with paler appearance at low magnification.

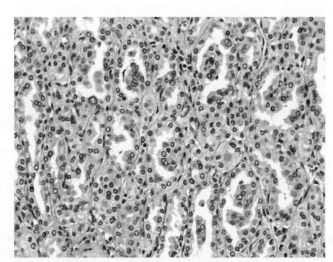

Figure 2.10.2   Same case as Figure 2.10.1 composed of stubby glomeruloid papillary structures lacking well-formed fibrovascular cores admixed with tubular proliferation. Epithelial cells with moderate amount of eosinophilic cytoplasm.

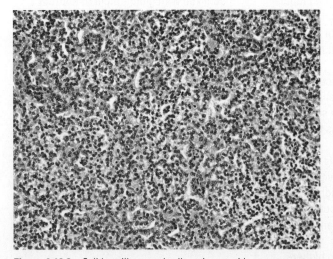

Figure 2.10.3   Solid papillary renal cell carcinoma with a more compact appearance.

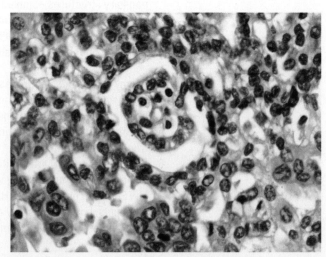

Figure 2.10.4   Same case as Figure 2.10.3 with occasional stubby glomeruloid papillary structures.

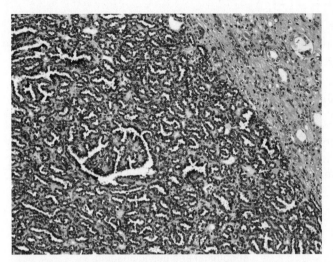

Figure 2.10.5   Metanephric adenoma showing "blue/basophilic" low-power appearance.

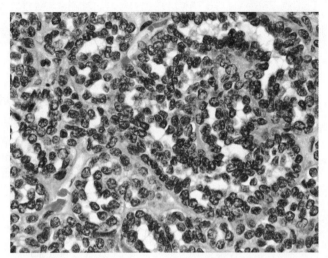

Figure 2.10.6   Same case as Figure 2.10.5 showing a very high N/C ratio with bland cytology.

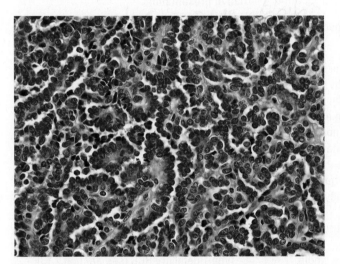

Figure 2.10.7   Metanephric adenoma with papillary formation.

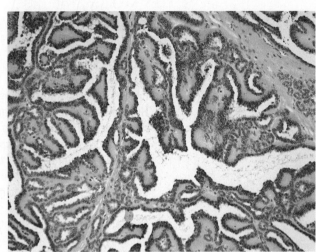

Figure 2.10.8   Metanephric adenoma with papillary formation. Note more typical small tubules in the wall.

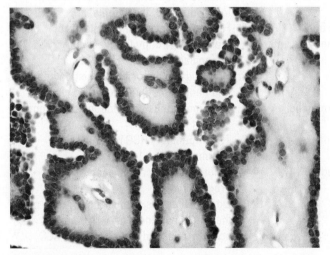

Figure 2.10.9   Same case as Figure 2.10.8 with bland cells with a high N/C ratio in myxoid stroma typical of metanephric adenoma.

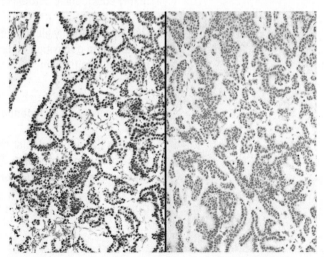

Figure 2.10.10   Metanephric adenoma positive for WT-1 (**left**) and negative for CK7 (**right**). Solid papillary RCC has the opposite immunohistochemical profile.

	Tubulopapillary Hyperplasia/Papillary Adenoma	Papillary Renal Cell Carcinoma
Age	Adults. Incidentally found in nephrectomies performed for papillary RCC (fifth to sixth decades) or end-stage kidney disease	Adults, peak incidence in fifth to sixth decades. Earlier incidence in hereditary renal carcinoma syndromes.
Location	Unifocal or multifocal	Usually unifocal. Multifocal and bilateral in hereditary papillary RCC
Symptoms	None	Currently, incidentally detected during abdominal and pelvic imaging
Signs	None	Pain, hematuria, flank mass are the classic triad of presentation
Etiology	Trisomy 7, 17, and loss of chromosome Y	Trisomy 7, 17, and loss of chromosome Y. (see Section 2.13)
Gross and Histology	1. Tubulopapillary renal hyperplasia/papillary renal adenoma are by definition unencapsulated and <0.5 cm in size. Hyperplasias are smaller than adenomas, nonspherical, and fit into the normal architecture, compared to spherical expansile adenomas *(Figs. 2.11.1 and 2.11.2)* 2. Cystic change, necrosis, and hemorrhage are not seen. Calcifications may be seen 3. Proliferation of tubular structures and/or papillary structures 4. Papillae and tubules lined by a single layer of polygonal epithelial cells with small to moderate amount of granular/foamy eosinophilic cytoplasm *(Figs. 2.11.3–2.11.6)* 5. Usually lack foamy histiocytes and hemosiderin deposition in histiocytes and neoplastic epithelium 6. Psammomatous calcifications may be seen 7. Nuclear size and nucleolar features are those of Fuhrman grades 1–2 8. Mitotic figures not encountered 9. Organ confined by definition	1. Grossly encapsulated with distinct pushing borders. Variable size; by definition if the lesion lacks malignant cytology it is >0.5 cm. Lesions less <0.5 cm are carcinomas only if have malignant cytology or vascular invasion 2. Cystic change, necrosis, and hemorrhage relatively common in larger masses. Calcifications are encountered 3. Composed of admixture of tubular and papillary proliferation 4. Type 1 papillary RCC (see Section 2.13). Papillae and tubules lined by single-layered polygonal epithelial cells with small to moderate amount of granular/foamy eosinophilic cytoplasm 5. Foamy histiocytes and cholesterol clefts may occupy fibrovascular cores of papillary structures *(Fig. 2.11.8)*. Hemosiderin deposition in histiocytes and neoplastic epithelium also typical 6. Psammomatous calcifications frequently present 7. Type 1 papillary RCC is generally Fuhrman grades 1–2 8. Mitotic figures can be seen in higher-grade lesions 9. Extrarenal extension including invasion of the renal sinus and renal vein branches may occur in locally advanced papillary RCC

	Tubulopapillary Hyperplasia/Papillary Adenoma	**Papillary Renal Cell Carcinoma**
Special studies	• Not helpful in this differential	• Not helpful in this differential
Treatment	None. Incidentally found in resection specimens done for other causes	Excision, partial, or radical nephrectomy
Prognosis	Benign	Primarily stage, grade, and clinical performance status dependent

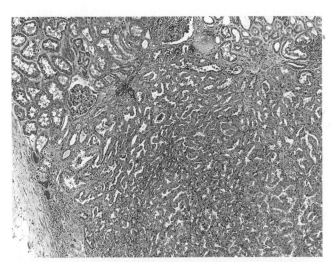

Figure 2.11.1   Papillary renal adenoma. Size of the lesion (<5 mm) differentiates from carcinoma as well as the lack of a capsule and nuclear atypia.

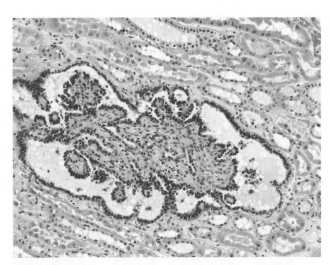

Figure 2.11.2   Tubulopapillary renal hyperplasia with a single dilated tubule containing papillary projections. The lesion is nonexpansile.

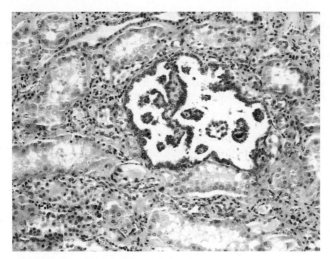

Figure 2.11.3   Tubulopapillary renal hyperplasia.

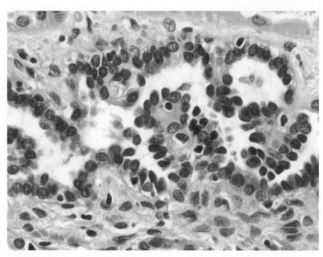

Figure 2.11.4   Tubulopapillary renal hyperplasia with bland cytology.

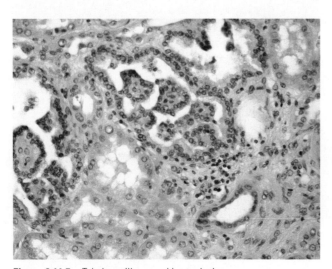

Figure 2.11.5   Tubulopapillary renal hyperplasia.

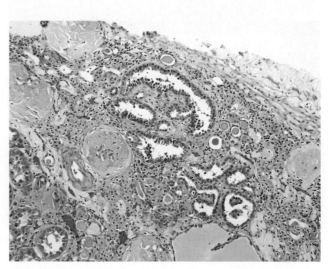

Figure 2.11.6   Tubulopapillary renal hyperplasia with predominant tubule formation.

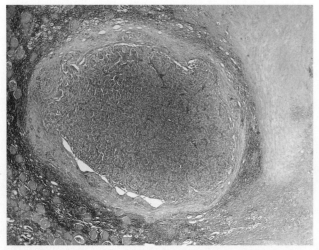

Figure 2.11.7   Expansile nodule (>0.5 cm) of papillary renal cell carcinoma with thickened capsule.

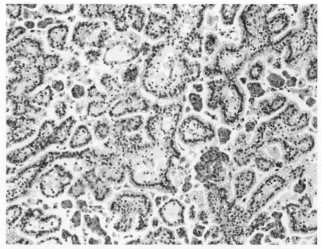

Figure 2.11.8   Complex papillary growth of papillary RCC with foamy histiocytes seen occupying fibrovascular cores.

	Mucinous Tubular Spindle Cell Carcinoma (MTSC)	Papillary Renal Cell Carcinoma
Age	Adults, second to ninth decades, peak incidence in sixth decade. Female predominance	Adults, peak incidence in fifth to sixth decades. Earlier (starting second decade) in hereditary renal carcinoma syndromes
Location	Usually unifocal	Usually unifocal. Multifocal and bilateral in hereditary papillary RCC
Symptoms	Mostly incidentally detected during abdominal and pelvic imaging	Currently, incidentally detected during abdominal and pelvic imaging
Signs	Occasionally pain, hematuria, flank mass	Pain, hematuria, flank mass are the classic triad of presentation
Etiology	Trisomy 7, 17, and loss of chromosome Y are not present. Wide range of chromosomal losses including chromosomes 1, 4, 6, 8, 9, 13, 14, 15, 18, 21, and 22	Trisomy 7, 17, and loss of chromosome Y are common
Gross and Histology	1. Grossly well-circumscribed solid tan mass with distinct borders. Variable size. Cystic change, necrosis, and hemorrhage not typically present 2. Admixture of compressed elongated tubular and spindle cells with light eosinophilic cytoplasm. In some cases, tubular, spindled, or mucinous features may be minor *(Figs. 2.12.1–2.12.4)* 3. Bland epithelial cells with small ovoid-round nuclei and inconspicuous nucleoli *(Fig. 2.12.5)* 4. Mitotic activity is low 5. Variable amount of stromal mucopolysaccharide present 6. Occasionally, a pseudopapillary appearance may result from separation of epithelial cells from surrounding myxoid stroma. Bona fide papillary structures with fibrovascular cores not seen. Variable presence of stromal foamy histiocytes and inflammatory infiltrates *(Fig. 2.12.6)* 7. Hemosiderin deposition not seen in epithelium 8. Psammomatous calcifications absent 9. Extrarenal extension invasion of renal vessels not seen	1. Grossly encapsulated with distinct pushing borders. Variable size. Cystic change, necrosis, and hemorrhage relatively common in larger masses. Calcifications are encountered 2. Composed of admixture of tubular and papillary proliferation. Papillae and tubules lined by a single layer of polygonal epithelial cells with small to moderate amount of granular/foamy eosinophilic cytoplasm *(Fig. 2.12.7)* 3. Nuclear features in type 1 papillary RCC are usually Fuhrman grades 1–2. Type 2 papillary RCC generally Fuhrman grades 3–4. Some papillary RCC can have slightly spindled cells or mucin or elongated tubules mimicking MTSC but have more nuclear atypia *(Figs. 2.12.8–2.12.12)* 4. Variable mitotic activity, increased in higher-grade lesions 5. Stromal mucopolysaccharide typically not present. No intratubular mucin 6. Foamy histiocytes and cholesterol clefts may occupy fibrovascular cores 7. Hemosiderin deposition in histiocytes and neoplastic epithelium typical 8. Psammomatous calcifications frequently present 9. Extrarenal extension including invasion of the renal sinus and renal vein branches may occur in locally advanced papillary RCC

	Mucinous Tubular Spindle Cell Carcinoma (MTSC)	Papillary Renal Cell Carcinoma
Special studies	Not helpful in this differential	Not helpful in this differential
Treatment	Partial or radical nephrectomy	Partial or radical nephrectomy
Prognosis	Excellent with only rare cases with metastases	Primarily stage, grade and, clinical performance status dependent

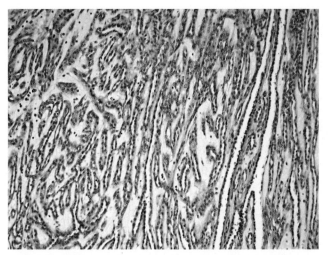

Figure 2.12.1   Classic MTSC with elongated tubules separated by mucin.

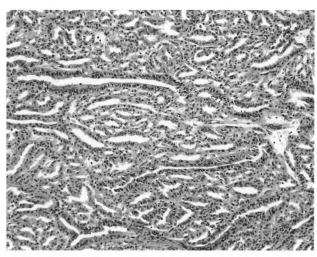

Figure 2.12.2   "Mucin-poor" MTSC with elongated to serpentine tubules.

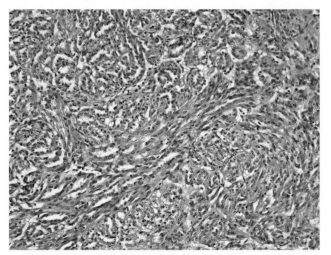

Figure 2.12.3   Transition between tubular and spindled morphology in MTSC.

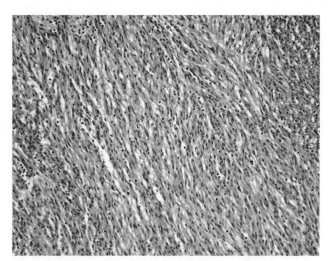

Figure 2.12.4   MTSC exhibiting spindle cell predominance.

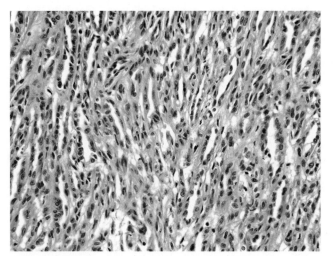

Figure 2.12.5   Transition between tubular and spindled morphology in MTSC. Note bland cytology.

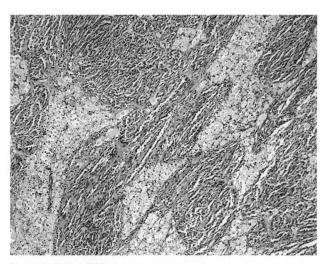

Figure 2.12.6   MTSC with foamy histiocytes in stroma.

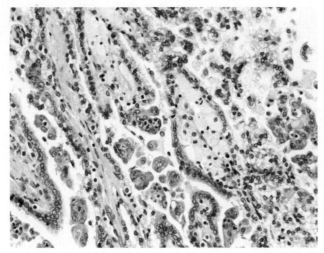

Figure 2.12.7   Papillary renal cell carcinoma with foamy histiocytes occupying fibrovascular cores.

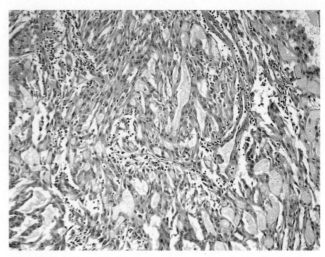

Figure 2.12.8   Unusual RCC with areas of tubules and spindling with mucin.

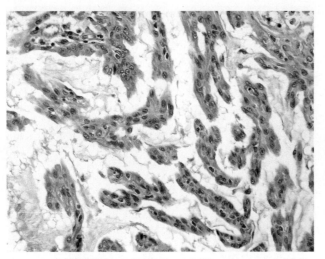

Figure 2.12.9   Same case as Figure 2.12.8 with more cytologic atypia than allowed for MTSC.

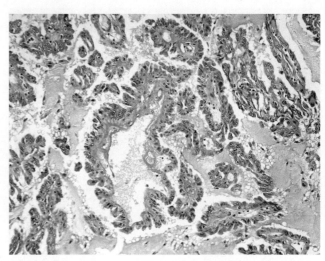

Figure 2.12.10   Same case as Figures 2.12.8 and 2.12.9 with true papillary fronds surrounded by mucin and more atypia than MTSC.

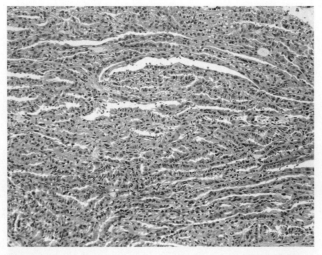

Figure 2.12.11   Elongated tubules in a renal tumor mimicking MTSC.

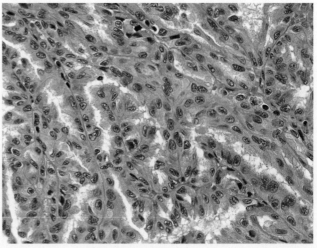

Figure 2.12.12   Same case as Figure 2.12.11 showing too much cytologic atypia and focal papillary fronds, ruling out MTSC.

	Clear Cell Papillary Carcinoma	Clear Cell Renal Cell Carcinoma
Age	Adults, mean age 61 y (33–87 y)	Adults, peak incidence in sixth decade. Earlier incidence in familial renal carcinoma syndromes such as vHL syndrome
Location	Cortical, unifocal. Multifocal in 25% of cases. Multifocality predominantly in the setting of end-stage kidney disease (ESKD)	Usually unifocal. Multifocal and bilateral in <5% of cases. The latter mainly in the familial syndromic setting
Symptoms	25% associated with ESKD, others incidentally found during imaging for unrelated causes	Currently, incidentally detected during abdominal and pelvic imaging
Signs	Abdominal mass	Pain, hematuria, flank mass are the classic triad of presentation
Etiology	Unknown. No evidence of somatic *vHL* gene inactivation or c-met oncogene alteration. Low-level chromosome 7 and 17 polysomy occasionally found	Somatic *vHL* gene inactivation in approximately two-thirds of sporadic cases. Inherited germ line *vHL* mutation (3p25-26) in vHL syndrome
Gross and Histology	1. Mean size 2 cm (0.2–7.5 cm). Cystic change almost always present. Solid areas typically white-pale yellow. Necrosis and hemorrhage not encountered 2. Spectrum of patterns in variable proportions. (a) Branched papillary structures with hypocellular fibrovascular cores lined by cuboidal to flat cells with optically clear cytoplasm project into cystic spaces. (b) Branched acinar structures lined by clear cells with characteristic luminal polarization of some of nuclei. (c) Other areas indistinguishable from clear cell RCC with intraacinar hemorrhage *(Figs. 2.13.1–2.13.8)* 3. Nuclear and nucleolar size almost always low Fuhrman grade (1–2) 4. Extrarenal extension including vascular invasion not seen	1. Mean size 7 cm (wide size range). Solid and cystic mass with distinct pushing borders. Solid areas typically golden to yellow. Associated necrosis and hemorrhage common in larger masses. Calcifications are encountered 2. Polygonal cells with optically clear to granular eosinophilic cytoplasm, arranged in acini, tubules, nests, or solid sheets. Nuclear polarization not a feature *(Figs. 2.13.9 and 2.13.10)*. Papillary structures typically not seen. Intratubular and intraacinar hemorrhage and rich vascular capillary stromal network common 3. Conspicuous to prominent nucleoli not seen in Fuhrman grade 1–2 tumors 4. Extrarenal extension including vascular invasion not typically seen in Fuhrman grade 1 and 2 tumors
Special studies	Distinctive CK7 and CAIX positive. CAIX membranous positive, yet not apically, resulting in a cup-shaped pattern	CK7 negative and CAIX positive circumferentially around cells
Treatment	Partial or radical nephrectomy is curative	Partial or radical nephrectomy for localized disease. Targeted therapy is increasingly used for metastatic disease
Prognosis	Vast majority stage T1 with excellent prognosis. No evidence of metastasis has been documented	Primarily stage, grade, and clinical performance status dependent

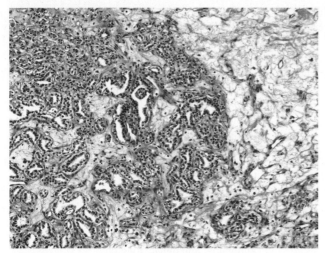

Figure 2.13.1 Clear cell papillary renal cell carcinoma with tubules in myxoid stroma.

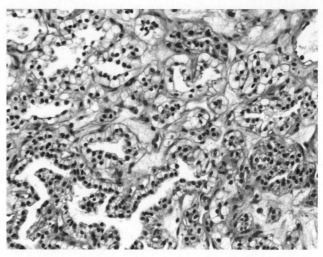

Figure 2.13.2 Same case as Figure 2.13.1 with tubules lined by clear cells.

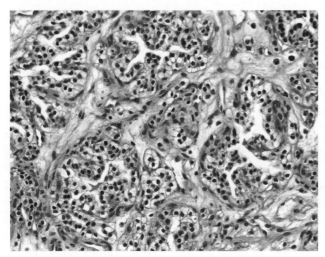

Figure 2.13.3 Same case as Figures 2.13.1 and 2.13.2 with papillary tufting lined by clear cells.

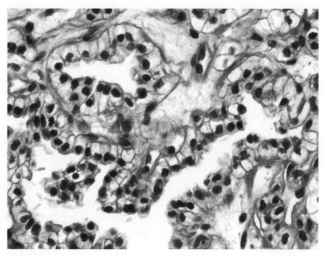

Figure 2.13.4 Same case as Figures 2.13.1–2.13.3 with tubules lined by cells with bland cytology with reversed polarity having subnuclear clear cytoplasm.

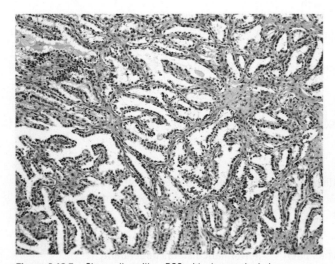

Figure 2.13.5 Clear cell papillary RCC with elongated tubules.

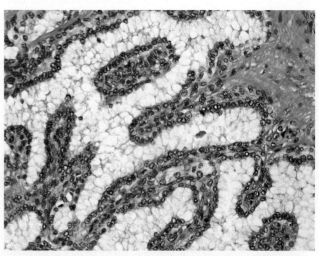

Figure 2.13.6 Same case as Figure 2.13.5 with cells having bland cytology and abundant clear cytoplasm. Focal papillary projections are noted.

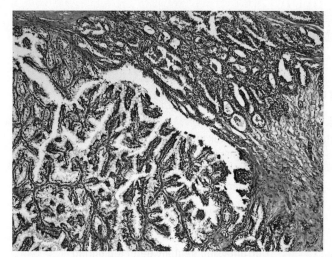

Figure 2.13.7 Clear cell papillary RCC with tubules (*upper right*) and papillary formation (*lower left*).

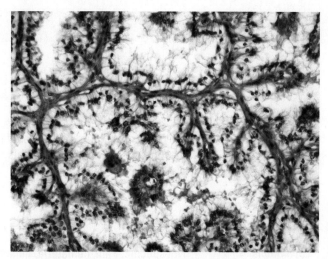

Figure 2.13.8 Same case as Figure 2.13.7 with papillary structures lined by cells with clear cytoplasm and reversed nuclear polarity.

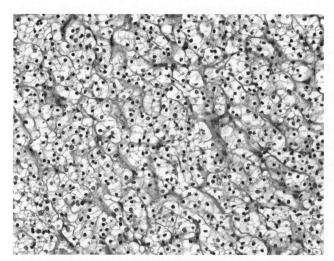

Figure 2.13.9 Clear cell renal cell carcinoma composed of cells with optically clear cytoplasm arranged in nests.

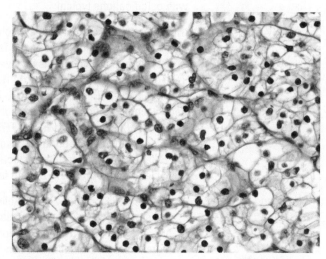

Figure 2.13.10 Same case as Figure 2.13.10 with bland cytology and lack of reversed nuclear polarity.

	miTF/TFE-Family Translocation Renal Cell Carcinoma (tRCC)	Clear Cell Renal Cell Carcinoma
Age	One-third of pediatric RCC. Also affects older patients with a strong female predominance	Adults, peak incidence in sixth decade. Earlier incidence (starting second decade) in familial renal carcinoma syndromes such as vHL syndrome
Location	Usually unifocal and cortical	Usually unifocal. Multifocal and bilateral in <5% of cases, mainly in familial syndromic setting
Symptoms	Not specific. Pain, hematuria, flank mass	Currently, incidentally detected during abdominal and pelvic imaging
Signs	Abdominal mass. Detectable on imaging with calcifications typical	Pain, hematuria, flank mass are the classic triad of presentation
Etiology	tRCC tumors bear gene fusions involving *miTF/TFE* transcription factor gene family. Most frequent translocations involve the *TFE3* gene at the Xp11 locus (Xp11 RCC) and include t(X;17) leading to *ASPL-TFE3* gene fusion (identical to alveolar soft part sarcoma); t(X;1) leading to *PRCC-TFE3* gene fusion. A second subset of tRCC involve the *TFEB* gene and result from translocation t(6;11) leading to *Alpha-TFEB* gene fusion	See Section 2.14
Gross and Histology	1. Mean size 6.8 cm (6.1–21 cm). Solid masses, golden to yellow. Associated necrosis and hemorrhage common in larger masses. Calcifications may be seen. 2. Xp11 RCC composed of clear/pale eosinophilic cells growing in a nested and papillary architecture *(Figs. 2.15.1–2.15.4)* 3. Calcifications in the form of psammoma bodies are frequent 4. t(6;11) carcinomas, in addition to larger polygonal clear or eosinophilic cells, have a biomorphic population of smaller cells clustered around hyaline *(Fig. 2.15.5)* 5. Nuclear and nucleolar feature predominantly Fuhrman grades 3 and 4 6. Extrarenal extension including vascular invasion not infrequent 7. Strong tendency to spread to perirenal lymph nodes	1. Solid and cystic mass with distinct pushing borders. Mean size 7 cm (wide size range). Nodular solid areas, typically golden to yellow in color. Associated necrosis and hemorrhage common in larger masses. Calcifications are encountered 2. Polygonal cells with optically clear to granular eosinophilic cytoplasm, arranged in acini, tubules, nests, or solid sheets *(Fig. 2.15.6)*. Papillary structures not seen. Intratubular and intraacinar hemorrhage and rich capillary network typical 3. Psammomatous calcifications not seen 4. Biomorphic cell appearance not present 5. Conspicuous to prominent nucleoli found in Fuhrman grade 3–4 carcinomas 6. Extrarenal extension including invasion of renal sinus and vascular invasion seen in locally advanced clear cell RCC 7. Spread to perirenal lymph nodes only in advanced high-grade tumors

	miTF/TFE-Family Translocation Renal Cell Carcinoma (tRCC)	Clear Cell Renal Cell Carcinoma
Special studies	• Epithelial markers EMA, AE1/AE3, and CAM5.2 usually negative as well as vimentin • TFE3 and cathepsin K are the most sensitive and specific markers of Xp11 RCC. TFEB and cathepsin K label tRCC TFEB t(6,11) carcinomas. t(X;17) leading to *ASPL-TFE3* gene fusion and t(6;11) involving the *Alpha-TFEB* gene can be documented by break-apart FISH	• Vimentin, AE1/AE3, and CAM5.2 positive • TFE3, TFEB, and cathepsin K expression is negative. FISH studies for Xp11 and TFEB translocations are negative
Treatment	Radical nephrectomy. Targeted therapy with mTOR inhibitors is considered in advanced disease	Partial or radical nephrectomy for localized disease. Targeted therapy is increasingly used for metastatic disease
Prognosis	Primarily stage dependent. Children have a better prognosis than do adults	Primarily stage, grade and clinical performance status dependent

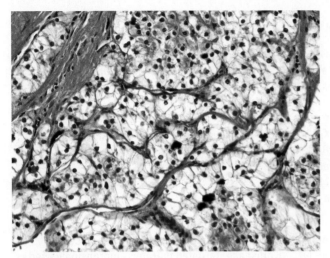

Figure 2.14.1 XP11 renal cell carcinoma composed of clear/pale cells growing in a nested architecture with calcifications.

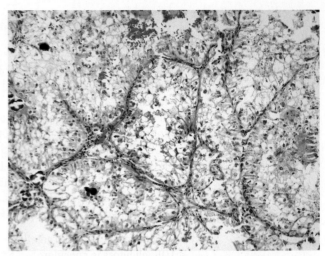

Figure 2.14.2 XP11 renal cell carcinoma composed of abundant clear/pale eosinophilic cells growing in a nested architecture with calcifications. (Courtesy of Dr. Peter Argani.)

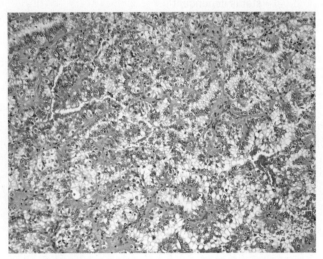

Figure 2.14.3 XP11 renal cell carcinoma composed of abundant clear/pale eosinophilic cells growing in a papillary architecture. (Courtesy of Dr. Peter Argani.)

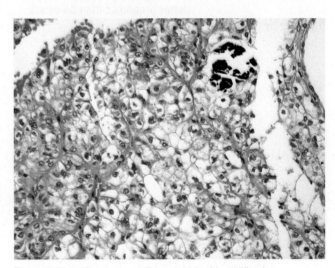

Figure 2.14.4 Same case as Figure 2.14.3 with calcification.

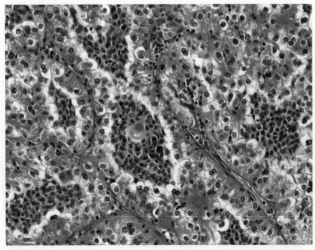

Figure 2.14.5 Translocation RCC harboring t(6;11)(p21;q12) leading to *Alpha-TFEB* with dual population of smaller cells. (Courtesy of Dr. Peter Argani.)

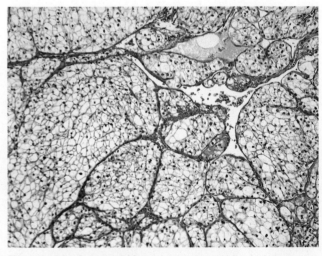

Figure 2.14.6 Clear cell RCC growing in a nested/alveolar pattern.

	Renal–Adrenal Fusion/Ectopic Intrarenal Adrenal Tissue	Clear Cell Renal Cell Carcinoma
Age	Any age. Rare. Usually incidentally in surgical specimens or at autopsy	Adults, peak incidence in sixth decade
Location	Almost all at the superior pole of the kidney. Varies from plaque, wedge-shaped, or spherical subcapsular lesions to irregular nests deep in the renal parenchyma	Usually unifocal. Multifocal and bilateral in <5% of cases, mainly in familial syndromic setting
Symptoms	Most detected at surgery for other reasons or incidentally during imaging	Currently, incidentally detected during abdominal and pelvic imaging
Signs	None	Pain, hematuria, flank mass are the classic triad of presentation
Etiology	Fusion from failure of retroperitoneal mesenchyme to stimulate adrenal capsule formation. Ectopic adrenal tissue when fragment of primitive adrenal gland sheds off during development and implants in the kidney	See Section 2.14
Histology	1. Variably incomplete or absent fibrous capsule separating from a normal kidney although uncommonly can be complete capsule at the base of the lesion *(Figs. 2.15.1 and 2.15.2)*	1. Capsule variable although typically not prominent
	2. In minority of cases, normal adrenal architecture is maintained. In remaining cases, small to intermediate solid nests or trabeculae of clear cells and eosinophilic cells with an intervening capillary network intermixed randomly without obvious zonation	2. Arranged in acini, tubules, nests, or solid sheets with rich vascular capillary stromal network, can be similar to intrarenal adrenal tissue
	3. Uncommon cases with irregular islands of clear cells deep in the kidney or lining a cyst *(Figs. 2.15.3 and 2.15.4)*	3. Can have multicystic clear cell RCC mimicking adrenal tissue next to cysts
	4. Cells can have pale or eosinophilic cytoplasm	4. Cells can have pale or eosinophilic cytoplasm
	5. Abundant microvesicular or spongy cytoplasm filled with lipid droplets *(Fig. 2.15.5)*	5. Clear cells have dissolved empty cytoplasm
	6. Yellow to light brown lipofuscin pigment commonly present	6. Lipofuscin typically absent
	7. Uniformly small round nuclei with no cytologic atypia or prominent nucleoli	7. May have small round nuclei with no cytologic atypia or prominent nucleoli
	8. May contain scattered mature adipocytes	8. Lacks mature adipocytes
	9. Cells can irregularly extend into renal parenchymal in an infiltrative manner	9. Most low-grade clear cell RCC not invade irregularly into surrounding the normal kidney
	10. Can extend beyond the renal capsule into perirenal adipose tissue without a surrounding fibrous capsule *(Fig. 2.15.6)*.	10. Unusual for low-grade clear cell RCC to extend out of the kidney

	Renal–Adrenal Fusion/Ectopic Intrarenal Adrenal Tissue	Clear Cell Renal Cell Carcinoma
Special studies	• Typically positive for inhibin and Melan A • Negative for PAX8, RCC, CD10, EMA, and pancytokeratin	• Typically negative for inhibin and Melan A • Positive for PAX8, RCC, CD10, EMA, and pancytokeratin.
Treatment	None	Partial or radical nephrectomy for localized disease. Targeted therapy is increasingly used for metastatic disease
Prognosis	Benign	Primarily stage, grade, and clinical performance status dependent

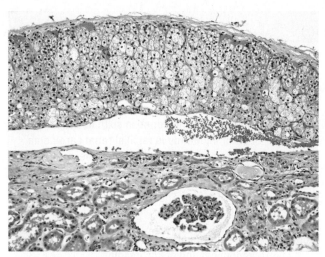

Figure 2.15.1   Lack of normal architecture of the adrenal gland in renal–adrenal fusion with no capsule separating the two components.

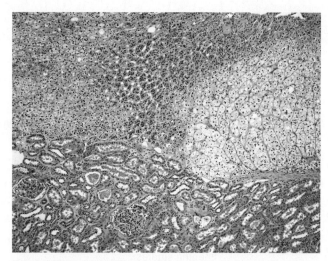

Figure 2.15.2   Adrenal tissue in direct contact with the renal cortex with no intervening fibrous capsule.

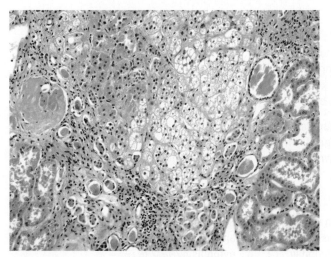

Figure 2.15.3   Renal–adrenal fusion with adrenal tissue extending into the renal cortex in an infiltrative manner.

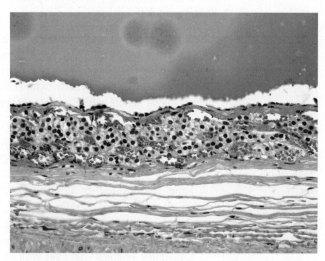

Figure 2.15.4   Renal–adrenal fusion with clear cells in the wall of a simple renal cyst, with a prominent vascular network similar to that seen in clear cell renal cell carcinoma.

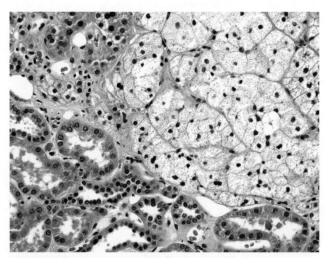

Figure 2.15.5   Renal–adrenal fusion with microvesicular cytoplasm of zona fasciculata cells.

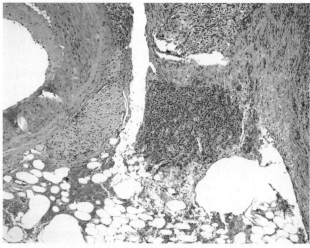

Figure 2.15.6   Ectopic adrenal tissue extending from the subcaspular region into perirenal adipose tissue, without a surrounding fibrous capsule.

	Chromophobe Renal Cell Carcinoma	Clear Cell Renal Cell Carcinoma
Age	Usually sixth and seventh decades (30–90 y)	Adults, peak incidence in sixth decade. Earlier incidence in familial renal carcinoma syndromes such as vHL syndrome
Location	Usually unifocal. Multifocal and bilateral in rare cases, mainly in familial syndromic setting (Birt-Hogg-Dubé syndrome [BHD])	Usually unifocal. Multifocal and bilateral in < 5% of cases. The latter mainly in the familial syndromic setting
Symptoms	Most asymptomatic and detected incidentally on imaging studies	Currently, incidentally detected during abdominal and pelvic imaging
Signs	Abdominal mass, detectable on imaging. Fibrofolliculomas, lung cysts, and pneumothorax features of BHD	Pain, hematuria, flank mass are the classic triad of presentation
Etiology	Unknown in sporadic cases. Possible loss of chromosomes 1, 6, 10, 13, 17, 21, and Y. Inherited germ line mutation in the folliculin gene with familial forms. Chromophobe RCC, oncocytoma, hybrid oncocytoma/chromophobe tumors in BHD with oncocytosis	See Section 2.14
Gross and Histology	1. Well-circumscribed unencapsulated tumors with distinct pushing borders. Size ranges from 2 to 22 cm (mean 8 cm). Solid light brown cut surface. Necrosis, hemorrhage, and cystic change infrequent 2. Classic type composed of large polygonal cells with pale and lightly reticulated cytoplasm. Commonly admixed with cells with eosinophilic cytoplasm, which if predominates termed "eosinophilic variant" *(Figs. 2.16.1 and 2.16.2)* 3. Cells arranged in nests or solid sheets with minor tubular structures *(Figs. 2.16.2–2.16.4)* 4. Intratubular and intraacinar hemorrhage not typical 5. Prominent, plant-like, thick cell membranes *(Figs. 2.16.2 and 2.16.5)* 6. Irregular, wrinkled, notched nuclei (raisenoid) and perinuclear halos *(Figs. 2.16.2, 2.16.5 and 2.16.6)* 7. Multinucleation frequent 8. Medium-sized vessels with eccentrically hyalinized walls 9. Nuclear and nucleolar features usually equivalent to Fuhrman grade 3 *(Figs. 2.16.2 and 2.16.5)*, yet Fuhrman grading not applicable given their overall indolent behavior 10. Extrarenal extension including vascular invasion only rarely seen	1. Encapsulated tumors with distinct pushing borders. Mean size 7 cm (wide size range). Cystic change is not uncommon. Solid areas typically golden to yellow with necrosis and hemorrhage in larger masses. Calcifications are encountered 2. Polygonal cells with distinct cell border and optically clear to granular eosinophilic cytoplasm *(Fig. 2.16.7)* 3. Cells arranged in acini, tubules, nests, or solid sheets 4. Intratubular and intraacinar hemorrhage typical 5. Cell borders not obvious 6. Raisenoid nuclei not seen and perinuclear clearing (halos) absent *(Fig. 2.16.8)* 7. Multinucleation only present in higher-grade (Fuhrman grade 4) lesions 8. Rich vascular capillary tumor stromal network is characteristic 9. Nuclear and nucleolar size varies according to tumor grade 10. Extrarenal extension including invasion of the renal sinus and renal vein branches is seen in locally advanced higher-grade tumors

	Chromophobe Renal Cell Carcinoma	**Clear Cell Renal Cell Carcinoma**
Special studies	• CK7 typically diffuse positive and CD117 membranous staining • CAIX negative • Hales colloidal iron positivity, typically in perinuclear distribution, yet stain is technically difficult, and in most institutions, stains are not specific	• CK7 and CD117 negative • CAIX positive • Hales colloidal iron negative
Treatment	Partial or radical nephrectomy for localized disease	Partial or radical nephrectomy for localized disease. Targeted therapy is increasingly used for metastatic disease
Prognosis	5-y survival >90%. Stage dependent. Rare high-grade nonsarcomatoid tumors with increased cellularity, necrosis, pleomorphism, and increased mitotic figures also with a worse prognosis	Primarily stage, grade, and clinical performance status dependent

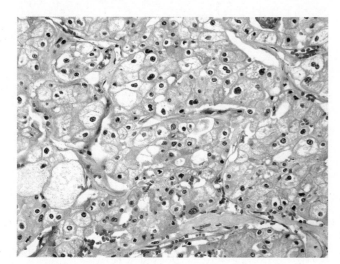

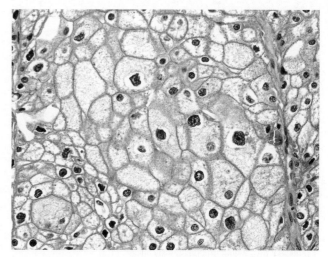

Figure 2.16.1   Chromophobe RCC with mixture of pale and lightly reticulated cytoplasm admixed with cells with granular eosinophilic cytoplasm.

Figure 2.16.2   Sheets of classic chromophobe RCC with pale and lightly reticulated cytoplasm. Cells have plant-like cytoplasm borders and raisenoid nuclei with perinuclear halos. Nuclei have irregular notches.

2 KIDNEY

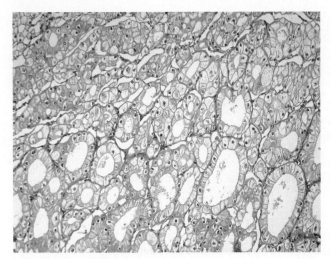

Figure 2.16.3   Tubular chromophobe RCC.

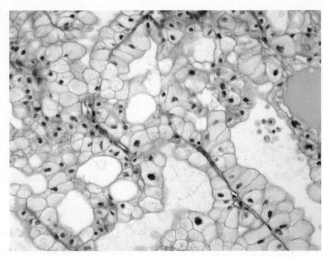

Figure 2.16.4   Same case as Figure 2.16.3 with pale, lightly reticulated cytoplasm.

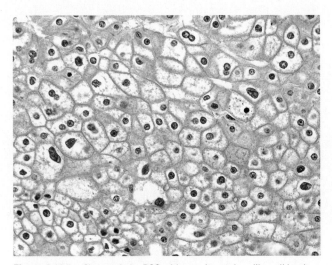

Figure 2.16.5   Chromophobe RCC with prominent plant-like cell borders and nuclear atypia with irregular crinkly nuclei.

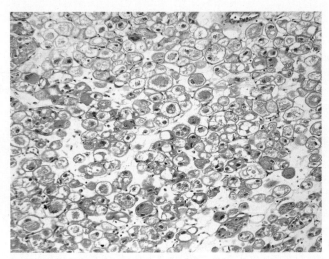

Figure 2.16.6   Chromophobe RCC with prominent plant-like cell borders.

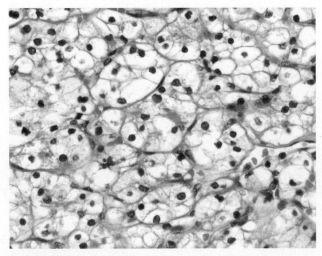

Figure 2.16.7   Low-grade clear cell RCC with optically clear cytoplasm.

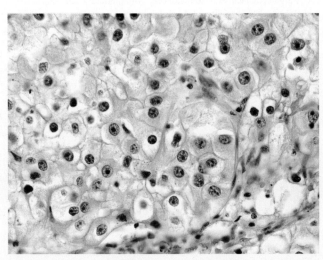

Figure 2.16.8   Clear cell RCC Fuhrman grade 3 with round nuclei and visible nucleoli.

	Oncocytoma	Chromophobe Renal Cell Carcinoma
Age	Mean age seventh decade. Wide age range	Usually sixth and seventh decades (30–90 y)
Location	Usually unifocal. Multifocal and bilateral tumors mainly in Birt-Hogg-Dubé syndrome (BHD)	Usually unifocal. Multifocal and bilateral in rare cases, mainly in BHD
Symptoms	Most asymptomatic and detected incidentally on imaging studies	Most asymptomatic and detected incidentally on imaging studies
Signs	Classic triad of hematuria, flank mass, and pain in rare cases. Fibrofolliculomas, lung cysts, and pneumothorax features of BHD	Abdominal mass, detectable on imaging
Etiology	Unknown in sporadic cases. Minimal cytogenetic alterations. Inherited germ line mutation in the folliculin gene on chromosome 17p11.2 associated with familial form	Multiple chromosomal loss (see Section 2.16).
Gross and Histology	1. Well-circumscribed unencapsulated tumor with pushing border. Size widely variable. Cystic change not common. Solid cut surface dark brown-mahogany. Hemorrhage in one-fifth of cases. Typical central scar in one-third of cases. Necrosis infrequent 2. Typically, cells are arranged in nests, acini, tubules, or microcysts in a fibromyxoid stroma *(Fig. 2.17.1)* 3. Large, round-to-polygonal cells with abundant eosinophilic cytoplasm *(Fig. 2.17.1)*. Also smaller tumor cells with scant granular cytoplasm and dense hyperchromatic nuclei termed "oncoblasts" *(Fig. 2.17.2)* 4. Well-preserved nuclei that with fine chromatin are uniformly round with variably sized nucleoli *(Fig. 2.17.3)*. Pyknotic dark nuclei with crenated irregular edges should be discounted *(Fig. 2.17.4)*. Scattered cells with degenerative nuclear atypia with multinucleation and pseudoinclusions can be seen, often clustered *(Figs. 2.17.5 and 2.17.6)* 5. Lacks prominent, plant-like, thick cell membranes 6. Extrarenal extension can be seen in 20% of cases and not an indication of malignancy *(Fig. 2.17.7)*. Invasion of the renal sinus and renal vein branches can rarely be seen in typical oncocytomas *(Figs. 2.17.8 and 2.17.9)*	1. Well-circumscribed but not encapsulated tumors with distinct pushing borders. Size ranges from 2–22 cm (mean, 8 cm). Solid light brown cut surface. Necrosis, hemorrhage, and cystic change infrequent 2. Cells arranged in compact nests or solid sheets with only minor tubular and acinar structures *(Figs. 2.17.10 and 2.17.11)*. Typically lacks fibromyxoid stroma 3. Classic type with large polygonal cells with pale and lightly reticulated cytoplasm. Commonly admixed with cells with eosinophilic cytoplasm, which if predominant termed "eosinophilic variant," likely to be confused with oncocytoma *(Figs. 2.17.10 and 2.17.11)* 4. Raisenoid nuclei with an irregular, wrinkled, notched nuclear membrane and perinuclear halos typical, yet not every cell will have irregular nuclei *(Figs. 2.17.10 and 2.17.12)* 5. Prominent, plant-like, thick cell membranes 6. Extrarenal extension including invasion of the renal sinus and renal vein branches uncommonly seen

	Oncocytoma	Chromophobe Renal Cell Carcinoma
Special studies	• Only helpful immunohistochemical stain is CK7. Patchy focal staining typical • Hales colloidal iron typically not that useful as difficult to achieve reliable results. If present in oncocytoma usually limited to luminal cytoplasm	• CK7 tends to be diffuse • Hales colloidal iron is often not specific, but in the classic case, shows diffuse cytoplasmic staining
Treatment	Excision or partial nephrectomy	Partial or radical nephrectomy for localized disease
Prognosis	Benign behavior even if lesion extends out of the kidney or has vascular invasion	5-y disease survival >90%. Primarily stage dependent. The rare presence of sarcomatoid or high-grade features (see Section 2.16) negatively impacts prognosis

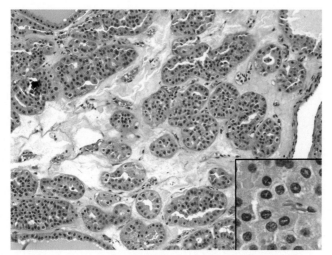

Figure 2.17.1 Oncocytoma containing eosinophilic cells arranged in nests and acini set in a fibromyxoid stroma. Cells have abundant dense eosinophilic cytoplasm with uniform round nuclei (**inset**).

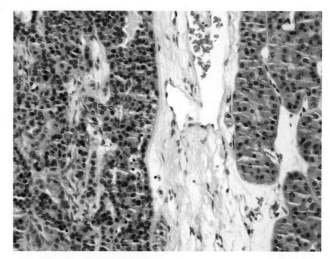

Figure 2.17.2 Oncocytoma with oncoblasts (*left*).

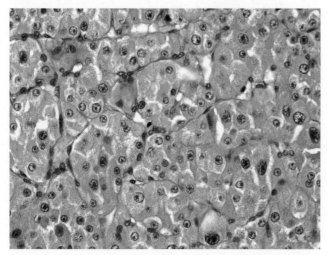

Figure 2.17.3 Oncocytoma with uniform nuclei with prominent nucleoli.

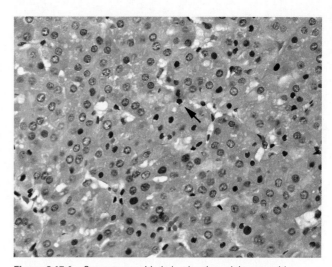

Figure 2.17.4 Oncocytoma with dark pyknotic nuclei, some with crenated irregular appearance. Background well-preserved nuclei are uniform and round.

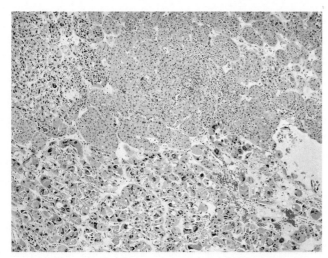

Figure 2.17.5 Oncocytoma with nodules of cells with degenerative atypia.

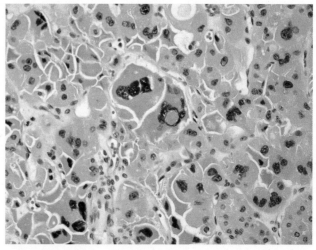

Figure 2.17.6 Same case as Figure 2.17.5 with degenerative atypia, multinucleation, and nuclear pseudoinclusions.

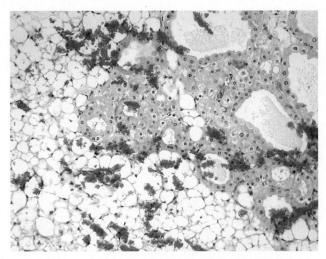

Figure 2.17.7   Oncocytoma involving perirenal adipose tissue.

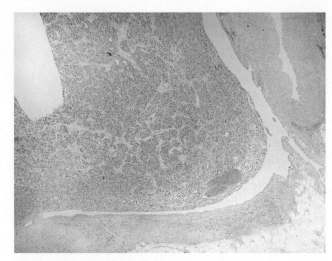

Figure 2.17.8   Oncocytoma invading a large vein.

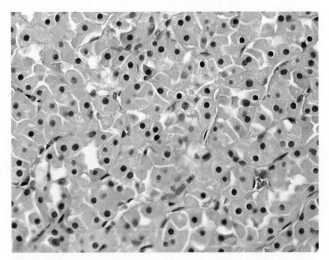

Figure 2.17.9   Same case as Figure 2.17.8 showing classic oncocytoma.

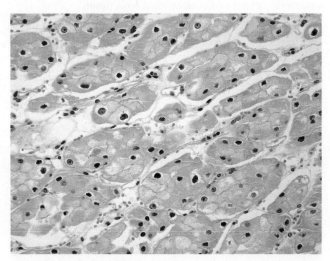

Figure 2.17.10   Chromophobe renal cell carcinoma composed almost exclusively of large polygonal cells with granular eosinophilic cytoplasm. Cells have plant-like cytoplasm borders and raisenoid nuclei with perinuclear halos.

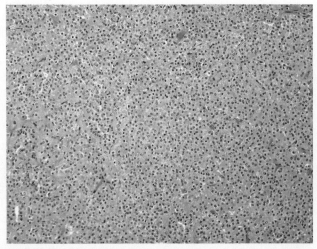

Figure 2.17.11   Chromophobe renal cell carcinoma with diffuse growth pattern that would be unusual in oncocytoma.

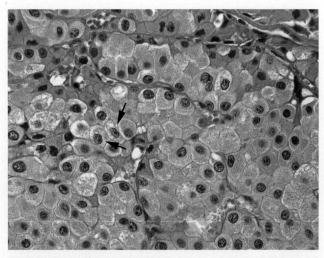

Figure 2.17.12   Same case as Figure 2.17.11 with occasional notched nuclei (*arrows*) diagnostic of chromophobe RCC.

	Oncocytoma	Oncocytic Papillary Renal Cell Carcinoma
Age	Mean age seventh decade. Wide age range	Adults, peak incidence in fifth to sixth decades
Location	Usually unifocal. Multifocal and bilateral tumors occur in rare cases, mainly in Birt-Hogg-Dubé syndrome	Usually unifocal
Symptoms	Most asymptomatic and detected incidentally on imaging studies	Currently, incidentally detected during abdominal and pelvic imaging
Signs	Classic triad of hematuria, flank mass, and pain in rare cases	Pain, hematuria, flank mass are the classic triad of presentation
Etiology	See Section 2.18	See Section 2.14
Gross and Histology	1. Well-circumscribed unencapsulated tumors with pushing borders. Size is widely variable. Cystic change not common. Solid cut surface is dark brown-mahogany. Hemorrhage in one-fifth of cases. Central scar in one-third of cases. Necrosis absent 2. Large, round-to-polygonal cells with abundant eosinophilic cytoplasm 3. Cells are arranged in nests, acini, tubules, or microcysts. Lacks papillary structures with rare exception of a few papillary projections into dilated cysts (*Fig. 2.18.1*) 4. Small tumor cells with scant granular cytoplasm and dense hyperchromatic nuclei termed "oncoblasts" may be seen 5. Uniformly round nuclei with inconspicuous nucleoli 6. Scattered degenerative nuclear atypia with multinucleation may be seen 7. Striking edematous hypocellular fibromyxoid stroma 8. Foamy histiocytes and cholesterol clefts are not present 9. Hemosiderin deposition in histiocytes and neoplastic epithelium not seen 10. Psammomatous calcifications are not present	1. Grossly encapsulated with distinct pushing borders. Variable size. Cystic change, necrosis, and hemorrhage relatively common in larger masses. Calcifications are encountered 2. Composed of large, round-to-polygonal cells with abundant eosinophilic cytoplasm 3. Composed of admixture of tubular and papillary proliferation (*Figs. 2.18.2–2.18.5*). Papillary structures are lined by multilayered columnar granular eosinophilic/oncocytic cell (type 2 papillary RCC) 4. "Oncoblasts" are not seen 5. Generally Fuhrman grades 3–4 with some nuclei showing nuclear irregularity (*Figs. 2.18.6 and 2.18.7*), although may have bland nuclei 6. Nuclear atypia not degenerative appearing but well-preserved nuclei 7. Myxoid hyalinized stromal not typically present 8. Foamy histiocytes and cholesterol clefts typically occupy papillary fibrovascular cores (*Figs. 2.18.8–2.18.10*) 9. Hemosiderin deposition in histiocytes as well and neoplastic epithelium (*Fig. 2.18.6*) 10. Psammomatous calcifications are frequently present
Special studies	CK7 shows focal patchy staining	Typically diffusely positive for CK7
Treatment	Partial nephrectomy	Partial or radical nephrectomy
Prognosis	Benign	Malignant with primarily stage, grade, and clinical performance status dependent

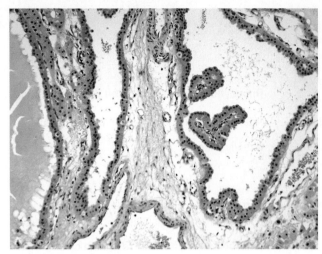

Figure 2.18.1   Oncocytoma with a few papillary projections into dilated cysts.

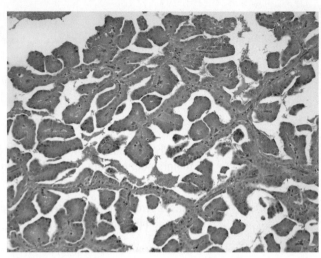

Figure 2.18.2   Oncocytic papillary renal cell carcinoma.

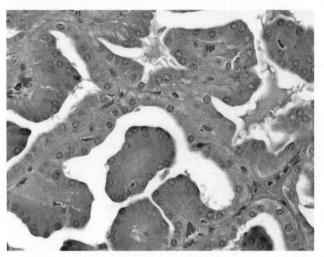

Figure 2.18.3   Higher magnification of case in Figure 2.18.2.

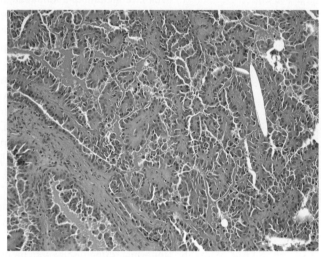

Figure 2.18.4   Oncocytic papillary renal cell carcinoma.

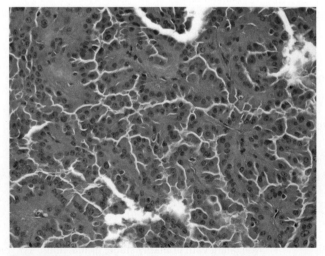

Figure 2.18.5   Higher magnification of case in Figure 2.18.4.

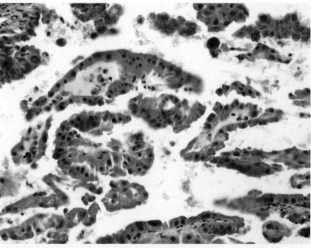

Figure 2.18.6   Oncocytic papillary renal cell carcinoma with hemosiderin deposition in tumor cells and histiocytes.

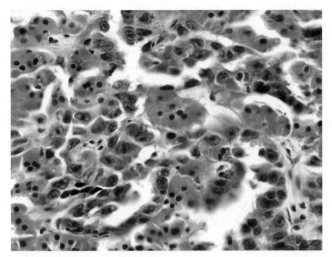

Figure 2.18.7 Same case as Figure 2.18.6 with nononcocytic cells with prominent atypia admixed with oncocytic appearing cells.

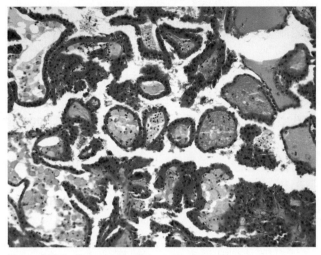

Figure 2.18.8 Oncocytic papillary renal cell carcinoma.

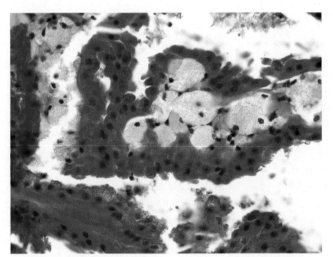

Figure 2.18.9 Same case as Figure 2.18.8 with foamy macrophages in stalks.

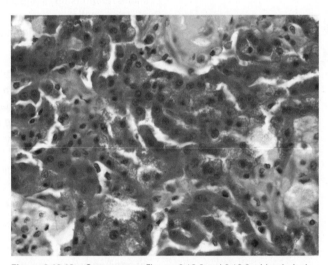

Figure 2.18.10 Same case as Figures 2.18.8 and 2.18.9 with relatively uniform nuclei with prominent nucleoli.

	Tubulocystic Carcinoma	Oncocytoma
Age	Adults. Mean age at diagnosis 57 y (30–80 y). Male predominant	Mean age seventh decade. Wide age range
Location	Usually unifocal. Cortical at times involving medullary region	Usually unifocal. Multifocal and bilateral tumors occur in BHD syndrome
Symptoms	Usually incidentally detected during imaging	Most asymptomatic and detected incidentally on imaging studies
Signs	Abdominal mass, detectable on imaging	Fibrofolliculomas, lung cysts, and pneumothorax seen in BHD
Etiology	Unknown. Trisomy 17 in some raising possible relationship to papillary RCC. Conflicting studies comparing gene expression between tubulocystic carcinoma and papillary RCC	See Section 2.17
Gross and Histology	1. Well-circumscribed unencapsulated tumors. Average size 4.3 cm (0.5–17.5 cm). Necrosis and hemorrhage not seen. Cut surface impart a unique sponge-like appearance. Lacks necrosis 2. Composed of small- to medium-sized cysts ranging from microscopic to 1 cm in diameter *(Figs. 2.19.1 and 2.19.2)* 3. Occasionally, can see minor component of papillary carcinoma *(Figs. 2.19.3–2.19.8)* 4. Large, round-to-polygonal cells with abundant eosinophilic cytoplasm 5. Cysts are lined by cells with hobnail appearance with vesicular nuclei and prominent nucleoli. Nuclei vary in shape and some have irregular shapes *(Fig. 2.19.2)* 6. Only occasional mitotic figures encountered 7. Intervening stroma is paucicellular fibrous and focally edematous 8. Typically organ confined with no associated renal sinus or renal vein invasion	1. Well-circumscribed but unencapsulated tumors with pushing borders. Size widely variable. Cystic change not common. Solid cut surface dark brown-mahogany. Hemorrhage in one-fifth of cases. Central scar in one-third of cases. Lacks necrosis 2. Variant that can be confused with tubulocystic carcinoma composed of tubules some with cystic dilatation *(Figs. 2.19.9–2.19.12)*. In addition, typically also some nests 3. Never see significant papillary component (see Section 2.18) 4. Large, round-to-polygonal cells with abundant eosinophilic cytoplasm 5. Tubules lined by well-preserved nuclei have fine chromatin and are uniformly round with variably sized nucleoli *(Figs. 2.19.11 and 2.19.12)* 6. Mitotic figures rare 7. Often abundant fibromyxoid stroma 8. Extrarenal extension in 20% of cases. Invasion of renal vessels can be rarely seen
Special studies	Not helpful in this differential	Not helpful in this differential
Treatment	Partial or simple nephrectomy	Excision or partial nephrectomy
Prognosis	Favorable with <10% rate of reported metastases	Benign behavior even if lesion extends out of the kidney or has vascular invasion

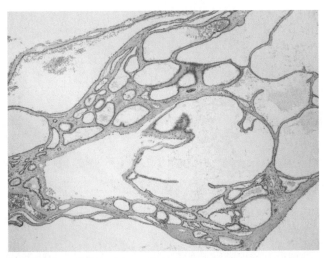

Figure 2.19.1   Tubulocystic carcinoma composed of small- to medium-sized cysts.

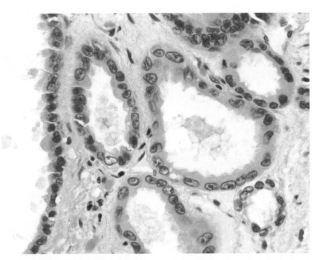

Figure 2.19.2   Same case as Figure 2.19.1 lined by large, round-to-polygonal cells with abundant eosinophilic cytoplasm and atypical irregular nuclei.

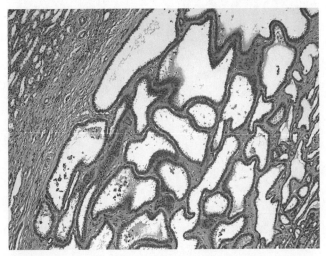

Figure 2.19.3   Tubulocystic carcinoma composed of small- to medium-sized cysts.

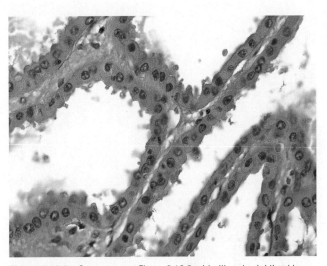

Figure 2.19.4   Same case as Figure 2.19.3 with dilated acini lined by cells with oncocytic cytoplasm and atypical nuclei.

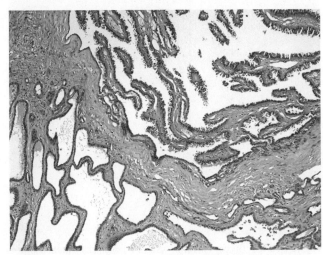

Figure 2.19.5   Same case as Figures 2.19.3 and 2.19.4 with a focal papillary component.

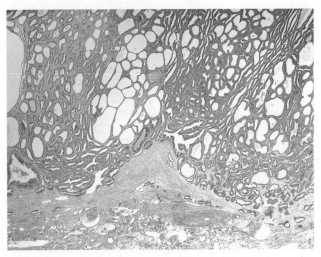

Figure 2.19.6   Tubulocystic carcinoma with well-circumscribed mass composed of small- to medium-sized cysts.

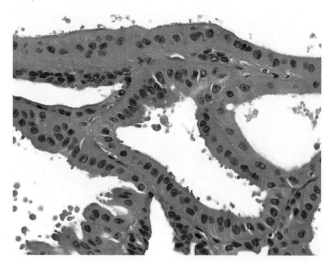

Figure 2.19.7 Same case as Figure 2.19.6 with oncocytic cells having atypical nuclei.

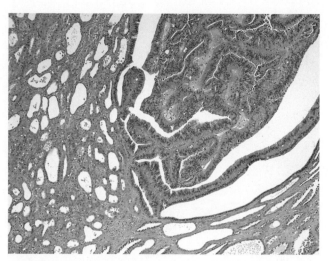

Figure 2.19.8 Same case as Figures 2.19.6 and 2.19.7 with a focal papillary component.

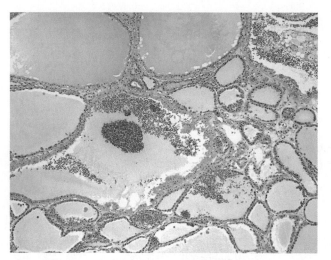

Figure 2.19.9 Oncocytoma with cystically dilated acini.

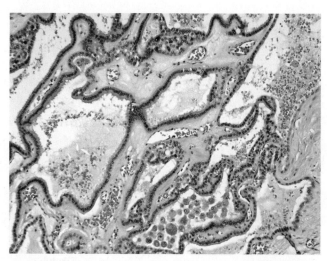

Figure 2.19.10 Same case as Figure 2.19.3 with variable-sized dilated acini.

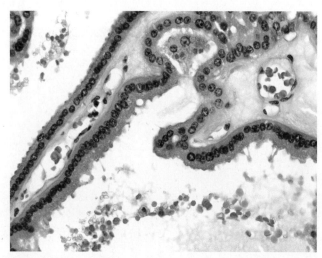

Figure 2.19.11 Same case as Figures 2.19.3 and 2.19.4 with bland, round nuclei and oncocytic cytoplasm.

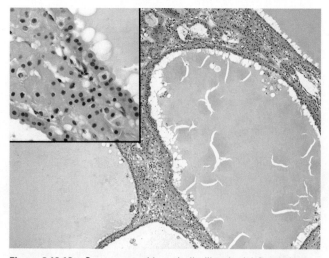

Figure 2.19.12 Oncocytoma with cystically dilated acini. **Inset** shows bland cytology of cells lining dilated acini with colloid secretions as well as small clusters of oncocytic cells between the cysts.

	Collecting Duct Carcinoma	Tubulocystic Carcinoma
Age	Adults. Mean age 55 y (13–83 y)	Adults. Mean age at diagnosis 57 y (30–80 y). Male predominant
Location	Usually unifocal. Medullary renal sinus mass	Usually unifocal. Cortical with at times involving medullary region
Symptoms	Pain, hematuria, flank mass. Some incidentally detected during imaging	Usually incidentally detected during abdominal and pelvic imaging. Pain, hematuria, flank mass only in rare cases
Signs	Abdominal mass, detectable on imaging	Abdominal mass, detectable on imaging
Etiology	Unknown. LOH 1q, 6p, 8p, 13q, and 21q. Deletion 1q23.1-32.2. HER 2neu amplification in up to 50% of cases	See Section 2.19
Gross and Histology	1. Large tumors often involving most of the kidney 2. Irregular infiltrative borders with satellite nodules (Figs. 2.20.1–2.20.4) 3. Solid gross appearance 4. Necrosis and hemorrhage relatively common 5. Tubulopapillary structures, cords, glandular, and/or solid sheets. Lacks cyst formation (Figs. 2.20.1–2.20.4) 6. Cells with moderate amount of basophilic or eosinophilic cytoplasm 7. Vesicular pleomorphic nuclei with prominent nucleoli (Fig. 2.20.4) 8. Frequent mitotic activity 9. Inflamed abundant dense desmoplastic stroma (Figs. 2.20.1–2.20.3) 10. Dysplastic medullary collecting duct structures and medullary intratubular colonization are distinctive features when present 11. Typically infiltrative into perirenal adipose tissue at time of diagnosis	1. Average size 4.3 cm (0.5–17.5 cm). 2. Well circumscribed (Figs. 2.20.5 and 2.20.6) 3. Typical multilocular cystic cut surface impart a unique sponge-like appearance 4. Necrosis and hemorrhage are not seen 5. Composed of small-sized cystic structures ranging from microscopic to 1 cm in diameter (Figs. 2.20.5, 2.20.7, and 2.20.8). Can have focal papillary component (see Section 2.19) 6. Cysts are lined by cells with moderate amount of amphophilic cytoplasm, some with hobnail appearance (Figs. 2.20.6, 2.20.9, and 2.20.10) 7. Vesicular nuclei with prominent nucleoli 8. Only occasional mitotic figures encountered 9. Intervening stroma is paucicellular fibrous and focally edematous 10. Lacks dysplastic medullary collecting duct structures and medullary intratubular colonization 11. Almost always organ confined with no associated renal sinus or renal vein invasion
Special studies	Not helpful in this differential	Not helpful in this differential
Treatment	Radical nephrectomy with adjuvant chemotherapy	Partial or simple nephrectomy
Prognosis	20% of patients alive 2 y postdiagnosis. At presentation, 50% with lymph node metastases; other common sites of spread include liver, lung, and bone	Good with <10% rate of reported metastases

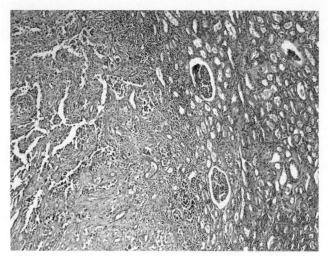

Figure 2.20.1   Collecting duct carcinoma with infiltrative edge.

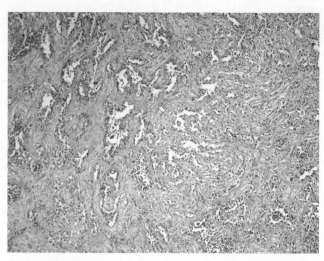

Figure 2.20.2   Same case as Figure 2.20.1 with infiltrating tubules in desmoplastic stroma.

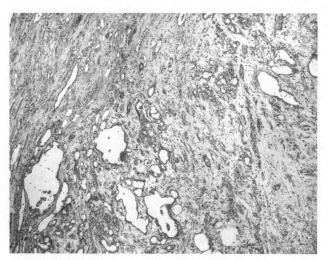

Figure 2.20.3   Collecting duct carcinoma with infiltrative edge with variably sized tubules, some dilated, associated with a desmoplastic stroma.

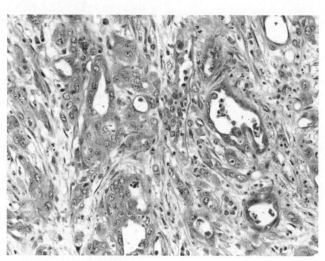

Figure 2.20.4   Same case as Figure 2.20.3 with tubules having significant cytologic atypia.

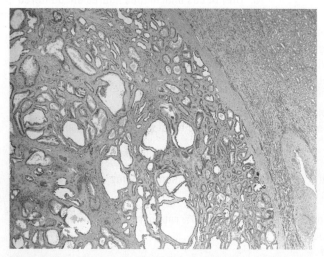

Figure 2.20.5   Well-circumscribed tubulocystic carcinoma with variably sized tubules and cysts.

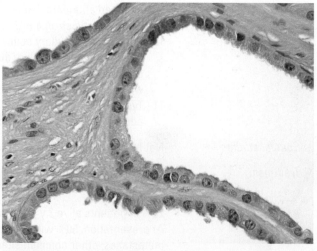

Figure 2.20.6   Same case as Figure 2.20.5 with nuclear atypia in tubules.

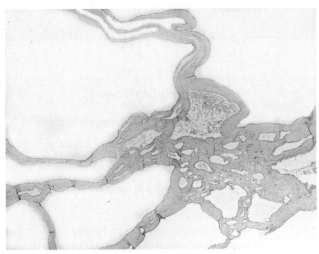

Figure 2.20.7 Tubulocystic carcinoma with markedly dilated cysts.

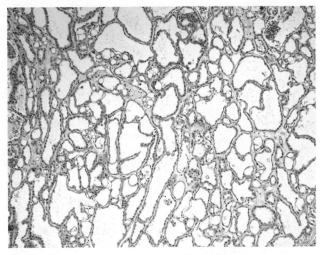

Figure 2.20.8 Tubulocystic carcinoma with smaller cysts.

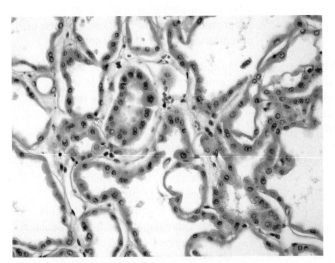

Figure 2.20.9 Same case as Figure 2.20.8 with nuclear atypia in tubules.

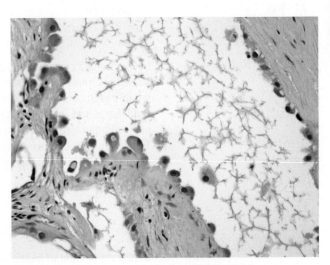

Figure 2.20.10 Tubulocystic carcinoma with hobnail cells.

	Collecting Duct Carcinoma	Renal Medullary Carcinoma
Age	Adults. Mean age 55 y (13–83 y). No race predilection	Young adults. Almost exclusively in black patients
Location	Usually unifocal. Medullary renal sinus mass	Usually unifocal. Medullary renal sinus mass
Symptoms	Pain, hematuria, flank mass. Some incidentally detected during imaging	Pain, hematuria, flank mass
Signs	Abdominal mass, detectable on imaging	Weight loss, symptoms, and signs associated with distant metastases. Mass detectable on imaging. Strong association with sickle cell trait/disease
Etiology	See Section 2.20	Unknown. Inactivation of the tumor suppressor gene *hSNF5/INI1* on long arm of chromosome 22 is frequently detected
Gross and Histology	1. Irregular infiltrative borders with satellite nodules. Usually centrally located with common involvement of the renal sinus and renal vein. Necrosis and hemorrhage relatively common 2. Tubulopapillary structures, cords, glandular, and/or solid sheets (*Fig. 2.21.1*) 3. Moderate amount of basophilic or eosinophilic cytoplasm 4. Vesicular pleomorphic nuclei with prominent nucleoli (*Fig. 2.21.2*) 5. Frequent mitotic activity 6. Typically lacks associated inflammation to the degree seen in renal medullary carcinoma; however, some cases with significant inflammation (*Fig. 2.21.3*) 7. Inflamed abundant dense desmoplastic stroma 8. Dysplastic medullary collecting duct structures and medullary intratubular colonization are distinctive features when present 9. Typically infiltrative into perirenal adipose tissue at time of diagnosis 10. Lacks sickled erythrocytes	1. Irregular infiltrative borders usually centered in medullary region with common involvement of the renal sinus and renal vein. Necrosis and hemorrhage common 2. Distinction from collecting duct carcinoma not possible on morphologic grounds alone. Tubulopapillary structures, cords, glandular, and/or solid sheets. Microcystic and reticular patterns somewhat similar to testicular yolk sac tumors (*Figs. 2.21.4 and 2.21.5*) 3. Moderate amount of basophilic or eosinophilic cytoplasm. Rhabdoid/plasmacytoid morphology can be present (*Figs. 2.21.6 and 2.21.7*) 4. Vesicular pleomorphic nuclei with prominent nucleoli 5. Frequent mitotic activity 6. Microabscess formation and diffuse infiltration by neutrophils within tumor epithelial sheets frequently found 7. Inflamed abundant dense desmoplastic stroma 8. Dysplastic medullary collecting duct structures and medullary intratubular colonization not typically seen 9. Typically infiltrative into perirenal adipose tissue at time of diagnosis 10. Occasionally, sickled erythrocytes can be identified (*Fig. 2.21.8*)

	Collecting Duct Carcinoma	**Renal Medullary Carcinoma**
Special studies	Both positive for PAX8 and cytokeratins. p63 and GATA3 usually negative. Loss of *hSNF5/INI1* can be seen in both	Not helpful in this differential
Treatment	Radical nephrectomy with adjuvant chemotherapy	Radical nephrectomy with adjuvant chemotherapy
Prognosis	20% of patients alive 2 y after diagnosis	Only rare reports of survival beyond 1st year post-diagnosis. Majority have lymph node metastases at time of diagnosis often with metastases to liver, lung, and bone

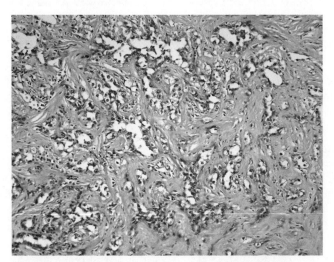

Figure 2.21.1   Collecting duct carcinoma with tubules infiltrating desmoplastic stroma.

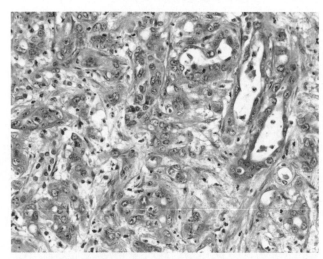

Figure 2.21.2   Collecting duct carcinoma with solid nests and tubules and prominent nuclear atypia.

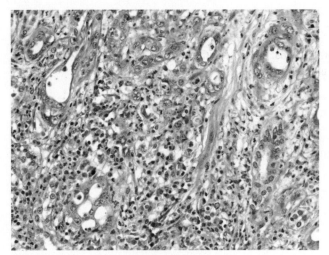

Figure 2.21.3   Collecting duct carcinoma with prominent acute inflammation.

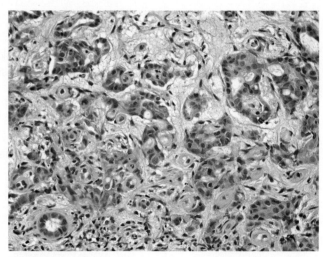

Figure 2.21.4   Renal medullary carcinoma composed of tubules in a myxoid stroma.

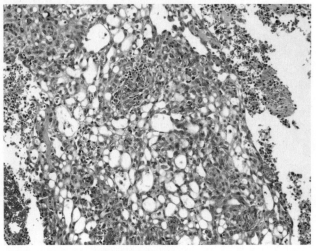

Figure 2.21.5   Renal medullary carcinoma with a prominent microcystic pattern.

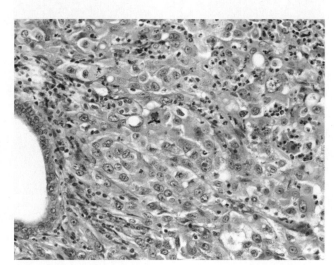

Figure 2.21.6   Renal medullary carcinoma with abundant cytoplasm, high-grade cytology, mitotic figures, and admixed acute inflammation.

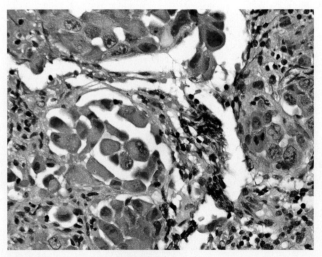

Figure 2.21.7   Renal medullary carcinoma with rhabdoid features.

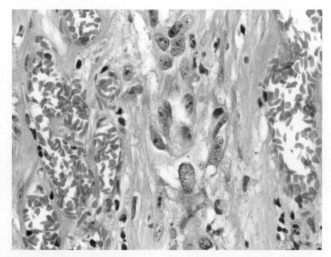

Figure 2.21.8   Sickle cells seen in medullary carcinoma.

	Collecting Duct Carcinoma	Invasive Urothelial Carcinoma of the Renal Pelvis
Age	Adults. Mean age 55 y (13–83 y). No race predilection	Adults. Peak incidence in sixth decade
Location	Usually unifocal. Medullary renal sinus mass	Medullary location. Usually associated with prior history of lower tract urothelial carcinoma
Symptoms	Pain, hematuria, flank mass. Some are incidentally detected imaging	Hematuria, flank pain secondary to obstruction
Signs	Abdominal mass, detectable on imaging	Hydronephrosis/pyelonephritis. Filling defect on imaging. Positive urine cytology
Etiology	See Section 2.20	Smoking history. Underlying molecular changes include p53, Rb, and cell cycle control alterations
Gross and Histology	1. Irregular infiltrative borders with satellite nodules. Usually centrally located with common involvement of the renal sinus and renal vein. Necrosis and hemorrhage relatively common	1. Infiltrative tumors with irregular borders. Although epicenter of tumor is usually at the renal sinus, involvement of cortex is found in higher stage disease. Residual papillary component within renal pelvis favors urothelial carcinoma. Necrosis and hemorrhage relatively common
	2. Tubulopapillary structures, cords, glandular, and/or solid sheets (*Figs. 2.22.1–2.22.4*)	2. Irregular nests. Cords, gland-like lumina, and solid sheets also can be seen (*Fig. 2.22.5*)
	3. Cells with moderate amount of basophilic or eosinophilic cytoplasm	3. Moderate amount of basophilic or eosinophilic cytoplasm and occasional squamous differentiation
	4. Vesicular pleomorphic nuclei with prominent nucleoli	4. Vesicular pleomorphic nuclei with prominent nucleoli
	5. Frequent mitotic activity	5. Frequent mitotic activity
	6. Inflamed abundant dense desmoplastic stroma	6. Inflamed abundant dense desmoplastic stroma
	7. Dysplastic medullary collecting duct structures and medullary intratubular colonization are distinctive features, yet not frequently seen	7. CIS may be present in renal pelvis (*Fig. 2.22.6*) and can colonize collecting ducts with solid nests as opposed to dysplastic glandular cells in collecting duct carcinoma (*Figs. 2.22.7 and 2.22.8*)
	8. Typically infiltrative into perirenal adipose tissue at time of diagnosis	8. Overall lower-stage disease at presentation
Special studies	• PAX8 positive • p63 and GATA3 are usually negative	• PAX8 variably positive • p63 and GATA3 are positive
Treatment	Radical nephrectomy with adjuvant chemotherapy	Radical nephroureterectomy. Adjuvant chemotherapy specific for urothelial carcinoma in advanced disease
Prognosis	Dismal with 20% of patients remaining alive 2 y after diagnosis	Stage dependent: 5-y survival <50% in pT3/pT4 disease

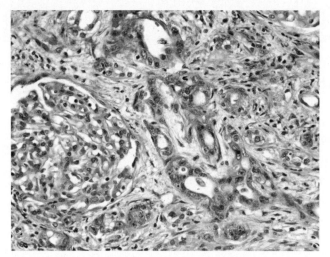

Figure 2.22.1   Collecting duct carcinoma with tubules infiltrating around the glomerulus.

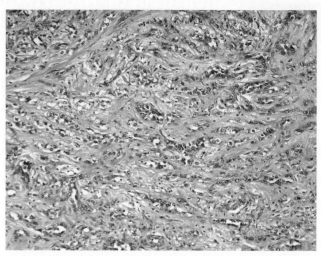

Figure 2.22.2   Collecting duct carcinoma composed of cords of cells in a desmoplastic stroma.

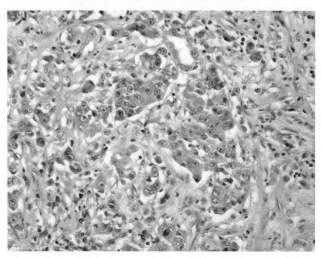

Figure 2.22.3   Collecting duct carcinoma with infiltrating nests of cells with prominent atypia.

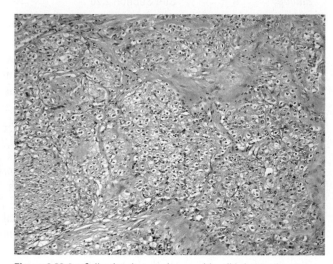

Figure 2.22.4   Collecting duct carcinoma with solid sheets of tumor.

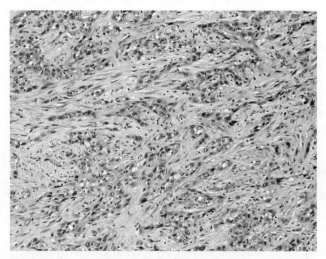

Figure 2.22.5   Invasive renal pelvic urothelial carcinomas with nests of cells in a desmoplastic stroma.

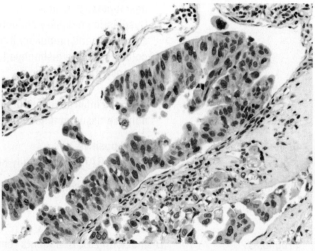

Figure 2.22.6   CIS within the renal pelvis in a patient with invasive urothelial carcinoma.

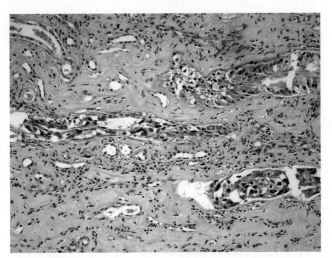

Figure 2.22.7   CIS of the renal pelvis with solid nests extending into collecting ducts.

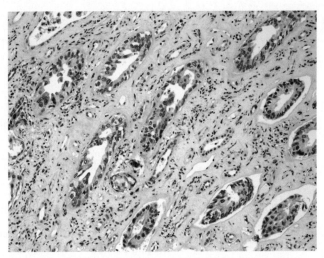

Figure 2.22.8   CIS colonizing collecting ducts with individual cells mimicking dysplastic glandular cells seen in some collecting duct carcinoma.

	Cystic Nephroma (CN)	Mixed Epithelial and Stromal Tumor (MEST)
Age	Middle-aged adults. Strong female predominance (8:1)	Middle-aged adults. Strong female predominance (8:1)
Location	Cortical or medullary. Unifocal	Cortical or medullary, some with herniation of a polypoid mass into the renal pelvis. Unifocal
Symptoms	Abdominal mass, hematuria, flank pain	Abdominal mass, hematuria, flank pain
Signs	Frequently asymptomatic and discovered on imaging studies	Frequently asymptomatic and discovered on imaging studies
Etiology	Unknown. Perimenopausal females or males endogenous or exogenous estrogenic treatment. Most experts consider MEST and CN part of the morphologic spectrum of the same lesion given shared clinicopathologic features	Unknown. Perimenopausal females or males endogenous or exogenous estrogenic treatment
Gross and Histology	1. Encapsulated variable-sized mass with variably sized macroscopic cysts filled with serous fluid *(Fig. 2.23.1)*. Lacks necrosis 2. Variably sized macroscopic cysts. Very thin septae without solid foci *(Fig. 2.23.2)* 3. Cysts lined by bland epithelial columnar/ cuboidal to flat cells with occasional hobnail appearance *(Fig. 2.23.3)*. Degenerative cytoplasmic clearing may be encountered but abundant clear cytoplasm not present. Significant epithelial atypia not present 4. Do not see small tubules or fibroadenomatoid pattern 5. Stroma has areas of hypercellularity acquiring ovarian-like appearance in female patients. Other areas have a more fibrous appearance 6. Confined to the kidney	1. Encapsulated variable-sized mass with solid and cystic areas. Lacks necrosis 2. Focally can have cysts indistinguishable from CN along with cysts with thickened septae to more solid areas with focal cysts *(Figs. 2.23.4–2.23.7)* 3. Epithelium lining cysts and tubules in MEST identical to those lining cysts in CN *(Fig. 2.23.8)* 4. Often proliferation of small tubules with thyroid-like secretions *(Fig. 2.23.9)*. Can be arranged in a fibroadenomatoid/phylloidal pattern *(Figs. 2.23.5, 2.23.10, and 2.23.11)* 5. Ovarian-like stroma, which can also show smooth muscle, fibrous, and adipose differentiation *(Figs. 2.23.9, 2.23.10, and 2.23.12)* 6. Other than occasionally projecting into renal sinus as polypoid mass, organ confined
Special studies	Stromal cells positive for ER, PR, and occasionally CD10, smooth muscle actin, and desmin. Cytokeratins, PAX8, PAX2 positivity in the epithelial cyst lining	Same as cystic nephroma
Treatment	Partial nephrectomy	Partial nephrectomy
Prognosis	Benign	Benign

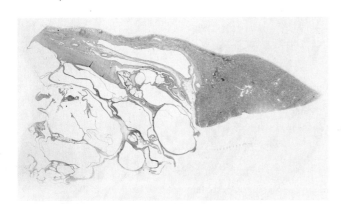

Figure 2.23.1   Scanning magnification of cystic nephroma with multiple cysts separated by thin septae without solid foci.

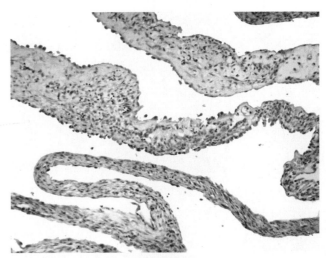

Figure 2.23.2   Cystic nephroma cysts vary minimally in thickness with some having cellular ovarian-like stroma.

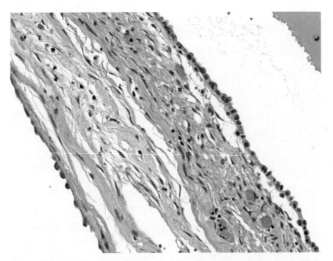

Figure 2.23.3   Cystic nephroma cysts lined by bland epithelial cuboidal-to-flat cells.

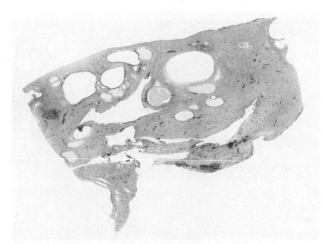

Figure 2.23.4   MEST with equal mixture of cysts and stroma.

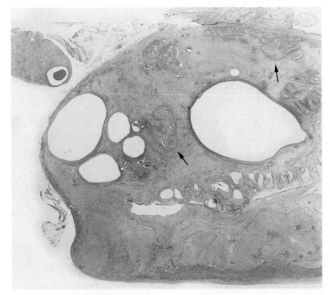

Figure 2.23.5   MEST with a more prominent stromal component including fibroadenomatoid foci (*arrows*).

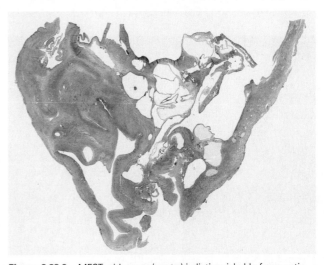

Figure 2.23.6   MEST with areas (*center*) indistinguishable from cystic nephroma.

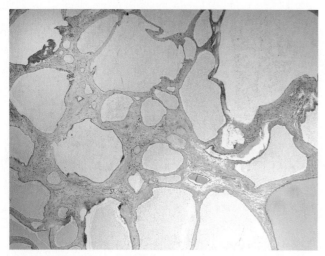

Figure 2.23.7   MEST with variably sized cysts separated by fibrous stroma, more than what is seen in cystic nephroma.

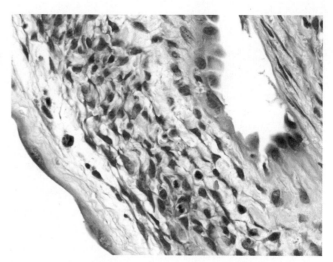

Figure 2.23.8   MEST with tubules with attenuated lining (*lower left*) and cuboidal epithelium surrounded by ovarian-like stroma.

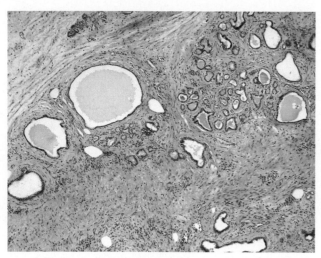

Figure 2.23.9   MEST with proliferation of small tubules containing dense colloid.

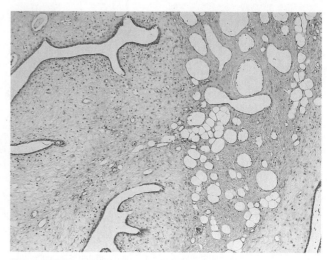

Figure 2.23.10   MEST with adipose tissue.

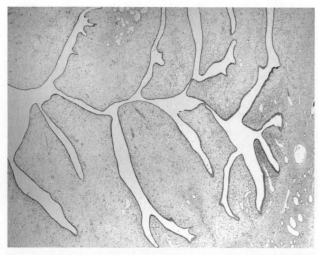

Figure 2.23.11   Same case as Figure 2.23.10 with a phylloidal pattern.

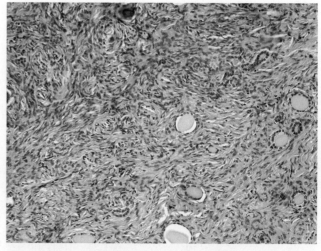

Figure 2.23.12   Solid MEST with extensive ovarian-like stroma and small tubules with colloid secretions.

	Sarcomatoid Renal Cell Carcinoma	Leiomyosarcoma of the Kidney
Age	Mean age 60 y	Mean age around 60 y (20s to elderly)
Location	Can be cortical or medullary. Often large involving both	Typically involves most of the kidney
Symptoms/Signs	Abdominal mass, hematuria, flank pain	Abdominal mass, hematuria, flank pain Mass on imaging
Etiology	Unknown	Most likely arises from either intrarenal blood vessels or muscle fibers of the renal pelvis *(Fig. 2.24.8)*
Gross and Histology	1. Grossly, large masses. Bulging, fleshy gray-white. May have necrosis 2. May be seen with any histologic subtype of RCC or can occur in pure form without recognizable histologic subtype of RCC *(Fig. 2.24.1)* 3. Arranged in haphazard spindle cells often lacking well-formed fascicles *(Fig. 2.24.2)* 4. Spindle cells are overtly atypical and can have pleomorphic giant cells *(Fig. 2.24.3)* 5. Frequent mitotic figures 6. Necrosis common *(Fig. 2.24.4)* 7. By definition high grade, Fuhrman grade 4 8. Typically infiltrates widely into adjacent renal parenchyma *(Fig. 2.24.5)*	1. Large masses (mean size 13.4 cm). Can be same as sarcomatoid RCC 2. Not associated with RCC 3. With rare exception, composed of well-formed fascicles *(Fig. 2.24.9)*. Occasional cases with areas of bizarre pleomorphic cells with haphazard growth pattern 4. Range of atypia from low-grade tumors with nuclear hyperchromasia, yet relatively uniform cytology to cases with more prominent atypia. Nuclei typically ovoid cigar shaped often with perinuclear vacuoles *(Fig. 2.24.10)*. Occasionally, marked pleomorphism *(Figs. 2.24.11 and 2.24.12)* 5. Range of mitotic activity but on average around 10 per 10 HPF 6. Necrosis common 7. All tumors high grade (grade 2 or grade 3) 8. Often a relatively well-circumscribed lesion without infiltration around preexisting glomeruli and renal tubules
Special studies	• PAX8 positive in approximately 70% of sarcomatoid areas • Pancytokeratin can also be positive to a lesser extent *(Figs. 2.24.6 and 2.24.7)* • Focal desmin can be uncommonly seen *(Fig. 2.24.7)*.	• PAX8 negative • Focal keratin can be seen • Typically diffuse desmin positive
Treatment	Radical nephrectomy	Radical nephrectomy
Prognosis	Approximately a 30% survival. Even focal sarcomatoid pattern associated with a poor prognosis and not necessary to quantify the percent of sarcomatoid growth pattern	Distant metastases identified in 90% of patients; 75% of all patients eventually died of tumor. Metastases most commonly seen in the lungs; other organs affected by metastases include liver, bone, and other random sites

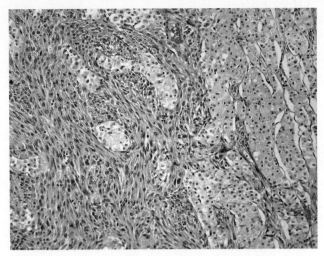

Figure 2.24.1   Sarcomatoid renal cell carcinoma composed of chromophobe RCC (*right*) and nonspecific malignant cells (*left*).

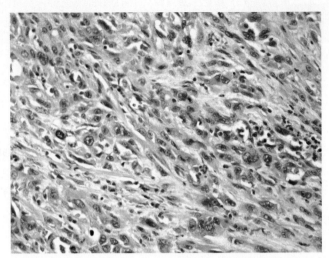

Figure 2.24.2   Sarcomatoid renal cell carcinoma with haphazard array of highly atypical spindle cells.

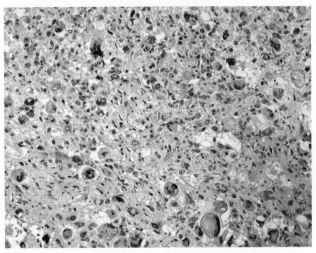

Figure 2.24.3   Sarcomatoid renal cell carcinoma with pleomorphic giant cells.

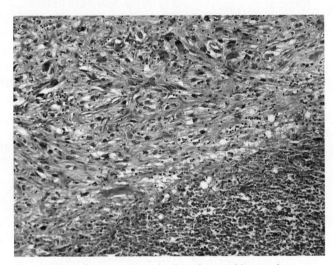

Figure 2.24.4   Sarcomatoid renal cell carcinoma with necrosis.

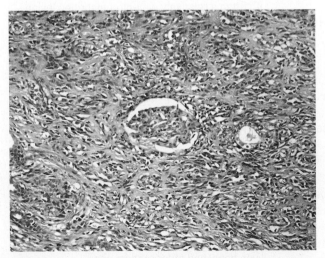

Figure 2.24.5   Sarcomatoid renal cell carcinoma infiltrating around normal kidney structures.

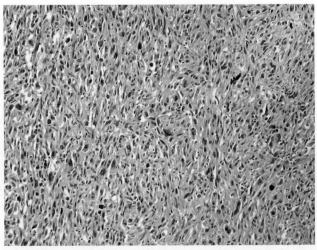

Figure 2.24.6   Sarcomatoid renal cell carcinoma with haphazard arrangement of highly atypical spindle cells.

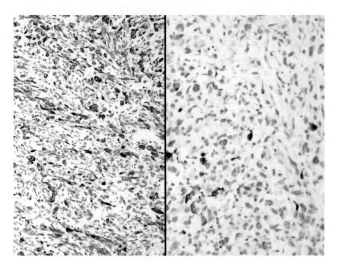

Figure 2.24.7   Same case as Figure 2.24.6 with pancytokeratin staining (**left**) and focal desmin staining (**right**).

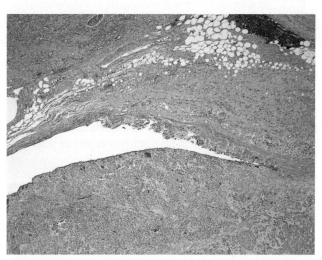

Figure 2.24.8   Leiomyosarcoma of the kidney arising from a large vessel in the renal hilum.

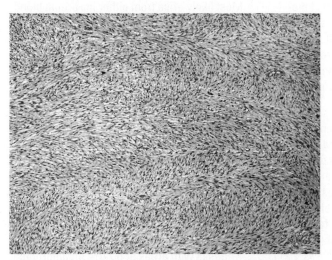

Figure 2.24.9   Same case as Figure 2.24.8 well formed with fascicles.

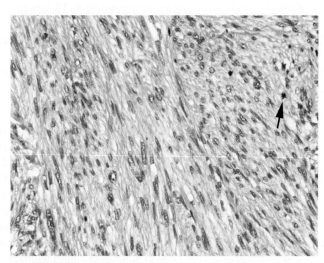

Figure 2.24.10   Same case as Figures 2.24.8 and 2.24.9 with cigar-shaped nuclei, perinuclear vacuoles, mitotic figures (*arrow*), and moderate nuclear pleomorphism.

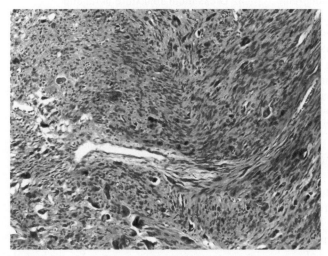

Figure 2.24.11   Leiomyosarcoma of the kidney with mixture of better differentiated areas and more atypical foci.

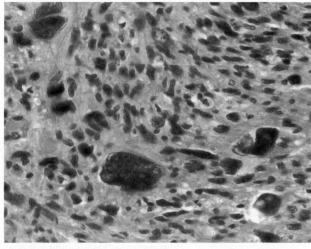

Figure 2.24.12   Same case as Figure 2.24.11 with focal pleomorphic tumor giant cells.

	Angiomyolipoma (AML)	Leiomyosarcoma of the Kidney
Age	Adults. Peak incidence in fifth decade. Earlier in the setting of tuberous sclerosis (TS). Female predilection	Mean age around 60 y (20s to elderly)
Location	Cortical or medullary. Unifocal in sporadic with multiple bilateral lesions in TS	Typically involves most of the kidney
Symptoms	Abdominal mass, hematuria, flank pain secondary to rupture/hemorrhage	Abdominal mass, hematuria, flank pain
Signs	In TS patients, AML are detected on imaging surveillance	Mass on imaging
Etiology	Unknown in sporadic. In TS, inactivation of the *TSC1/2* (hamartin/tuberin) tumor suppressor gene. Autosomal dominant. In addition to AML, also see renal cysts, rarely clear cell RCC, pancreatic cysts, pulmonary lymphangioleiomyoma, cutaneous angiofibroma, and CNS tubers and subependymal giant cell astrocytomas	Most likely arise from either intrarenal blood vessels or renal pelvis muscle
Gross and Histology	1. Grossly, well circumscribed with minimal infiltrative borders. Hemorrhage and cyst formation common. Gross depends on proportions of fat, smooth muscle, and vascular components. Surgically resected AML tend to resemble smooth muscle tumors 2. Smooth muscle component can be fascicular indistinguishable from smooth muscle tumor and in other areas more haphazard *(Figs. 2.25.1 and 2.25.2)* 3. In some areas, spindle cells radiate off of the vessel walls *(Fig. 2.25.3)* 4. May see focal admixture of fat and abnormal vascular structures *(Figs. 2.25.1 and 2.25.4)* 5. Smooth muscle cells have identical nuclei to those in low-grade leiomyosarcomas yet the cytoplasm is looser and filamentous 6. Spindle cells can show focal nuclear atypia *(Figs. 2.25.5 and 2.25.6)*. Epithelioid areas with bizarre nuclei can also be seen less frequently (see Section 2.26) 7. Hyalinized collagen common *(Figs. 2.25.7 and 2.25.8)* 8. Necrosis, increased mitoses, and atypical mitoses typically with epithelioid variant 9. Extrarenal extension and involvement of perirenal lymph node not evidence of malignant behavior	1. Large masses (mean size 13.4 cm). Grossly, encapsulated variable-sized mass with solid and cystic areas 2. With rare exception, composed of well-formed fascicles *(Fig. 2.25.9)*. Occasional cases with areas of bizarre pleomorphic cells with haphazard growth pattern 3. Can arise off of large vessels in the hilum of the kidney but within the tumor 4. Lacks focal admixture of fat and abnormal vascular structures 5. Nuclei are cigar shaped with cytoplasm lacking the filamentous appearance seen in AML *(Fig. 2.25.10)* 6. Range of atypia from low-grade tumors with nuclear hyperchromasia yet relatively uniform to cases with more prominent atypia. Occasionally, marked pleomorphism and epithelioid morphology 7. Hyalinized collagen uncommon 8. Range of mitotic activity but on average around 10 per 10HPF. Necrosis common. All tumors high grade (grade 2/3 or grade 3/3) 9. Often involves perirenal soft tissue

	Angiomyolipoma (AML)	Leiomyosarcoma of the Kidney
Special studies	• Positive for HMB-45, Melan A, and tyrosinase. S100 protein can be positive • Smooth muscle actin and desmin often also positive • Cytokeratins negative in spindle cells • PAX8 negative in spindle cells	• HMB-45, Melan A, tyrosinase, and S100 protein negative • Typically diffuse desmin positive • Focal keratin positivity can be seen • PAX8 negative
Treatment	Partial or radical nephrectomy	Radical nephrectomy
Prognosis	Benign unless atypical and epithelioid (see Section 2.26)	Distant metastases in 90% of patients; 75% of all patients eventually died of tumor. Metastases most commonly seen in the lungs. Other organs affected by metastases include liver, bone, and other random sites

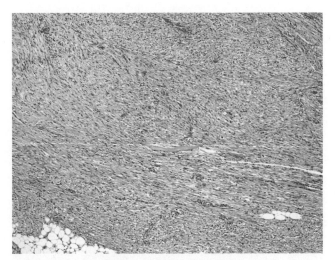

Figure 2.25.1   Angiomyolipoma (AML) composed primarily of fascicles of smooth muscle with a focal adipose component (*bottom left*).

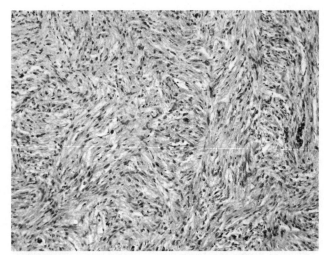

Figure 2.25.2   AML with more haphazard array of smooth muscle with less fascicular growth pattern.

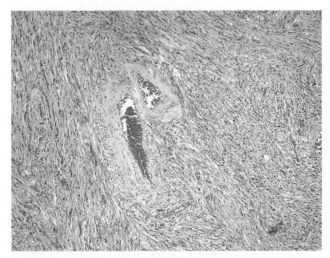

Figure 2.25.3   AML with a smooth muscle component radiating off of vessels.

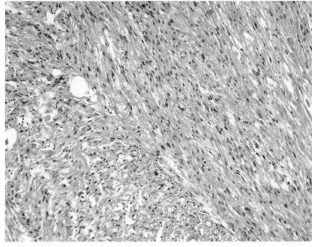

Figure 2.25.4   AML with fascicles of smooth muscle cut in different planes. Note rare adipocytes (*upper left*).

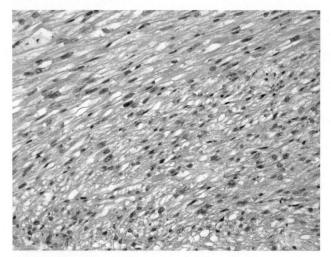

Figure 2.25.5   AML with focal nuclear enlargement and hyperchromasia.

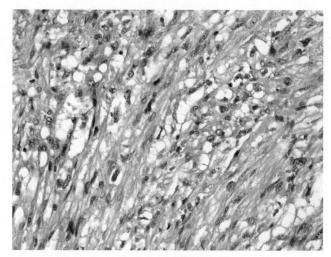

Figure 2.25.6   AML with focal mild nuclear atypia.

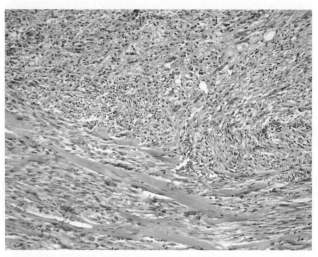

Figure 2.25.7   AML with focal bands of hyalinized collagen.

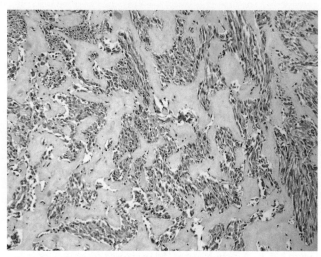

Figure 2.25.8   AML with abundant hyalinized collagen.

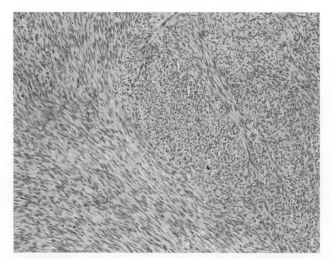

Figure 2.25.9   Leiomyosarcoma of the kidney showing typical anastomosing bundle architecture.

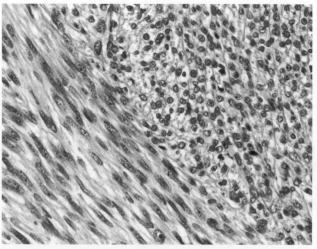

Figure 2.25.10   Same case as Figure 2.25.9 with cigar-shaped nuclei and lack of pale filamentous cytoplasm.

	Epithelioid Angiomyolipoma with Atypia	Renal Cell Carcinoma, Unclassified Type
Age	Adults. Peak incidence in fourth decade. Earlier in setting of tuberous sclerosis (TS)	Adults, peak incidence in sixth decade
Location	Cortical or medullary. Unifocal in sporadic. Multiple, bilateral in TS	Usually unifocal
Symptoms	Frequently presents with abdominal mass, hematuria, or flank pain secondary to rupture/hemorrhage	Pain, hematuria, flank mass. Less likely to be incidentally detected during abdominal and pelvic imaging
Signs	In TS patients, detected on imaging surveillance	Abdominal mass, detectable on imaging
Etiology	See Section 2.25	Unknown
Gross and Histology	1. Large, grossly infiltrative tumors with extrarenal extension and renal vessels invasion. Usually tan solid with areas of hemorrhage and necrosis 2. Epithelioid cells have an overall high N/C ratio with a variable amount of pale clear to eosinophilic cytoplasm. Often has population of pleomorphic cells with multinucleation and abundant cytoplasm termed "amoeboid cells" *(Figs. 2.26.1–2.26.5)* 3. In some cases, ordinary AML with adipose cells and abnormal vessels may be present 4. May show high mitotic activity and atypical mitotic forms *(Fig. 2.26.6)* 5. Areas of necrosis are frequently present 6. May have vascular invasion *(Figs. 2.26.7 and 2.26.8)* 7. Extrarenal extension is often encountered in malignant examples	1. Variable morphology not conforming to those of typical RCC subtypes. If high grade, solid masses usually with pushing borders often with necrosis and hemorrhage 2. May be composed of sheets of anaplastic polygonal cells with eosinophilic cytoplasm lacking acinar or tubular arrangement. Prominent nucleoli, large nuclei with multinucleated tumor cells are found (Fuhrman grades 3–4) *(Figs. 2.26.9 and 2.26.10)* 3. Lacks features of usual AML 4. Mitotic figures increased in high grade lesions 5. Necrosis common 6. Vascular invasion common 7. Extrarenal extension including vascular invasion often seen in high-grade tumors
Special studies	• Typically positive for HMB-45, Melan A, tyrosinase *(Fig. 2.26.4)* • Cytokeratins and PAX8 negative	• HMB-45, Melan A, tyrosinase negative • Cytokeratins and PAX8 positive
Treatment	Nephrectomy	Partial or radical nephrectomy for localized disease
Prognosis	In one-third of cases, recurrence and metastasis. Malignant behavior correlated with presence of three of the four following features: (a) >70% atypical epithelioid areas, (b) ≥2 mitoses per 10 HPF, (c) atypical mitotic figures, or (d) necrosis	Primarily stage, grade, and clinical performance status dependent

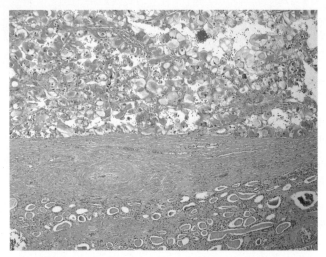

Figure 2.26.1   Epithelioid angiomyolipoma (AML) with atypia consisting of sheets of cells.

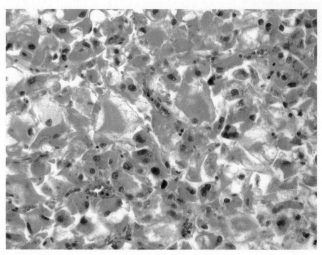

Figure 2.26.2   Same case as Figure 2.26.1 with sheets of large cells with abundant densely eosinophilic cytoplasm.

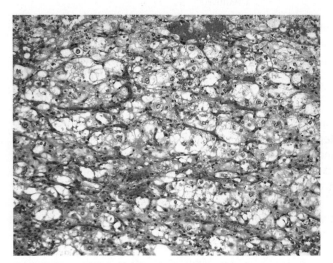

Figure 2.26.3   Epithelioid AML with nests of clear cells mimicking clear cell RCC.

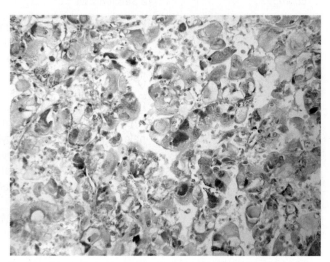

Figure 2.26.4   Same case as Figures 2.26.1 and 2.26.2 positive for HMB-45.

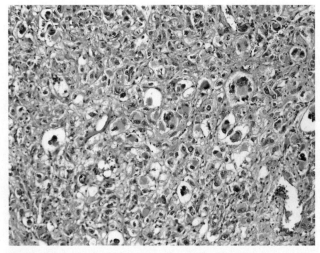

Figure 2.26.5   Epithelioid AML with numerous pleomorphic tumor giant cells.

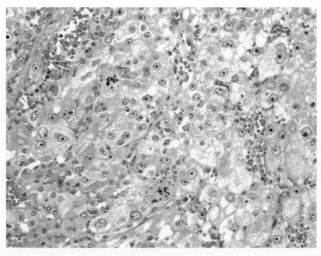

Figure 2.26.6   Epithelioid AML with atypical mitotic figures.

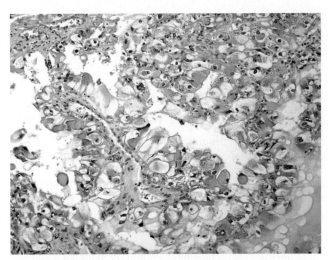

Figure 2.26.7   Epithelioid AML with atypia consisting of large pleomorphic cells with both dense eosinophilic and paler cytoplasm.

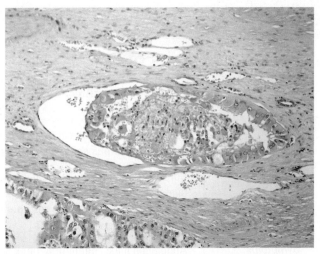

Figure 2.26.8   Same case as Figure 2.26.7 with vascular invasion.

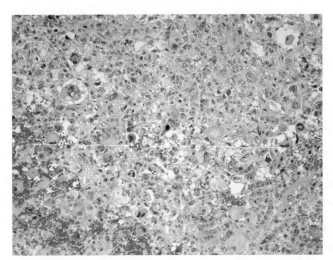

Figure 2.26.9   Renal cell carcinoma, unclassified type with numerous pleomorphic tumor giant cells.

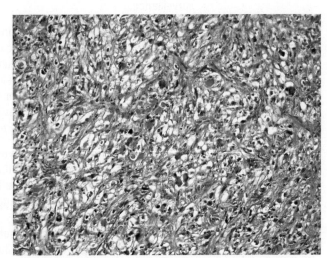

Figure 2.26.10   Clear cell carcinoma Fuhrman grade 4 with slight spindling of clear cells and tumor giant cells with eosinophilic cytoplasm.

2 KIDNEY

	Angiomyolipoma (AML)	Lipoma/Normal Retroperitoneal Adipose Tissue
Age	Adults. Peak incidence in fifth decade. Earlier in the setting of tuberous sclerosis (TS). Female predilection	Typically biopsied in adults
Location	Cortical or medullary. Unifocal in sporadic. Multiple bilateral renal AMLs in 70% of TS patients. Can extend from surface of cortex into retroperitoneum where manifests as a perirenal mass	Either in the kidney or in perirenal tissue
Symptoms	Abdominal mass, hematuria, flank pain secondary to rupture/hemorrhage	Flank pain secondary to hemorrhage into retroperitoneal fat
Signs	In TS patients, AML are detected on imaging surveillance	Lipomas may be seen on imaging
Etiology	Unknown in sporadic. In TS, inactivation of the *TSC1/2* (hamartin/tuberin) tumor suppressor gene on 9q34/16p13. Autosomal dominant. In addition to multiple bilateral renal AML, renal cysts, rarely clear cell RCC, pancreatic cysts, pulmonary lymphangioleiomyoma, cutaneous angiofibroma and central nervous system tubers, and subependymal giant cell astrocytoma tumors	Unknown in lipoma. Retroperitoneal hemorrhage due to multiple etiologies could mimic hemorrhage into fat-predominant AML
Gross and Histology	1. Well-circumscribed masses with minimal infiltrative borders. Cut surface with fat-predominant AML resembles a lipoma. Retroperitoneal fat-predominant AML with hemorrhage difficult to recognize grossly as a tumor 2. Vast majority of the lesion can resemble normal adipose tissue. Occasional expanded space between adipocytes containing cells with lightly eosinophilic filamentous cytoplasm *(Figs. 2.27.1–2.27.4)*. Hemorrhage can mask the tumor cells *(Fig. 2.27.5)* 3. Occasional small- to medium-sized vessels where the outer border of the vessel is not well defined and PEComa cells radiate off the vessel into surrounding adipose tissue	1. Intrarenal lipoma indistinguishable from other lipomas. Hemorrhage into retroperitoneal adipose tissue difficult to distinguish from fat-predominant AML with hemorrhage 2. Normal adipose tissue lacking subtle PEComa filamentous cells 3. Lacks spindle cells radiating off of the vessel walls
Special studies	• Spindle cell component positive for HMB-45, Melan A, tyrosinase • Smooth muscle actin and desmin often also positive • S100 can be positive	• Negative for HMB-45, Melan A, tyrosinase • Negative for smooth muscle actin and desmin • S100 positive
Treatment	Partial or radical nephrectomy or excision of retroperitoneal lesion	None
Prognosis	Benign although can involve lymph nodes *(Fig. 2.27.6)*. Can have significant morbidity and even mortality due to massive retroperitoneal hemorrhage	If lipoma of the kidney, benign. If retroperitoneal hemorrhage, then prognosis depends on the extent of hemorrhage and etiology

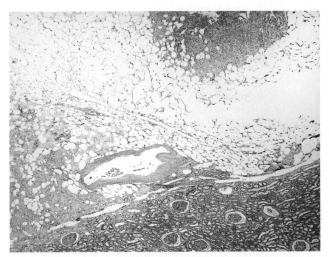

Figure 2.27.1   Angiomyolipoma (AML) predominantly composed of adipose tissue arising from cortical surface of the kidney.

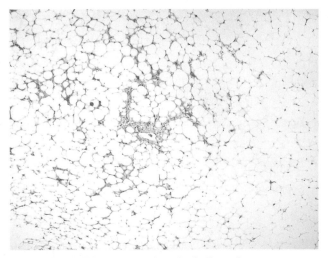

Figure 2.27.2   AML composed of mostly of adipose tissue.

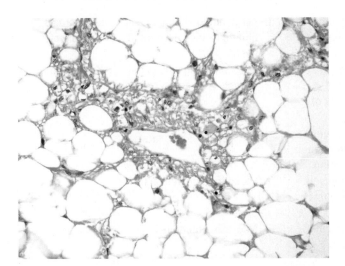

Figure 2.27.3   Same case as Figure 2.27.2 with focal vessel PECOMA smooth muscle spindling off a small vessel.

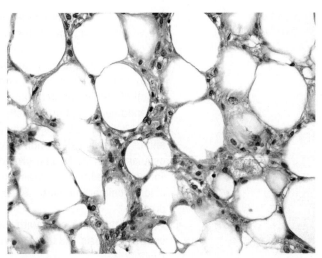

Figure 2.27.4   Same case as Figures 2.27.2 and 2.27.3 with PECOMA cells interspersed between adipose tissue. Cells have delicate fibrillar cytoplasm.

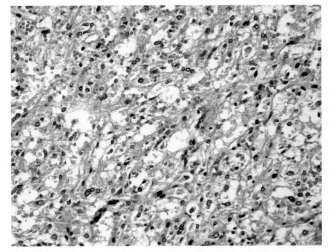

Figure 2.27.5   Fat-predominant AML with hemorrhage, which masks the tumor cells.

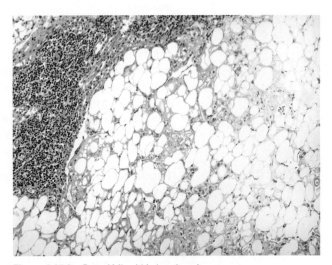

Figure 2.27.6   Fatty AML within lymph node.

	Anastomosing Hemangioma	Angiosarcoma
Age	No sex predominance. Adults from 40s to elderly	Male predominance. Typically in adults, mean age around 60 y
Location	Cortical. Unifocal	Cortical. Unifocal
Symptom	Usually none	Flank pain, mass, hematuria. May have cachexia with weight loss and fever. Symptoms from metastases at time of presentation
Signs	Often detected on imaging done for other reasons	Large mass on imaging
Etiology	Unknown	Some associated with immunosuppression
Gross and Histology	1. Grossly, well-demarcated mahogany brown with spongy consistency. Typically 1–2 cm 2. Anastomosing sinusoidal capillary-sized vessels with scattered hobnail endothelial cells within a framework of nonendothelial supporting cells *(Figs. 2.28.1–2.28.4)*. Loose stromal edema and/or stromal hyalinization between the cellular zones of vascular proliferation 3. Tortuous "feeding" and draining vessels of large caliber (both arteries and veins) present 4. Vascular thrombi typical with zones of central sclerosis and focal necrosis *(Fig. 2.28.5)* 5. Lacks cellular atypia, multilayering of endothelial cells, and apoptotic figures with only rare mitotic activity *(Figs. 2.28.3 and 2.28.4)* 6. Prominent extramedullary hematopoiesis and striking hyaline globules reminiscent of those seen in Kaposi sarcoma in a minority of cases *(Figs. 2.28.6 and 2.28.7)* 7. Minor extension into adjacent adipose tissue and rarely can predominantly grow within the renal vein *(Figs. 2.28.7 and 2.28.8)*	1. Large hemorrhagic masses with necrosis and infiltrative borders into perirenal soft tissue 2. Anastomosing sinusoidal capillary-sized vessels with scattered hobnail endothelial cells 3. Lacks feeding vessels 4. Necrosis common 5. Prominent atypia with highly cellular, malignant-appearing, mitotically active endothelial cells showing at least focal formation of vascular channels. Solid epithelioid areas and areas of spindle cell morphology frequently present 6. Can see extramedullary hematopoiesis and hyaline globules in some angiosarcomas 7. Typically invades adjacent adipose tissue
Special studies	• Positive for CD34, CD31, and other vascular markers • Negative for keratin AE1/3	• Positive for CD34, CD31, and other vascular markers • Epithelioid variant can be keratin positive
Treatment	Partial or radical nephrectomy or excision of retroperitoneal lesion	Surgery and chemotherapy with radiotherapy tailored to the individual case
Prognosis	Benign	Poor with average survival 6–7 mo

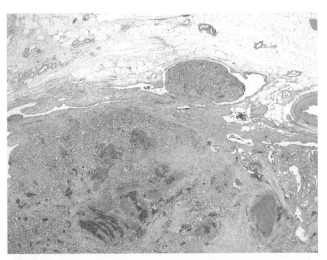

Figure 2.28.1   Low magnification of an anastomosing hemangioma of the renal pelvis. The lesion has an overall lobulated appearance, and there is a nearby medium-sized vein into which the lesion has extended.

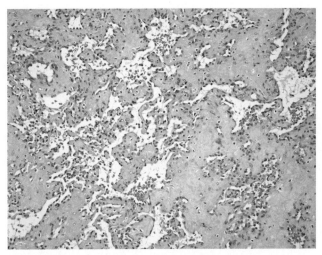

Figure 2.28.2   Anastomosing vessels of anastomosing hemangioma.

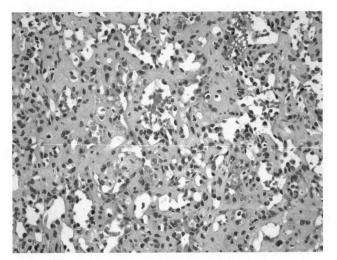

Figure 2.28.3   Same case as Figure 2.28.2 with bland cytology.

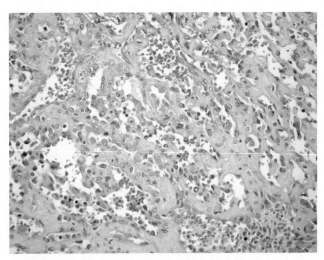

Figure 2.28.4   Same case as Figures 2.28.2 and 2.28.3 with intravascular tufting.

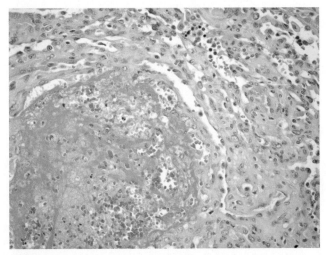

Figure 2.28.5   Anastomosing hemangioma with thrombi.

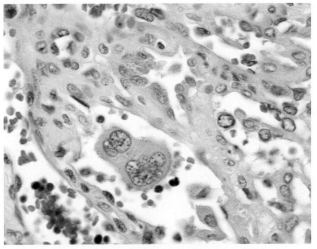

Figure 2.28.6   Anastomosing hemangioma with cytoplasmic hyaline globules and megakaryocyte as evidence of extramedullary hematopoiesis.

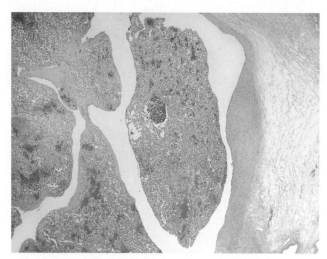

Figure 2.28.7   Renal vein involvement by an anastomosing hemangioma.

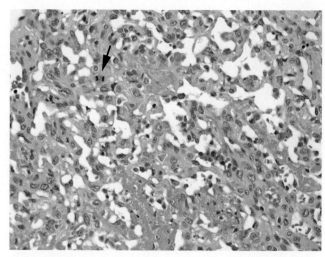

Figure 2.28.8   Same case as Figure 2.28.7 with anastomosing channels lined by bland endothelium containing fibrin. A rare mitotic figure is noted (*arrow*).

SUGGESTED READINGS

2.1–2.7

Ellison DA, Parham DM, Bridge J, Beckwith JB. Immuno-histochemistry of primary malignant neuroepithelial tumors of the kidney: a potential source of confusion? A study of 30 cases from the national wilms tumor study pathology center. *Hum Pathol.* 2007;38:205–211.

Gadd S, Beezhold P, Jennings L, et al. Mediators of receptor tyrosine kinase activation in infantile fibrosarcoma: a children's oncology group study. *J Pathol.* 2012;228:119–130.

Parham DM. Neuroectodermal and neuroendocrine tumors principally seen in children. *Am J Clin Pathol.* 2001;115(Suppl): S113–S128.

2.8–2.9

Moch H. Cystic renal neoplasms: new entities and molecular findings. *Pathologe.* 2010;31(Suppl 2):239–243.

Srigley JR, Delahunt B, Eble JN, et al. The international society of urological pathology (ISUP) vancouver classification of renal neoplasia. *Am J Surg Pathol.* 2013;37:1469–1489.

Suzigan S, Lopez-Beltran A, Montironi R, et al. Multilocular cystic renal cell carcinoma : a report of 45 cases of a kidney tumor of low malignant potential. *Am J Clin Pathol.* 2006;125:217–222.

2.10–2.11

Al-Ahmadie HA, Alden D, Fine SW, et al. Role of immunohisto-chemistry in the evaluation of needle core biopsies in adult renal cortical tumors: an ex vivo study. *Am J Surg Pathol.* 2011;35:949–961.

Tan PH, Cheng L, Rioux-Leclercq N, et al. Renal tumors: diagnostic and prognostic biomarkers. *Am J Surg Pathol.* 2013;37:1518–1531.

Tickoo SK, Reuter VE. Differential diagnosis of renal tumors with papillary architecture. *Adv Anat Pathol.* 2011;18:120–132.

2.12

Argani P, Netto GJ, Parwani AV. Papillary renal cell carcinoma with low-grade spindle cell foci: a mimic of mucinous tubular and spindle cell carcinoma. *Am J Surg Pathol.* 2008;32:1353–1359.

Fine SW, Argani P, DeMarzo AM, et al. Expanding the histologic spectrum of mucinous tubular and spindle cell carcinoma of the kidney. *Am J Surg Pathol.* 2006;30:1554–1560.

2.13

Gobbo S, Eble JN, Grignon DJ, et al. Clear cell papillary renal cell carcinoma: a distinct histopathologic and molecular genetic entity. *Am J Surg Pathol.* 2008;32:1239–1245.

Tickoo SK, dePeralta-Venturina MN, Harik LR, et al. Spectrum of epithelial neoplasms in end-stage renal disease: an experience from 66 tumor-bearing kidneys with emphasis on histologic patterns distinct from those in sporadic adult renal neoplasia. *Am J Surg Pathol.* 2006;30:141–153.

Williamson SR, Eble JN, Cheng L, Grignon DJ. Clear cell papillary renal cell carcinoma: differential diagnosis and extended immunohistochemical profile. *Mod Pathol.* 2013;26:697–708.

2.14

Argani P, Hicks J, De Marzo AM, et al. Xp11 translocation renal cell carcinoma (RCC): extended immunohistochemical profile emphasizing novel RCC markers. *Am J Surg Pathol.* 2010;34:1295–1303.

Argani P, Olgac S, Tickoo SK, et al. Xp11 translocation renal cell carcinoma in adults: expanded clinical, pathologic, and genetic spectrum. *Am J Surg Pathol.* 2007;31:1149–1160.

Argani P, Yonescu R, Morsberger L, et al. Molecular confirmation of t(6;11)(p21;q12) renal cell carcinoma in archival paraffin-embedded material using a break-apart TFEB FISH assay expands its clinicopathologic spectrum. *Am J Surg Pathol.* 2012;36:1516–1526.

2.15

Murphy WM, Grignon DJ, Perlman EJ. *Tumors of the Kidney, Bladder, and Related Urinary Structures.* Washington, DC: American Registry of Pathology; 2004.

Sangoi AR, Fujiwara M, West RB, et al. Immunohistochemical distinction of primary adrenal cortical lesions from metastatic clear cell renal cell carcinoma: a study of 248 cases. *Am J Surg Pathol.* 2011;35:678–686.

Ye H, Yoon GS, Epstein JI. Intrarenal ectopic adrenal tissue and renal-adrenal fusion: a report of nine cases. *Mod Pathol.* 2009;22:175–181.

2.16–2.18

Al-Ahmadie HA, Alden D, Fine SW, et al. Role of immunohisto-chemistry in the evaluation of needle core biopsies in adult renal cortical tumors: an ex vivo study. *Am J Surg Pathol.* 2011;35:949–961.

Przybycin CG, Cronin AM, Darvishian F, et al. Chromophobe renal cell carcinoma: a clinicopathologic study of 203 tumors in 200 patients with primary resection at a single institution. *Am J Surg Pathol.* 2011;35:962–970.

Tan PH, Cheng L, Rioux-Leclercq N, et al. Renal tumors: diagnostic and prognostic biomarkers. *Am J Surg Pathol.* 2013;37:1518–1531.

Wang HY, Mills SE. KIT and RCC are useful in distinguishing chromophobe renal cell carcinoma from the granular variant of clear cell renal cell carcinoma. *Am J Surg Pathol.* 2005;29:640–646.

2.19–2.22

Albadine R, Schultz L, Illei P, et al. PAX8 (+)/p63 (-) immunostaining pattern in renal collecting duct carcinoma (CDC): a useful immunoprofile in the differential diagnosis of CDC versus urothelial carcinoma of upper urinary tract. *Am J Surg Pathol.* 2010;34:965–969.

Liu Q, Galli S, Srinivasan R, et al. Renal medullary carcinoma: molecular, immunohistochemistry, and morphologic correlation. *Am J Surg Pathol.* 2013;37:368–374.

MacLennan GT, Farrow GM, Bostwick DG. Low-grade collecting duct carcinoma of the kidney: report of 13 cases of low-grade mucinous tubulocystic renal carcinoma of possible collecting duct origin. *Urology.* 1997;50:679–684.

Srigley JR, Delahunt B, Eble JN, et al. The international society of urological pathology (ISUP) vancouver classification of renal neoplasia. *Am J Surg Pathol.* 2013;37:1469–1489.

2.23

Adsay NV, Eble JN, Srigley JR, et al. Mixed epithelial and stromal tumor of the kidney. *Am J Surg Pathol.* 2000;24:958–970.

Srigley JR, Delahunt B, Eble JN, et al. The international society of urological pathology (ISUP) vancouver classification of renal neoplasia. *Am J Surg Pathol.* 2013;37:1469–1489.

Zhou M, Kort E, Hoekstra P, et al. Adult cystic nephroma and mixed epithelial and stromal tumor of the kidney are the same disease entity: molecular and histologic evidence. *Am J Surg Pathol.* 2009;33:72–80.

2.24–2.27

Brimo F, Robinson B, Guo C, et al. Renal epithelioid angiomyolipoma with atypia: a series of 40 cases with emphasis on clinicopathologic prognostic indicators of malignancy. *Am J Surg Pathol.* 2010;34:715–722.

Chang A, Brimo F, Montgomery EA, Epstein JI. Use of PAX8 and GATA3 in diagnosing sarcomatoid renal cell carcinoma and sarcomatoid urothelial carcinoma. *Hum Pathol.* 2013;44(8):1563–1568.

Miller JS, Zhou M, Brimo F, et al. Primary leiomyosarcoma of the kidney: a clinicopathologic study of 27 cases. *Am J Surg Pathol.* 2010;34:238–242.

Nese N, Martignoni G, Fletcher CD, et al. Pure epithelioid PEComas (so-called epithelioid angiomyolipoma) of the kidney: a clinicopathologic study of 41 cases: detailed assessment of morphology and risk stratification. *Am J Surg Pathol.* 2011;35:161–176.

2.28

Montgomery E, Epstein JI. Anastomosing hemangioma of the genitourinary tract: a lesion mimicking angiosarcoma. *Am J Surg Pathol.* 2009;33:1364–1369.

Zenico T, Saccomanni M, Salomone U, Bercovich E. Primary renal angiosarcoma: case report and review of world literature. *Tumori.* 2011;97:e6–e9.

3

Bladder

	Normal Urothelium	Urothelial Dysplasia
Age	Any age, but typically biopsied in adults	Typically adults
Location	Not pertinent	Anywhere with urothelial lining
Symptoms	Asymptomatic	Asymptomatic
Signs	None. Although biopsy typically done either during follow-up of prior urothelial neoplasia or for mapping at the time of biopsy of urothelial carcinoma to determine multifocality	None. Although biopsy typically done either during follow-up of prior urothelial neoplasia or for mapping at the time of biopsy of urothelial carcinoma to determine multifocality
Etiology	Not pertinent	Precursor in some cases to urothelial carcinoma *in situ* (CIS). Can also be seen adjacent to noninvasive low-grade papillary urothelial carcinoma
Histology	1. Normal thickness consisting of 6–7 cell layers, yet no need to count *(Figs. 3.1.1–3.1.3)* 2. Cohesive cells 3. Umbrella cells present 4. Uniform cells without enlarged hyperchromatic nuclei 5. Mitotic figures typically absent 6. Polarity maintained	1. Range from normal thickness to hyperplastic *(Figs. 3.1.4–3.1.6)* 2. Cohesive cells 3. Umbrella cells present 4. Scattered cells with scattered, slightly enlarged hyperchromatic nuclei *(Figs. 3.1.4–3.1.6)* 5. Mitotic figures typically absent but if few present still consistent with diagnosis *(Fig. 3.1.5)* 6. Polarity in general maintained although slight loss may be present
Special studies	CK20 stains the umbrella cell layer only	CK20 stains full thickness of the urothelium, although exceptions occur
Treatment	Not applicable	Typically, dysplasia itself not treated. Patients followed more closely with shorter-interval cystoscopy and may undergo additional tissue sampling, urine cytology, and urine FISH studies to evaluate for CIS
Prognosis	Not applicable	Increased risk of CIS either concurrently or subsequently, although accurate data on the magnitude of risk are lacking, hampered by poor interobserver reproducibility of diagnosing dysplasia. Studies cite 5%–19% risk of progressing to urothelial carcinoma

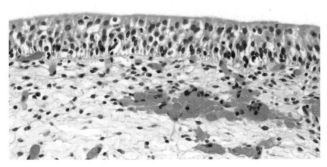

Figure 3.1.1   Normal urothelium.

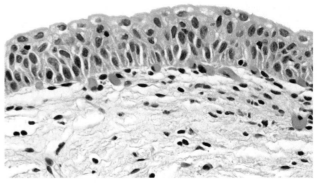

Figure 3.1.2   Urothelium with slight variation in nuclear size still consistent with normal.

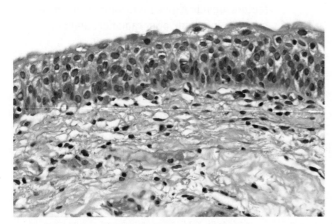

Figure 3.1.3   Normal urothelium with slight variation in polarity but lacking nuclear atypia.

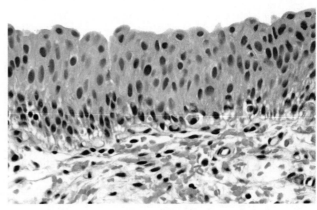

Figure 3.1.4   Dysplasia with scattered mildly enlarged hyperchromatic nuclei.

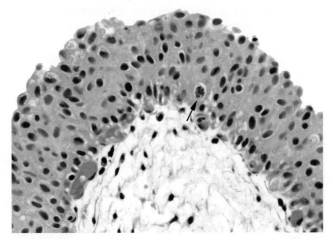

Figure 3.1.5   Dysplasia with scattered mildly enlarged hyperchromatic nuclei and mitotic figures (*arrow*).

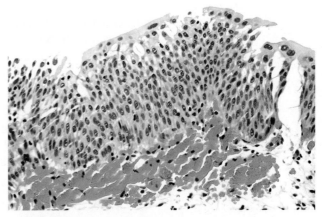

Figure 3.1.6   Dysplasia with a thickened urothelium and diffuse mildly enlarged hyperchromatic nuclei.

	Urothelial Dysplasia	Carcinoma *In Situ* (CIS)
Age	Typically adults	Typically adults
Location	Anywhere with urothelial lining	Anywhere with urothelial lining
Symptoms	Asymptomatic	Asymptomatic or symptoms identical to that seen with urinary tract infections
Signs	None. Although biopsy typically done either during follow-up of prior urothelial neoplasia or for mapping at the time of biopsy of urothelial carcinoma to determine multifocality	None or hematuria, typically microscopic
Etiology	Precursor in some cases to urothelial CIS. Can also be seen adjacent to noninvasive low-grade papillary urothelial carcinoma	Most common is smoking, accounting for 60% and 30% of all urothelial carcinomas in males and females, respectively. Other risk factors include exposure to various chemicals, heredity, infection, prior radiation, and prior cyclophosphamide chemotherapy
Histology	1. Range from normal thickness to hyperplastic 2. Cohesive cells 3. Umbrella cells present 4. Scattered cells with scattered, slightly enlarged hyperchromatic nuclei *(Figs. 3.2.1–3.2.4)* 5. Prominent nucleoli typically absent 6. Relatively uniform nuclear size and shape without irregular nuclei 7. Mitotic figures typically absent 8. Typically abundant cytoplasm 9. Polarity in general maintained although slight loss may be present	1. Varies from a single cell layer to normal thickness to hyperplastic 2. Often dyscohesive cells 3. Umbrella cells typically absent, but in some cases present 4. Markedly enlarged hyperchromatic nuclei (the largest nucleus 5× size of lamina propria lymphocyte nuclei) *(Figs. 3.2.5–3.2.8)* 5. Some cases may show prominent nucleoli *(Fig. 3.2.7)* 6. Variability of nuclear size and shape with scattered, irregular nuclei *(Figs. 3.2.5–3.2.8)* 7. Mitotic figures, sometimes frequent, may be present 8. Cytoplasm ranges from abundant to scant with marked variation of the nuclear-to-cytoplasmic (N:C) ratio 9. Polarity lost resulting in cellular disorder
Special studies	• CK20 stains abnormal cells, although exceptions occur • p53 typically negative • UroVysion FISH may demonstrate aneusomy for chromosomes 3,7,17 or loss of 9p, yet with less frequency than CIS	• CK20 stains abnormal cells, although exceptions occur • p53 may be positive, yet only intense diffuse staining present specific • UroVysion FISH demonstrates aneusomy for chromosomes 3,7,17 or loss of 9p. Sensitivity and specificity are close to 100% for the diagnosis of CIS

	Urothelial Dysplasia	**Carcinoma *In Situ* (CIS)**
Treatment	Typically, dysplasia itself not treated. The patient followed more closely with shorter-interval cystoscopy and may undergo additional tissue sampling, urine cytology to evaluate for CIS	Initial diagnosis of CIS typically treated with a course of intravesicular BCG. If CIS recurs following a complete course of BCG, some authorities recommend immediate cystectomy
Prognosis	Increased risk of CIS either concurrently or subsequently, although accurate data on the magnitude of risk are lacking, hampered by poor interobserver reproducibility of diagnosing dysplasia. Studies cite 5%–19% risk of progressing to urothelial neoplasia	Evolution from CIS to invasion highly variable with some cases having rapid progression and others a more protracted time course. Overall, invasive carcinoma develops in up to 50% of patients within 5 y. The initial tumor-free response with BCG is as high as 84%. Approximately 50% show a durable response for a median of 4 y

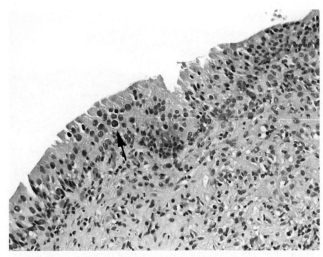

Figure 3.2.1 Dysplasia with scattered, mildly enlarged hyperchromatic nuclei (*arrow*).

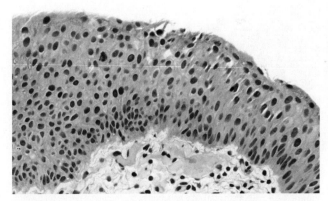

Figure 3.2.2 Dysplasia with scattered, mildly enlarged hyperchromatic nuclei.

3 BLADDER

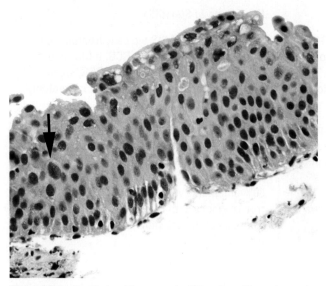

Figure 3.2.3   Dysplasia with scattered, mildly enlarged hyperchromatic nuclei (*arrow*).

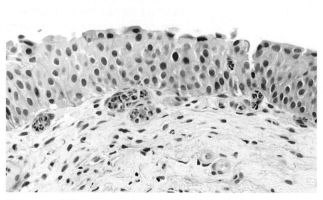

Figure 3.2.4   Dysplasia with scattered, mildly enlarged hyperchromatic nuclei.

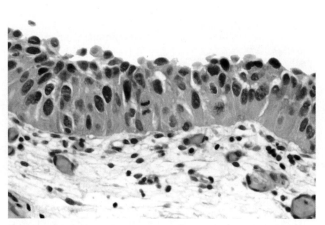

Figure 3.2.5   CIS with markedly enlarged hyperchromatic nuclei relative to stromal lymphocytes. Cells have abundant cytoplasm and a mitotic figure.

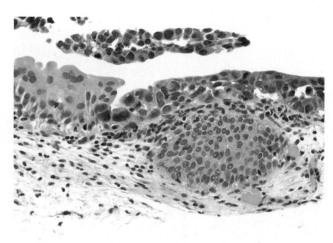

Figure 3.2.6   CIS with markedly enlarged hyperchromatic nuclei relative to the normal urothelium in von Brunn nest.

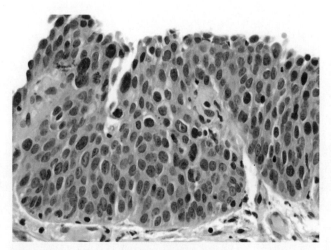

Figure 3.2.7   CIS with variably sized and shaped nuclei. Largest nuclei are markedly enlarged relative to stromal lymphocytes.

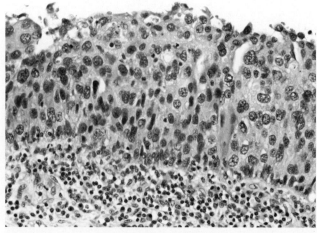

Figure 3.2.8   CIS with a thickened urothelium with diffusely enlarged and hyperchromatic nuclei.

	Normal Urothelium on Frozen Sections of the Ureter	Carcinoma *In Situ* (CIS) on Frozen Sections of the Ureter
Age	Adults	Typically adults
Location	Distal ureter	Distal ureter
Symptoms	None	Asymptomatic in this setting
Signs	None	None in this setting
Etiology	Frozen sections of the ureter margin typically done at the time of cystectomy for urothelial carcinoma	Frozen sections of the ureter margin typically done at the time of cystectomy for urothelial carcinoma
Histology	1. Using the 10× lens, nuclei should appear very small and do not stand out as abnormal. Appears almost the same size as lymphocyte nuclei *(Figs. 3.3.1–3.3.4)* 2. Normal thickness consisting of six to seven cell layers, yet no need to count 3. Cohesive cells, yet difficult to evaluate with a frozen-section artifact 4. Umbrella cells present, yet hard to appreciate on frozen section 5. Mitotic figures typically absent 6. At most minimal variability of nuclear size and shape, yet variability can be exaggerated at high magnification on frozen section	1. Using the 10× lens, some nuclei appear large and abnormal *(Figs. 3.3.5–3.3.8)* 2. May vary from just a single cell layer to normal thickness to hyperplastic 3. Often dyscohesive cells ranging from cells just starting to detach from each other, to clusters of cells lifting off the basement membrane, to more widely dispersed individual cells 4. Umbrella cells typically absent, but in some cases present 5. Mitotic figures may be present 6. Some variability of nuclear size and shapes among abnormal cells with scattered irregular nuclei
Special studies	Not pertinent	Not pertinent
Treatment	No need to take an additional section of the ureter	Urologist will take an additional section of the ureter closer to the kidney and submit for another frozen section. If there is persistent CIS close to the kidney, most urologists will not perform a nephrectomy to obtain negative margins. The contralateral renal pelvis and ureter are also at increased risk of developing urothelial carcinoma, and renal preservation is critical given the morbidity and mortality of renal dialysis in the situation of bilateral nephrectomies
Prognosis	Still at risk of developing multifocal urothelial neoplasia in the ipsilateral renal pelvis and remaining ureter, as well as rest of the urothelial tract	If CIS is left at a margin and there is recurrence of urothelial carcinoma, it is typically not at the site of the resection but elsewhere in the urothelial tract

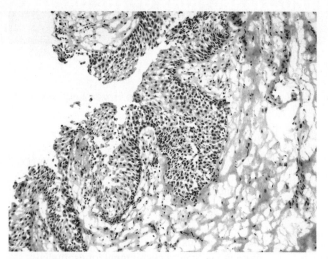

Figure 3.3.1   Benign ureteral margin at frozen section. All images in this chapter are taken at the same magnification of 10× lens.

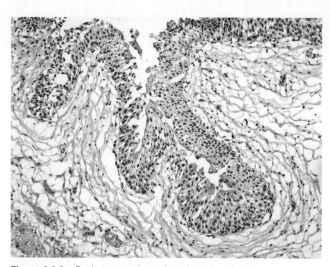

Figure 3.3.2   Benign ureteral margin at frozen section.

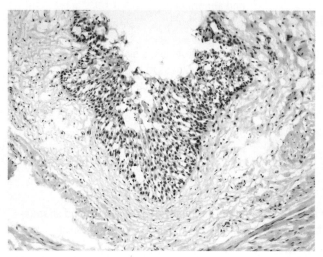

Figure 3.3.3   Benign ureteral margin at frozen section with hyperplastic appearance possibly due to tangential sectioning.

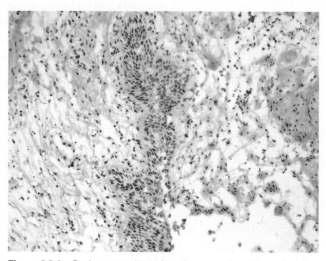

Figure 3.3.4   Benign ureteral margin at frozen section with an air-drying artifact giving rise to an appearance of slightly enlarged nuclei.

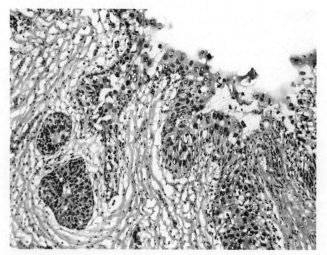

Figure 3.3.5   CIS with overtly enlarged and hyperchromatic nuclei.

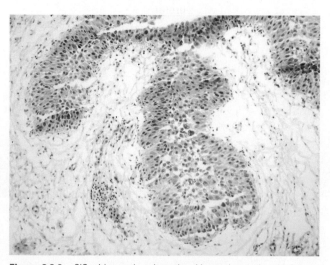

Figure 3.3.6   CIS with overtly enlarged and hyperchromatic nuclei.

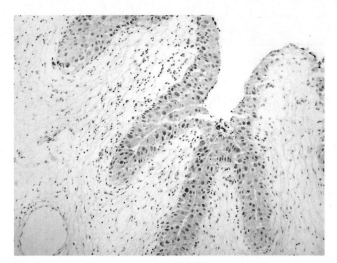

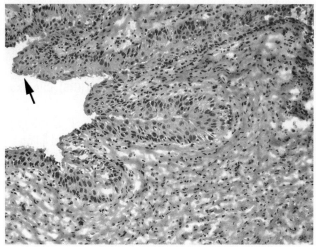

Figure 3.3.7   CIS with overtly enlarged and hyperchromatic nuclei.

Figure 3.3.8   More difficult case where it is borderline CIS, but there is still sufficient nuclear enlargement compared to the more normal urothelium (*arrow*) to ask the urologist to resect more ureter in an attempt to obtain a normal urothelium.

	Carcinoma *In Situ* (CIS), Clinging Type	Denuded Urothelium
Age	Typically adults	Any age, but typically biopsied in adults
Location	Anywhere with urothelial lining	Anywhere with urothelial lining
Symptoms	May be asymptomatic or can have symptoms identical to that associated with urinary tract infections	Asymptomatic
Signs	May be none or can be associated with hematuria, typically microscopic	None. Although biopsy typically done either during follow-up of prior urothelial neoplasia or for mapping at the time of biopsy of urothelial carcinoma to determine multifocality
Etiology	See Section 3.5	May result from instrumentation or shedding of CIS cells
Histology	1. Areas of the specimen lack the urothelium 2. Single cells either resting on the basement membrane or dyscohesive *(Figs. 3.4.1–3.4.5)* 3. Markedly enlarged hyperchromatic nuclei visibly abnormal using the 10× lens with the largest nucleus 5× size of lamina propria lymphocyte nuclei *(Figs. 3.4.1–3.4.5)* 4. Some variability of nuclear size and shapes among abnormal cells with scattered irregular nuclei 5. Mitotic figures, sometimes frequent, may be present	1. Areas of the specimen lack the urothelium 2. May have areas of a preserved cohesive normal urothelium or single cells resting on the basement membrane 3. Preserved urothelium appears like small dots using 10× lens with the largest nucleus 2–3× size of lamina propria lymphocyte nuclei *(Fig. 3.4.6)* 4. Uniform cells without enlarged hyperchromatic nuclei 5. Mitotic figures typically absent unless accompanied by inflammation and reactive changes
Special studies	• CK20 stains abnormal cells, although exceptions occur • p53 may be positive, yet only intense diffuse staining present, specific for CIS • UroVysion FISH demonstrates aneusomy for chromosomes 3, 7, 17 or loss of 9p	• CK20 negative in cells, as the only positive cells are umbrella cells, which are absent in areas of denudation • p53 negative yet false positive occurs with weak to moderate nuclear staining • UroVysion FISH demonstrates lack of aneusomy for chromosomes 3,7,17 or loss of 9p. Sensitivity and specificity are close to 100% for the diagnosis of CIS
Treatment	Same treatment as usual CIS (see Section 3.2)	Denudation is an abnormal finding especially if biopsy taken without the use of cautery. Urinary cytology and close follow-up recommended due to the associated finding of denudation with concurrent or subsequent CIS

	Carcinoma *In Situ* (CIS), Clinging Type	Denuded Urothelium
Prognosis	Same prognosis as usual CIS (see Section 3.2)	In the setting of denuded biopsies, CIS develops within 24 mo in 45% of patients where specimens obtained by cold cup biopsy compared to none obtained by hot wire loop biopsy. CIS develops within 24 mo in 75% of patients if in addition to cold cup biopsy there is a history of CIS vs. 29% if cold cup biopsy and no history of CIS

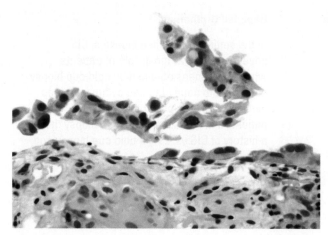

Figure 3.4.1   CIS with lifting of the urothelium from the basement membrane.

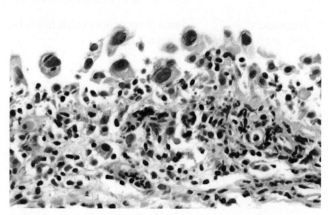

Figure 3.4.2   CIS with loosely cohesive cells with markedly enlarged hyperchromatic nuclei.

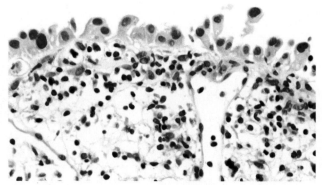

Figure 3.4.3   CIS with loosely cohesive cells with markedly enlarged hyperchromatic nuclei. The largest nucleus (*left*) is four to five times the size of lymphocytes.

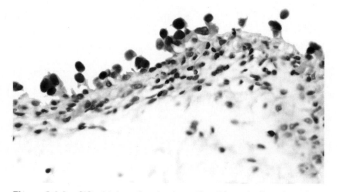

Figure 3.4.4   CIS with loosely cohesive cells with markedly enlarged hyperchromatic nuclei.

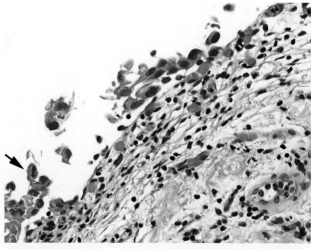

Figure 3.4.5   CIS with loosely cohesive cells with markedly enlarged hyperchromatic nuclei and mitotic figures (*arrow*).

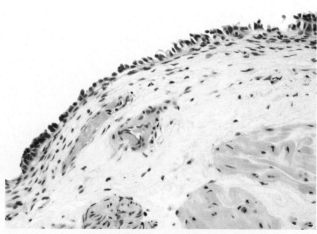

Figure 3.4.6   Benign urothelium with denudation. The remaining urothelium consists of cells with relatively small uniform nuclei.

	Carcinoma *In Situ* (CIS)	Reactive Urothelium
Age	Typically adults	Any age, but typically biopsied in adults
Location	Anywhere with urothelial lining	Anywhere with urothelial lining
Symptoms	May be asymptomatic or can have symptoms identical to that associated with urinary tract infections	Asymptomatic or may be associated symptoms relating to specific etiology
Signs	May be none or can be associated with hematuria, typically microscopic	Associated signs relating to any condition that irritates the bladder.
Etiology	Numerous environmental risk factors. Most common is history of smoking, accounting for 60% and 30% of all urothelial carcinomas in males and females, respectively. Other risk factors include exposure to various chemicals (especially aromatic amines), heredity, infection, prior radiation, and prior chemotherapy with cyclophosphamide	Some of the more common situations resulting in a reactive urothelium include urinary calculi, colovesical fistula, infection, and instrumentation
Histology	1. The urothelium may be thin, hyperplastic, or of normal thickness 2. Most cases have cells with markedly enlarged nuclei. Visibly abnormal using 10× lens with the largest nucleus 5× size of lamina propria lymphocyte nuclei 3. Nuclei typically very hyperchromatic although occasionally with prominent nucleoli *(Figs. 3.5.1–3.5.3)* 4. Nuclei are often irregular *(Figs. 3.5.1–3.5.3)* 5. Mitotic figures, sometimes frequent, may be present 6. Most cases lack inflammation within the urothelium, although exceptions occur *(Figs. 3.5.1–3.5.3)*	1. The urothelium may be thin, hyperplastic, or of normal thickness 2. Enlarged nuclei, may be as large as CIS 3. Nuclei vesicular with central prominent nucleoli *(Figs. 3.5.4–3.5.7)* 4. Nuclei uniform in size and shape 5. Mitotic figures may be numerous *(Fig. 3.5.5)* 6. Degree of reactive changes proportional to the extent of intramucosal inflammation. Both acute and chronic inflammation within the urothelium can result in reactive changes. Even a few inflammatory cells in the urothelium can lead to reactive changes. There are always some lymphocytes in the lamina propria, which by themselves are not enough to give rise to reactive atypia

	Carcinoma *In Situ* (CIS)	Reactive Urothelium
Special studies	• CK20 stains abnormal cells, although exceptions occur • p53 may be positive, yet only intense diffuse staining present is specific for CIS • CD44 supposed to label the basal cell layer or absent • Ki-67 is increased but not specific for CIS • UroVysion FISH demonstrates aneusomy for chromosomes 3,7,17 or loss of 9p. Sensitivity and specificity are close to 100% for the diagnosis of CIS	• CK20 labels only umbrella cells, although not 100% sensitive or specific *(Fig. 3.5.8)* • p53 negative, yet false positive occurs with weak to moderate nuclear staining *(Fig. 3.5.9)* • CD44 supposed to label full thickness, although not as widely used as CK20 • Ki-67 may be increased in the reactive urothelium to the same extent as CIS *(Fig. 3.5.10)* • UroVysion FISH demonstrates lack of aneusomy for chromosomes 3,7,17 or loss of 9p
Treatment	See Section 3.2	Tailored to the specific etiology
Prognosis	See Section 3.2	Treatment of the underlying cause resolves reactive changes

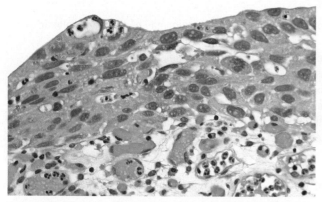

Figure 3.5.1   CIS with inflammation. Cells show marked nuclear pleomorphism.

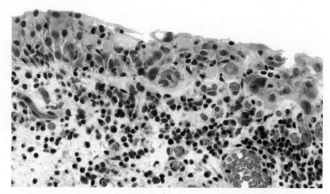

Figure 3.5.2   CIS with inflammation. Cells show marked nuclear pleomorphism.

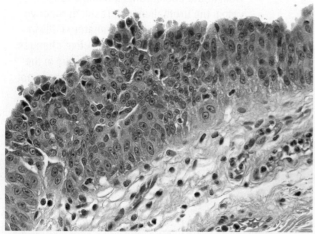

Figure 3.5.3   CIS with prominent nucleoli. In contrast to reactive changes, there is no inflammation in the urothelium, and nuclei are variable in size and shape.

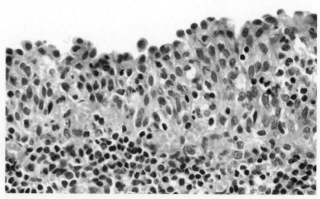

Figure 3.5.4   Reactive changes with numerous intramucosal lymphocytes and vesicular nuclei with visible nucleoli.

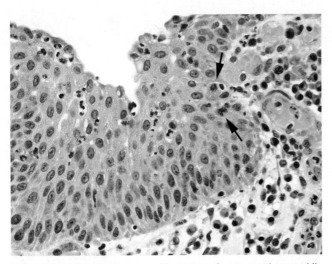

Figure 3.5.5 Reactive changes with numerous intramucosal neutrophils and vesicular nuclei with prominent nucleoli and mitotic figures (*arrows*).

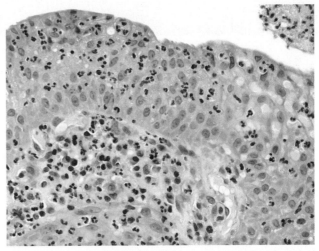

Figure 3.5.6 Reactive changes with numerous intramucosal neutrophils and vesicular nuclei with prominent nucleoli. Nuclei are uniformly enlarged and lack variation in shape.

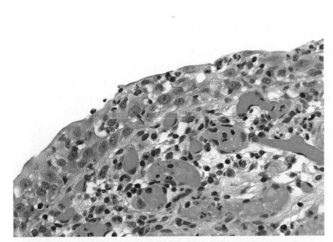

Figure 3.5.7 Reactive changes with numerous intramucosal neutrophils and eosinophils. Nuclei are vesicular with prominent nucleoli and are uniformly enlarged without pleomorphism.

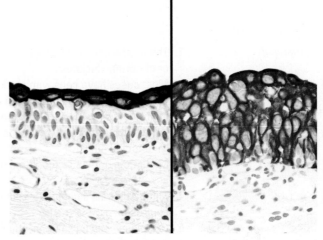

Figure 3.5.8 CK20 typically stains umbrella cells only in the normal and reactive urothelium (**left**) with diffuse CK20 immunoreactivity in dysplasia and CIS (**right**).

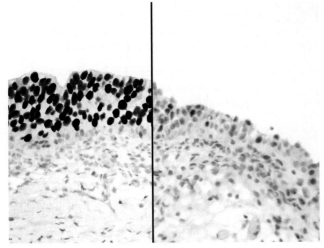

Figure 3.5.9 Diffuse strong p53 staining in CIS (**left**) compared to weak and moderate patchy p53 labeling (**right**) that is not diagnostic for CIS.

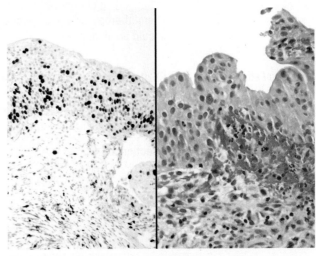

Figure 3.5.10 Reactive urothelium (**right**) with a marked increase in Ki-67 labeling (**left**).

	Carcinoma *In Situ* (CIS)	**Radiation/Chemotherapy Urothelial Atypia**
Age	Typically adults	Any age, but typically biopsied in adults
Location	Anywhere with urothelial lining	Anywhere with urothelial lining
Symptoms	May be asymptomatic or can have symptoms identical to that associated with urinary tract infections	Asymptomatic or may be associated irritative symptoms
Etiology	Prior irradiation or cyclophosphamide can predispose to development of CIS, typically years after therapy	Intravesical chemotherapy with mitomycin typically only affects morphology of umbrella cells. Cyclophosphamide and radiation can cause changes mimicking CIS. Changes in the urothelium lining the lumen should not persist beyond 1 year after cessation of radiation/chemotherapy. Radiation/chemotherapy atypia within von Brunn nests, the urothelium can persist for years
Histology	1. The urothelium may be thin, hyperplastic, or of normal thickness 2. Most cases have cells with markedly enlarged hyperchromatic nuclei visibly abnormal using 10× lens with the largest nucleus 5× size of lamina propria lymphocyte nuclei 3. Multinucleated and vacuolated nuclei absent *(Fig. 3.6.1)* 4. Mitotic figures, sometimes frequent, may be present *(Fig. 3.6.1)* 5. Cytoplasm may be scant or abundant, but not spindled or excessive 6. In some cases, CIS is not distinguishable from radiation/chemotherapy atypia. In the setting of prior radiation/chemotherapy, only unequivocal CIS should be diagnosed.	1. The urothelium may be thin, hyperplastic, or of normal thickness 2. Enlarged nuclei, as large seen in CIS, are vesicular with central prominent nucleoli 3. Nuclei are bizarre with multinucleation and vacuolization *(Figs. 3.6.2–3.6.6)* 4. Mitotic figures are absent 5. Cytoplasm typically abundant and often spindled with strap-like cells *(Figs. 3.6.2, 3.6.3, and 3.6.6)* 6. In some cases with urothelial atypia and a short (<1 y) interval between end of radiation/chemotherapy, the histologic distinction between CIS is not clear and close follow-up and repeat biopsy with a longer follow-up are recommended
Special studies	• CK20 stains abnormal cells, although exceptions occur • p53 may be positive, yet only intense diffuse staining is more specific for CIS	• Data not definitive on CK20 in radiation/chemotherapy atypia • p53 negative, yet false positive occurs with weak to moderate nuclear staining
Treatment	See Section 3.2	No treatment needed unless other side effects from the prior therapy such as hemorrhagic cystitis
Prognosis	See Section 3.2	Prior irradiation or systemic cyclophosphamide therapy associated with an increased risk of CIS years after treatment

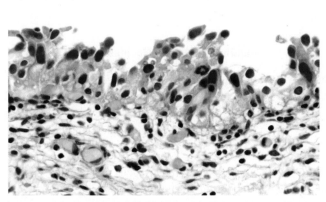

Figure 3.6.1   CIS with markedly enlarged hyperchromatic nuclei and mitotic figures and modest amount of cytoplasm.

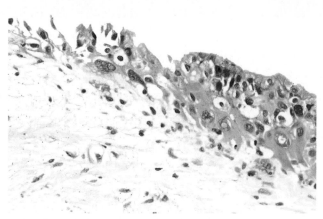

Figure 3.6.2   Radiation atypia with enlarged nuclei with a degenerative appearance with nuclear vesicles. Cells also have abundant spindled cytoplasm.

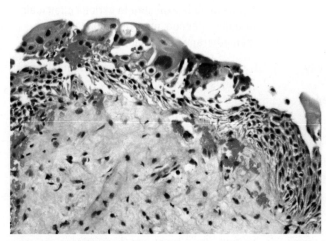

Figure 3.6.3   Radiation atypia with degenerative nuclear atypia and abundant cytoplasm.

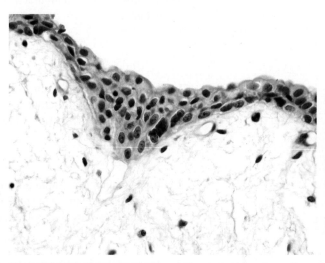

Figure 3.6.4   Radiation atypia with a multinucleated hyperchromatic nucleus.

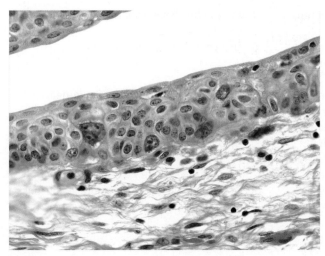

Figure 3.6.5   Radiation atypia with a multinucleated nucleus.

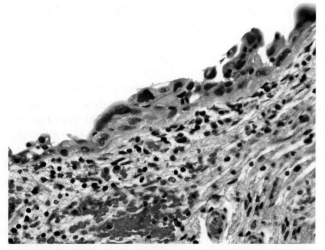

Figure 3.6.6   Radiation atypia with degenerative nuclear atypia and abundant cytoplasm.

3 BLADDER

	Polypoid Cystitis	Papillary Urothelial Neoplasm
Age	Any age, but typically biopsied in adults	Any age, but typically biopsied in adults
Location	Anywhere with urothelial lining	Anywhere with urothelial lining
Symptoms	Asymptomatic or may be associated symptoms relating to specific etiology	Typically gross or microscopic hematuria
Signs	Associated signs relating to any condition that irritates the bladder. At cystoscopy, the lesion is often clearly reactive to the urologist	At cystoscopy, the urologist can usually recognize that a lesion is a papillary urothelial neoplasm as opposed to polypoid cystitis
Etiology	Most often cited is indwelling catheter but others include urinary calculi, colovesical fistula, infection, instrumentation, and prior irradiation	Numerous environmental risk factors. Most common is history of smoking, accounting for 60% and 30% of all urothelial carcinomas in males and females, respectively. Other risk factors include exposure to various chemicals, heredity, infection, prior radiation, and prior chemotherapy with cyclophosphamide
Histology	1. Simple folds of urothelium in continuity with the underlying bladder *(Figs. 3.7.1–3.7.3)*. Rare fronds may appear to be free floating or branching 2. Stroma within fronds appears pale as a result of edema with scattered inflammatory cells *(Figs. 3.7.1–3.7.3)*. 3. Stroma within fronds may in later stages appear more dense pink as a result of fibrosis with scattered lymphocytes *(Figs. 3.7.4–3.7.7)* 4. Stalks typically lack prominent numerous small capillaries 5. In majority of cases, some of the fronds will have broad base although others in the same case may be narrow 6. Reactive urothelium may be seen, including mitotic figures (see Section 3.5) *(Fig. 3.7.8)* 7. In about one-third of cases may be focal or diffuse thickening of the urothelium. Most normal thickness *(Figs. 3.7.1, 3.7.2, and 3.7.4–3.7.8)* 8. At low magnification, >90% of the lesion has features of polypoid cystitis, yet there may be isolated fronds that out of context could be interpreted as a low-grade papillary urothelial neoplasm *(Figs. 3.7.2, 3.7.6, and 3.7.8)*	1. As a result of complex branching papillary fronds, most of the papillary structures in a given plane of section appear to be free floating detached from the underlying bladder surrounded on the slide by white space *(Fig. 3.7.9)* 2. Stalks may occasionally appear clear at low power, usually due to dilated lymphatics but occasionally due to stromal edema. Inflammatory cells within stalks are typically absent or minimal *(Fig. 3.7.10)*. 3. Stalks have loose connective tissue with delicate light eosinophilic appearance 4. Stalks often have numerous small capillaries *(Fig. 3.7.9)* 5. Base of fronds typically narrow 6. Urothelial atypia consists of enlarged variably sized hyperchromatic nuclei 7. With the exception of papilloma, the urothelium thickened *(Fig. 3.7.9)* 8. At low magnification, the entire lesion looks like a papillary urothelial neoplasm

	Polypoid Cystitis	**Papillary Urothelial Neoplasm**
Special studies	Not helpful in this differential	Not helpful in this differential
Treatment	Tailored to the specific etiology	Tailored to the tumor's grade, size, multifocality and whether the lesion is a recurrence or primary lesion (see Sections 3.9–3.11)
Prognosis	Treatment of the underlying cause resolves the reactive changes	See Sections 3.9–3.11

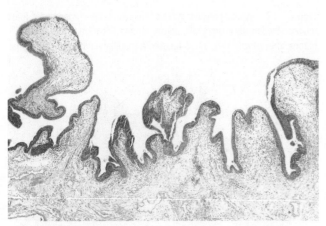

Figure 3.7.1   Polypoid cystitis with simple folds of pale, edematous urothelium.

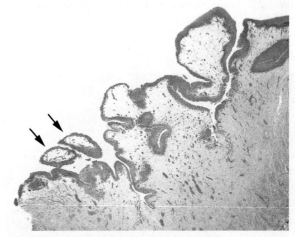

Figure 3.7.2   Polypoid cystitis with mostly simple folds with wide base but occasional smaller edematous papillary structures (*arrows*) that could be misdiagnosed as a papillary urothelial neoplasm.

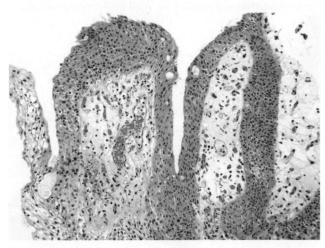

Figure 3.7.3   Polypoid cystitis with simple folds of pale edematous urothelium containing inflammatory cells.

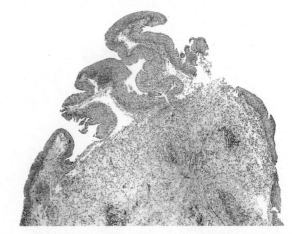

Figure 3.7.4   Polypoid cystitis with simple folds and densely fibrotic and inflamed stroma.

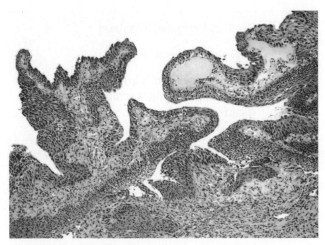

Figure 3.7.5   Polypoid cystitis with occasional branching folds and densely fibrotic and inflamed stroma.

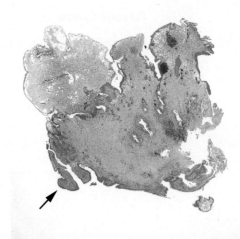

Figure 3.7.6   Typical polypoid cystitis (*top*) with simple broad based folds replaced by densely eosinophilic fibrotic stroma. Focal small fronds with fibrous cores (*arrow*) were misdiagnosed as papillary urothelial carcinoma.

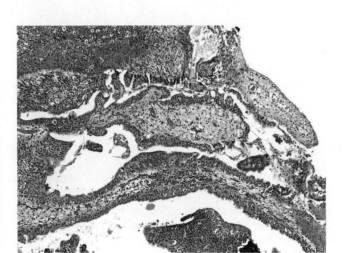

Figure 3.7.7   Unusual case of polypoid cystitis with long simple folds containing abundant inflammation and fibrous tissue.

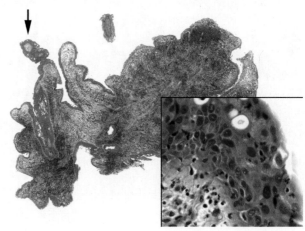

Figure 3.7.8   Polypoid cystitis with areas showing simple broad based folds with intense inflammation. Focal small fronds (*arrow*) were misdiagnosed as papillary urothelial carcinoma. **Inset** shows an inflamed reactive urothelium.

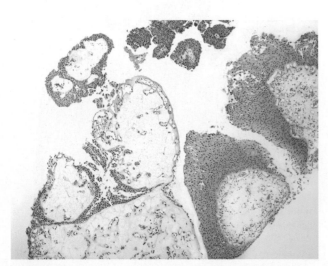

Figure 3.7.9   Low-grade papillary urothelial carcinoma with edematous yet not inflamed stalks containing numerous prominent capillaries. Focally, the urothelium is markedly thickened.

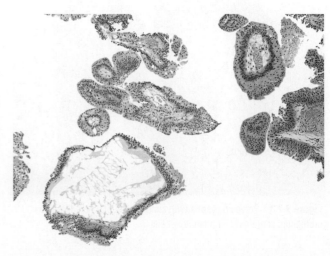

Figure 3.7.10   Low-grade papillary urothelial carcinoma with dilated lymphatic in stalk. Lesion has multiple "free-floating" fronds indicative of a complex branching papillary lesion.

	Papillary Urothelial Hyperplasia	Urothelial Papilloma
Age	Mean age mid-late 50s with wide range	Mean age mid-late 50s with wide range. Can rarely be seen in children
Location	Anywhere with urothelial lining	Anywhere with urothelial lining
Symptoms	Most commonly asymptomatic detected at cystoscopy for follow-up of prior urothelial neoplasms. Next most commonly presents with hematuria	Typically gross or microscopic hematuria
Signs	At cystoscopy, the lesion is subtle and in order of decreasing frequency thought to be a papillary neoplasm, papillary irregularity, or irregular mucosa	At cystoscopy, delicate papillary lesion, typically solitary and relatively small
Etiology	A subset of papillary urothelial hyperplasia demonstrates loss of chromosomal arm 9q, which is among the earliest event in bladder cancer progression, demonstrating that some cases of papillary hyperplasia are precancerous lesions of the bladder	Thought to be the same as urothelial carcinoma
Histology	1. Simple folds of the urothelium in continuity with the underlying bladder *(Figs. 3.8.1–3.8.4)*	1. As a result of complex branching papillary fronds, most of the papillary structures in a given plane of section appear to be free floating detached from the underlying bladder surrounded on the slide by white space *(Figs. 3.8.5 and 3.8.6)*
	2. May see subtle slight branching of folds at the tips of papillary folds	2. In a minority of cases, can see secondary branching of smaller fronds from larger ones
	3. In most cases, there is thickening of the urothelium	3. The urothelium is normal thickness
	4. Cytology is normal. In some cases, there is the architecture of papillary urothelial hyperplasia yet with marked cytologic atypia, which is termed *CIS with early papillary formation*	4. Cytology is normal
	5. Umbrella cells inconspicuous	5. Umbrella cells vary from inconspicuous to apocrine to having prominent degenerative atypia
	6. Base of the papillae may show collection of dilated capillaries	6. Within the papillae are often a collection of small congested capillaries
Special studies	Not helpful in this differential	Not helpful in this differential
Treatment	Typically, not treated but patients closely followed. In cases of *CIS with early papillary formation*, treated as CIS	Typically, resected by TUR and not treated with adjuvant therapy

	Papillary Urothelial Hyperplasia	**Urothelial Papilloma**
Prognosis	60% have a history of prior urothelial neoplasms, 80% of which are low grade. The 5-y actuarial risk of subsequently developing an urothelial neoplasm in the setting of papillary urothelial hyperplasia is 28% and 50% for those without and with a history of prior papillary urothelial neoplasms. In two-thirds of cases, the subsequent neoplasm is low grade (papilloma, PUNLMP, low-grade carcinoma). All together two-thirds of patients with papillary urothelial hyperplasia have a history of prior, concurrent, or subsequent urothelial neoplasms	In most cases once resected, the lesion does not recur. In about 10% of cases, the lesion recurs as papilloma and in 10% as low-grade papillary carcinoma or PUNLMP. Only rare cases in patients with immunosuppression progress to high-grade papillary or invasive carcinoma

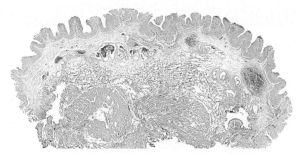

Figure 3.8.1   Papillary urothelial hyperplasia with thickened folds of the urothelium.

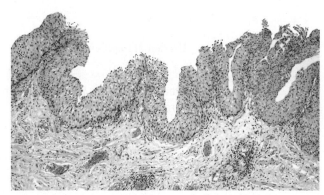

Figure 3.8.2   Papillary urothelial hyperplasia with thickened folds of the urothelium.

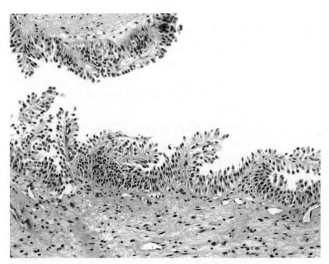

Figure 3.8.3   Papillary lesion that is borderline between papillary urothelial hyperplasia and early papilloma.

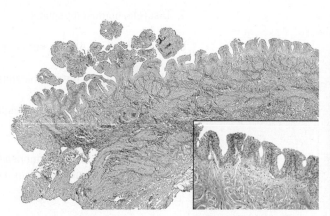

Figure 3.8.4   Papillary urothelial hyperplasia (*right* and **inset**) with adjacent papilloma (*left*).

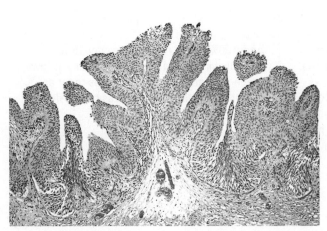

Figure 3.8.5   Early papilloma with branching and beginning of "detached" papillary fronds.

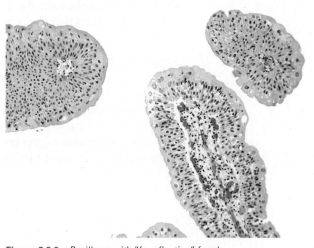

Figure 3.8.6   Papilloma with "free-floating" fronds.

3   BLADDER

	Urothelial Papilloma	Papillary Urothelial Neoplasm of Low Malignant Potential
Age	Mean age mid-late 50s with wide range. Can rarely be seen in children	Mean age mid-60s with wide range. Can rarely be seen in children
Location	Anywhere with urothelial lining	Anywhere with urothelial lining
Symptoms	Typically gross or microscopic hematuria	Typically gross or microscopic hematuria
Signs	At cystoscopy, delicate papillary lesion, typically solitary and relatively small	At cystoscopy, papillary lesion, typically solitary with wide range in size
Etiology	Thought to be the same as urothelial carcinoma	Thought to be the same as urothelial carcinoma
Histology	1. Typically small lesion that fits on one slide 2. Discrete, nonfused papillae 3. Inverted growth pattern not common 4. The urothelium is normal thickness *(Figs. 3.9.1 and 3.9.2)* 5. Cytology is normal with some cells having nuclear grooves 6. Umbrella cells vary from inconspicuous to apocrine to prominent degenerative atypia 7. Mitotic figures absent.	1. Ranges in size but can be large requiring multiple slides to totally submit 2. Usually discrete, nonfused papillae but some may be fused 3. Often with a prominent inverted growth pattern 4. The urothelium is overtly thick, even at low magnification *(Figs. 3.9.3 and 3.9.4)* 5. Cytology is normal or at most slightly enlarged nuclei with some cells having nuclear grooves *(Fig. 3.9.5)* 6. Umbrella cells inconspicuous. 7. Mitotic figures virtually absent or at most rarely seen toward the basement membrane.
Special studies	Not helpful in this differential.	Not helpful in this differential.
Treatment	Typically, resected by TUR and not treated with adjuvant therapy. Urologists recommend routine cystoscopies for life, although if after many years there is no recurrence, patients typically stop coming back for follow-up	Typically, resected by TUR and not treated with adjuvant therapy. Followed for life with routine cystoscopy
Prognosis	In most cases once resected, the lesion does not recur. In about 10% of cases, the lesion recurs as papilloma and in 10% as low-grade papillary carcinoma or PUNLMP. Only rare cases in the literature in patients with immunosuppression progress to high-grade papillary or invasive carcinoma	About 30% risk of recurrence over 15 years, typically as PUNLMP but occasionally as low-grade carcinoma. Only rare cases recur as higher-grade cancer with invasion. No deaths due to bladder cancer

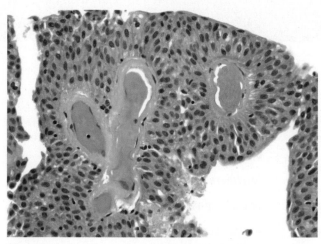

Figure 3.9.1   Papilloma with the urothelium of normal thickness and cytology.

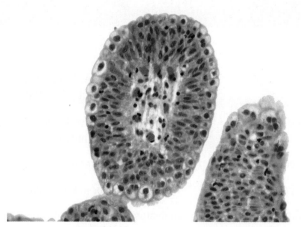

Figure 3.9.2   Papilloma.

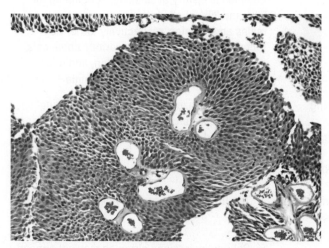

Figure 3.9.3   PUNLMP with the overtly thickened urothelium.

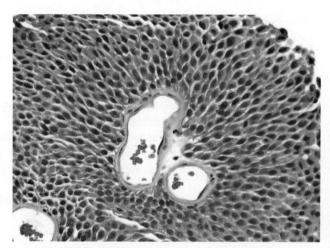

Figure 3.9.4   Same case as Figure 3.9.3 with benign cytology.

3   BLADDER

	Papillary Urothelial Neoplasm of Low Malignant Potential (PUNLMP)	Low-Grade Papillary Urothelial Carcinoma
Age	Mean age mid-60s with wide range. Can rarely be seen in children	Mean age mid-60s with wide range. Can rarely be seen in children
Location	Anywhere with urothelial lining	Anywhere with urothelial lining
Symptoms	Typically gross or microscopic hematuria	Typically gross or microscopic hematuria
Signs	At cystoscopy, papillary lesion. May be solitary or multifocal	At cystoscopy, papillary lesion, typically solitary or multifocal
Etiology	Thought to be the same as urothelial carcinoma	Numerous environmental risk factors. Most common is history of smoking, accounting for 60% and 30% of all urothelial carcinomas in males and females, respectively. Other risk factors include exposure to various chemicals, heredity, infection, prior radiation, and prior chemotherapy with cyclophosphamide
Histology	1. Ranges in size. Can be large requiring multiple slides to totally submit 2. Usually discrete, nonfused papillae but some may be fused 3. Often with a prominent inverted growth pattern 4. The urothelium is overtly thick, even at low magnification (Figs. 3.10.1–3.10.4) 5. Polarity strictly maintained 6. Cytology is normal or at most slightly enlarged nuclei some with nuclear grooves (Figs. 3.10.1–3.10.4) 7. Every microscopic field is monotonous with uniformly sized and shaped nuclei having light chromatin 8. Nucleoli indistinct 9. Mitotic figures virtually absent or at most rarely seen toward the basement membrane	1. Ranges in size but can be large requiring multiple slides to totally submit 2. Usually discrete, nonfused papillae but some may be fused 3. Often with a prominent inverted growth pattern 4. The urothelium is typically overtly thickened 5. Polarity maintained although may not appear quite as regular as in PUNLMP 6. Cytology is mostly normal with scattered slightly enlarged hyperchromatic nuclei that stand out even at lower magnification. Nuclear grooves not as common 7. Scattered larger hyperchromatic nuclei with minimal variation in shape. Lacks the uniformity of PUNLMP (Figs. 3.10.5–3.10.8) 8. Nucleoli range from indistinct to small but visible 9. Mitotic figures range from uncommon to scattered seen at all layers of the urothelium
Special studies	Not helpful in this differential	Not helpful in this differential

	Papillary Urothelial Neoplasm of Low Malignant Potential (PUNLMP)	**Low-Grade Papillary Urothelial Carcinoma**
Treatment	Typically, resected by TUR and not treated with adjuvant therapy. Followed for life with routine cystoscopy	Typically, resected by TUR with immediate instillation of intravesical chemotherapy recommended even for lesions with low risk of recurrence. Intravesical BCG not used for initial therapy, yet potentially used in patients with recurrent low-grade papillary urothelial carcinoma. Followed for life with routine cystoscopy
Prognosis	At 5 and 15 y, 10% and 30% risk of recurrence, respectively, typically as PUNLMP but occasionally as low-grade carcinoma. Only rare cases recur as higher-grade cancer with invasion. No deaths due to bladder cancer	At 5 and 15 y, 30% and 40% risk of recurrence, respectively, typically as low-grade carcinoma but occasionally as higher-grade carcinoma. Higher rate of recurrence vs. PUNLMP. 10% of cases recur as higher-grade cancer with invasion, higher rate than in PUNLMP. 1%–2% of patients eventually die due to bladder cancer

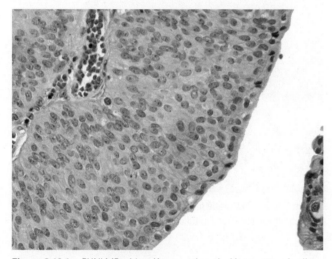

Figure 3.10.1 PUNLMP with uniform cytology, lacking scattered cells with nuclear hyperchromasia.

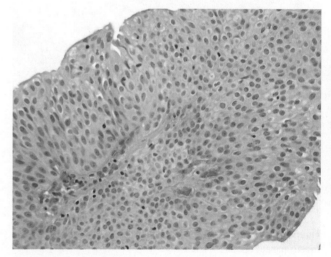

Figure 3.10.2 PUNLMP.

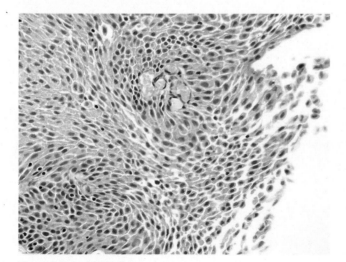

Figure 3.10.3 PUNLMP.

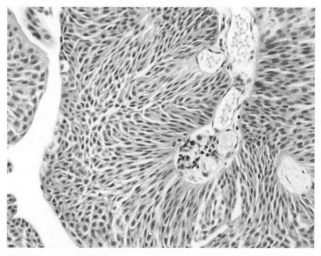

Figure 3.10.4 PUNLMP.

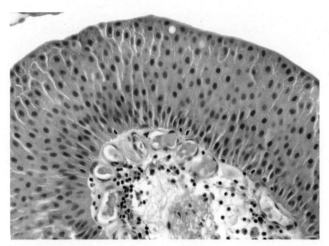

Figure 3.10.5 Low-grade papillary urothelial carcinoma with scattered hyperchromatic nuclei.

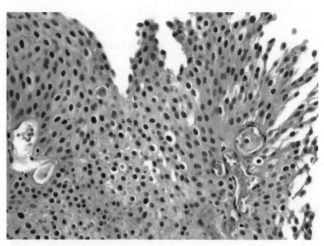

Figure 3.10.6 Low-grade papillary urothelial carcinoma with scattered hyperchromatic nuclei.

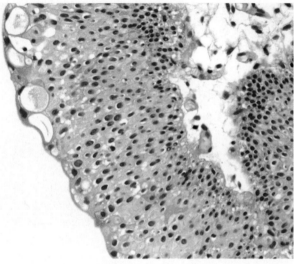

Figure 3.10.7 Low-grade papillary urothelial carcinoma with scattered hyperchromatic nuclei.

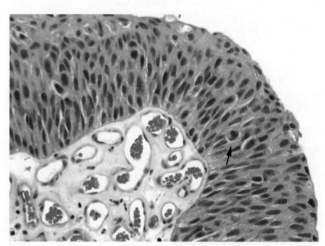

Figure 3.10.8 Low-grade papillary urothelial carcinoma with scattered hyperchromatic nuclei and mitotic figures (*arrow*).

	Low-Grade Papillary Urothelial Carcinoma	High-Grade Papillary Urothelial Carcinoma
Age	Mean age mid-60s with wide range. Can rarely be seen in children	Mean age mid-60s with wide range. Not as common as lower-grade papillary urothelial neoplasms under 20 y of age
Location	Anywhere with urothelial lining	Anywhere with urothelial lining
Symptoms	Typically gross or microscopic hematuria	Typically gross or microscopic hematuria
Signs	At cystoscopy, papillary lesion, solitary or multifocal	Same as low-grade papillary carcinoma, yet increased likelihood of sessile growth
Etiology	See Section 3.10	See Section 3.10
Histology	1. Ranges in size, but can be large requiring multiple slides to totally submit 2. Usually discrete, nonfused papillae but some may be fused 3. Often with a prominent inverted growth pattern 4. The urothelium is overtly thick, even at low magnification 5. Polarity maintained with evenly space nuclei that are regularly distributed in an orderly almost row-like fashion *(Figs. 3.11.1–3.11.3)* 6. Cytology is mostly normal with scattered slightly enlarged hyperchromatic nuclei visible at lower magnification, comparable to nuclei of dysplasia *(Figs. 3.11.1–3.11.3)* 7. Nucleoli range from indistinct to small but visible 8. Mitotic figures uncommon to scattered, seen in all layers of the urothelium. 9. Cells typically cohesive 10. Umbrella cells usually present 11. Uncommon tumors where vast majority is low grade and <5% high grade. Controversial whether to call "high grade," or "low grade with very focal high grade" adding a comment that the significance of this finding is unknown	1. Ranges in size, but can be large requiring multiple slides to totally submit 2. May have discrete, nonfused papillae but often fused 3. Often with a prominent inverted growth pattern 4. The urothelium is typically thickened 5. Loss of polarity (irregular spacing of cells) or spindling of cells or irregular overlapping of nuclei *(Fig. 3.11.4)* 6. Cytology is mostly abnormal with markedly enlarged hyperchromatic nuclei that stand out even at lower magnification, comparable to nuclei of CIS *(Figs. 3.11.4 and 3.11.5)* 7. Nucleoli range from indistinct to small but visible. In some cases, diffuse very prominent nucleoli *(Fig. 3.11.6)* 8. Mitotic figures frequent, seen in all layers of the urothelium *(Figs. 3.11.4 and 3.11.6)*. 9. Dyscohesive cells frequent *(Fig. 3.11.7)* 10. Umbrella cells usually absent 11. Uncommon cases with mixed low- and high-grade morphology. If high grade >5%, uniformly accepted should be called "high grade" *(Fig. 3.11.8)*
Special studies	Not helpful in this differential	Not helpful in this differential

	Low-Grade Papillary Urothelial Carcinoma	**High-Grade Papillary Urothelial Carcinoma**
Treatment	Typically, resected by TUR with immediate instillation of intravesical chemotherapy, even for lesions with low risk of recurrence. Intravesical BCG not used for initial therapy, yet potentially used with recurrent low-grade papillary urothelial carcinoma. Followed for life with routine cystoscopy	Typically, resected by TUR and then treated with intravesical BCG therapy. Followed for life with routine cystoscopy
Prognosis	At 5 y, 30% risk of recurrence, typically as low-grade carcinoma but occasionally as higher-grade carcinoma. 10% of cases recur as higher-grade cancer with invasion. 1%–2% of patients eventually die of disease	At 5 y, 30% risk of recurrence, typically as high-grade carcinoma. 30% of cases recur with invasion. 15% of patients eventually die of bladder cancer

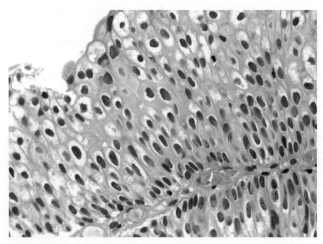

Figure 3.11.1　Low-grade papillary urothelial carcinoma with uniform polarity and scattered minimally enlarged hyperchromatic nuclei.

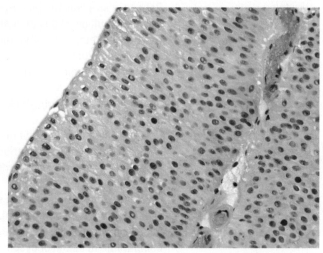

Figure 3.11.2　Low-grade papillary urothelial carcinoma with uniform polarity and scattered minimally enlarged hyperchromatic nuclei.

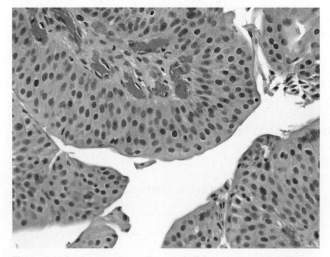

Figure 3.11.3　Low-grade papillary urothelial carcinoma with uniform polarity and scattered minimally enlarged hyperchromatic nuclei.

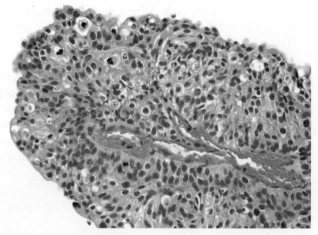

Figure 3.11.4　High-grade papillary urothelial carcinoma with loss of polarity with nuclei not lining up in uniform spatial arrangement. Numerous mitotic figures noted.

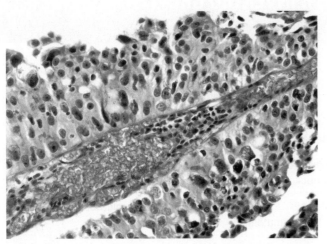

Figure 3.11.5   High-grade papillary urothelial carcinoma with marked pleomorphism.

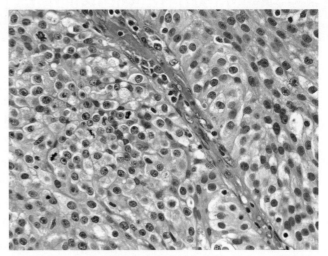

Figure 3.11.6   High-grade papillary urothelial carcinoma with diffuse prominent nucleoli and numerous mitotic figures.

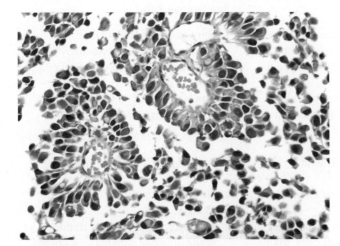

Figure 3.11.7   High-grade papillary urothelial carcinoma with dyscohesive cells with hyperchromatic nuclei.

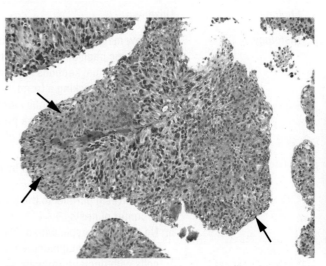

Figure 3.11.8   High-grade papillary carcinoma with areas showing more uniform cytology and preserved polarity (*arrows*) with rest of the tumor high grade.

	Inverted Urothelial Papilloma	Noninvasive Urothelial Carcinoma with Inverted Growth Pattern
Age	Mean age mid-late 50s–60s with wide range	Mean age mid-60s with wide range
Location	Occurs at any location in the urothelial tract, yet most the common trigone or bladder neck	Anywhere with urothelial lining
Symptoms	Typically gross or microscopic hematuria, obstructive or irritative lower urinary tract symptoms	Typically gross or microscopic hematuria
Signs	At cystoscopy, polypoid with smooth surface. Over 95% unifocal. Usually <3 cm, but wide range in size	At cystoscopy, papillary lesion with delicate coral-like surface. Solitary or multifocal with wide range in size
Etiology	Unknown	See Section 3.10
Histology	1. At low magnification, surface is smooth without exophytic papillary fronds, with exception of rare tangential sections resulting in a polypoid structure mimicking a frond *(Figs. 3.12.1–3.12.7)* 2. In some areas in continuity with surface but in most without, the lamina propria filled with anastomosing thin columns of the urothelium *(Figs. 3.12.1–3.12.5)* 3. Periphery of columns lined by cells with a palisading appearance *(Fig. 3.12.8)* 4. Cells stream parallel to the basement membrane in center of nests *(Fig. 3.12.8)* 5. No cytologic atypia with only rare cases showing bland multinucleated giant cells. Many cells with nuclear grooves 6. Mitotic figures rare and when present only at the periphery of columns 7. Cyst formation filled with eosinophilic secretions common *(Fig. 3.12.3)* 8. Intervening stroma delicate with lack of inflammation	1. Rare to have papillary urothelial neoplasm without any exophytic component, although uncommonly it occurs 2. The lamina propria filled with large rounded nests of the urothelium *(Figs. 3.12.9 and 3.12.10)* 3. Lack of palisading at periphery of nests 4. No streaming of cells in center of nests 5. Cytologic atypia depends on the grade. Inverted pattern of exophytic papilloma or PUNLMP may have no atypia *(Figs. 3.12.9 and 3.12.11)*. Inverted pattern of low-grade carcinoma with scattered hyperchromatic enlarged nuclei *(Figs. 3.12.10 and 3.12.12)*. Inverted pattern of high-grade carcinoma with marked cytologic atypia. Nuclear grooves seen in inverted pattern of exophytic papilloma and PUNLMP and less in low-grade and not in high-grade carcinoma 6. Mitotic figures vary in frequency depending on the grade 7. Cyst formation filled with eosinophilic secretions uncommon, although may see smaller gland-like lumina or true gland formation 8. Intervening stroma may have inflammation
Special studies	Not helpful in this differential	Not helpful in this differential

	Inverted Urothelial Papilloma	**Noninvasive Urothelial Carcinoma with Inverted Growth Pattern**
Treatment	Resected by TUR. Controversial whether to recommend follow-up cystoscopy. If so, can be done less frequently than that for urothelial carcinoma and for only 3 y	Typically, resected by TUR with adjuvant therapy depending on the grade (see Sections 3.8–3.11). Followed for life with routine cystoscopy
Prognosis	No risk of recurrence. No risk of progression to urothelial carcinoma. 1%–2% have prior history, synchronous, or subsequent urothelial carcinoma	Risk of recurrence, progression, and death varies according to grade (see Sections 3.8–3.11)

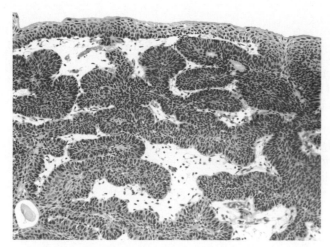

Figure 3.12.1   Inverted papilloma with anastomosing columns of the urothelium beneath the smooth surface.

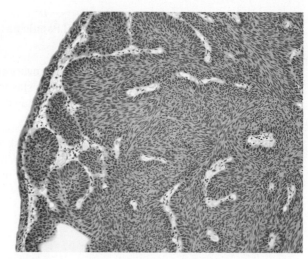

Figure 3.12.2   Inverted papilloma with anastomosing columns of the urothelium beneath the smooth surface.

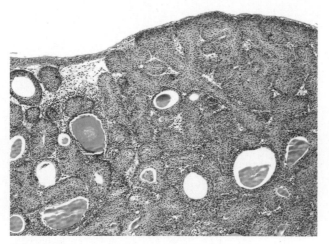

Figure 3.12.3   Inverted papilloma with colloid-filled cysts.

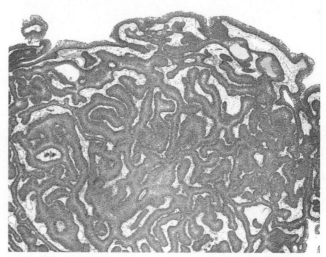

Figure 3.12.4   Inverted papilloma with anastomosing columns of the urothelium beneath the slightly polypoid surface. Rare fronds (*left*) in the setting of typical inverted papilloma do not change the diagnosis.

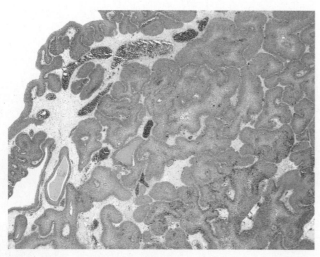

Figure 3.12.5   Typical inverted papilloma.

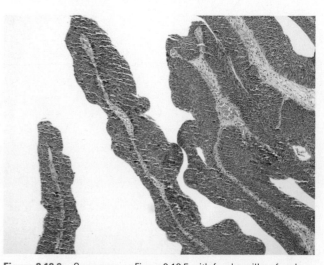

Figure 3.12.6   Same case as Figure 3.12.5 with focal papillary fronds.

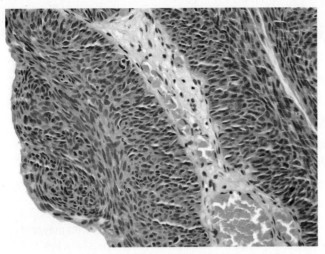

Figure 3.12.7   Higher magnification of Figure 3.12.6 with papillary fronds having the same spindled urothelium seen in the inverted portion of the tumor, still consistent with inverted papilloma.

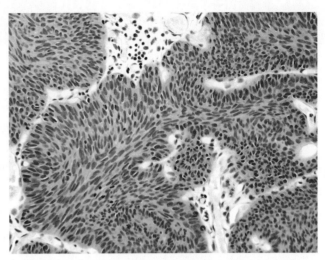

Figure 3.12.8   Inverted papilloma with streaming of nuclei parallel to columns.

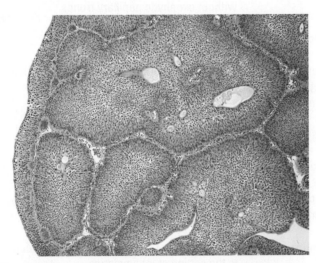

Figure 3.12.9   Inverted growth of PUNLMP with large rounded nests.

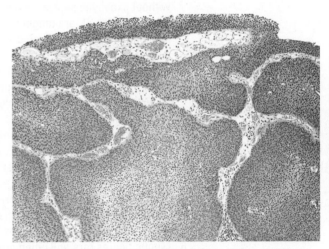

Figure 3.12.10   Inverted growth of low-grade papillary urothelial carcinoma with large rounded nests.

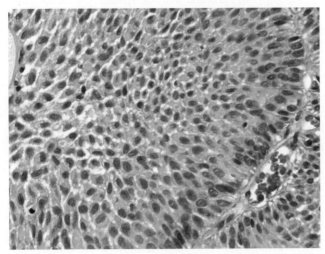

Figure 3.12.11   Same case as Figure 3.12.9 with bland cytology.

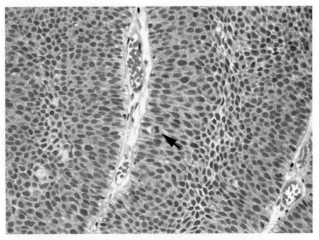

Figure 3.12.12   Same case as Figure 3.12.10 with scattered hyperchromatic nuclei and mitotic figures (*arrow*).

3 BLADDER

	Inverted Urothelial Papilloma	Florid von Brunn Nest Proliferation
Age	Mean age mid-late 50s–60s with wide range	Wide age range
Location	Occurs at any location in the urothelial tract, yet most common the trigone or bladder neck	Occurs at any location in the urothelial tract with the ureter and renal pelvis as common sites
Symptoms	Typically gross or microscopic hematuria	Typically gross or microscopic hematuria
Signs	At cystoscopy, polypoid with smooth surface. Almost always solitary. Usually <3 cm, but wide range in size	At cystoscopy, can be tumor-like with polypoid mass with smooth surface. Almost always solitary. Usually <3 cm
Etiology	Unknown	Unknown
Histology	1. At low magnification, surface is smooth without exophytic papillary fronds, with exception of rare tangential section resulting in a polypoid structure mimicking a frond 2. In some areas in continuity with surface but in most without, the lamina propria filled with anastomosing thin columns of the urothelium *(Figs. 3.13.1–3.13.3)* 3. Periphery of columns lined by cells with a palisading appearance *(Fig. 3.13.3)* 4. Cells stream parallel to the basement membrane in center of nests *(Fig. 3.13.3)* 5. No cytologic atypia with only rare cases showing bland multinucleated giant cells. Many cells with nuclear grooves 6. Mitotic figures rare and when present only at the periphery of columns 7. Cyst formation filled with eosinophilic secretions common 8. Intervening stroma delicate with lack of inflammation	1. At low magnification, surface is smooth without exophytic papillary fronds 2. The lamina propria filled with large rounded nests of the urothelium *(Figs. 3.13.4–3.13.8)* 3. Variable palisading at periphery of nests 4. No streaming of cells in center of nests 5. No cytologic atypia. May have nuclear grooves 6. Mitotic figures rare and when present seen in the setting of inflammation 7. Cyst formation filled with eosinophilic secretions common in the bladder and less in the ureter and renal pelvis *(Figs. 3.13.4–3.13.6)* 8. Intervening stroma may have inflammation that can cause reactive cytologic changes (see Section 3.5)
Special studies	Not helpful in this differential	Not helpful in this differential
Treatment	Resected by TUR. Controversial whether to recommend follow-up cystoscopy. If so, can be done less frequently than that for urothelial carcinoma and for only 3 y	Resected by TUR

	Inverted Urothelial Papilloma	Florid von Brunn Nest Proliferation
Prognosis	No risk of recurrence. No risk of progression to urothelial carcinoma. 1%–2% have prior history, synchronous, or subsequent urothelial carcinoma	Not a neoplasm and no risk of recurrence or progression. Not related to inverted papilloma with exception of uncommon cases in the renal pelvis and ureter where there are multifocal lesions with some having morphology of inverted papilloma and other von Brunn nests. Typically, these uncommon cases are treated by nephroureterectomy based on the radiologic and ureteroscopic appearance. Given that major surgery has already been performed, these cases are best diagnosed as inverted papillomas with areas resembling von Brunn nests. The relationship of these overlap lesions with other urothelial neoplasms is unknown.

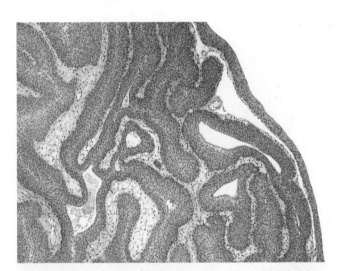

Figure 3.13.1 Inverted papilloma with smooth surface and underlying anastomosing thin columns of urothelium.

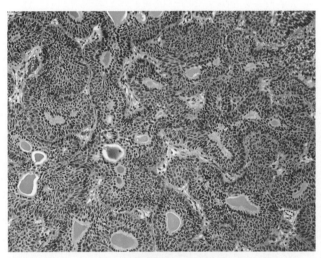

Figure 3.13.2 Inverted papilloma with anastomosing thin columns of urothelium with colloid cysts.

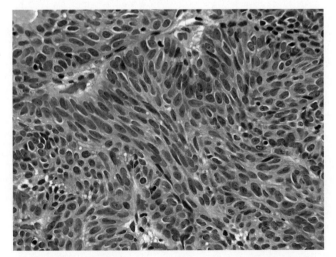

Figure 3.13.3 Inverted papilloma with streaming of nuclei parallel to columns and peripheral palisading of nuclei at epithelial–stromal interface.

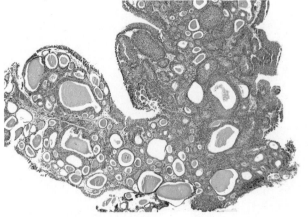

Figure 3.13.4 Polypoid florid proliferation of von Brunn nests mimicking a tumor.

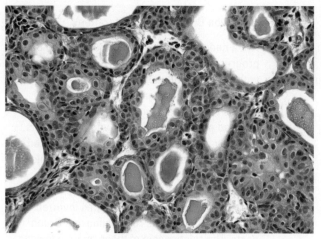

Figure 3.13.5 Same case as Figure 3.13.4 with rounded colloid-filled nests.

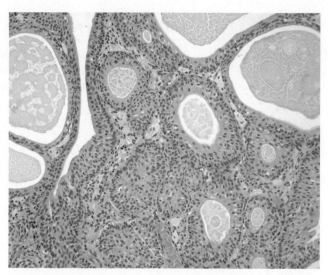

Figure 3.13.6 Rounded von Brunn nests with colloid.

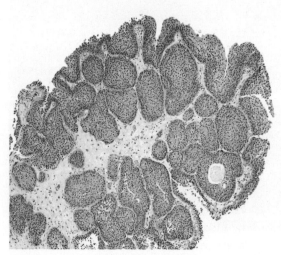

Figure 3.13.7 Florid proliferation of von Brunn nests resulting in a tumor-like lesion.

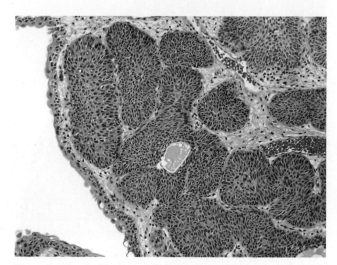

Figure 3.13.8 Proliferation of rounded von Brunn nests.

	Florid von Brunn Nest Proliferation	Nested Urothelial Carcinoma
Age	Wide age range	Mean age mid-60s with wide range. Uncommon in females
Location	Occurs at any location in the urothelial tract with the ureter and renal pelvis as common sites	Typically the bladder, with only rare cases in the renal pelvis or ureter
Symptoms	Typically gross or microscopic hematuria	Typically gross or microscopic hematuria
Signs	At cystoscopy, can be tumor-like with polypoid mass with smooth surface. Almost always solitary. Usually <3 cm, but wide range in size	At cystoscopy, nodular surface typically without an exophytic papillary component. Usually solitary. Wide range in size
Etiology		See Section 3.10
Histology	1. At low magnification, surface is smooth without exophytic papillary fronds	1. At low magnification, surface is typically smooth without exophytic papillary fronds *(Figs. 3.14.6 and 3.14.7)*. Uncommon cases where surface shows CIS or papillary urothelial carcinoma
	2. The lamina propria filled with large rounded nests of the urothelium in the bladder *(Fig. 3.14.1)*. In the ureter and renal pelvis and uncommonly in the bladder, small rounded nests *(Figs. 3.14.2–3.14.5)*	2. The lamina propria filled with small crowded nests of the urothelium in the classic variant and large irregular nests in the large nested variant *(Figs. 3.14.7 and 3.14.8)*
	3. In resection specimens, can appreciate that the nests are linear or lobular without an infiltrative lower border (i.e., can mentally draw a straight line at the base of the lesion) *(Figs. 3.14.2–3.14.4)*	3. Has an irregular base with infiltrative nests extending to different depths *(Figs. 3.14.6 and 3.14.9)*. Diagnosis should not be made on biopsy of the ureter or renal pelvis in the absence of the muscularis propria invasion, since cannot appreciate infiltrative border and overlapping morphologic features with von Brunn nests in these sites
	4. Nests evenly spaced	4. Nests often very crowded, back to back *(Figs. 3.14.8 and 3.14.10)*
	5. Never invades the muscularis propria	5. Often invades the muscularis propria *(Figs. 3.14.6, 3.14.9, and 3.14.10)*
	6. No cytologic atypia unless inflamed with reactive changes where mitotic figures may be seen (see Section 3.5)	6. No cytologic atypia in areas, yet deeper nests may have prominent nucleoli and occasional mitotic figures *(Figs. 3.14.7–3.14.10)*
	7. No stromal reaction	7. Typically, no stromal reaction in usual variant but variable desmoplastic stroma with variable inflammatory response in large nested variant
	8. Cyst formation filled with eosinophilic secretions common in the bladder and less in the ureter and renal pelvis *(Fig. 3.14.1)*	8. Can see small cyst formation
	9. Lack of tubular formation although can see gland-like lumina and cystitis glandularis toward centers of nests	9. Some cases have tubular differentiation. If predominant, called tubular variant of urothelial carcinoma (see Section 3.16)

	Florid von Brunn Nest Proliferation	**Nested Urothelial Carcinoma**
Special studies	Most cases with low Ki-67 rate	Most cases with low Ki-67 rate, with only a few cases with rate >20%
Treatment	Resected by TUR	Radical surgery typically required as usually invades the muscularis propria
Prognosis	No risk of recurrence or progression	Aggressive behavior comparable to invasive high-grade urothelial carcinoma

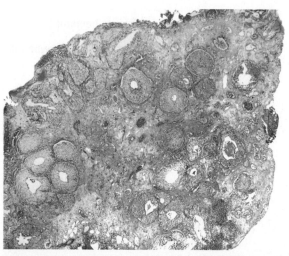

Figure 3.14.1 Proliferation of von Brunn nests in the bladder consisting of large uniform nests with central cyst formation.

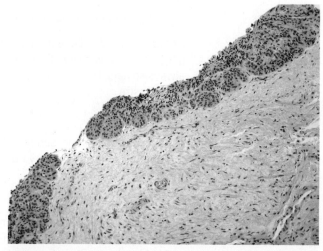

Figure 3.14.2 Proliferation of von Brunn nests in the bladder with small nests. The nests have a noninfiltrative base and cluster just beneath the surface.

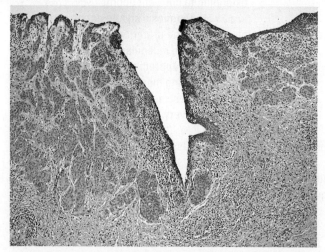

Figure 3.14.3 Proliferation of von Brunn nests in the bladder with small nests. The nests have a noninfiltrative base and cluster just beneath the surface.

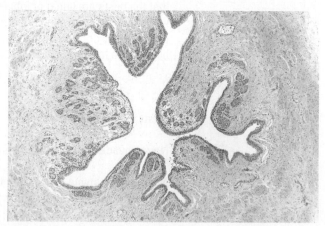

Figure 3.14.4 Proliferation of von Brunn nests in the bladder with small nests arranged in a lobular and linear array beneath the urothelium. Nests are circumferential around the ureter and are noninfiltrative.

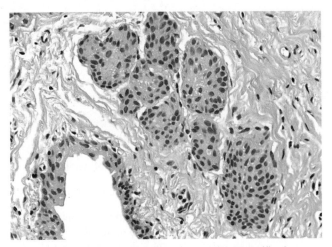

Figure 3.14.5   Same case as Figure 3.14.4 at higher magnification.

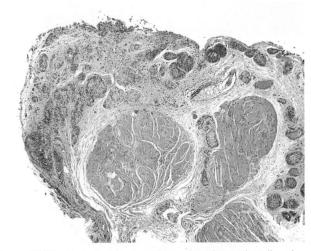

Figure 3.14.6   Nested carcinoma with smooth surface and small- and medium-sized nests infiltrating the muscularis propria.

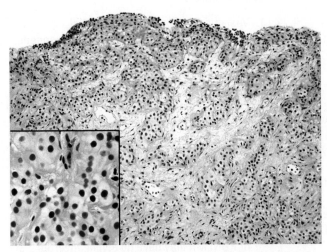

Figure 3.14.7   Nested carcinoma with smooth surface and small nests irregularly infiltrating lamina propria. **Inset** shows bland cytology.

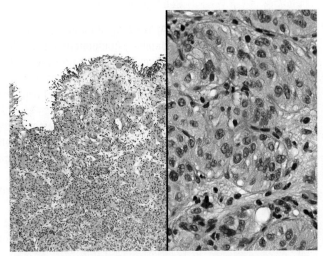

Figure 3.14.8   Nested carcinoma with crowded small nests filling the lamina propria (**left**) having minimal cytologic atypia (**right**).

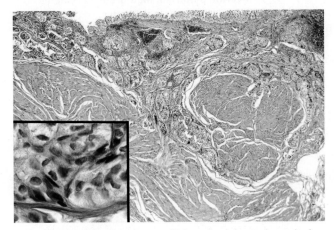

Figure 3.14.9   Nested carcinoma with irregular downward growth of small nests invading the muscularis propria. **Inset** shows no atypia.

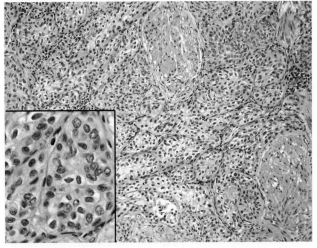

Figure 3.14.10   Nested carcinoma with back-to-back small nests invading the muscularis propria. Cells resemble normal urothelial cells with some even having nuclear grooves (**inset**).

3 BLADDER

	Nested Urothelial Carcinoma, Large Nest Variant	Noninvasive Carcinoma with Inverted Growth Pattern
Age	Mean age mid-60s with wide range	Mean age mid-60s with wide range
Location	Most commonly the bladder	Occurs at any location in the urothelial tract
Symptoms	Typically gross or microscopic hematuria	Typically gross or microscopic hematuria
Signs	At cystoscopy, an exophytic papillary component is present in the majority of cases corresponding to a low-grade papillary carcinoma component. Usually solitary. Wide range in size	At cystoscopy, papillary lesion with delicate coral-like surface. Solitary or multifocal with wide range in size. Rare cases with purely inverted growth pattern without an exophytic component
Etiology	See Section 3.10	See Section 3.10
Histology	1. At low magnification, surface has a papillary component in over 80% of cases, the vast majority low-grade papillary urothelial carcinoma 2. The lamina propria filled with large, irregularly shaped nests *(Figs. 3.15.1–3.15.3)* 3. Has an irregular base with infiltrative nests extending to different depths 4. Nests can be crowded but typically irregularly spaced apart 5. Often invades the muscularis propria *(Figs. 3.15.1–3.15.3)* 6. No cytologic atypia in areas, yet deeper nests may have prominent nucleoli *(Figs. 3.15.4–3.15.6)* 7. Mitotic figures average 1 to 2 per HPF 8. Variable desmoplastic stroma with variable inflammatory response *(Figs. 3.15.3 and 3.15.4)* 9. Necrosis in one-third of cases	1. Vast majority of papillary urothelial neoplasms have some exophytic component, although uncommonly entire lesion is inverted 2. The lamina propria filled with large, rounded nests of the urothelium *(Figs. 3.15.7 and 3.15.8)* 3. Nests lack an infiltrative border at the base of the lesion 4. Nests crowded with more uniform spacing *(Figs. 3.15.7 and 3.15.8)* 5. Does not involve the muscularis propria 6. Cytologic atypia depends on the grade. Inverted pattern of exophytic papilloma or PUNLMP may have no atypia. Inverted pattern of low-grade carcinoma with scattered hyperchromatic enlarged nuclei. Inverted pattern of high-grade carcinoma with marked cytologic atypia 7. Mitotic figures vary in frequency depending on the grade 8. Lacks desmoplastic stroma 9. Lacks necrosis
Special studies	Most cases would be expected to have low Ki-67 rate, yet no studies on this issue	Ki-67 varies depending on the grade of the tumor
Treatment	Radical surgery typically required as usually invades the muscularis propria	Typically, resected by TUR with adjuvant therapy depending on the grade (see Sections 3.8–3.11). Followed for life with routine cystoscopy
Prognosis	Limited number of cases with follow-up, yet capable of metastatic behavior and death	Risk of recurrence, progression, and death varies according to grade (see Sections 3.8–3.11)

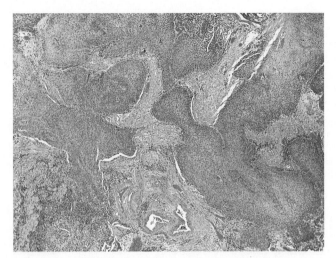

Figure 3.15.1   Large nested carcinoma with irregular large nests invading the muscularis propria associated with an inflammatory response.

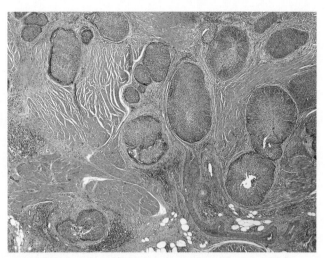

Figure 3.15.2   Large nested carcinoma with variably sized nests invading through the muscularis propria.

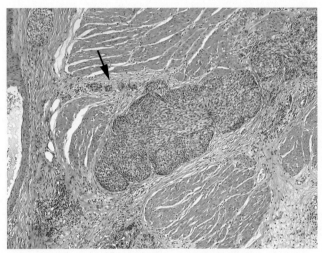

Figure 3.15.3   Same case as Figure 3.15.2 with desmoplastic stromal reaction. Also present are small nests of infiltrating carcinoma (*arrow*).

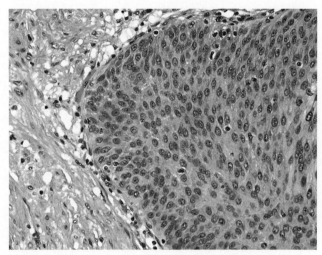

Figure 3.15.4   Same case as Figure 3.15.1 with minimal atypia and no stromal reaction.

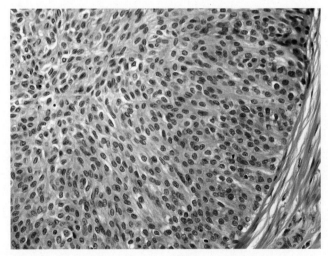

Figure 3.15.5   Same case as Figure 3.15.2 with minimal atypia.

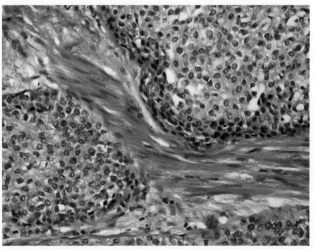

Figure 3.15.6   Same case as Figures 3.15.2, 3.15.3, and 3.15.5 with bland nests of the urothelium invading the muscularis propria.

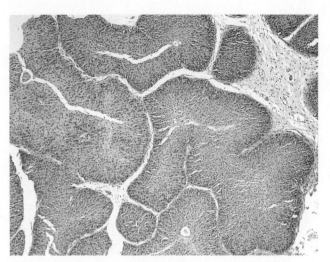

Figure 3.15.7 Noninvasive low-grade papillary urothelial carcinoma with noninfiltrative evenly spaced nests.

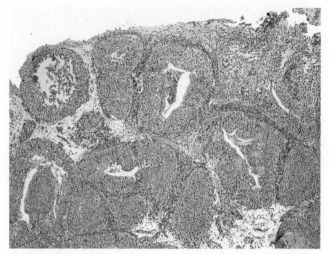

Figure 3.15.8 Noninvasive low-grade papillary urothelial carcinoma with uniform rounded nests.

	Tubular Carcinoma	Nephrogenic Adenoma
Age	Mean age mid-60s. Very uncommon in women	Mean age 40s with wide range. Twice as common in men
Location	Anywhere with urothelial lining	Anywhere with urothelial lining
Symptoms	Typically gross or microscopic hematuria	Typically gross or microscopic hematuria
Signs	At cystoscopy, nodular surface typically lacking an exophytic papillary component, although uncommon cases may have a papillary low-grade carcinoma surface lesion. Usually solitary. Wide range in size	At cystoscopy, variably papillary or nodular. 20% multifocal. Although most <1 cm, can be up to 7 cm
Etiology	Considered a variant of nested urothelial carcinoma	Results from shed renal tubular cells implanting into areas of prior injured urothelial mucosa. Often, history of prior surgery, instrumentation, calculi, or infection
Histology	1. At low magnification, surface is typically smooth without exophytic papillary fronds 2. Uncommon cases with surface showing CIS or papillary urothelial carcinoma 3. The lamina propria filled with small crowded tubules and often focal small nests *(Figs. 3.16.1 and 3.16.2)* 4. Lacks vascular-like structures lined by flattened epithelial cells or signet ring cell–like tubules 5. Lacks peritubular hyaline connective tissue sheath 6. Lacks dense eosinophilic thyroid-like secretions 7. No cytologic atypia in areas, yet deeper nests may have prominent nucleoli 8. Occasional mitotic figures 9. Irregular base with infiltrative tubules extending to different depths 10. Often invades the muscularis propria 11. Usually lacks desmoplastic stroma and inflammatory response	1. At low magnification, surface is typically smooth yet can have focal exophytic papillary fronds 2. If surface papillary, lined by cuboidal epithelium 3. Although tubules often present, solid nests are absent 4. In addition to tubules, vascular-like structures lined by flattened epithelial cells or signet ring cell–like tubules *(Figs. 3.16.3 and 3.16.4; also see Section 3.17)* 5. Some tubules surrounded by hyaline connective tissue sheath *(Fig. 3.16.4)* 6. Some tubules with dense eosinophilic thyroid-like secretions *(Fig. 3.16.4; also see Section 3.17)* 7. May have prominent nucleoli. Only atypia is in hobnail cells lining vascular-like structures 8. Mitotic figures either absent or extremely rare 9. May have an irregular base with infiltrative tubules extending to different depths 10. Can uncommonly involve superficial muscle in the bladder neck (see Section 3.17) 11. Associated with acute and chronic inflammation

	Tubular Carcinoma	**Nephrogenic Adenoma**
Special studies	• Most cases with low Ki-67 rate, with only a few cases with rate >20% • PAX8 negative	• Low Ki-67 rate • PAX8 positive
Treatment	Radical surgery typically required as usually invades the muscularis propria	Benign, no treatment needed
Prognosis	Aggressive behavior comparable to invasive high-grade urothelial carcinoma	Benign although can be multifocal and can "recur" following biopsy and reinjury of the urothelium

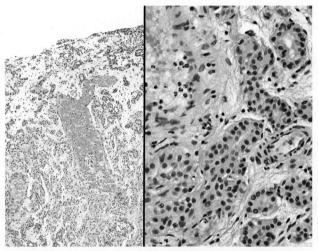

Figure 3.16.1   Tubular carcinoma with nests and tubules filling the lamina propria (*left*). Lesion consists of a mixture of nests (*lower left of* **left panel**) and tubules (*upper right of* **left panel**) with bland cytology.

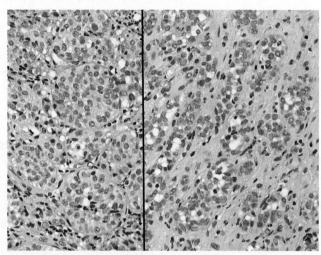

Figure 3.16.2   Tubular carcinoma with crowded cytologically bland nests (**left**) and tubules (**right**) invading the lamina propria.

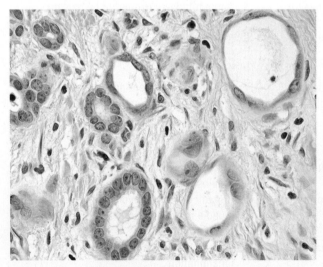

Figure 3.16.3   Nephrogenic adenoma composed of tubules lined by cuboidal cells with prominent nucleoli. Some tubules lined by flattened epithelium resembling vessels.

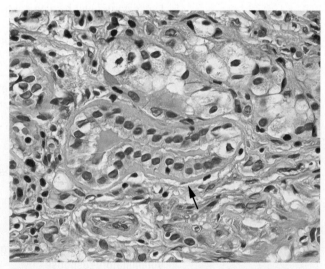

Figure 3.16.4   Nephrogenic adenoma composed of tubules lined by cuboidal cells. Tubule contains dense colloid and is surrounded by collagen rim (*arrow*).

	Nephrogenic Adenoma	Clear Cell Adenocarcinoma
Age	Mean age 40s with wide range. Twice as common in men	Mean age mid-late 50s–60s. Uncommon in males
Location	Anywhere with urothelial lining	The bladder or urethra. Predilection for urethral diverticula
Symptoms	Typically gross or microscopic hematuria	Typically gross or microscopic hematuria
Signs	At cystoscopy, variably papillary or nodular. 20% multifocal. Although most <1 cm, can be up to 7 cm	At cystoscopy, typically a large unifocal exophytic tumor
Etiology	Results from shed renal tubular cells implanting into areas of prior injured urothelial mucosa. Often, history of prior surgery, instrumentation, calculi, or infection	Some cases associated with endometriosis and others with urothelial carcinoma
Histology	1. Tubules, papillary, vascular-like, and signet ring cell–like patterns. Lacks solid foci *(Figs. 3.17.1–3.17.3)* 2. Eosinophilic cytoplasm with at most only rare focal clear cytoplasm *(Fig. 3.17.4)* 3. Some tubules surrounded by hyaline connective tissue sheath *(Fig. 3.17.3)* 4. Some tubules with dense eosinophilic thyroid-like secretions *(Fig. 3.17.5)* 5. May have prominent nucleoli. Pleomorphism only in hobnail cells lining vascular-like structures 6. Lacks hyperchromatic nuclei even in hobnail cells *(Figs. 3.17.1–3.17.3)* 7. Mitotic figures either absent or extremely rare 8. Necrosis absent 9. Can uncommonly involve superficial muscle in the bladder neck *(Fig. 3.17.5)*	1. Solid, tubular, and papillary patterns *(Figs. 3.17.7–3.17.10)* 2. Variably eosinophilic and/or clear cytoplasm *(Fig. 3.17.11)* 3. Tubules lack hyaline connective tissue sheath 4. Tubules lack dense eosinophilic thyroid-like secretions 5. Prominent cytologic atypia, although foci and rare cases may have relatively minimal atypia 6. Hyperchromatic nuclei, even in the rare cases with relatively bland nuclei *(Figs. 3.17.7–3.17.9)* 7. Mitotic figures common 8. Necrosis common 9. Deeply invasive into the muscularis propria, although not evident on limited biopsy *(Fig. 3.17.12)*
Special studies	• Low Ki-67 rate *(Fig. 3.17.6)* • PAX8 positive	• Ki-67 typically >20% *(Fig. 3.17.6)* • PAX8 positive
Treatment	Benign, no treatment needed	Typically requires radical cystectomy. Unclear if radiotherapy or chemotherapy helpful
Prognosis	Benign although can be multifocal and can "recur" following biopsy and reinjury of the urothelium	In general, more aggressive than urothelial carcinoma. Lymph nodes and bone most common sites of metastases

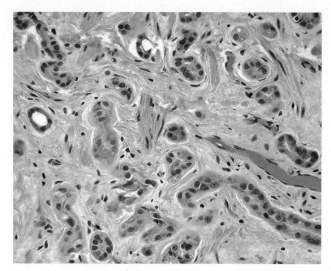

Figure 3.17.1 Tubules of nephrogenic adenoma with visible nucleoli but lacking nuclear hyperchromasia.

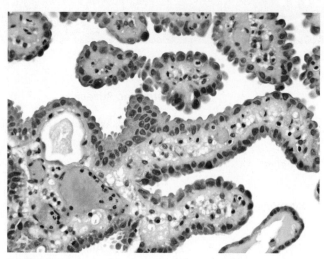

Figure 3.17.2 Papillary nephrogenic adenoma lined by bland cuboidal epithelium.

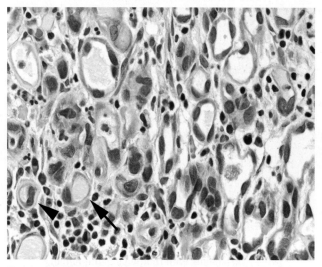

Figure 3.17.3 Nephrogenic adenoma with attenuated epithelium resembling vessels and signet ring cells with mucin (*arrow*). Peritubular hyaline rim of collagen is seen in some small tubules (*arrowhead*).

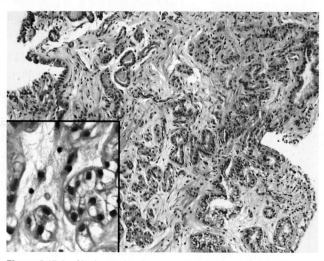

Figure 3.17.4 Nephrogenic adenoma with focal dense thyroid-like secretions (*upper left*) and focal clear cells (*lower right* and **inset**).

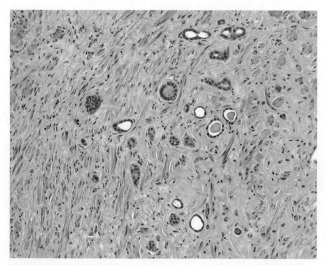

Figure 3.17.5 Nephrogenic adenoma with dense thyroid-like secretions invading the superficial muscularis propria. Cells lack nuclear hyperchromasia.

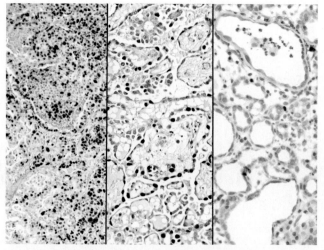

Figure 3.17.6 Low Ki-67 in nephrogenic adenoma (**right**) compared to solid clear cell adenocarcinoma (**left**) and papillary clear cell adenocarcinoma (**center**).

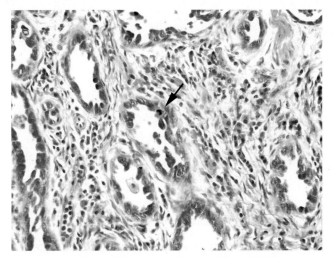

Figure 3.17.7 Clear cell adenocarcinoma with tubules lined by hyperchromatic hobnail nuclei with mitotic figures (*arrow*).

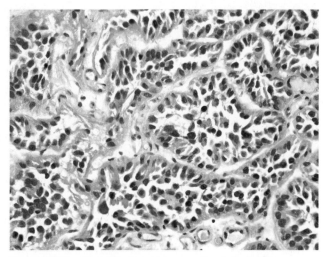

Figure 3.17.8 Clear cell adenocarcinoma with tubules lined by hyperchromatic hobnail nuclei.

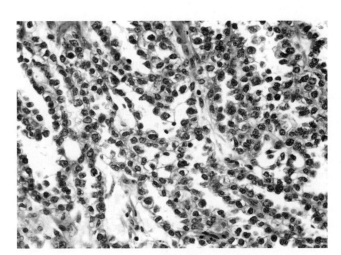

Figure 3.17.9 Clear cell adenocarcinoma with tubules lined by hyperchromatic nuclei surrounded by clear cytoplasm.

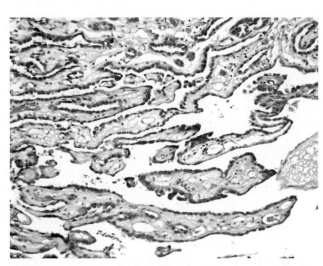

Figure 3.17.10 Clear cell adenocarcinoma with papillary fronds lined by hyperchromatic nuclei.

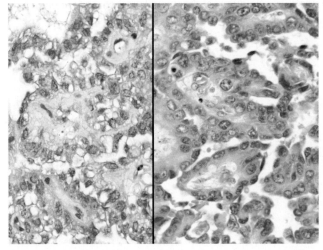

Figure 3.17.11 Clear cell adenocarcinoma lined by either clear (**left**) or eosinophilic (**right**) cytoplasm.

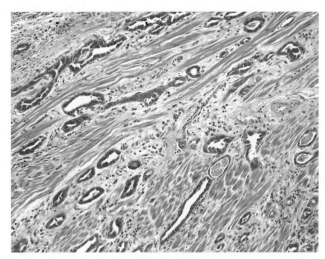

Figure 3.17.12 Clear cell adenocarcinoma with tubules invading the muscularis propria.

	Clear Cell Adenocarcinoma	Urothelial Carcinoma, Clear Cell Differentiation
Age	Mean age mid-late 50s–60s. Marked female predominance	Mean age mid-late 60s. Male > female
Location	The bladder or urethra. Predilection for urethral diverticula	Anywhere with urothelial lining
Symptoms	Typically gross or microscopic hematuria	Typically gross or microscopic hematuria
Signs	At cystoscopy, typically a large unifocal exophytic tumor	At cystoscopy, varies depending on the stage of the tumor
Etiology	Some cases associated with endometriosis and others with urothelial carcinoma	Same as usual urothelial carcinoma
Histology	1. Solid, tubular, and papillary patterns *(Figs. 3.18.1 and 3.18.2)* 2. Variably eosinophilic and/or clear cytoplasm 3. Prominent cytologic atypia, although foci and rare cases may have relatively minimal atypia *(Figs. 3.18.1 and 3.18.2)* 4. Deeply invasive into the muscularis propria, although not evident on limited biopsy	1. Nests and sheets of cells in infiltrating carcinoma *(Fig. 3.18.3)*. Clear cell differentiation also seen in noninvasive papillary carcinoma *(Fig. 3.18.4)* 2. Ranging from focal to extensive clear cytoplasm. Elsewhere more typical of usual urothelial carcinoma with eosinophilic cytoplasm 3. Variable cytologic atypia depending on the grade 4. Invasive carcinoma usually deeply invasive into the muscularis propria
Special studies	PAX8 positive	PAX8 negative
Treatment	Typically requires radical cystectomy	Depends on stage and grade, no different than usual urothelial carcinoma
Prognosis	In general, more aggressive than urothelial carcinoma. Lymph nodes and bone, the most common sites of metastases	No different than usual urothelial carcinoma

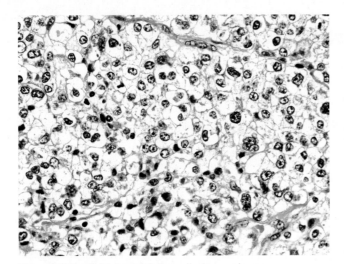

Figure 3.18.1   Solid sheets of clear cell adenocarcinoma.

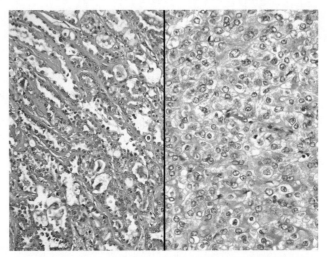

Figure 3.18.2   Clear cell adenocarcinoma with tubules (**left**) and solid sheets (**right**).

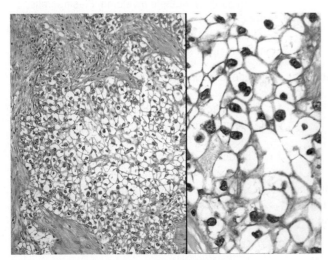

Figure 3.18.3   Nests of clear cell urothelial carcinoma.

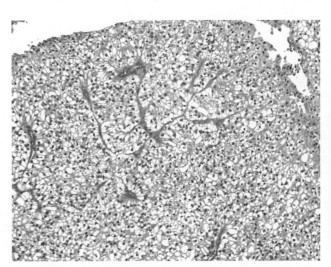

Figure 3.18.4   Papillary urothelial carcinoma with clear cytoplasm.

	Plasmacytoid Urothelial Carcinoma	**Plasmacytoma/Normal Plasma Cells**
Age	Mean age mid-60s. Male > female	Middle age to elderly for plasmacytoma
Location	Anywhere with urothelial lining	No preference
Symptoms	Typically gross or microscopic hematuria	Typically gross or microscopic hematuria for plasmacytoma. Patients could have systemic symptoms if part of multiple myeloma
Signs	At cystoscopy, tumors often do not make a large exophytic mass but are more infiltrative	At cystoscopy, variable appearance for plasmacytoma
Etiology	Same as usual urothelial carcinoma	Plasmacytoma can be isolated or as a component of multiple myeloma. Plasma cells are a common component of usual chronic inflammatory infiltrate seen nonspecifically in many bladder specimens
Histology	1. Infiltrating loosely cohesive individual cells *(Fig. 3.19.1)* 2. Plasmacytoid cytoplasm *(Fig. 3.19.2)* 3. Hyperchromatic nuclei *(Fig. 3.19.2)* 4. Coexistence with other morphologies that have loosely cohesive cells, including rhabdoid and bland cells resembling infiltrating lobular carcinoma with occasional signet ring cells 5. May coexist with usual urothelial carcinoma 6. Invasive carcinoma usually deeply invasive into the muscularis propria in a pattern similar to signet-ring cell carcinoma with a linitis plastica pattern	1. Loosely cohesive individual cells *(Fig. 3.19.3)* 2. Plasmacytoid cytoplasm *(Fig. 3.19.4)* 3. Plasmacytoma typically not pleomorphic, resembling normal plasma cells although binucleated plasma cells may be present *(Fig 3.19.4)*. Typically not hyperchromatic nuclei 4. Rhabdoid and lobular carcinoma-like patterns absent 5. No relationship to urothelial carcinoma 6. Typically not that deeply infiltrative but clustered under the urothelium
Special studies	• CD138 positive • CK7 and GATA3 positive • If plasma cells present, polyclonal	• CD138 positive • CK7 and GATA3 negative • Polyclonal population of kappa- and lambda-positive cells with reactive plasma cells. Clonal population with typically lambda light chain restriction in plasmacytoma

	Plasmacytoid Urothelial Carcinoma	Plasmacytoma/Normal Plasma Cells
Treatment	Depends on stage and grade, no different than usual urothelial carcinoma	Treatment for plasmacytoma depends if localized to the bladder or part of multiple myeloma. If localized can be treated with radiotherapy. Common to see normal plasma cells and lymphocytes in bladder biopsies in the absence of clinical cystitis. Consequently, the presence of these inflammatory cells should not be histologically diagnosed as "chronic cystitis"
Prognosis	No different than usual urothelial carcinoma	Only rare cases of plasmacytoma of the bladder reported with worse prognosis for patients with systemic multiple myeloma

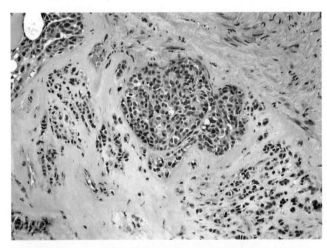

Figure 3.19.1   Nests of urothelial carcinoma with plasmacytoid features.

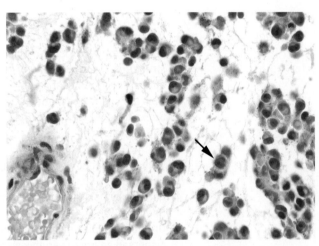

Figure 3.19.2   Same case as Figure 3.19.1 consisting of cells with hyperchromatic nuclei and plasmacytoid cytoplasm. Some nuclei have prominent nucleoli (*arrow*).

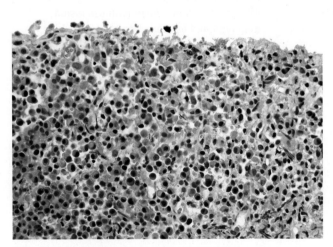

Figure 3.19.3   Plasmacytoma involving the bladder.

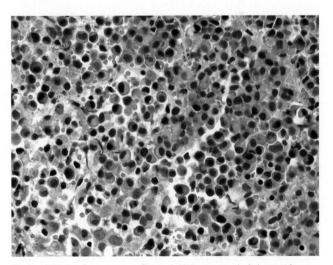

Figure 3.19.4   Same case as Figure 3.19.3 composed of sheets of mature plasma cells.

3 BLADDER

	Low-Grade Papillary Urothelial Carcinoma	Condyloma
Age	Any age, but typically biopsied in adults	Any age, but typically biopsied in adults
Location	Anywhere with urothelial lining	Anywhere with urothelial lining
Symptoms	Typically gross or microscopic hematuria	Typically gross or microscopic hematuria
Signs	At cystoscopy, the urologist typically cannot distinguish a papillary urothelial neoplasm from a condyloma	Papillary neoplasm
Etiology	See Section 3.10	HPV related. Typically has concurrent or history of condylomas on the external genitalia
Histology	1. As a result of complex branching papillary fronds, most of the papillary structures in a given plane of section appear to be free floating detached from the underlying bladder *(Fig. 3.20.1)* 2. Stalks typically well developed with fibrovascular cores *(Fig. 3.20.1)* 3. With the exception of papilloma, a thickened urothelium 4. Rare for cytoplasm to be clear (see Section 3.18) 5. Urothelial atypia consists of randomly dispersed enlarged variably sized hyperchromatic nuclei *(Fig. 3.20.2)* 6. Mitotic figures present in increasing number from low- to high-grade papillary urothelial carcinoma 7. Inverted growth pattern common 8. May be associated with invasive urothelial carcinoma	1. Verrucous folds of epithelium with thin fibrovascular cores, lacking "free-floating" papillary fronds *(Figs. 3.20.3 and 3.20.4)* 2. Lacks well-formed stalks, showing only capillaries in the middle of folds of epithelium *(Figs. 3.20.3 and 3.20.4)* 3. Thickened nonkeratinizing squamous epithelium *(Fig. 3.20.5)* 4. Cytoplasmic clearing around nuclei (koilocytosis) *(Figs. 3.20.5 and 3.20.6)* 5. Atypia consists of crinkly mostly small nuclei, lacking hyperchromasia unless accompanied by moderate to severe dysplasia. With increasing dysplasia, zone of cells with a higher nuclear-to-cytoplasmic ratio and nuclear hyperchromasia proliferating off the basal cell layer *(Fig. 3.20.6)* 6. Mitotic figures uncommon unless lesion accompanied by moderate to severe dysplasia 7. Inverted growth pattern common 8. May be associated with invasive squamous cell carcinoma
Special studies	*In situ* hybridization negative for HPV. Immunohistochemistry for p16 may be positive	*In situ* hybridization in condyloma without dysplasia variably positive for low-risk (HPV 6/11) HPV. In cases with moderate to severe dysplasia increasingly positive for high-risk HPV (HPV 16/18 and others). *In situ* hybridization may be negative for wide spectrum HPV but positive for individual HPV stains. Immunohistochemistry for p16 positive.

	Low-Grade Papillary Urothelial Carcinoma	**Condyloma**
Treatment	Tailored to the tumor's grade, size, and multifocality and whether the lesion is a recurrence or primary lesion (see Sections 3.10 and 3.11)	Resected or fulgurated
Prognosis	See Sections 3.10 and 3.11	Difficult to eradicate due to multifocality. Increased risk of developing squamous cell carcinoma of the bladder

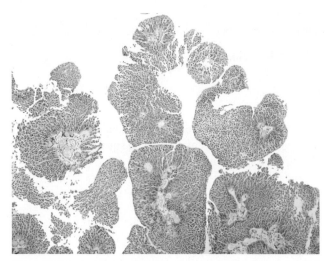

Figure 3.20.1 Isolated papillary fronds of low-grade papillary urothelial carcinoma.

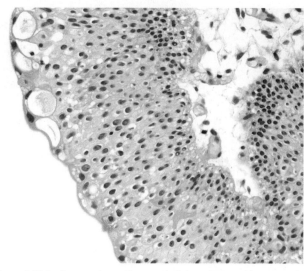

Figure 3.20.2 Low-grade papillary urothelial carcinoma with scattered slightly enlarged hyperchromatic nuclei.

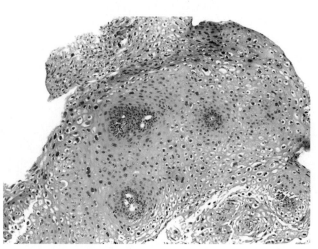

Figure 3.20.3 Bladder condyloma with verrucous folds of epithelium with thin fibrovascular cores, lacking "free-floating" papillary fronds.

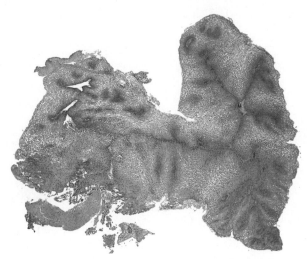

Figure 3.20.4 Condyloma of the bladder with verrucous folds of epithelium with thin fibrovascular cores.

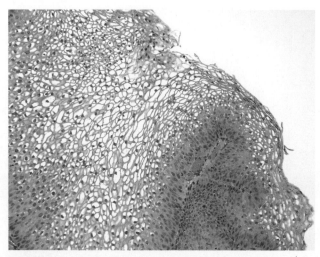

Figure 3.20.5 Condyloma involving the bladder with squamous epithelium with abundant clear cytoplasm.

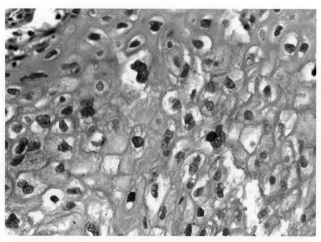

Figure 3.20.6 Bladder condyloma with crinkly irregular nuclei in cells with koilocytosis.

	Condyloma	Squamous Papilloma
Age	Any age, but typically biopsied in adults	Any age, but typically biopsied in adults
Location	Anywhere with urothelial lining	Anywhere with urothelial lining
Symptoms	Typically gross or microscopic hematuria	Typically gross or microscopic hematuria
Signs	Typically has concurrent or history of condylomas on the external genitalia. Often multifocal	Squamous papillomas typically a solitary lesion unassociated with lesions on the external genitalia
Etiology	HPV related	Unrelated to HPV. No known risk factor
Histology	1. Verrucous folds of epithelium with thin fibrovascular cores, mostly lacking "free-floating" papillary fronds *(Fig. 3.21.1)* 2. Lacks stalks showing only capillaries in the middle of folds of epithelium *(Fig. 3.21.1)* 3. Thickened nonkeratinizing squamous epithelium 4. Cytoplasmic clearing around nuclei (koilocytosis) *(Fig. 3.2.2)* 5. Atypia consists of crinkly mostly small nuclei, lacking hyperchromasia unless accompanied by moderate to severe dysplasia. With increasing dysplasia, zone of cells with a higher nuclear-to-cytoplasmic ratio and nuclear hyperchromasia proliferating off the basal cell layer *(Fig. 3.21.2)* 6. Mitotic figures uncommon unless lesion accompanied by moderate to severe dysplasia 7. Inverted growth pattern common 8. May be associated with invasive squamous cell carcinoma	1. "Free-floating" papillary fronds *(Figs. 3.21.3 and 3.21.4)* 2. Well-established stalks with fibrovascular cores *(Figs. 3.21.3–3.21.6)* 3. Thickened nonkeratinizing squamous epithelium *(Figs. 3.21.5 and 3.21.6)* 4. Cytoplasm lightly eosinophilic lacking koilocytosis *(Figs. 3.21.5 and 3.21.6)* 5. Lacks atypia *(Figs. 3.21.5 and 3.21.6)* 6. Mitotic figures uncommon 7. Lacks an inverted growth pattern 8. Not associated with invasive squamous cell carcinoma
Special studies	*In situ* hybridization in condyloma without dysplasia variably positive for low-risk (HPV 6/11) HPV. In cases with moderate to severe dysplasia, increasingly positive for high-risk HPV (HPV 16/18 and others). *In situ* hybridization may be negative for wide spectrum HPV but positive for individual HPV stains. Immunohistochemistry for p16 positive	Not associated with HPV
Treatment	Resected or fulgurated	Resected or fulgurated
Prognosis	Difficult to eradicate due to multifocality. Increased risk of developing squamous cell carcinoma of the bladder	Once resected, lesion does not recur. No increased risk of developing squamous cell carcinoma of the bladder

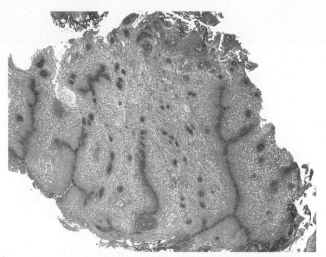

Figure 3.21.1   Condyloma involving the bladder with verrucous folds of epithelium with thin fibrovascular cores, mostly lacking "free-floating" papillary fronds.

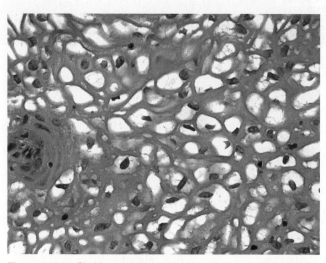

Figure 3.21.2   Bladder condyloma with koilocytosis and crinkly nuclei.

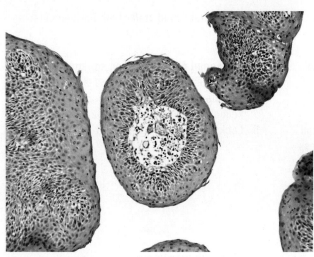

Figure 3.21.3   Bladder squamous papilloma composed of papillary fronds lined by squamous epithelium.

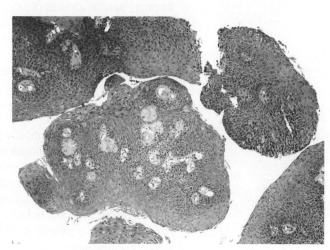

Figure 3.21.4   Bladder squamous papilloma composed of papillary fronds lined by squamous epithelium.

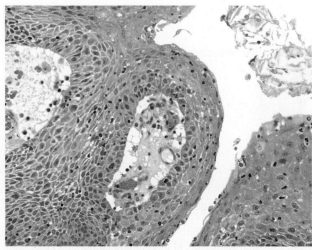

Figure 3.21.5   Squamous papilloma of the bladder lined by inflamed benign squamous epithelium.

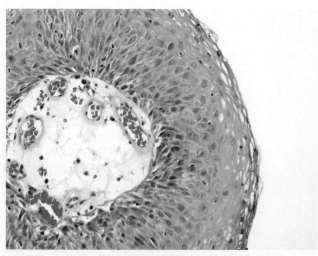

Figure 3.21.6   Squamous papilloma of the bladder lined by benign squamous epithelium lacking koilocytosis and viral atypia.

	Fibroepithelial Polyp	Urothelial Papilloma
Age	Wide range from children to adults. Marked male predominance. More than half in neonates or children, some with urogenital malformations	Mean age mid-late 50s with wide range
Location	Anywhere with urothelial lining	Anywhere with urothelial lining
Symptoms	Urinary obstruction, urinary hesitancy, dysuria, enuresis, hematuria, flank pain, or infection	Typically gross or microscopic hematuria
Signs	At cystoscopy, variably sized polypoid mass typically at the verumontanum or bladder neck. Typically solitary	At cystoscopy, delicate papillary lesion, typically solitary and relatively small
Etiology	Unknown	See Section 3.10
Histology	1. Overall architecture is polypoid fibrous lesion with papillary or finger-like projections from the surface. Another pattern is polypoid growth with florid cystitis cystica *(Figs. 3.22.1–3.22.4)* 2. Dense fibrous stroma *(Figs. 3.22.1–3.22.4)* 3. The urothelium is normal thickness *(Figs. 3.22.1, 3.22.2, and 3.22.4)*. Occasionally lined by glandular lining *(Fig. 3.22.3)* 4. Cytology is normal 5. Umbrella cells vary from inconspicuous to apocrine to prominent degenerative atypia	1. As a result of complex branching papillary fronds, most of the papillary structures in a given plane of section appear to be free floating detached from the underlying bladder *(Figs. 3.22.5 and 3.22.6)* 2. Delicate loose connective tissue stalks *(Figs. 3.22.5 and 3.22.6)* 3. The urothelium is normal thickness *(Figs. 3.22.5 and 3.22.6)* 4. Cytology is normal 5. Umbrella cells not prominent
Special studies	Not helpful in this differential diagnosis	Not helpful in this differential.
Treatment	Resected by TUR. No need for routine follow-up with cystoscopy	Resected by TUR. Patients followed for life with cystoscopy for possible recurrent urothelial neoplasia
Prognosis	Benign	In most cases once resected, the lesion does not recur. In about 10% of cases, the lesion recurs as papilloma and in 10% as low-grade papillary carcinoma or PUNLMP. Only rare cases in the literature in patients with immunosuppression progress to high-grade or invasive carcinoma.

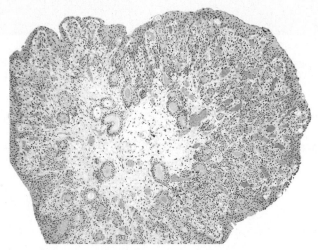

Figure 3.22.1 Fibroepithelial polyp with polypoid growth and underlying florid cystitis cystica.

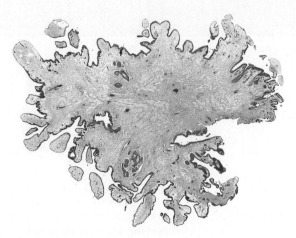

Figure 3.22.2 Fibroepithelial polyp with finger-like projections from the surface.

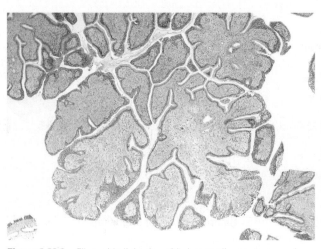

Figure 3.22.3 Fibroepithelial polyp with dense collagen stroma and lined by both the urothelium and glandular epithelium.

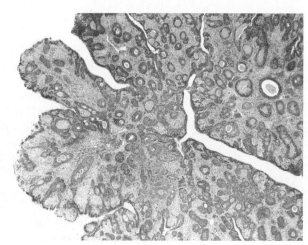

Figure 3.22.4 Club-shaped fibroepithelial polyp with stroma containing florid cystitis cystica.

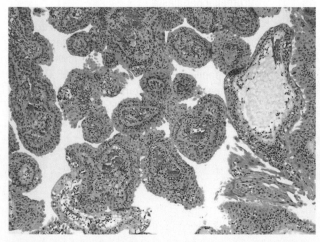

Figure 3.22.5 Papilloma with delicate "free-floating" papillary fronds lined by the normal-thickness urothelium.

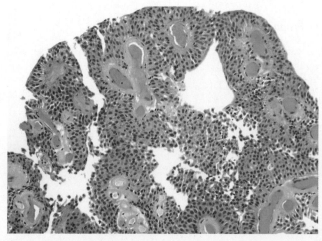

Figure 3.22.6 Isolated papillary fronds of papilloma lined by the normal-cytology and normal-thickness urothelium.

	Malakoplakia	Poorly Differentiated Urothelial Carcinoma
Age	Middle age. Female predominance with a 4:1 ratio	Mean age mid-late 50s–60s with wide range
Location	The bladder, the most common site	Anywhere with urothelial lining
Symptoms	Typically gross or microscopic hematuria. Patients may have disabilities, immunosuppressed, or other chronic illnesses	Typically gross or microscopic hematuria
Signs	Cystoscopy reveals mucosal plaques and nodules that occasionally become larger masses	At cystoscopy, typically large exophytic often ulcerative mass. Occasionally, more subtle with a linitis plastica diffuse infiltrative appearance
Etiology	Bacteria or bacterial fragments form a nidus for the calcium phosphate crystals that laminate the Michaelis-Gutmann bodies. Associated with a defect in the intraphagosomal digestion, which accounts for the unusual immune response	See Section 3.10
Histology	1. Sheets or nests of cells *(Fig. 3.23.1)* 2. Can form large masses with destruction of the muscularis propria 3. Large fairly cohesive cluster of histiocytes with eosinophilic cytoplasm (von Hansemann cells) with small basophilic extracytoplasmic or intracytoplasmic calculopherules resembling bull's-eyes on a target (Michaelis-Gutmann bodies). Variable numbers of Michaelis-Gutmann bodies present in a given case *(Figs. 3.23.2 and 3.23.3)* 4. Relatively bland histiocytic appearing nuclei 5. Occasional benign multinucleated giant cells 6. Later lesions can be associated with fibrosis *(Fig. 3.23.4)*	1. Sheets or nests of cells *(Fig. 3.23.5)* 2. Can form large masses with destruction of the muscularis propria 3. Typically cohesive, yet can be loosely cohesive cells with abundant pale eosinophilic cytoplasm resembling histiocytes *(Fig. 3.23.6)* 4. Nuclei are typically but not always pleomorphic *(Fig. 3.23.6)* 5. Lacks benign multinucleated giant cells 6. More cellular desmoplastic response may be seen
Special studies	• Michaelis-Gutmann bodies positive for calcium stains (von Kossa) and iron stains (Prussian blue) • Cells positive for histiocyte markers (i.e., CD68) • Negative for keratins	• Negative for calcium and iron stains • Negative for CD68 • Positive for keratins, especially CK7

	Malakoplakia	**Poorly Differentiated Urothelial Carcinoma**
Treatment	Primarily based on controlling the urinary tract infections, which stabilizes the disease. Adding bethanechol, a cholinergic agent thought to increase the intracellular cyclic guanosine monophosphate levels considered to be the defect-causing macrophage dysfunction, may also be useful. Surgery may be necessary as the disease progresses, despite antimicrobial treatment	Stage dependent
Prognosis	Excellent	Stage dependent

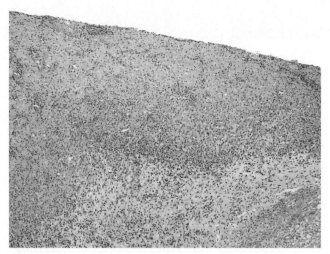

Figure 3.23.1   Malakoplakia consisting of sheets of histiocytes.

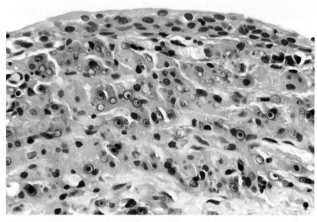

Figure 3.23.2   Numerous Michaelis-Gutmann bodies in malakoplakia.

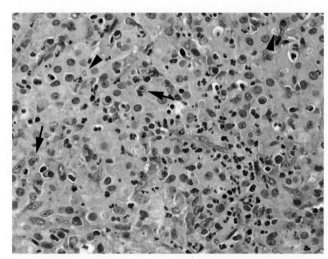

Figure 3.23.3   Malakoplakia with targetoid Michaelis-Gutmann bodies (*arrows*). Depending on the plane of section, the bull's-eye appearance is not apparent (*arrowheads*).

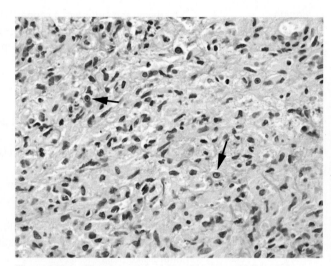

Figure 3.23.4   Fibrosing malakoplakia with scattered Michaelis-Gutmann bodies (*arrows*).

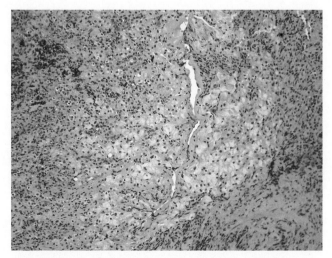

Figure 3.23.5   Urothelial carcinoma with cohesive nests of cells resembling histiocytes.

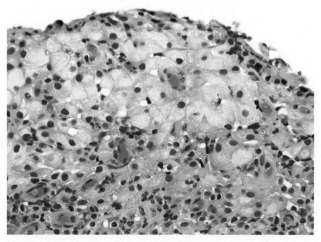

Figure 3.23.6   Same case as Figure 3.23.5 composed of cohesive cells with abundant pale cytoplasm and relatively uniform nuclei.

	Biopsy Site Reaction	Residual Urothelial Carcinoma
Age	Mean age mid-60s with wide range	Mean age mid-60s with wide range
Location	Anywhere with urothelial lining, typically the bladder	Anywhere with urothelial lining
Symptoms	May be persistent hematuria or asymptomatic with rebiopsy for staging purposes	May be persistent hematuria or mass or asymptomatic with rebiopsy for staging purposes
Signs	At cystoscopy, prior biopsy site with ulceration where it can be impossible to distinguish vs. residual cancer	At cystoscopy, may be obvious residual tumor, but in other cases, indistinguishable from a prior biopsy site
Etiology	Typically in the setting of a repeat TUR to assess for muscularis propria invasion following an initial biopsy showing invasive urothelial carcinoma	Where this differential diagnosis exists is in the setting of a repeat TUR to assess for muscularis propria invasion following an initial biopsy showing invasive urothelial carcinoma
Histology	1. May be nests of histiocytes *(Figs. 3.24.1–3.24.3)* 2. Often multinucleated giant cells present *(Fig. 3.24.1)* 3. Histiocytes have abundant cytoplasm with bland nuclei 4. Cellular myofibroblastic reaction	1. Nests of cells 2. Multinucleated giant cells may be in adjacent tissue 3. Cells can have abundant cytoplasm and pleomorphic, hyperchromatic nuclei 4. Cellular desmoplastic response may be seen
Special studies	Immunohistochemistry positive for pancytokeratin in bundles of smooth muscle cells *(Fig. 3.24.4)* and in myofibroblastic tissue culture–like cells *(Fig. 3.24.5)*	Positive for keratins, especially CK7, in epithelioid single cells, cell clusters, rows of cells, or nests of carcinoma *(Fig. 3.24.6)*
Treatment	Depends on the stage of the tumor on the initial biopsy	If muscularis propria invasion present typically radical cystectomy
Prognosis	Depends on the stage of the tumor on the initial biopsy	Stage dependent

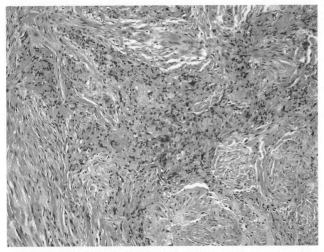

Figure 3.24.1   Bladder biopsy site with a cluster of epithelioid histiocytes resembling carcinoma. Scattered multinucleated giant cells are present.

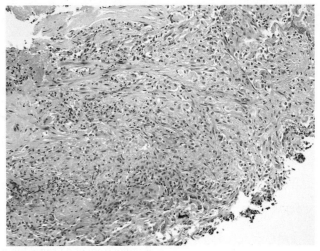

Figure 3.24.2   Exuberant biopsy site reaction.

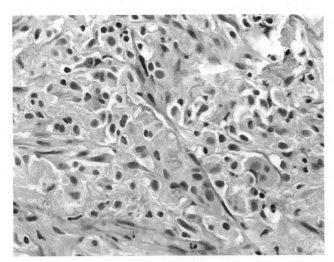

Figure 3.24.3   Same case as Figure 3.24.2 with bland nests of histiocytes.

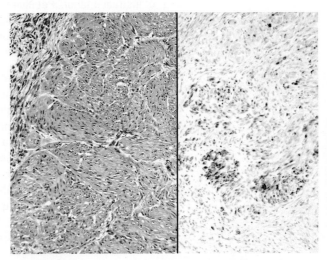

Figure 3.24.4   Smooth muscle from biopsy site (**left**) with keratin positivity (**right**).

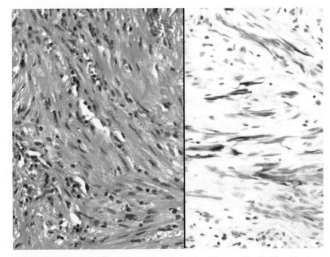

Figure 3.24.5   Myofibroblastic reactive from biopsy site (**left**) with keratin positivity (**right**).

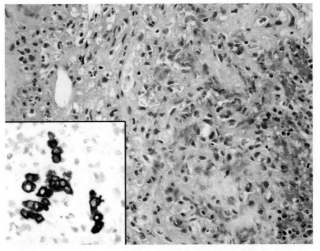

Figure 3.24.6   Biopsy site which on H&E is difficult to identify carcinoma. **Inset** shows clusters of epithelioid keratin-positive cells consistent with residual carcinoma.

	Fibromyxoid Nephrogenic Adenoma	Collagen Injection
Age	Mid-60s to late 70s. Male predominance	Wide range
Location	Anywhere with urothelial lining	Typically around the urethra or ureteral orifices
Symptoms	Typically gross or microscopic hematuria	Hematuria or obstructive symptoms
Signs	No information	At cystoscopy, nodular submucosal nodule in area of prior implantation
Etiology	Results from shed renal tubular cells implanting into areas of prior injured mucosa. Often, history of prior surgery or instrumentation. Peculiar fibromyxoid pattern may be treatment related as most men have history of bladder or prostate carcinoma typically treated by irradiation	Prior history of urethral collagen injection to treat urinary incontinence or subureteral collagen injection for vesicoureteral reflux
Histology	1. Focal usual nephrogenic adenoma typically present consisting of atrophic tubules or vascular-like tubules lined by hobnail cells with a minority of cases having flat or papillary surface lined by cuboidal epithelium 2. Pale eosinophilic fibromyxoid deposits containing compressed tubules resembling small vessels or fibroblasts *(Figs. 3.25.1 and 3.25.2)* 3. No surrounding giant cell reaction 4. Surrounding tissue may have associated with acute and chronic inflammation	1. Lacks usual nephrogenic adenoma 2. Pale acellular eosinophilic fibromyxoid deposits *(Figs. 3.25.3 and 3.25.4)* 3. Typically lacks foreign body giant cell reaction 4. No associated inflammatory tissue reaction *(Figs. 3.25.3 and 3.25.4)*
Special studies	• Keratin, PAX8, and AMACR positive in entrapped compressed tubules *(Fig. 3.25.1)*. Many more epithelial structures identified with keratin than appreciated on H&E-stained sections • Background matrix positive for periodic acid–Schiff with focal staining for mucicarmine • Congo red negative	• Keratin, PAX8, and AMACR negative • Can stain pink with periodic acid–Schiff with negative mucicarmine • Congo red negative
Treatment	Benign, no treatment needed	Benign, treatment only required if collagen migrates leading to obstruction or irritative symptoms
Prognosis	Benign although can be multifocal and can "recur" following biopsy and reinjury of the urothelium	Relates to the initial reason for the injection

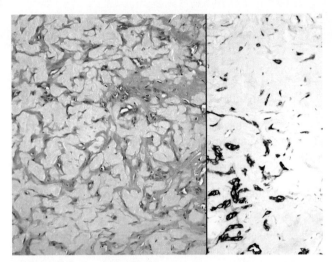

Figure 3.25.1 Fibromyxoid nephrogenic adenoma with entrapped tubules highlighted by keratin (**right**).

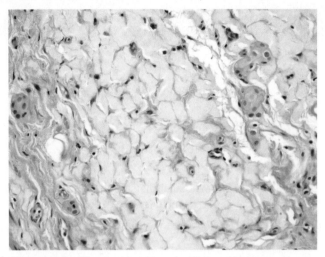

Figure 3.25.2 Fibromyxoid nephrogenic adenoma with entrapped tubules (*right*).

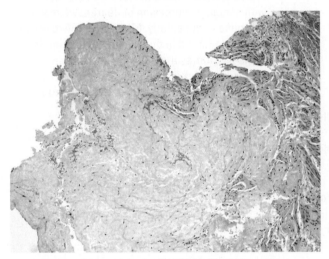

Figure 3.25.3 Collagen injection into the bladder with amorphous eosinophilic deposits.

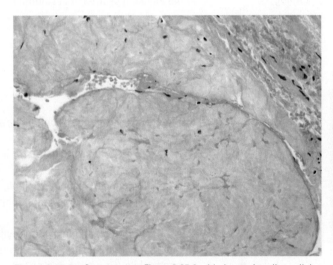

Figure 3.25.4 Same case as Figure 3.25.3 with dense virtually acellular collagen and lack of stromal response.

	Lymphoepithelioma-like Carcinoma	Large Cell Lymphoma
Age	Mean around 70 y (range 50s–80s)	Typically middle age to elderly. More common in females, typically middle aged
Location	Anywhere with urothelial lining	Anywhere with urothelial lining
Symptoms	Usually hematuria. May have obstructive symptoms	Hematuria or obstructive symptoms
Signs	Mass, as with usual urothelial carcinoma	Exophytic mass that could be indistinguishable from carcinoma. Large cell lymphoma is the most common secondary lymphoma or systemic lymphoma presenting first in the bladder
Etiology	Same as usual urothelial carcinoma	Typically none, although may be associated with immunosuppression or decreased immune response of the elderly. May be classified as (a) primary localized in the bladder; (b) presenting in the bladder as the first sign of systemic disease; and (c) recurrent in patients with a history of lymphoma (secondary lymphoma)
Histology	1. Sheets, cords, and trabeculae of cells *(Figs. 3.26.1–3.26.4)* 2. Cells can be cohesive clusters or individual cells *(Figs. 3.26.1–3.26.4)* 3. Large nuclei with multiple nucleoli, abundant eosinophilic to amphophilic cytoplasm *(Figs. 3.26.1 and 3.26.2)* 4. Associated brisk benign lymphocytic infiltrate with occasional more prominent neutrophils *(Figs. 3.26.1–3.26.4)* 5. May have associated CIS or usual infiltrating urothelial carcinoma 6. May have ulceration	1. Nests or sheets of cells 2. Cells typically loosely cohesive *(Figs. 3.26.5 and 3.26.6)* 3. Large nuclei with multiple nucleoli, abundant eosinophilic to amphophilic cytoplasm *(Figs. 3.26.5 and 3.26.6)* 4. May have associated small lymphocytic infiltrate where the small lymphocytes are irregular or regular 5. Lacks CIS or usual urothelial carcinoma 6. May have ulceration
Special studies	• Positive for keratins, especially CK7 *(Fig. 3.26.1)* • Negative for CD45 and CD20 in large, atypical cells • EBV negative	• Negative for keratins • Large atypical lymphoma cells positive for CD45 and usually CD20 *(Fig. 3.26.5)* • EBV may be positive if associated with immunosuppression or in some elderly patients
Treatment	If pure lymphoepithelioma-like carcinoma may respond to chemotherapy such that cystectomy can be avoided. Otherwise, if muscularis propria invasion present, radical cystectomy	TUR followed by chemotherapy and/or radiation therapy
Prognosis	When mixed with conventional urothelial carcinoma, their outcome is similar to that for conventional urothelial carcinoma and depends on the stage of the associated carcinoma. If pure, potentially better outcome when treated with chemotherapy	Recurrent lymphoma has the worst prognosis, often measured in months, as it is a sign of widely disseminated disease resistant to therapy

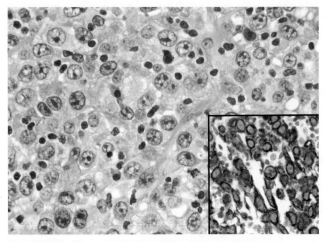

Figure 3.26.1 Lymphoepithelioma-like carcinoma with relatively uniform nuclei and prominent nucleoli intimately admixed with lymphocytes. Large cells are positive for keratin 7 (**inset**).

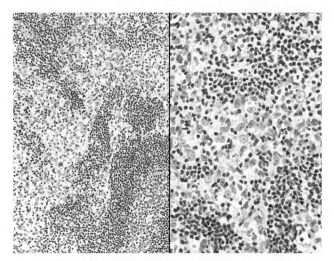

Figure 3.26.2 Lymphoepithelioma-like carcinoma with nests of tumor separated by dense collection of lymphocytes (**left**). Tumor cells have prominent nucleoli and abundant pale cytoplasm (**right**).

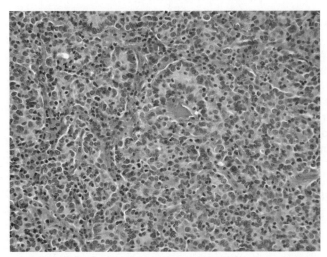

Figure 3.26.3 Lymphoepithelioma-like carcinoma with ribbons of tumor containing scattered lymphocytes.

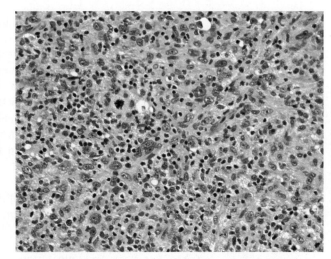

Figure 3.26.4 Lymphoepithelioma-like carcinoma with individual pleomorphic tumor cells showing numerous mitotic figures infiltrated by lymphocytes.

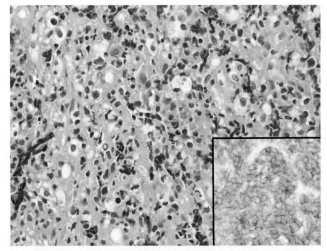

Figure 3.26.5 Large cell lymphoma of the bladder positive for CD20 (**inset**).

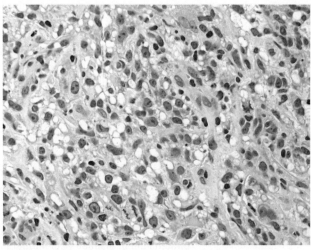

Figure 3.26.6 Large cell lymphoma of the bladder with numerous mitotic figures.

3 BLADDER

	Undifferentiated Urothelial Carcinoma with Osteoclasts	Undifferentiated Carcinoma or Sarcoma
Age	Majority 60s or older	In cases with this differential diagnosis, adults
Location	Anywhere with urothelial lining, yet more frequently see around the renal pelvis	Anywhere with urothelial lining
Symptoms	Usually hematuria. May have obstructive symptoms	Usually hematuria. May have obstructive symptoms
Signs	Large masses, 5 to 11 cm. Occasionally, an associated papillary urothelial component	Mass usually indistinguishable from infiltrating urothelial carcinoma
Etiology	Unknown	See Section 3.10 for urothelial carcinoma. Unknown for sarcoma
Histology	1. Sheets of epithelioid cells, yet can be spindled *(Figs. 3.27.1 and 3.27.2)* 2. Mononuclear epithelioid cells have varying degrees of cytologic atypia, with many relatively bland nuclei *(Figs. 3.27.3 and 3.27.4)* 3. Admixed osteoclastic giant cells with numerous small bland nuclei. Number of giant cells range in frequency from sparse to numerous, indistinguishable from giant cell tumor of bone *(Figs. 3.27.3 and 3.27.4)* 4. Necrosis common 5. Mitoses may be common in an epithelioid mononuclear component, yet not in osteoclastic giant cells 6. Very infiltrative growth 7. May have associated CIS, papillary, or usual infiltrating urothelial carcinoma	1. Sheets of spindle or epithelioid cells *(Fig. 3.27.6)* 2. If more epithelioid, typically pleomorphic 3. Tumor giant cells with pleomorphic nuclei *(Fig. 3.27.6)* 4. Necrosis common 5. Frequent mitotic activity both in spindle cells and tumor giant cells 6. Very infiltrative growth 7. If sarcoma, not associated with CIS, papillary, or usual infiltrating urothelial carcinoma. If large cell undifferentiated urothelial carcinoma may be associated with more recognizable urothelial carcinoma
Special studies	• Mononuclear cells are variably positive for keratins, in some cases only rare positive cells and other cases keratin negative *(Fig. 3.27.5)* • Osteoclastic giant cells CD68, CD51, and CD54 positive and negative for keratin • Ki-67 elevated in mononuclear cells *(Fig. 3.27.5)*	• Sarcoma negative for keratins with undifferentiated urothelial carcinoma keratin positive • CD68 typically negative • Ki-67 elevated
Treatment	Same as urothelial carcinoma. Often arises in the renal pelvis, necessitating nephroureterectomy. Same chemotherapy as for urothelial carcinoma	Typically radical cystectomy
Prognosis	Aggressive often with advanced stage. Most patients die of disease with metastases within a few years	Most undifferentiated sarcomas or carcinomas present with large advanced stage disease. Associated with a poor prognosis

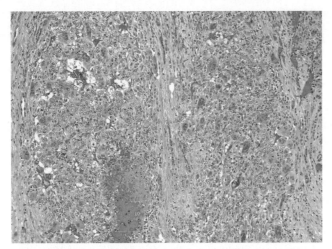

Figure 3.27.1 Undifferentiated urothelial carcinoma composed of sheets of mononuclear cells with numerous osteoclastic giant cells.

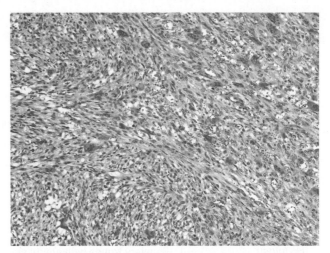

Figure 3.27.2 Undifferentiated urothelial carcinoma with osteoclastic giant cells with spindled mononuclear cells.

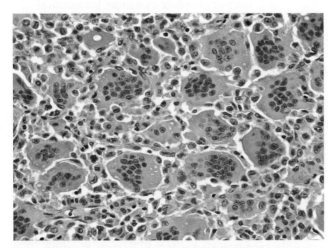

Figure 3.27.3 Undifferentiated urothelial carcinoma composed of bland mononuclear cells with numerous osteoclastic giant cells.

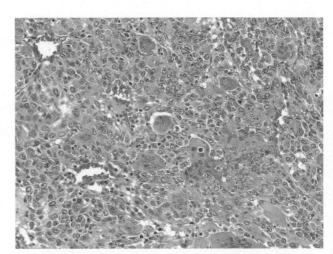

Figure 3.27.4 Undifferentiated urothelial carcinoma composed of cellular sheets of bland mononuclear cells with numerous osteoclastic giant cells.

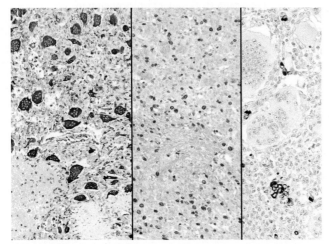

Figure 3.27.5 Undifferentiated urothelial carcinoma with osteoclastic giant cells where giant cells are positive for CD68 (**left**) and scattered mononuclear cells are pancytokeratin positive (**right**). Mononuclear cells show a high Ki-67 proliferation rate (**center**).

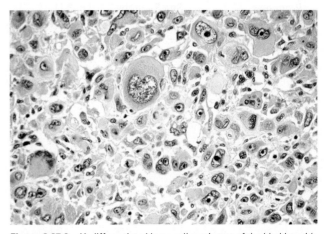

Figure 3.27.6 Undifferentiated large cell carcinoma of the bladder with pleomorphic tumor giant cells.

3 BLADDER

	Noninvasive Urothelial Carcinoma	Superficially Invasive Urothelial Carcinoma
Age	Mean age mid-60s with wide age range	Mean age mid-60s with wide age range
Location	Anywhere with urothelial lining	Anywhere with urothelial lining
Symptoms	Usually hematuria	Usually hematuria
Signs	Similar to cases with superficial invasion	Similar to cases with no invasion
Etiology	See Section 3.10	See Section 3.10
Histology	1. Papillary fronds with empty stalks or base of tumor with sharp straight demarcation between stroma and epithelium 2. Large rounded nests in the lamina propria with no retraction artifact 3. Lack of individual cells in lamina propria 4. Lack of inflammatory stromal reaction	1. Stalks of papillary fronds or base of tumor with the lamina propria containing clusters or tongues of cells, often with more eosinophilic cytoplasm (paradoxical differentiation) (Figs. 3.28.1–3.28.5) 2. Small irregular nests in the lamina propria with retraction artifact (Figs. 3.28.6–3.28.8) 3. Individual cells in the lamina propria (Figs. 3.28.9 and 3.28.10) 4. Occasional inflammatory stromal reaction
Special studies	Keratin stains fail to identify individual cells in stroma	Occasionally, keratin stains helpful to confirm individual tumor cells in lamina propria
Treatment	See Sections 3.4, 3.8–3.11	Initial TUR. If multifocal superficially invasive tumor, associated CIS, lymphovascular invasion, or unresectable tumors, cystectomy may be recommended. In the absence of these adverse parameters, a repeat TUR is recommended prior to BCG, since there is a 20% risk of understaging. If tumor does not completely respond in 3 mo, then possibly another course of BCG or cystectomy
Prognosis	See Sections 3.4, 3.8–3.11	Following BCG, risk of progression to muscularis propria invasion is around 12%

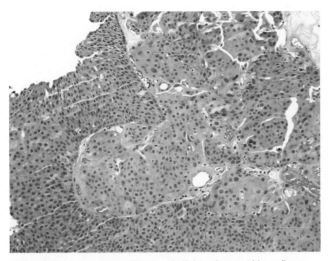

Figure 3.28.1   Invasive papillary urothelial carcinoma with confluent nests of tumor with abundant eosinophilic cytoplasm filling the stalks.

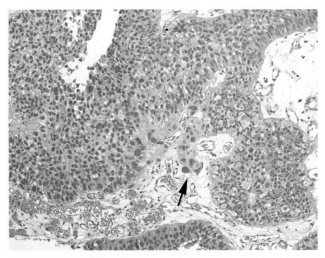

Figure 3.28.2   Invasive papillary urothelial carcinoma with paradoxical differentiation of advancing edge of an invasive tumor (*arrow*).

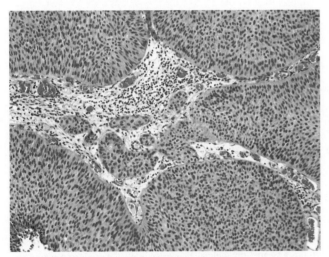

Figure 3.28.3   Invasive papillary urothelial carcinoma with small irregular nests of invasive carcinoma within the stalk as opposed to large, even straight border of adjacent noninvasive.

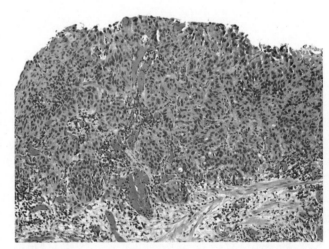

Figure 3.28.4   Invasive urothelial carcinoma with numerous small crowded nests of carcinoma within the lamina propria.

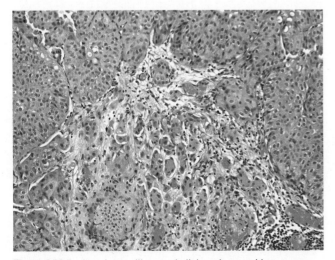

Figure 3.28.5   Invasive papillary urothelial carcinoma with numerous small crowded nests of carcinoma within the lamina propria at base of the tumor.

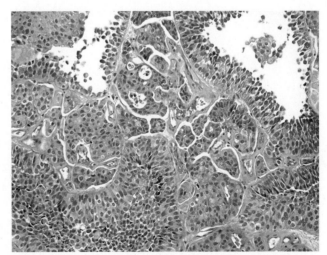

Figure 3.28.6   Invasive papillary urothelial carcinoma with numerous small nests of invasive carcinoma surrounded by retraction artifact filling up the stalk.

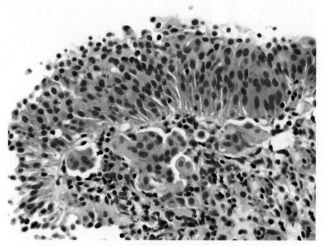

Figure 3.28.7   Superficially infiltrating urothelial carcinoma with small nests in the lamina propria with retraction artifact.

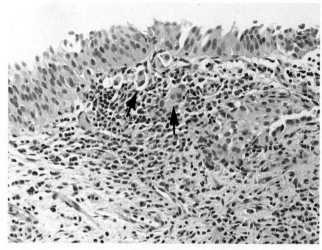

Figure 3.28.8   Superficially infiltrating urothelial carcinoma with small nests in the lamina propria with retraction artifact (*arrows*).

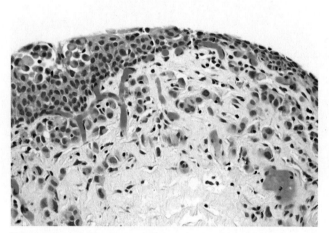

Figure 3.28.9   Infiltrating urothelial carcinoma with individual tumor cells in the lamina propria. The overlying urothelium is normal.

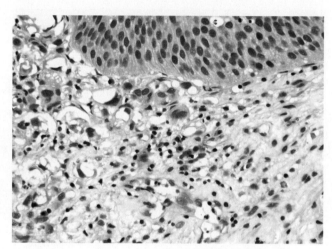

Figure 3.28.10   CIS with microinvasive urothelial carcinoma in the lamina propria.

	Muscularis Propria Invasion	Muscularis Mucosae Invasion
Age	Mean age mid-60s with wide age range	Mean age mid-60s with wide age range
Location	Anywhere along urothelial tract	Anywhere along urothelial tract
Symptoms	Usually hematuria	Usually hematuria
Signs	Imaging studies can identify muscularis propria invasion if fairly extensive, although treatment for muscularis propria invasion typically requires histologic confirmation	Imaging studies not sensitive to differentiate extensive lamina propria vs. superficial muscularis propria invasion
Etiology	See Section 3.10	See Section 3.10
Histology	1. Tumor-infiltrating thick muscle bundles *(Fig. 3.29.1)* 2. Invaded muscle not associated with row of dilated veins 3. Although each muscle bundle is thin, there are numerous thin muscles invaded by extensive solid sheets of tumor *(Figs. 3.29.2–3.29.5)* 4. Tumor infiltrates multiple small regular rows of muscle bundles, characteristic of the muscularis propria at the trigone and bladder neck *(Fig. 3.29.6)*	1. Limited tumor infiltrating thin superficial muscle bundles *(Fig. 3.29.9)* 2. Tumor invading thin muscle associated with row of dilated veins corresponding to the midlevel of the lamina propria *(Fig. 3.29.10)* 3. Only a few thin muscle bundles invaded by extensive solid sheets of tumor may be indeterminate between muscularis mucosae and muscularis propria invasion 4. In the trigone and bladder neck, there is no muscularis mucosae
Special studies	• Desmin may highlight numerous small muscle bundles associated with extensive tumor, consistent with the muscularis propria being fragmented by carcinoma *(Figs. 3.29.4, 3.29.5, and 3.29.7)* • Keratin can highlight crushed or cauterize tumor in thick muscle bundles of the muscularis propria *(Fig. 3.29.8)*	• Desmin staining is not specific for the muscularis propria vs. muscularis mucosae. Smoothelin supposed to weakly label the muscularis mucosae and strongly the muscularis propria. However, due to a lot of overlap not useful in practice • Keratin-positive tumor in muscle can be the muscularis mucosae or can be muscularis propria invasion
Treatment	Typically radical cystectomy	See Section 3.28
Prognosis	Following muscularis propria invasion on TURB and subsequent radical cystectomy, the 5-y disease-specific survivals are 81%–90%, 70%–80%, and 40%–52%, if tumor in the corresponding radical cystectomy extends into the lamina propria, muscularis propria, and perivesical tissue, respectively	See Section 3.28

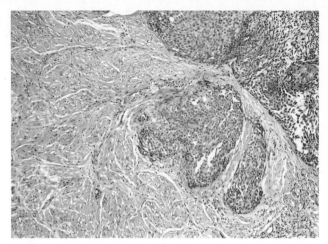

Figure 3.29.1   Straightforward case of the muscularis propria with a large muscle bundle invaded by carcinoma.

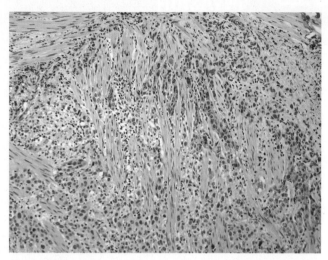

Figure 3.29.2   Muscularis propria large muscle bundle being split by invasive carcinoma.

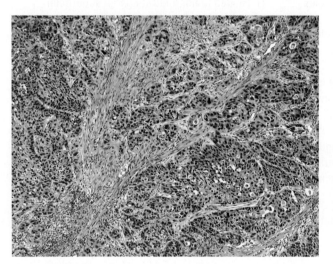

Figure 3.29.3   Muscularis propria large muscle bundle being split by invasive carcinoma.

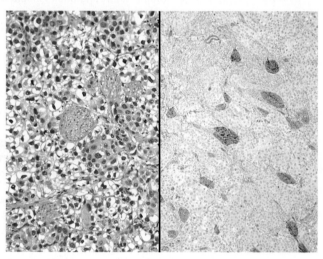

Figure 3.29.4   Numerous small fascicles of muscle invaded by carcinoma consistent with the muscularis propria being dissected by carcinoma (**left**) with muscle highlighted by desmin (**right**).

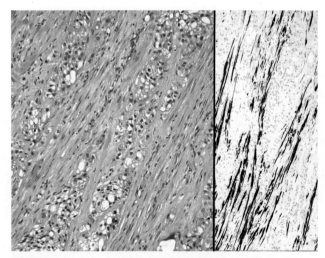

Figure 3.29.5   Numerous small bundles invaded by carcinoma consistent with the muscularis propria being dissected by carcinoma (**left**) with muscle highlighted by desmin (**right**).

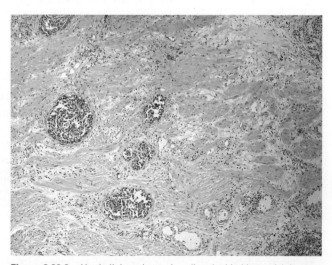

Figure 3.29.6   Urothelial carcinoma invading the bladder neck/trigone-layered smaller muscle bundles of the muscularis propria.

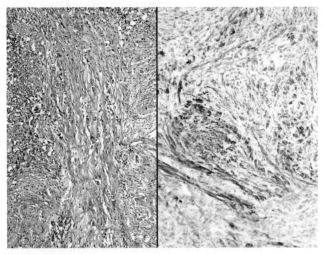

Figure 3.29.7   Individual cells of high-grade urothelial carcinoma invading spindle cells where it is difficult to distinguish between fibrosis and muscle (**left**). Desmin positivity (**right**) is diagnostic of muscularis propria invasion.

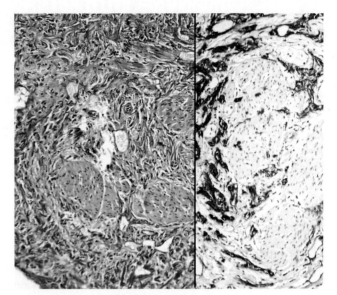

Figure 3.29.8   Heavily cauterized cellular infiltrate surrounds the muscularis propria (**left**). Keratin positivity (**right**) is diagnostic of muscularis propria invasion.

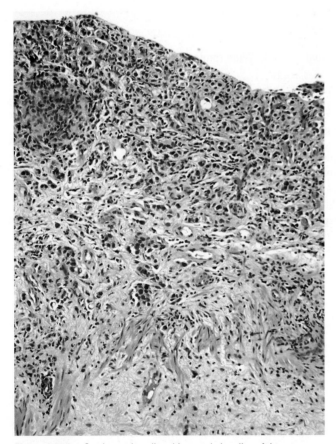

Figure 3.29.9   Carcinoma invading thin muscle bundles of the muscularis mucosae.

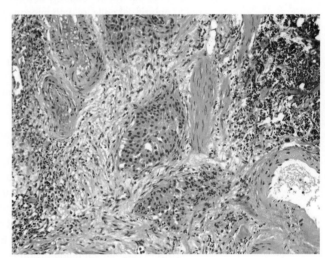

Figure 3.29.10   Muscularis mucosae invasion with thin muscle bundles associated with dilated veins.

	Infiltrating Micropapillary Carcinoma	Infiltrating Carcinoma with Retraction Artifact
Age	Mean age mid-60s with wide age range	Mean age mid-60s with wide age range
Location	Anywhere along urothelial tract	Anywhere along urothelial tract
Symptoms	Usually hematuria	Usually hematuria
Signs	None specific	None specific
Etiology	See Section 3.10	See Section 3.10
Histology	1. Multiple uniformly sized nests within a single lacuna or sometimes numerous uniform nests each within a single lacuna *(Figs. 3.30.1–3.30.5)* 2. Shapes of nests do not necessarily conform to the shape of the space 3. May but not necessarily see reverse polarity of cells as with micropapillary carcinoma in other organs *(Figs. 3.30.1, 3.30.3, and 3.30.5)* 4. Typically extensive tumor with frequent muscularis propria invasion 5. Some cases associated with noninvasive micropapillary carcinoma	1. Variably sized nests, each surrounded by a single space *(Fig. 3.30.6)* 2. Shapes of nests conform to the shape of the space *(Fig. 3.30.6)* 3. Not see reverse polarity of cells 4. Wide range in tumor extent and stage 5. Typically not associated with noninvasive micropapillary carcinoma
Special studies	Not useful in this differential diagnosis	Not useful in this differential diagnosis
Treatment	As micropapillary carcinomas are typically associated with muscularis propria invasion, some have advocated cystectomy even if only lamina propria invasion is identified on initial TURB. Others recommend repeat TURB if lamina propria invasion on initial TURB to rule out sampling artifact with potential of initial understaging	Depends on the stage. See Sections 3.28 and 3.29
Prognosis	See Section 3.28	See Section 3.28

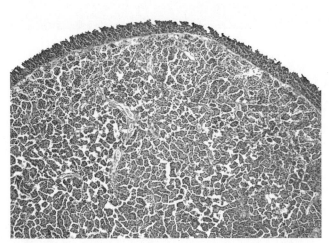

Figure 3.30.1   Low magnification of invasive micropapillary urothelial carcinoma.

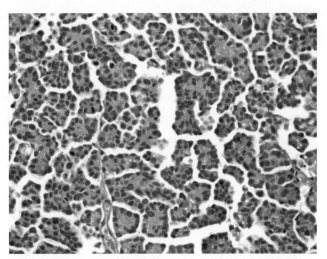

Figure 3.30.2   Same as Figure 3.30.1 with numerous uniformly sized nests of carcinoma with peripheral localization of nuclei and central cytoplasm in a large lacuna.

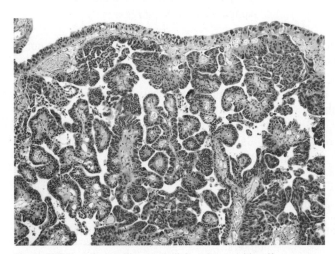

Figure 3.30.3   Micropapillary urothelial carcinoma with uniform nests of carcinoma with peripheral localization of nuclei and central cytoplasm in a large lacuna. Overlying CIS.

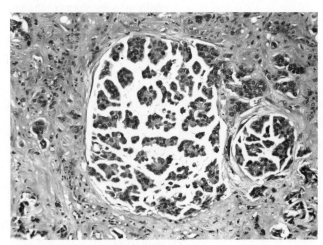

Figure 3.30.4   Micropapillary urothelial carcinoma with uniform nests of carcinoma in a large lacuna.

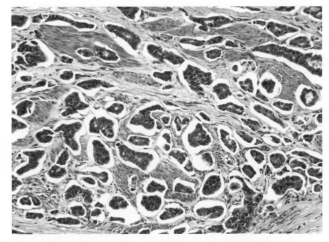

Figure 3.30.5   Micropapillary urothelial carcinoma invading the muscularis propria with numerous uniform nests of carcinoma with peripheral localization of nuclei and central cytoplasm, each in their own lacuna.

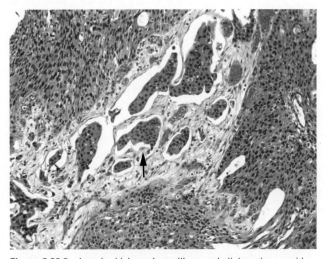

Figure 3.30.6   Invasive high-grade papillary urothelial carcinoma with retraction artifact. Nests are variably sized with each surrounded by a similar shaped lacuna (*arrow*).

3   BLADDER

	Infiltrating Urothelial Carcinoma with Vascular Invasion	Infiltrating Urothelial Carcinoma with Retraction Artifact
Age	Mean age mid-60s with wide age range	Mean age mid-60s with wide age range
Location	Anywhere along urothelial tract	Anywhere along urothelial tract
Symptoms	Usually hematuria	Usually hematuria
Signs	None specific	None specific
Etiology	See Section 3.10	See Section 3.10
Histology	1. Nests of carcinoma within spaces lined by endothelial cells (Figs. 3.31.1 and 3.31.2) 2. Shapes of nests do not necessarily conform to the shape of the space (Figs. 3.31.1 and 3.31.2) 3. Shape and size of nests within space differ from surrounding infiltrating tumor (Fig. 3.31.2) 4. Typically not numerous foci within a limited area, as inconsistent with the distribution of vessels 5. Can be seen in the lamina propria or muscularis propria 6. Lymphatic invasion may be present localized to a cluster of lymphatics around blood vessels (Figs. 3.31.3 and 3.31.4)	1. Nests within spaces lacking endothelial cell lining (Figs. 3.31.5 and 3.31.6) 2. Shapes of nests conform to the shape of the space (Figs. 3.31.5 and 3.31.6) 3. Shape and size of nests within space do not differ from surrounding infiltrating tumor 4. Can see virtually every nest within a limited area surrounded by a space (Fig. 3.31.6) 5. Can be seen in the lamina propria or muscularis propria 6. Not localized around blood vessels
Special studies	Vessels highlighted by CD31, ERG, factor VIII, and D240 (Figs. 3.31.3 and 3.31.4)	Immunohistochemistry negative for vascular markers
Treatment	Vascular invasion in the setting of superficial infiltrating high-grade carcinoma is one of the factors in deciding whether to proceed to cystectomy	Does not affect treatment
Prognosis	Worse prognosis when associated with muscularis propria invasion. Conflicting studies as to the effect of vascular invasion with lamina propria invasion	Does not affect prognosis

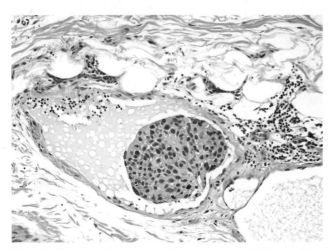

Figure 3.31.1 Vascular invasion with nest of tumor within lymphatic vessel filled with pale serous fluid and lined by endothelium. The nest's shape is different from the shape of the vessel.

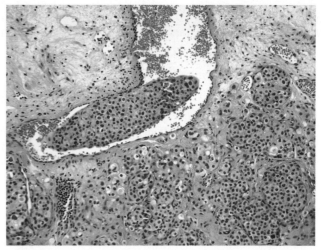

Figure 3.31.2 Vascular invasion within a blood vessel. The intravascular nest's shape is different from the shape of the vessel and from the surrounding infiltrating tumor.

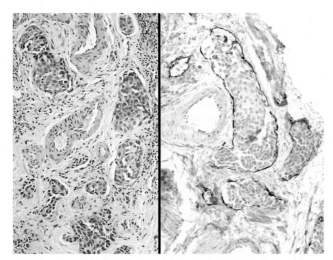

Figure 3.31.3 Vascular invasion surrounding clusters of blood vessels (**left**) with vascular invasion proven by CD31 labeling (**right**).

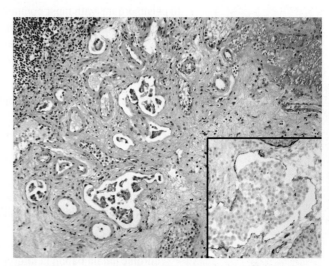

Figure 3.31.4 Numerous foci of vascular invasion surrounding clusters of blood vessels with vascular invasion proven by CD31 labeling (**inset**).

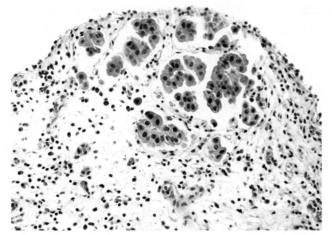

Figure 3.31.5 Infiltrating urothelial carcinoma with retraction artifact. The spaces lack an endothelial lining and are the same shape as the nests of carcinoma.

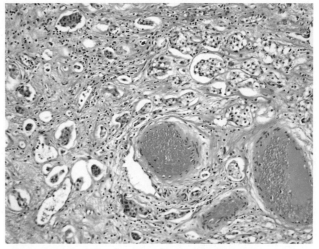

Figure 3.31.6 Infiltrating urothelial carcinoma with retraction artifact. Almost every nest of carcinoma is surrounded by a space.

3 BLADDER

	Pseudocarcinomatous Urothelial Hyperplasia	Superficially Invasive Urothelial Carcinoma
Age	Mean age mid-60s with wide age range. Males predominate	Mean age mid-60s with wide age range
Location	Typically the bladder	Anywhere along urothelial tract
Symptoms	Usually hematuria	Usually hematuria
Signs	Most commonly, cystoscopy shows localized erythematous lesion although can also appear as polypoid mass	Cystoscopy typically shows a mass lesion
Etiology	Late reactive process to bladder ischemia. In most cases, several years following radiation to pelvic organs with most common history of prior irradiation for prostate cancer. Less frequently history of systemic chemotherapy, severe systemic ischemic disease, indwelling catheter, or sickle cell disease	See Section 3.10
Histology	1. Nests of urothelial cells in lamina propria 2. Lack of overlying CIS or papillary carcinoma 3. Background stroma with numerous vessels having fibrin thrombi *(Figs. 3.32.1–3.32.8)* 4. Stroma with recent hemorrhage and extensive hemosiderin deposition *(Figs. 3.32.1–3.32.8)* 5. Most cases with prominent acute and chronic inflammation in intervening stroma *(Figs. 3.32.5, 3.32.6, and 3.32.8)* 6. Edema and vascular congestion common 7. The urothelium with mild to moderate nuclear pleomorphism *(Figs. 3.32.4 and 3.32.6)* 8. Mitotic figures in 25% of cases 9. Ulceration in 40% of cases 10. Vascular changes associated with prior irradiation often found	1. Nests of urothelial cells in lamina propria 2. May have overlying CIS or papillary carcinoma, yet not always present 3. Uncommon to have fibrin thrombi in surrounding vessels 4. Hemorrhage and hemosiderin deposition uncommon 5. Stroma may have inflammatory response yet typically absent or minimal 6. Edema and vascular congestion uncommon 7. The urothelium typically with moderate to marked nuclear pleomorphism, yet occasional cases with mild atypia 8. Mitotic figures can be seen 9. Ulceration uncommon 10. Lacks vascular changes seen with prior irradiation
Special studies	Not helpful in this differential	Not helpful in this differential

	Pseudocarcinomatous Urothelial Hyperplasia	**Superficially Invasive Urothelial Carcinoma**
Treatment	TUR without additional therapy	Initial TUR. If multifocal superficially invasive tumor, associated CIS, lymphovascular invasion, or unresectable tumors, cystectomy may be recommended. In the absence of these adverse parameters, a repeat TUR is recommended prior to BCG, since there is a 20% risk of understaging. If tumor does not completely respond in 3 mo, then possibly another course of BCG or cystectomy
Prognosis	Benign with no risk of developing urothelial carcinoma	Following BCG, risk of progression to muscularis propria invasion is around 12%

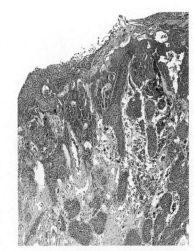

Figure 3.32.1   Pseudocarcinomatous urothelial hyperplasia with irregular nests protruding into the lamina propria. Between the nests are numerous dilated blood vessels.

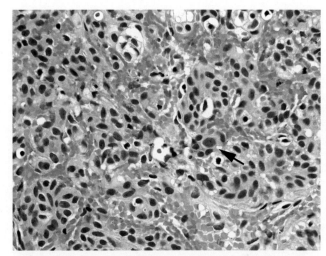

Figure 3.32.2   Same case as Figure 3.32.1 with nests showing focal moderate nuclear atypia (*arrow*) among extensive recent hemorrhage.

3   BLADDER

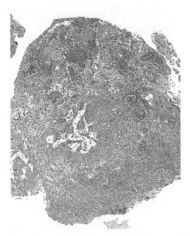

Figure 3.32.3 Pseudocarcinomatous urothelial hyperplasia with nests involving the lamina propria associated with dilated blood vessels (*top*) and extensive fibrin deposition (*bottom*).

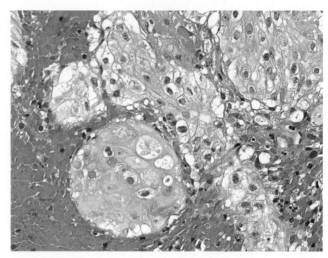

Figure 3.32.4 Same case as Figure 3.32.3 with nests showing focal moderate nuclear atypia with prominent nucleoli among extensive recent hemorrhage.

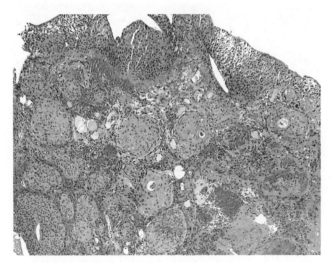

Figure 3.32.5 Pseudocarcinomatous urothelial hyperplasia with nests involving the lamina propria associated with dilated blood vessels, extravasated blood, and fibrin deposition (*lower right*).

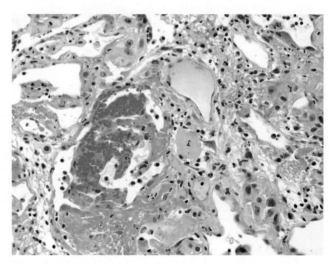

Figure 3.32.6 Pseudocarcinomatous urothelial hyperplasia with nests surrounding fibrin, extravasated blood with admixed acute and chronic inflammation. Moderate nuclear pleomorphism is present.

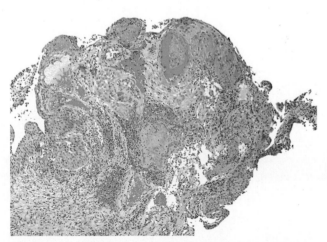

Figure 3.32.7 Pseudocarcinomatous urothelial hyperplasia with nests involving the lamina propria associated with dilated blood vessels, extravasated blood, inflammation, and fibrin deposition (*top*).

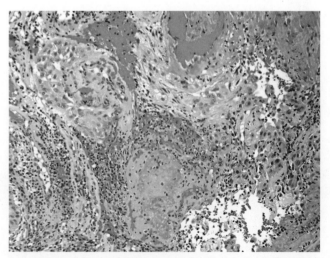

Figure 3.32.8 Same case as Figure 3.32.7 with nests associated with dilated blood vessels, extravasated blood, inflammation, and fibrin.

	Normal Fragmented Renal Ureter/Pelvis Urothelium	Low-Grade Papillary Urothelial Neoplasm
Age	Mean age mid-60s with wide age range	Mean age mid-60s with wide age range
Location	The ureter and renal pelvis	Anywhere along urothelial tract
Symptoms	Variable with some having hematuria, others follow-up for abnormal cytology or abnormal urinary FISH results	Typically gross or microscopic hematuria
Signs	At ureteroscopy, usually no mass seen	At ureteroscopy, papillary lesion, typically solitary or multifocal with wide range in size
Etiology	Due to the difficulty of obtaining biopsies of the ureter and renal pelvis, tissue is very limited and distorted	See Section 3.10
Histology	1. Strips of the urothelium that occasionally can partially round up to mimic a papillary frond *(Figs. 3.33.1–3.33.3)* 2. Normal-thickness urothelium *(Figs. 3.33.1 and 3.33.3)* 3. Cytology is normal often with nuclear grooves 4. If the urothelium inflamed can be reactive changes *(Fig. 3.33.4)* (see Section 3.5) 5. Mitotic figures absent unless the urothelium inflamed	1. Papillary fronds with fibrovascular cores surrounded by the urothelium *(Figs. 3.33.5–3.33.7)* 2. Typically overt thickened urothelium *(Figs. 3.33.5, 3.33.6, and 3.33.8)*. Only papilloma with the normal-thickness urothelium and papilloma in these sites is very rare 3. Cytology is mostly normal with scattered slightly enlarged hyperchromatic nuclei that stand out even at lower magnification *(Fig. 3.33.6)*. Nuclear grooves not as common 4. Inflammation in the urothelium of urothelial tumors uncommon 5. Mitotic figures range from uncommon to scattered seen at all layers of the urothelium
Special studies	Not helpful in this differential	Not helpful in this differential
Treatment	None	Typically, resected by TUR and immediate instillation of intravesical chemotherapy recommended even for lesions with low risk of recurrence. Intravesical BCG not used for initial therapy, yet potentially used in patients with recurrent low-grade papillary urothelial carcinoma. Followed for life with routine cystoscopy
Prognosis	Occasional cases with normal epithelium on biopsy of the renal pelvis or ureter have urothelial carcinoma on subsequent specimens, as it may be difficult to obtain diagnostic biopsies in these areas via ureteroscopy	See Sections 3.9 and 3.10. Even a diagnosis of papilloma will result in a patient being followed for life with routine cytology and cystoscopy because of the risk of recurrent urothelial neoplasms. Also a diagnosis of urothelial neoplasm in the renal pelvis and ureter sometimes results in a radical nephrectomy since difficult to visualize by imaging and ureteroscopy and may be worse disease than on biopsy

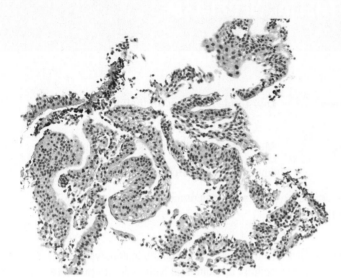

Figure 3.33.1   Strips of normal urothelium from biopsy of the renal pelvis.

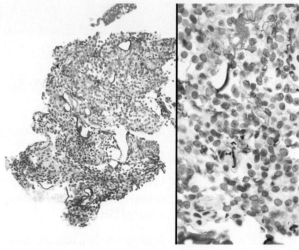

Figure 3.33.2   Strips of compressed normal urothelium from biopsy of the renal pelvis (**left**) with lack of papillary formation. Cytology is normal (**right**).

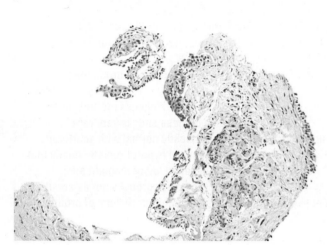

Figure 3.33.3   Normal biopsy of the renal pelvis with a detached strip of a benign urothelium mimicking a papillary urothelial tumor.

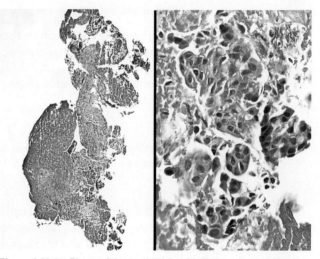

Figure 3.33.4   Biopsy of the renal pelvis with fibrin and recent blood and detached urothelial clusters (**left**). Higher magnification (**right**) with benign cytology and reactive changes.

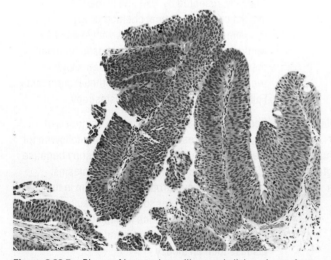

Figure 3.33.5   Biopsy of low-grade papillary urothelial carcinoma from the renal pelvis.

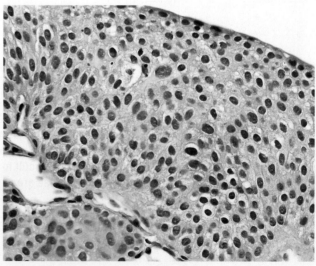

Figure 3.33.6   Same case as Figure 3.33.5 with scattered enlarged and hyperchromatic nuclei.

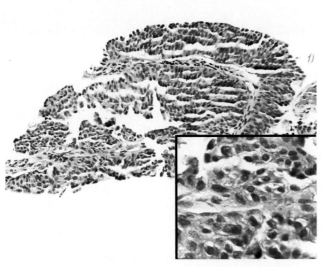

Figure 3.33.7   Biopsy of the renal pelvis showing low-grade papillary urothelial carcinoma with minimal variation in size and shape of nuclei (**inset**).

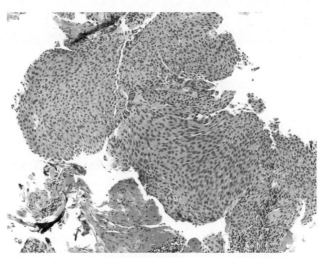

Figure 3.33.8   Markedly thickened strip of a urothelium consistent with low-grade papillary urothelial carcinoma.

	Bladder Adenocarcinoma and Villous Adenoma	Secondary Involvement by Extravesical Adenocarcinoma
Age	Adults, typically over 50 y of age	Adults, typically over 50 y of age
Location	Nonurachal adenocarcinoma: typically the posterior wall and trigone. Urachal adenocarcinoma: dome. Villous adenoma: the urachus and trigone	Colon carcinoma: the posterior bladder wall. Prostate adenocarcinoma: the bladder neck and trigone
Symptoms	Usually hematuria. Occasionally mucusuria	Usually hematuria. Occasionally mucusuria
Signs	Adenocarcinoma: mass. Villous adenoma: papillary lesion	Cystoscopy usually shows mass
Etiology	Nonurachal: arises through a process of glandular metaplasia of surface urothelium. Urachal: arises from glandular metaplasia in urachal remnants	Colon carcinoma can involve the bladder either via direct invasion or via metastases. Prostate adenocarcinoma typically directly invades the bladder
Histology	1. Identical to intestinal adenocarcinoma, including signet ring cells, colloid carcinoma with mucinous cells lining mucinous lakes, and enteric nonmucinous carcinoma *(Figs. 3.34.1–3.34.3)* 2. In some cases, can see mixed urothelial and adenocarcinoma *(Fig. 3.34.4)* 3. Adenocarcinoma typically high grade. Mucinous adenocarcinomas can show variable cytologic atypia yet in some areas will be overtly malignant 4. Typically not extensive undermining of the normal urothelium 5. Surface mucosa with *in situ* adenocarcinoma, villous adenoma, or urothelial carcinoma. Villous adenomas are identical to gastrointestinal tract lesions with potential for high-grade dysplasia and infiltrating carcinoma *(Figs. 3.34.5 and 3.34.6)* 6. Urachal adenocarcinoma by definition involves the dome	1. Colon carcinoma no different than bladder adenocarcinoma. Prostate mucinous adenocarcinoma contains cribriform and single glands floating in mucin *(Fig. 3.34.7)* 2. Not see admixed urothelial carcinoma 3. Secondary involvement by prostate and pancreas cancer may have bland cytology *(Figs. 3.34.8–3.34.10)* 4. Tumor often undermines the normal urothelium *(Figs. 3.34.9, 3.34.11, and 3.34.12)* 5. Secondary adenocarcinomas can colonize the surface mimicking *in situ* adenocarcinoma and villous adenoma *(Figs. 3.34.8, 3.34.10, and 3.34.12)* 6. Secondary adenocarcinoma typically does not involve the dome
Special studies	• CDX2 and CEA can be positive • Nuclear beta-catenin negative • Focal ER and PR can be seen. GCDFP and mammaglobin negative. GATA3 positive in adenocarcinomas with signet ring cells	• Gastrointestinal tumors, CDX2 and CEA positive • Nuclear beta-catenin positive • In uterine or breast adenocarcinomas, ER, PR, variably positive. In breast adenocarcinomas, GCDFP, mammaglobin, and GATA3 usually positive

	Bladder Adenocarcinoma and Villous Adenoma	**Secondary Involvement by Extravesical Adenocarcinoma**
Treatment	Adenocarcinoma usually requires radical cystectomy. If tumor is present in the dome and not that large can be treated with a partial cystectomy. Adjuvant chemotherapy and radiotherapy may be given depending on the extent of tumor. Villous adenoma treated by TUR. Before diagnosing primary bladder adenocarcinoma, recommended to clinically rule out colorectal primary	Cystectomy not performed. Systemic and local therapy tailored to the specific primary tumor
Prognosis	Adenocarcinoma: 5-y survival rates between 18% and 47%. Villous adenoma: Cured if totally resected, yet needs to be completely sampled to exclude associated invasive adenocarcinoma. On TURB, should be called "villous adenomatous lesion" commenting that this most likely represents a primary villous adenoma of the bladder but cannot exclude spread from an extravesical adenocarcinoma with clinical correlation required	Regardless of the primary site, reflects advanced disease with a poor prognosis

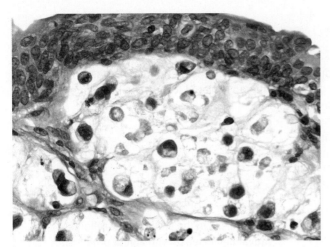

Figure 3.34.1   Signet-ring cell adenocarcinoma of the bladder.

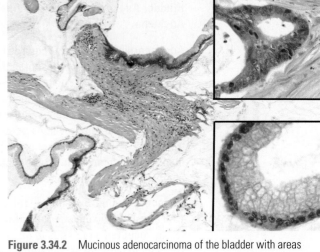

Figure 3.34.2   Mucinous adenocarcinoma of the bladder with areas showing bland cytology (**bottom inset**) and overtly malignant cytology (**top inset**).

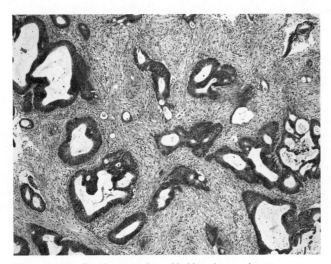

Figure 3.34.3   Enteric nonmucinous bladder adenocarcinoma.

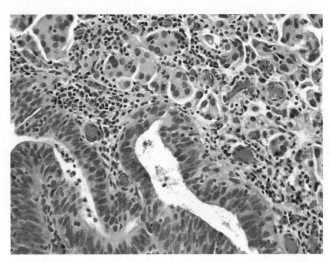

Figure 3.34.4   Mixed bladder adenocarcinoma (*bottom*) and urothelial carcinoma (*top*).

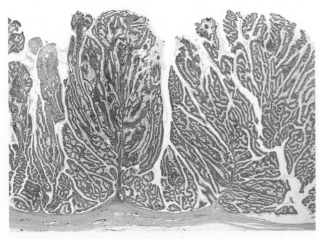

Figure 3.34.5   Villous adenoma of the bladder.

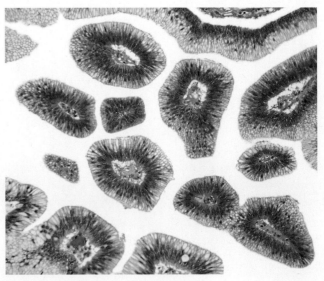

Figure 3.34.6   Same case as Figure 3.34.5.

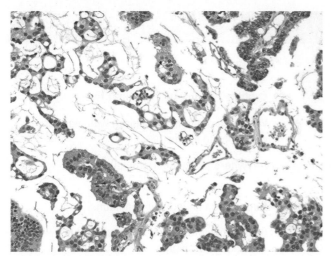

Figure 3.34.7 Mucinous adenocarcinoma of the prostate with cribriform, papillary, and single glands with bland cytology floating in mucin.

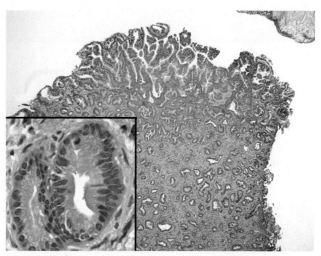

Figure 3.34.8 Metastatic pancreas cancer to the bladder with the surface showing papillary fronds. **Inset** shows bland cytology of infiltrating glands.

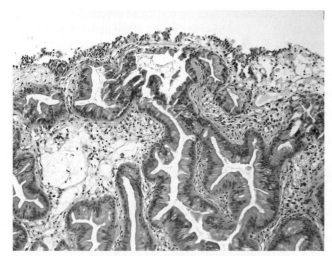

Figure 3.34.9 Same case as Figure 3.34.8 with bland irregular mucinous glands undermining the urothelium.

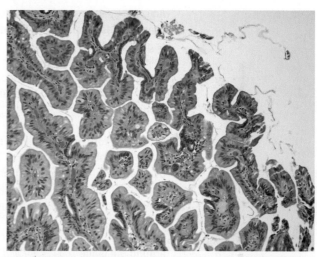

Figure 3.34.10 Same case as Figures 3.34.8 and 3.34.9 with a surface papillary component mimicking a primary villous adenoma of the bladder.

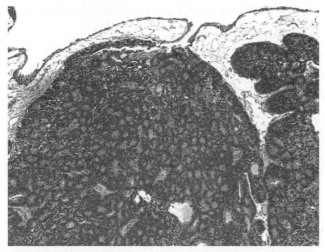

Figure 3.34.11 Prostate adenocarcinoma undermining the bladder urothelium.

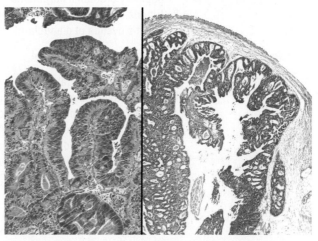

Figure 3.34.12 Colon adenocarcinoma involving the bladder with surface papillary fronds mimicking a primary villous adenoma (**left**) and adenocarcinoma undermining the bladder urothelium (**right**).

	Bladder Adenocarcinoma	Cystitis Glandularis, Intestinal Type
Age	Adults, typically over 50 y of age	Wide age range from children with bladder exstrophy to adults
Location	Urachal tumor in dome. Nonurachal tumors, typically the posterior wall and trigone	Anywhere along the urothelial tract
Symptoms	Usually hematuria. Occasionally mucusuria	Depends on underlying conditions
Signs	Typically, a large mass	Cystoscopy often shows a mass lesion mimicking carcinoma
Etiology	Either arises from intestinal metaplasia or from urachal remnants	Exstrophy, neurogenic bladder, and other causes of chronic irritation of the bladder such as indwelling catheter or calculi
Histology	1. Any of the patterns that may be seen in intestinal adenocarcinoma, including signet ring cells, colloid carcinoma with mucinous cells lining and floating with lakes of mucin, and enteric nonmucinous carcinoma 2. Typically high-grade and only rarely low-grade cytology *(Figs. 3.35.1 and 3.35.2)* 3. Lacks well-formed glands lined by numerous goblet cells 4. If extracellular mucin present, lined by and often floating malignant cells 5. May invade the muscularis propria 6. Often desmoplastic stromal reaction around the gland *(Figs. 3.35.1 and 3.35.2)* 7. Occasionally *in situ* adenocarcinoma, overlying villous adenoma, CIS, or papillary urothelial carcinoma 8. Glands do not merge with nonintestinal cystitis cystica et glandularis	1. Resembles normal colon crypts *(Figs. 3.35.3 and 3.35.4)*. Lacks any of the patterns that may be seen in intestinal adenocarcinoma 2. In almost all cases, nuclei cytologically bland *(Fig. 3.35.4)*. Only rare cases with dysplasia involving cystitis glandularis *(Figs. 3.35.5–3.35.7)* 3. Cells typically lined by goblet cells 4. May have acellular extracellular mucin adjacent to epithelium *(Figs. 3.35.8 and 3.35.9)* 5. Occasionally can involve the muscularis propria *(Figs. 3.35.8 and 3.35.9)* 6. Lacks desmoplastic stromal reaction around the glands *(Figs. 3.35.8 and 3.35.9)* 7. No *in situ* adenocarcinoma, overlying villous adenoma, CIS, or papillary urothelial carcinoma 8. Glands merge with nonintestinal cystitis cystica et glandularis *(Fig. 3.35.10)*
Special studies	Not helpful in this differential	Not helpful in this differential
Treatment	Usually requires radical cystectomy. However if tumor is present in the dome or anterior wall and not that large can be treated with a partial cystectomy. Adjuvant chemotherapy and radiotherapy may be given depending on the extent of tumor	Typically treated by TUR
Prognosis	Five-year survival rates between 18% and 47%	Benign and despite "recurrence/persistence" on subsequent TUR does not need further treatment. No increased risk of adenocarcinoma, except for increased risk of adenocarcinoma in exstrophy patients. Prognosis unknown for cases with associated dysplasia

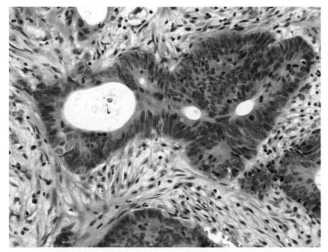

Figure 3.35.1   Bladder adenocarcinoma with overt cytologic atypia and inflamed desmoplastic stroma.

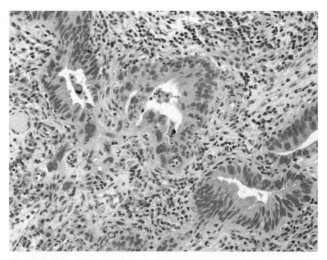

Figure 3.35.2   Bladder adenocarcinoma with pleomorphism and inflamed desmoplastic stroma.

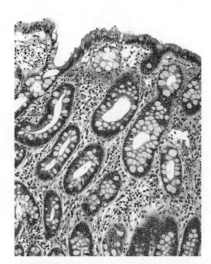

Figure 3.35.3   Bladder with intestinal metaplasia resembling the colon.

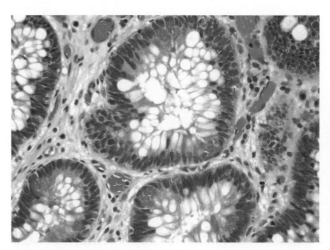

Figure 3.35.4   Intestinal metaplasia with goblet cells and no cytologic atypia.

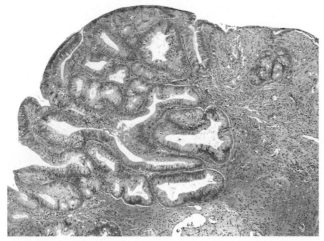

Figure 3.35.5   Intestinal metaplasia in the bladder with moderate dysplasia.

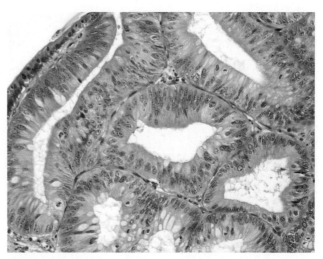

Figure 3.35.6   Same case as Figure 3.35.5 with loss of mucin and stratification of nuclei.

3   BLADDER

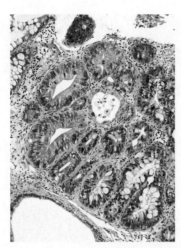

Figure 3.35.7   Intestinal metaplasia of the bladder with high-grade dysplasia.

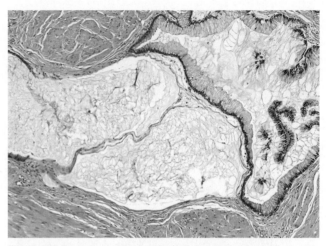

Figure 3.35.8   Intestinal metaplasia of the bladder with mucin extravasation involving the muscularis propria.

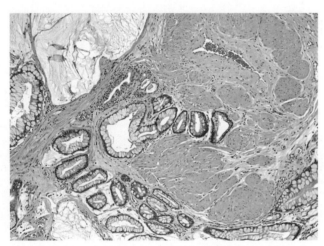

Figure 3.35.9   Intestinal metaplasia of the bladder with mucin extravasation (*upper left*) involving the muscularis propria. The gland do not elicit a stromal reaction.

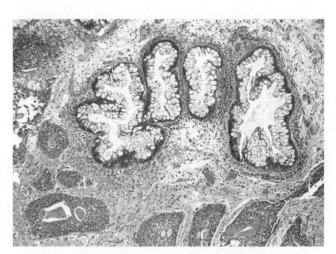

Figure 3.35.10   Intestinal metaplasia (*top*) with cystitis cystica et glandularis (*bottom*).

	Endometriosis/Endosalpingiosis	Bladder Adenocarcinoma
Age	Females, usually in 30s to 40s	Males or females, typically over 50 y of age
Location	Posterior wall	Urachal tumor in dome. Nonurachal tumors, typically the posterior wall and trigone
Symptoms	Pelvic pain, frequency, dysuria, hematuria, dyspareunia, dysmenorrhea	Usually hematuria. Occasionally mucusuria
Signs	Cystoscopy may show hemorrhagic spots and mass with endometriosis yet no pigmentation in endosalpingiosis. May be as large as 5 cm	Typically, large mass
Etiology	Displaced and implanted endometrial cells	Either arises from intestinal metaplasia or from urachal remnants
Histology	1. Glands lined by endometrial cells, cuboidal cells, or endocervical cells (Figs. 3.36.1–3.36.5). Can be dilated glands 2. Cytologically bland with rare exceptions showing focal reactive changes (Figs. 3.36.2 and 3.36.3) 3. Lacks extracellular mucin 4. May involve the muscularis propria and perivesical adipose tissue (Figs. 3.36.2, 3.36.3, and 3.36.5) 5. May have fibrosis around burnt out endometrial glands. Endocervicosis usually lacks stromal fibrosis (Fig. 3.36.2) although exceptions occur (Fig. 3.36.5) 6. Endometriosis often has hemorrhage and hemosiderin deposition in the stroma around glands 7. Endometriosis in most cases has cuff of cellular stroma surrounding glands 8. Lacks *in situ* adenocarcinoma, overlying villous adenoma, CIS, or papillary urothelial carcinoma	1. Any of the patterns that may be seen in intestinal adenocarcinoma, including signet ring cells, colloid carcinoma with mucinous cell lining and floating with lakes of mucin, and enteric nonmucinous carcinoma 2. Typically high-grade and only rarely low-grade cytology (Fig. 3.36.6) 3. If extracellular mucin present, lined by and often floating malignant cells 4. May invade the muscularis propria 5. Often desmoplastic stromal reaction around glands 6. Typically lacks stromal hemorrhage and hemosiderin deposition 7. Lacks endometrial stroma 8. Occasionally *in situ* adenocarcinoma, overlying villous adenoma, CIS, or papillary urothelial carcinoma
Special studies	• Glands positive for PAX8, ER, and PR • Endometrial stroma CD10 positive	• Glands negative for PAX8, ER, and PR • Stroma CD10 negative
Treatment	Once diagnosis made, can sometimes be treated hormonally. In some cases, partial cystectomy required to control local symptoms not responding to medical therapy	Usually requires radical cystectomy. However, if tumor is present in the dome or anterior wall and not that large can be treated with a partial cystectomy. Adjuvant chemotherapy and radiotherapy may be given depending on the extent of tumor
Prognosis	Benign. No increased risk of adenocarcinoma. Rare cases associated with clear cell adenocarcinoma	Five-year survival rates between 18% and 47%

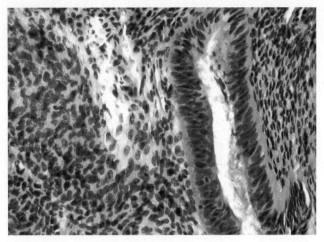

Figure 3.36.1 Endometriosis of the bladder with stroma that typically does not mimic adenocarcinoma.

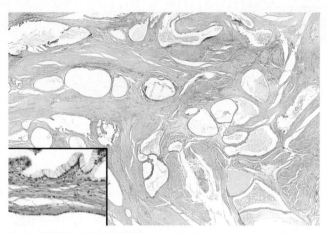

Figure 3.36.2 Endosalpingiosis that mimics adenocarcinoma with irregular infiltration of the muscularis propria. Glands lack a stromal reaction and are benign cytologically (**inset**).

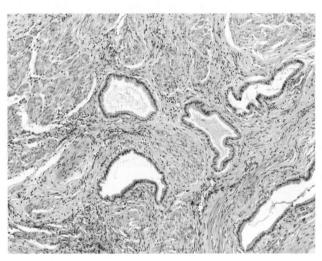

Figure 3.36.3 Endosalpingiosis involving the bladder without eliciting a stromal reaction.

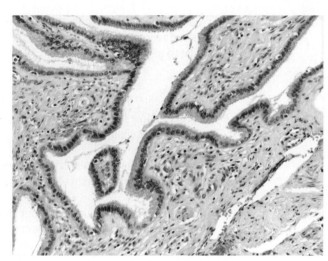

Figure 3.36.4 Same case as Figure 3.36.3 with benign cytology.

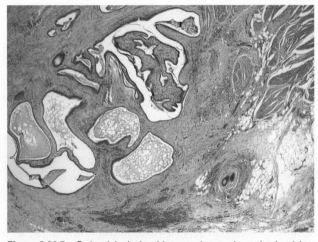

Figure 3.36.5 Endosalpingiosis with unusual stromal reaction involving the muscularis propria and perivesical adipose tissue.

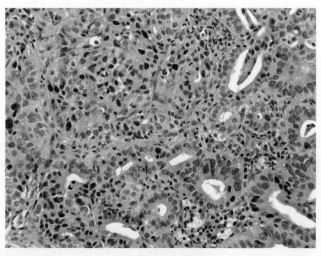

Figure 3.36.6 Bladder adenocarcinoma with overt cytologic atypia.

	Carcinoid Tumor	Cystitis Glandularis, Nonintestinal Type
Age	Middle-aged adults, range 30–73 y	Wide age range from children with bladder exstrophy to adults
Location	Often at the trigone or bladder neck	Anywhere along the urothelial tract
Symptoms	Usually hematuria	Depends on underlying conditions
Signs	Usually small (mean 5 mm, range 2–12 mm). Often appear as polypoid or smooth-surfaced submucosal nodule, sometimes associated with changes suggestive of an inflammatory process	Cystoscopy often shows a mass lesion mimicking carcinoma
Etiology	Unknown	Not necessarily a reaction to injury as can be seen in normal bladders in neonates
Histology	1. Uniform cuboidal or columnar cells forming pseudoglandular structures, including acini and cribriform glands *(Figs. 3.37.1–3.37.5)* 2. Nuclei with finely stippled chromatin, inconspicuous nucleoli *(Fig. 3.37.4)* 3. Moderate to abundant cytoplasm most often amphophilic but ranging from eosinophilic to basophilic 4. Basally located intracytoplasmic eosinophilic granules 5. Mitotic figures absent 6. Accompanied by cystitis glandularis, nonintestinal type *(Fig. 3.37.2)*	1. Nests of the urothelium with inner lining of columnar cells *(Fig. 3.37.2)*. Can form cribriform structures *(Fig. 3.37.6)* 2. In almost all cases, nuclei cytologically bland consisting of small round nuclei, although lacking stippled chromatin 3. Variable cytoplasm, yet typically eosinophilic 4. Lacks intracytoplasmic eosinophilic granules 5. Mitotic figures absent 6. Identical to cystitis glandularis seen adjacent to carcinoid tumors
Special studies	• Chromogranin and synaptophysin positive *(Fig. 3.37.5)* • CK7 positive	• Chromogranin and synaptophysin negative • CK7 positive
Treatment	Typically treated by TUR	Typically treated by TUR
Prognosis	Typically, small lesion cured by excision or biopsy. Rarely can be large more invasive tumor with a more unpredictable prognosis	Benign and despite "recurrence/persistence" on subsequent TUR does not need further treatment. No increased risk of adenocarcinoma, except for increased risk of adenocarcinoma in exstrophy patients

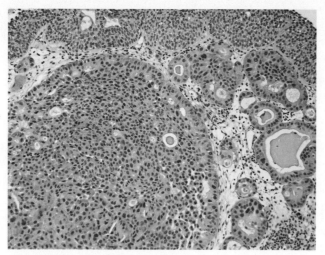

Figure 3.37.1   Carcinoid tumor with cribriform and focal glandular differentiation undermining the urothelium.

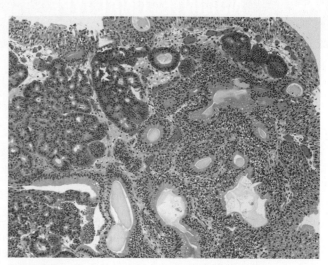

Figure 3.37.2   Carcinoid tumor with cribriform differentiation undermining urothelium. Adjacent cystitis cystica et glandularis (*right*).

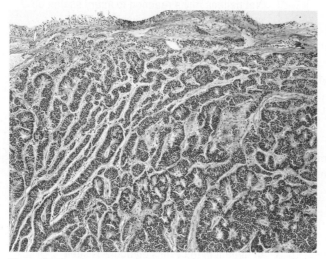

Figure 3.37.3   Carcinoid tumor composed of ribbons undermining the urothelium.

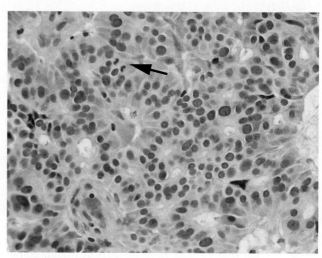

Figure 3.37.4   Bladder carcinoid with nuclei showing delicate chromatin and occasional enlargement and a mitotic figure (*arrow*).

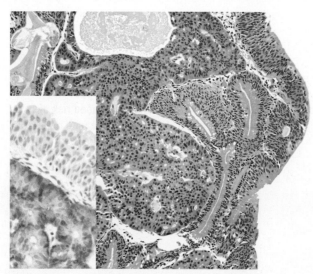

Figure 3.37.5   Bladder carcinoid with a strong chromogranin immunoreactivity (**inset**).

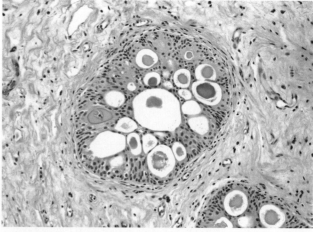

Figure 3.37.6   Cystitis cystica et glandularis.

	Paraganglioma	Invasive Urothelial Carcinoma
Age	Mean age 41 y, range 10–88 y	Mean age mid-late 50s–60s
Location	Mostly located in the trigone or dome	Anywhere along the urothelial tract. Mostly located in the posterior wall or trigone
Symptoms	Hematuria. Micturition attacks consisting of syncope, headache, hypertension, palpitation, blurred vision, and/or sweating following straining when urinating. Two-thirds of patients have hypertension	Usually hematuria
Signs	Most are exophytic with an intact smooth mucosa unless ulcerated. Varies from several millimeters to 10 cm. Most are solitary	Exophytic with irregular mucosa if accompanied by the overlying papillary carcinoma. Wide range in size. Multifocal tumors common
Etiology	Origin from normal paraganglia	See Section 3.10
Histology	1. Uniformly sized and shaped nests delineated by delicate fibrovascular septae *(Figs. 3.38.1 and 3.38.2)*. Crush artifact can obscure the nesting pattern *(Fig. 3.38.3)*. Can also less commonly see small nests in dense collagen *(Fig. 3.38.4)* 2. Uncommonly, can have foci of more diffuse growth where nesting pattern is not as evident *(Fig. 3.3.5)* 3. Abundant amphophilic granular cytoplasm *(Figs. 3.38.3–3.38.6)* yet also can be eosinophilic *(Fig. 3.38.2)* 4. Nuclei typically uniform, small, and round with uniform chromatin *(Fig. 3.38.2)*. Occasional scattered pleomorphic enlarged nuclei, most with a degenerative appearance consisting of smudgy indistinct chromatin *(Figs. 3.38.5 and 3.38.7)* 5. Mitotic figures uncommon 6. May have necrosis 7. Can invade the muscularis propria *(Figs. 3.38.8 and 3.38.9)*	1. Irregularly sized and shaped nests not intimately surrounded by delicate fibrovascular septae 2. Diffuse growth in addition to nests not uncommon 3. Typically eosinophilic cytoplasm lacking granular appearance 4. Most nuclei atypical with hyperchromatic nuclei and well-preserved chromatin detail 5. Mitotic figures common 6. May have necrosis 7. Can invade the muscularis propria
Special studies	• Cytokeratin negative • Synaptophysin and chromogranin positive *(Fig. 3.38.10)* • In some cases, S100 highlights sustentacular cells surrounding tumor nests *(Fig. 3.38.10)*	• Cytokeratin positive • Synaptophysin and chromogranin negative • Lacks S100 cells surrounding tumor nests

	Paraganglioma	Invasive Urothelial Carcinoma
Treatment	Initial TUR. Depending on the location and size of the tumor, final treatment could be only the initial TUR, repeat TUR, partial or radical cystectomy	If muscularis propria invasion present, cystectomy typically performed
Prognosis	10% are malignant, which cannot be predicted based on the morphology	See Section 3.29

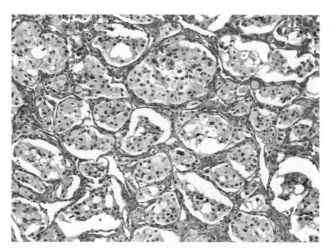

Figure 3.38.1   Nesting pattern of bladder paraganglioma.

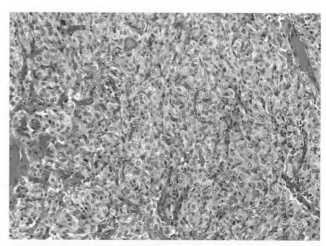

Figure 3.38.2   Bladder paraganglioma with ill-defined nests separated by a thin vascular network.

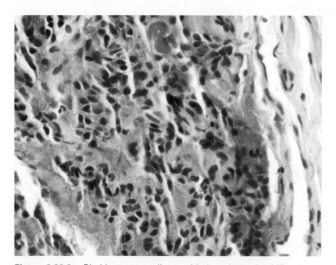

Figure 3.38.3   Bladder paraganglioma with densely amphophilic granular cytoplasm with crush artifact.

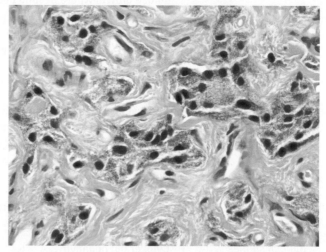

Figure 3.38.4   Small nests of paraganglioma in dense collagen.

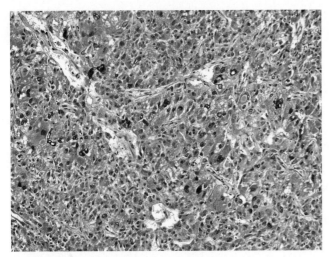

Figure 3.38.5   Sheets of bladder paraganglioma with densely amphophilic granular cytoplasm and degenerative atypia.

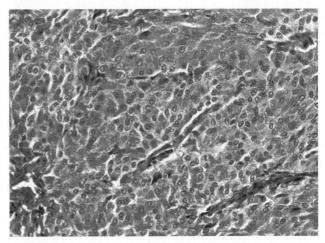

Figure 3.38.6   Nesting pattern of bladder paraganglioma with densely amphophilic granular cytoplasm and uniform nuclei.

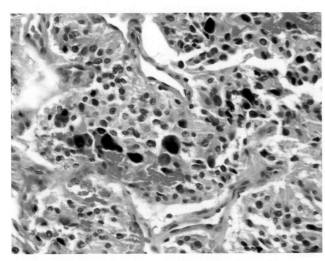

Figure 3.38.7   Nesting pattern of bladder paraganglioma with degenerative atypia.

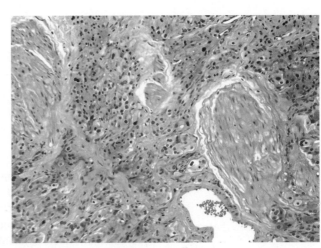

Figure 3.38.8   Paraganglioma invading the muscularis propria.

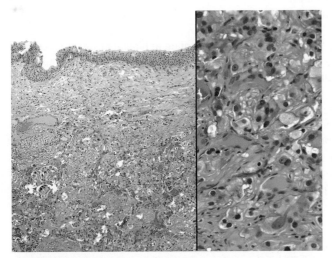

Figure 3.38.9   Paraganglioma invading the muscularis propria (**left**). Higher magnification shows small nests of cells with amphophilic granular cytoplasm.

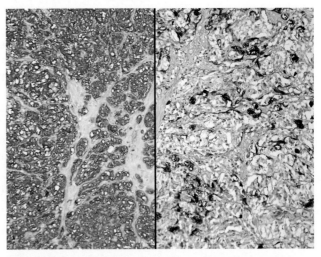

Figure 3.38.10   Paraganglioma with diffuse synaptophysin positivity (**left**) and S100 protein–positive sustentacular cells (**right**).

BLADDER

3

	Small Cell Carcinoma	Invasive Urothelial Carcinoma
Age	Mean age late-60s	Mean age mid-60s with wide age range
Location	Mostly located in the lateral wall or dome	Anywhere along the urothelial tract
Symptoms	Usually hematuria. Occasional paraneoplastic syndromes (peripheral neuropathy, hypercalcemia, hypophosphatemia, ectopic secretion of ACTH)	Usually hematuria
Signs	Large polypoid mass at cystoscopy. Typically unifocal	Mostly located in the posterior wall or trigone. Exophytic with irregular mucosa if accompanied by overlying papillary carcinoma. Wide range in size. Multifocal tumors common
Etiology	High-grade neuroendocrine differentiation from progression of urothelial carcinoma	See Section 3.10
Histology	1. At low magnification has a very "dark blue" appearance *(Fig. 3.39.1)* 2. Typically sheets of cells 3. Large areas of geographic necrosis seen at low magnification *(Fig. 3.39.1)* 4. Classic pattern with high nuclear-to-cytoplasmic ratio, nuclear molding, hyperchromatic nuclei without prominent nucleoli, numerous apoptotic bodies, and/or frequent mitotic figures *(Fig. 3.39.2)*. Can see spectrum with visible yet not huge nucleoli and slight cytoplasm, yet other features of small cell carcinoma present *(Fig. 3.39.3)* 5. In approximately 50% of cases, mixed histology with *in situ* or invasive urothelial, squamous, or glandular carcinoma components *(Figs. 3.39.4–3.39.6)*. Non–small cell components often stand out with abrupt demarcation from "bluer" small cell carcinoma background. Usually, a small cell carcinoma component predominates 6. Usually invades the muscularis propria	1. At low magnification has a more eosinophilic appearance 2. Most common pattern is irregularly sized and shaped nests although can be sheets in poorly differentiated tumors 3. Necrosis may be seen although typically focal 4. Enlarged nuclei with prominent nucleoli, abundant cytoplasm, frequent mitotic activity, infrequent apoptotic bodies 5. The presence of typical *in situ* or invasive urothelial carcinoma does not rule out a small cell carcinoma component 6. Can invade the muscularis propria

	Small Cell Carcinoma	Invasive Urothelial Carcinoma
Special studies	• Cytokeratin positive • Synaptophysin and CD56 usually positive. Chromogranin variably and focally positive. Even if tumor lacks immunohistochemical evidence of neuroendocrine differentiation, if morphology typical can still be diagnosed as small cell carcinoma • Ki-67 often >80% of cells positive	• Cytokeratin positive • Synaptophysin and chromogranin negative • Ki-67 usually not as high as in small cell carcinoma
Treatment	Initially treated with same chemotherapy as small cell carcinoma of lung. If tumor responds but local disease persists, could be followed by radical cystectomy	If muscularis propria invasion present, cystectomy typically performed
Prognosis	Tumor often initially responds but then quickly relapses with a 5-y survival rate of <15%	Following radical cystectomy, the 5-y disease-specific survivals are 81%–90%, 70%–80%, and 40%–52%, if tumor in the corresponding radical cystectomy extends into the lamina propria, muscularis propria, and perivesical tissue, respectively.

3 BLADDER

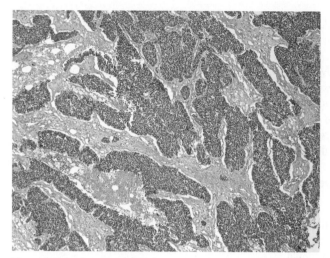

Figure 3.39.1   Low power "blue" appearance of small cell carcinoma of the bladder with necrosis (*lower left*).

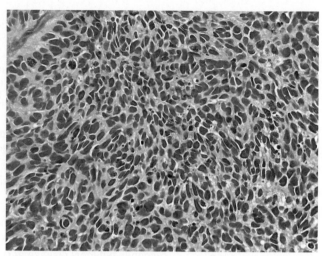

Figure 3.39.2   Classic small cell carcinoma with numerous apoptotic bodies and mitotic figures.

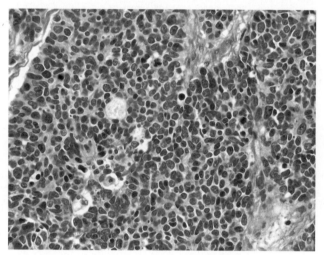

Figure 3.39.3   Small cell carcinoma of the bladder with some cells having somewhat more open chromatin. Cells still have scant cytoplasm, apoptosis, mitotic figures, and nuclear molding.

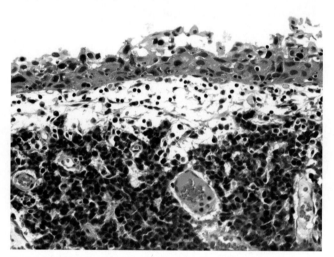

Figure 3.39.4   CIS with underlying small cell carcinoma.

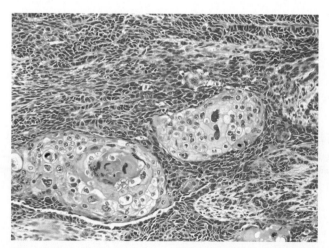

Figure 3.39.5   Small cell carcinoma with squamous cell carcinoma.

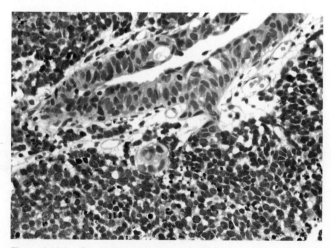

Figure 3.39.6   Small cell carcinoma with urothelial carcinoma.

	Choriocarcinoma	Urothelial Carcinoma with Trophoblastic Differentiation
Age	Rare with <10 cases. Wide age range from 19 years old to elderly. Mean 62 y	Mean age 65 y, range 23–85 y
Location	No predilection for specific location	No predilection for specific location
Symptoms	Hematuria, pelvic pain, urinary obstructive symptoms, symptoms relating to metastases at the time of presentation, or gynecomastia	Hematuria, pelvic pain, urinary obstructive symptoms, symptoms relating to metastases at the time of presentation, or gynecomastia
Signs	Usually large exophytic mass at cystoscopy	Cystoscopic appearance depends on the stage of disease
Etiology	Unknown	Assumed to be trophoblastic differentiation from urothelial stem cells
Histology	1. Dimorphic population of cytotrophoblasts and intimately admixed syncytiotrophoblasts *(Fig. 3.40.1)*. In rare cases, classic choriocarcinoma admixed with urothelial carcinoma or sarcomatoid urothelial carcinoma	1. May be invasive high-grade urothelial or squamous cell carcinoma with or without syncytiotrophoblasts. May be noninvasive papillary urothelial carcinoma of various grades with syncytiotrophoblasts *(Fig. 3.40.2)*
Special studies	• Cytokeratin positive • HCG-positive syncytiotrophoblasts	• Cytokeratin positive • In high-grade pleomorphic urothelial or squamous cell carcinoma, HCG can be present in tumor cells or elevated in the serum that lack the histologic features of syncytiotrophoblasts *(Figs. 3.40.3 and 3.40.4)*. In other cases, can see scattered classic HCG-positive syncytiotrophoblasts among HCG-negative urothelial carcinoma *(Fig. 3.40.2)*
Treatment	Treated with radical cystectomy and chemotherapy	Variable depending on the stage and grade of tumor
Prognosis	Poor prognosis with most patients dead within several years	Variable depending on the stage and grade of tumor

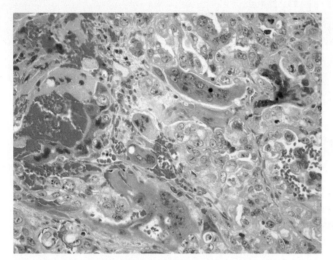

Figure 3.40.1   Choriocarcinoma of the bladder with dimorphic population of cytotrophoblasts and syncytiotrophoblasts.

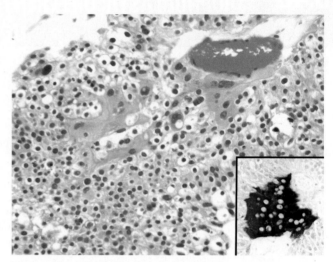

Figure 3.40.2   High-grade papillary urothelial carcinoma with syncytiotrophoblasts that are HCG positive (**inset**).

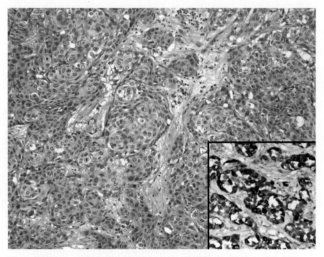

Figure 3.40.3   Infiltrating high-grade urothelial carcinoma with diffuse HCG immunoreactivity (**inset**).

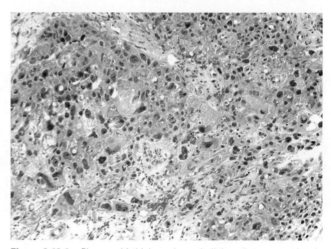

Figure 3.40.4   Pleomorphic high-grade urothelial carcinoma associated with markedly elevated serum HCG levels.

	Sarcomatoid Carcinoma (Carcinosarcoma)	Sarcoma
Age	Mean age mid-late 50s–60s, same age as urothelial carcinoma	Adults
Location	Mostly located in the posterior wall or trigone	No predilection for specific location in the bladder
Symptoms	Usually hematuria	Hematuria or urinary obstructive symptoms
Signs	Large exophytic masses	Usually large exophytic mass at cystoscopy. In certain sarcomas, may be more specific gross findings such as ossification or calcification in osteosarcoma or hemorrhage in angiosarcoma
Etiology	Biphasic tumor with differentiation toward mesenchymal lines from pluripotential stem cells in a carcinoma. Also known as "carcinosarcoma," so both terms should be included in the pathology report. Increased risk of developing several years following pelvic irradiation	Most common sarcoma in the bladder in adults is leiomyosarcoma. Much less commonly seen in adults are rhabdomyosarcoma, angiosarcoma, with other sarcomas exceedingly rare. Increased risk of developing following pelvic irradiation
Histology	1. An epithelial component recognizable on H&E stain is present in many but not all cases *(Figs. 3.41.1–3.41.3)*. Usually urothelial carcinoma, but can be squamous cell carcinoma, adenocarcinoma, or small cell carcinoma. Only epithelial differentiation may be CIS or papillary urothelial carcinoma 2. Mesenchymal differentiation may be nonspecific consisting of undifferentiated malignant spindle cells or can show specific (heterologous) mesenchymal features, most commonly osteogenic sarcoma, chondrosarcoma, rhabdomyosarcoma, or angiosarcoma *(Figs. 3.41.3 and 3.41.4)*. Typically not seen leiomyosarcoma as a component. Cases showing osteogenic sarcoma, chondrosarcoma, or a nonspecific malignant spindle cell tumor that might be classified as malignant fibrous histiocytoma most likely represent sarcomatoid carcinoma 3. Even in the absence of a carcinomatous component on either H&E stains or special studies, a history of urothelial carcinoma strongly favors sarcomatoid carcinoma 4. Usually deeply invasive, but some are polypoid into the bladder with superficial invasion	1. Lacks an epithelial component 2. Leiomyosarcoma consists of interlacing bundles of smooth muscle cells with eosinophilic cytoplasm with variable pleomorphism, mitotic activity, and necrosis *(Fig. 3.41.6)*. Even high-grade leiomyosarcomas usually have areas recognizable as classic smooth muscle differentiation. Other sarcomas are the same as in other sites 3. With a history of urothelial carcinoma, a definitive diagnosis of sarcoma should not usually be made 4. Usually invades the muscularis propria

	Sarcomatoid Carcinoma (Carcinosarcoma)	**Sarcoma**
Special studies	• Best epithelial marker is high molecular weight cytokeratin. Immunohistochemical evidence of epithelial differentiation in nonspecific malignant spindle cells is diagnostic of sarcomatoid carcinoma *(Fig. 3.41.5).* Can also highlight epithelial components • p63 also a sensitive marker yet not as specific • Specific mesenchymal components immunohistochemically identical to pure sarcomas	• Some sarcomas are focally cytokeratin positive, including leiomyosarcoma and angiosarcoma • p63 can focally label some sarcomas • Immunohistochemical results same as in other sites
Treatment	If muscularis propria invasion present, cystectomy typically performed. Typically, also treated with adjuvant chemotherapy	Usually treated with cystectomy with adjuvant chemotherapy tailored to the specific sarcoma
Prognosis	Poor prognosis with 70% dead within 2 y of diagnosis. Compared to patients with urothelial carcinoma alone, greater risk of death even after adjusting for stage at prognosis. Conflicting data whether heterologous elements are associated with a worse prognosis	High-grade leiomyosarcoma associated with a 40%–50% mortality. Other sarcomas, such as adult rhabdomyosarcoma and angiosarcoma, have a worse prognosis with most patients dead within a year

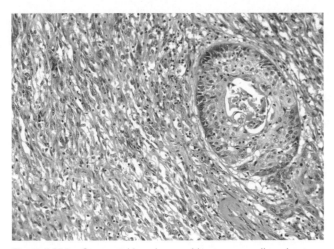

Figure 3.41.1 Sarcomatoid carcinoma with squamous cell carcinoma and spindle cell sarcoma.

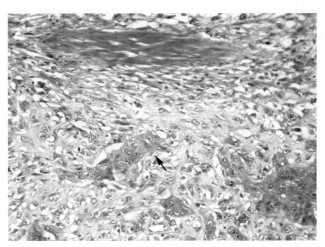

Figure 3.41.2 Sarcomatoid carcinoma with urothelial carcinoma (*arrow*) and sarcomatous stroma invading the muscularis propria.

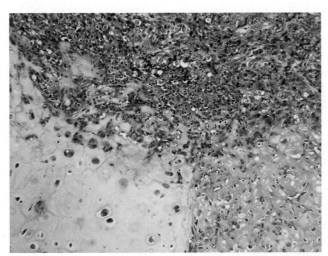

Figure 3.41.3 Sarcomatoid carcinoma with undifferentiated carcinoma (*top*) that was keratin positive and a chondrosarcomatous component.

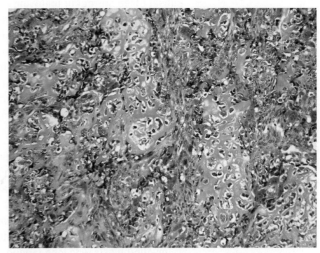

Figure 3.41.4 Sarcomatoid carcinoma with an osteosarcomatous component (epithelial component not shown).

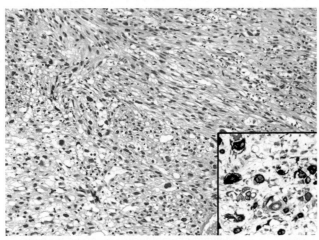

Figure 3.41.5 Sarcomatoid carcinoma with spindle cell sarcoma where an epithelial component is highlighted by pancytokeratin positivity (**inset**).

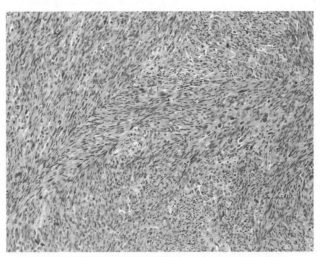

Figure 3.41.6 Leiomyosarcoma of the bladder composed of long fascicles of eosinophilic spindle cells cut in different planes of sections.

3 BLADDER

	Inflammatory Myofibroblastic Tumor (IMT)	Leiomyosarcoma
Age	Wide age range from children to adults	Mean age 58 y (29–84 y)
Location	No site predilection	No predilection for specific location
Symptoms	Hematuria or urinary obstructive symptoms	Hematuria or urinary obstructive symptoms
Signs	Often pedunculated mass at cystoscopy. Wide size ranges from <1 cm to >9 cm. Can invade perivesical adipose tissue	Usually large exophytic mass at cystoscopy
Etiology	Also known as pseudosarcomatous fibromyxoid tumor, pseudosarcomatous myofibroblastic tumor, and inflammatory pseudotumor. A smaller subset of lesions occur following recent TUR for benign bladder disease, designated by some as "postoperative spindle cell nodule." Regardless of whether there is or not a prior history of instrumentation, lesions have overlapping morphologic, immunohistochemical, and molecular features, demonstrate the same clinical behavior and should be considered the same entity	Most common sarcoma in the bladder in adults
Histology	1. May focally have fascicles of spindle cells with variable amounts of eosinophilic cytoplasm, yet typically haphazard without organized fascicles *(Fig. 3.42.1)* 2. Plump, stellate, or elongated spindle cells. Often cells have tissue culture–like myofibroblasts with long tapering cytoplasm on both sides of the nuclei *(Figs. 3.42.2 and 3.42.3)* 3. Often myxoid stromal background *(Figs. 3.42.1 and 3.42.2)* 4. Prominent vascularity with extravasated erythrocytes *(Figs. 3.42.4 and 3.42.5)* 5. Interspersed acute and chronic inflammatory cells *(Figs. 3.42.2, 3.42.3, and 3.42.6)* 6. Variable mitotic activity but can be numerous, yet no atypical ones *(Fig. 3.42.7)* 7. Nuclei enlarged yet relatively uniform in size and shape with vesicular chromatin and one to two distinct nucleoli *(Figs. 3.42.3–3.42.7)* 8. Can invade the muscularis propria *(Fig. 3.42.8)*	1. Fascicles of spindle cells cut longitudinally and in parallel with variable amounts of eosinophilic cytoplasm 2. Compact spindle cells that lack a tissue culture–like fibroblast appearance 3. Rarely, can be myxoid *(Figs. 3.42.9 and 3.42.10)* 4. Prominent vascularity not a notable feature 5. Lacks associated inflammation *(Figs. 3.42.9 and 3.42.10)* 6. Variable mitotic activity but can be numerous, including atypical ones 7. Nuclei enlarged with pleomorphism and scattered hyperchromatic nuclei *(Fig. 3.42.10)* 8. Can invade the muscularis propria
Special studies	• Two-thirds positive for ALK *(Fig. 3.42.8)* • Pancytokeratin positive in 81%, often diffusely • Commonly actin and desmin positive	• ALK negative • Cytokeratin positive in 25%–50% of cases • Actin and desmin usually positive
Treatment	Initially treated only by TUR. May necessitate cystectomy due to local tumor growth. Close follow-up is recommended	Usually treated with cystectomy with adjuvant chemotherapy reserved for high-grade lesions

	Inflammatory Myofibroblastic Tumor (IMT)	**Leiomyosarcoma**
Prognosis	Typically once resected, even incompletely, tumors tend to regress or stay stable. However, incomplete surgical resection may lead to recurrence in approximately one quarter of cases. A unique malignant case has been described with many morphologic features of IMT and an ALK rearrangement, yet overtly sarcomatous	High-grade leiomyosarcoma associated with a 40%–50% mortality. In cases with low cellularity and no mitotic activity, yet degenerative atypia, a diagnosis of symplastic leiomyoma can be made

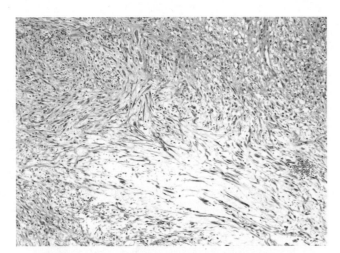

Figure 3.42.1   IMT with haphazard proliferation of spindle cells in a myxoid background.

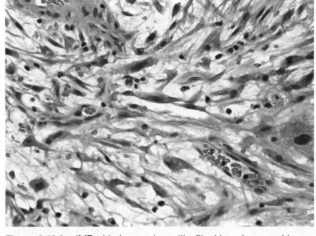

Figure 3.42.2   IMT with tissue culture–like fibroblasts in a myxoid background with inflammatory cells.

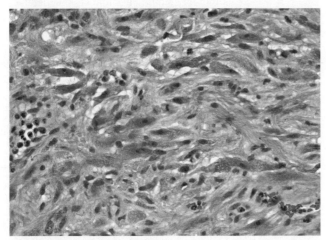

Figure 3.42.3   IMT with tissue culture–like fibroblasts with prominent nucleoli and scattered neutrophils.

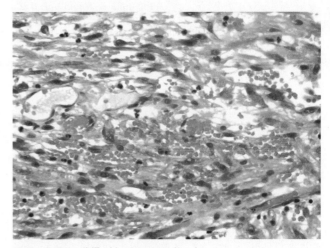

Figure 3.42.4   IMT with extravasated erythrocytes.

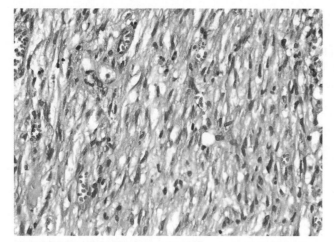

Figure 3.42.5   Numerous capillaries in IMT.

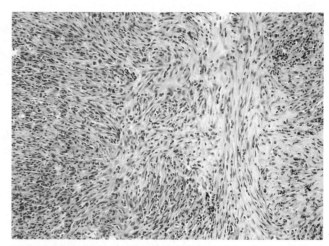

Figure 3.42.6   IMT with prominent inflammation.

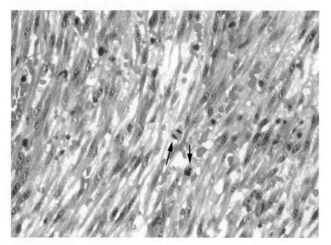

Figure 3.42.7   IMT with multiple mitotic figures (*arrows*) and extravasated erythrocytes.

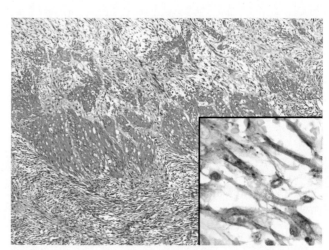

Figure 3.42.8   IMT involving the muscularis propria. **Inset** shows ALK immunoreactivity.

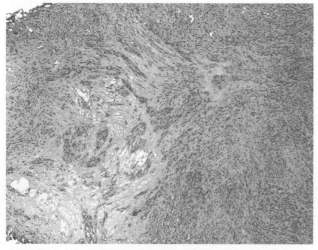

Figure 3.42.9   Myxoid bladder leiomyosarcoma composed of cellular fascicles of spindle cells. The tumor lacks associated inflammation, extravasated erythrocytes, or prominent capillaries.

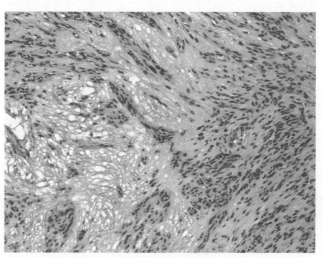

Figure 3.42.10   Same case as Figure 3.42.9 with cellular hyperchromatic nuclei.

	Leiomyoma	The Muscularis Propria
Age	Mean age 52 y (23–77 y)	Any age
Location	No predilection for specific location	Normal finding
Symptoms	Hematuria or urinary obstructive symptoms	Normal finding
Signs	Mean size 4.5 cm (0.7–15 cm)	Normal finding
Histology	1. Spindle cells cut longitudinally and in parallel with variable amounts of eosinophilic cytoplasm 2. Noninfiltrative nodular pattern *(Fig. 3.43.1)*. Large sheets and compact bundles of intersecting smooth muscle fascicles *(Figs. 3.43.1–3.43.4)* 3. Can have myxoid features, necrosis, or extensive hyalinization 4. No mitotic activity 5. Nuclei typically bland resembling normal smooth muscle cells. Occasional case with degenerative-looking nuclear atypia without mitotic activity or hypercellularity	1. Fascicles of spindle cells cut longitudinally and in parallel with variable amounts of eosinophilic cytoplasm 2. Well-formed separate bundles of smooth muscle *(Figs. 3.43.3 and 3.43.4)* 3. Lacks myxoid features, necrosis, or extensive hyalinization 4. No mitotic activity 5. Nuclei bland
Special studies	Special studies not helpful	Not helpful in this differential
Treatment	TUR is sufficient	Not pertinent
Prognosis	Few cases will have residual leiomyoma on repeat TUR. No risk of progression to leiomyosarcoma. If the lesion looks like leiomyoma on TUR, there is no risk of lesional heterogeneity where they may be unsampled leiomyosarcoma. Consequently, a diagnosis of leiomyoma can be established with certainty on TUR	Not pertinent

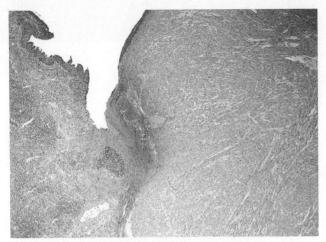

Figure 3.43.1 Bladder leiomyoma with well-circumscribed nodule of intersecting smooth muscle bundles.

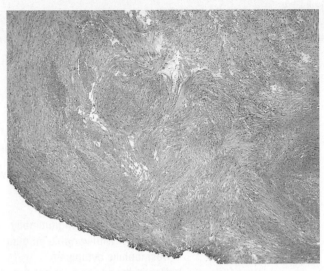

Figure 3.43.2 Bladder leiomyoma with compact intersecting smooth muscle bundles arranged in a haphazard array.

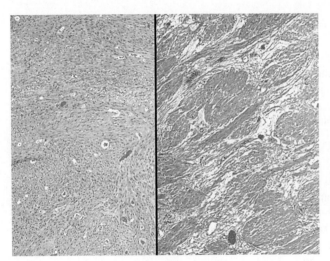

Figure 3.43.3 Bladder leiomyoma (**left**) with compact irregular muscle bundles cut in different planes of section contrasted to the normal muscularis propria (**right**) with well-formed discrete longitudinal muscle bundles.

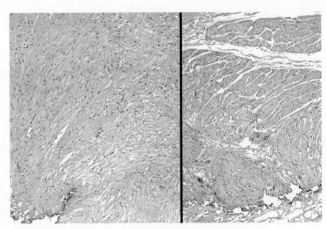

Figure 3.43.4 Bladder leiomyoma (**left**) with compact irregular muscle bundles cut in different planes of section contrasted to the normal muscularis propria (**right**) with well-formed discrete muscle bundles cut in cross section.

	Leiomyoma	Leiomyosarcoma
Age	Mean age 52 y (23–77 y)	Mean age 58 y (29–84 y)
Location	No predilection for specific location	No predilection for specific location
Symptoms	Hematuria or urinary obstructive symptoms	Hematuria or urinary obstructive symptoms
Signs	Mean size 4.5 cm (range 0.7–15 cm)	Usually large exophytic mass at cystoscopy. Mean size 4.9 cm (1.0–10 cm)
Etiology	Unknown	Unknown
Histology	1. Fascicles of spindle cells cut longitudinally and in parallel with variable amounts of eosinophilic cytoplasm *(Figs. 3.44.1 and 3.44.2)* 2. Noninfiltrative nodular pattern 3. Lacks epithelioid features 4. Can have myxoid features, uncommonly focal necrosis, or extensive hyalinization *(Fig. 3.44.3)*. Lacks mucosal ulceration 5. No mitotic activity 6. Nuclei typically bland, resembling normal smooth muscle cells. Occasional case with degenerative-looking nuclear atypia without mitotic activity or hypercellularity *(Fig. 3.44.4)* 7. Low cellularity *(Figs. 3.44.1 and 3.44.2)*	1. Fascicles of spindle cells cut longitudinally and in parallel with variable amounts of eosinophilic cytoplasm 2. An infiltrative border can be appreciated in two-thirds of high-grade and one-half of low-grade tumor 3. One quarter with epithelioid features 4. Can have myxoid features, necrosis, and mucosal ulceration 5. Mitotic activity ranges from 1 to 17/10 HPF (mean and median 7) *(Fig. 3.44.5)* 6. Nuclei enlarged with pleomorphism and hyperchromatic nuclei. Range of atypia based on grade, but even low-grade tumors have more atypia and cellularity than leiomyoma 7. Hypercellular *(Fig. 3.44.6)*
Special studies	Not helpful in this differential	Not helpful in this differential
Treatment	TUR is sufficient	High-grade leiomyosarcoma treated by cystectomy with adjuvant chemotherapy. Low-grade leiomyosarcoma may be treated by partial or radical cystectomy depending on the tumor size and location
Prognosis	Few cases will have residual leiomyoma on repeat TUR. No risk of progression to leiomyosarcoma. If the lesion looks like leiomyoma on TUR, there is no risk of lesional heterogeneity where they may be unsampled leiomyosarcoma. Consequently, a diagnosis of leiomyoma can be established with certainty	High-grade leiomyosarcoma associated with a 40%–50% mortality. Low-grade leiomyosarcoma cured by cystectomy. Uncommonly, there is lesional heterogeneity such that there is low-grade leiomyosarcoma on TUR yet high-grade sarcoma in the resection specimen

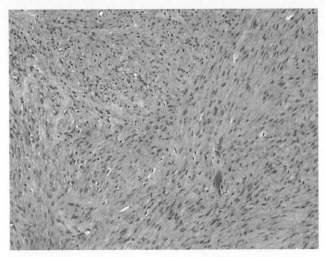

Figure 3.44.1   Bladder leiomyoma with low cellularity and bland cytology.

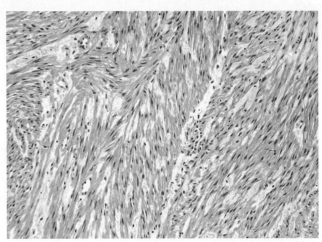

Figure 3.44.2   Bladder leiomyoma with low cellularity and bland cytology.

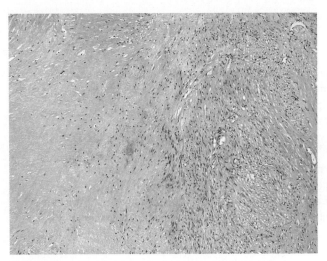

Figure 3.44.3   Bladder leiomyoma with low cellularity and bland cytology and hyalinization.

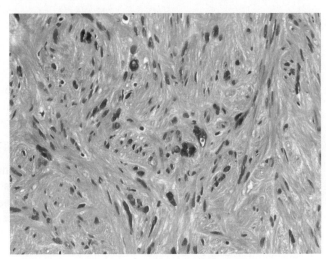

Figure 3.44.4   Bladder leiomyoma with low cellularity and degenerative atypia.

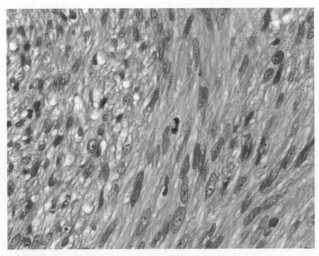

Figure 3.44.5   Low-grade bladder leiomyosarcoma with increased cellularity and mitotic activity.

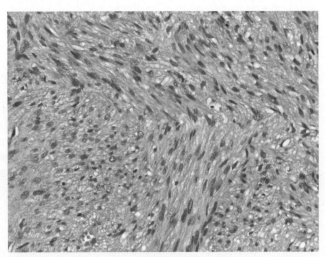

Figure 3.44.6   Low-grade bladder leiomyosarcoma with increased cellularity.

	Diffuse Neurofibroma	Normal Lamina Propria
Age	Range 22–48 y	Any age
Location	No site predilection	Normal finding
Symptoms	Hematuria, recurrent infection, irritative symptoms	Normal finding
Signs	Often multifocal	Normal finding
Etiology	On the basis of limited cases, it seems that diffuse neurofibromas in the bladder lack a close relationship to neurofibromatosis in contrast to plexiform neurofibroma. Nevertheless, reasonable for patients with diffuse neurofibroma to be evaluated for neurofibromatosis	Normal finding
Histology	1. Expansion of the lamina propria with occasional case superficially extending into the muscularis propria 2. Densely compact eosinophilic tissue (Fig. 3.45.1) 3. Paucicellular haphazardly arranged, uniform to stellate spindle cells in a delicate collagenous stroma (Fig. 3.45.2) 4. No mitotic activity 5. Wagner-Meissner bodies range from absent to focal to extensive (Fig. 3.45.3)	1. The lamina propria not expanded 2. Loose delicate collagen with intervening clear space (Fig. 3.45.4) 3. Paucicellular fibroblasts in a looser connective tissue matrix 4. No mitotic activity 5. No Wagner-Meissner bodies
Special studies	Diffuse S100 protein positive	S100 protein negative
Treatment	TUR is sufficient	None
Prognosis	Does not undergo malignant transformation	Not pertinent

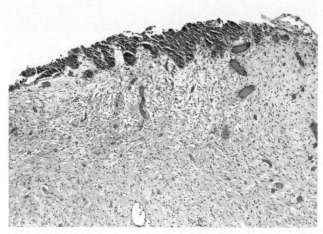

Figure 3.45.1   Diffuse neurofibroma with densely compact eosinophilic tissue filling the lamina propria.

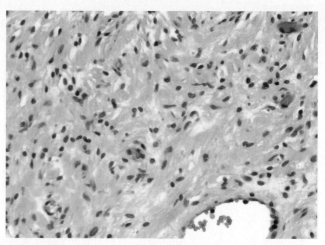

Figure 3.45.2   Same case as Figure 3.45.1 with paucicellular haphazardly arranged, uniform to stellate spindle cells in a compact stroma.

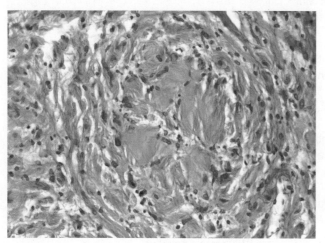

Figure 3.45.3   Bladder diffuse neurofibroma with Wagner-Meissner bodies.

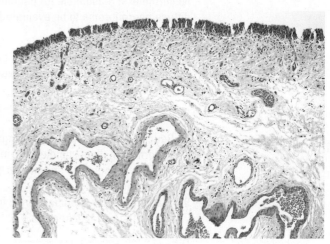

Figure 3.45.4   Normal lamina propria with delicate loose collagen.

SUGGESTED READINGS

3.1–3.6

Amin MB, McKenney JK. An approach to the diagnosis of flat intraepithelial lesions of the urinary bladder using the world health organization/international society of urological pathology consensus classification system. *Adv Anat Pathol.* 2002;9:222–232.

Cheng L, Cheville JC, Neumann RM, et al. Natural history of urothelial dysplasia of the bladder. *Am J Surg Pathol.* 1999;23:443–447.

Harnden P, Eardley I, Joyce AD, et al. Cytokeratin 20 as an objective marker of urothelial dysplasia. *Br J Urol.* 1996;78:870–875.

Levi AW, Potter SR, Schoenberg MP, et al. Clinical significance of denuded urothelium in bladder biopsy. *J Urol.* 2001;166:457–460.

McKenney JK, Desai S, Cohen C, et al. Discriminatory immunohistochemical staining of urothelial carcinoma in situ and non-neoplastic urothelium: an analysis of cytokeratin 20, p53, and CD44 antigens. *Am J Surg Pathol.* 2001;25:1074–1078.

Milord RA, Lecksell K, Epstein JI. An objective morphologic parameter to aid in the diagnosis of flat urothelial carcinoma in situ. *Hum Pathol.* 2001;32:997–1002.

Murphy WM, Soloway MS. Urothelial dysplasia. *J Urol.* 1982;127:849–854.

Parwani AV, Levi AW, Epstein JI, et al. Urinary bladder biopsy with denuded mucosa: denuding cystitis-cytopathologic correlates. *Diagn Cytopathol.* 2004;30:297–300.

Zuk RJ, Rogers HS, Martin JE, et al. Clinicopathological importance of primary dysplasia of bladder. *J Clin Pathol.* 1988;41:1277–1280.

3.7

Cina SJ, Epstein JI, Endrizzi JM, et al. Correlation of cystoscopic impression with histologic diagnosis of biopsy specimens of the bladder. *Hum Pathol.* 2001;32:630–637.

Lane Z, Epstein JI. Polypoid/papillary cystitis: a series of 41 cases misdiagnosed as papillary urothelial neoplasia. *Am J Surg Pathol.* 2008;32:758–764.

Young RH. Papillary and polypoid cystitis. A report of eight cases. *Am J Surg Pathol.* 1988;12:542–546.

3.8

Chow NH, Cairns P, Eisenberger CF, et al. Papillary urothelial hyperplasia is a clonal precursor to papillary transitional cell bladder cancer. *Int J Cancer.* 2000;89:514–518.

Swierczynski SL, Epstein JI. Prognostic significance of atypical papillary urothelial hyperplasia. *Hum Pathol.* 2002;33:512–517.

Taylor DC, Bhagavan BS, Larsen MP, et al. Papillary urothelial hyperplasia. A precursor to papillary neoplasms. *Am J Surg Pathol.* 1996;20:1481–1488.

3.9–3.11

Fine SW, Humphrey PA, Dehner LP, et al. Urothelial neoplasms in patients 20 years or younger: a clinicopathological analysis using the world health organization 2004 bladder consensus classification. *J Urol.* 2005;174:1976–1980.

Epstein JI, Amin MB, Reuter VR, et al. The World Health Organization/International Society of Urological Pathology consensus classification of urothelial (transitional cell) neoplasms of the urinary bladder. Bladder Consensus Conference Committee. *Am J Surg Pathol.* 1998;22:1435–1448.

Gonul II, Poyraz A, Unsal C, et al. Comparison of 1998 WHO/ISUP and 1973 WHO classifications for interobserver variability in grading of papillary urothelial neoplasms of the bladder. Pathological evaluation of 258 cases. *Urol Int.* 2007;78:338–344.

Holmang S, Hedelin H, Anderstrom C, et al. Recurrence and progression in low grade papillary urothelial tumors. *J Urol.* 1999;162:702–707.

Holmang S, Johansson SL. Urothelial carcinoma of the upper urinary tract: comparison between the WHO/ISUP 1998 consensus classification and WHO 1999 classification system. *Urology.* 2005;66:274–278.

McKenney JK, Amin MB, Young RH. Urothelial (transitional cell) papilloma of the urinary bladder: a clinicopathologic study of 26 cases. *Mod Pathol.* 2003;16:623–629.

Magi-Galluzzi C, Epstein JI. Urothelial papilloma of the bladder: a review of 34 de novo cases. *Am J Surg Pathol.* 2004;28:1615–1620.

Pan CC, Chang YH, Chen KK, et al. Prognostic significance of the 2004 WHO/ISUP classification for prediction of recurrence, progression, and cancer-specific mortality of non-muscle-invasive urothelial tumors of the urinary bladder: a clinicopathologic study of 1,515 cases. *Am J Clin Pathol.* 2010;133:788–795.

Pich A, Chiusa L, Formiconi A, et al. Biologic differences between noninvasive papillary urothelial neoplasms of low malignant potential and low-grade (grade 1) papillary carcinomas of the bladder. *Am J Surg Pathol.* 2001;25:1528–1533.

Samaratunga H, Makarov DV, Epstein JI. Comparison of WHO/ISUP and WHO classification of noninvasive papillary urothelial neoplasms for risk of progression. *Urology.* 2002;60:315–319.

Yin H, Leong AS. Histologic grading of noninvasive papillary urothelial tumors: validation of the 1998 WHO/ISUP system by immunophenotyping and follow-up. *Am J Clin Pathol.* 2004;121:679–687.

3.12–3.13

Amin MB, Gomez JA, Young RH. Urothelial transitional cell carcinoma with endophytic growth patterns: a discussion of patterns of invasion and problems associated with assessment of invasion in 18 cases. *Am J Surg Pathol.* 1997;21:1057–1068.

Eiber M, van Oers JM, Zwarthoff EC, et al. Low frequency of molecular changes and tumor recurrence in inverted papillomas of the urinary tract. *Am J Surg Pathol.* 2007;31:938–946.

Fine SW, Chan TY, Epstein JI. Inverted papillomas of the prostatic urethra. *Am J Surg Pathol.* 2006;30:975–979.

Fine SW, Epstein JI. Inverted urothelial papillomas with foamy or vacuolated cytoplasm. *Hum Pathol.* 2006;37:1577–1582.

Jones TD, Zhang S, Lopez-Beltran A, et al. Urothelial carcinoma with an inverted growth pattern can be distinguished from inverted papilloma by fluorescence in situ hybridization, immunohistochemistry, and morphologic analysis. *Am J Surg Pathol.* 2007;31:1861–1867.

Picozzi S, Casellato S, Bozzini G, et al. Inverted papilloma of the bladder: a review and an analysis of the recent literature of 365 patients. *Urol Oncol.* 2012 (epub ahead of print).

3.14–3.16

Cox R, Epstein JI. Large nested variant of urothelial carcinoma: 23 cases mimicking von Brunn nests and inverted growth pattern of noninvasive papillary urothelial carcinoma. *Am J Surg Pathol.* 2011;35:1337–1342.

Dhall D, Al-Ahmadie H, Olgac S. Nested variant of urothelial carcinoma. *Arch Pathol Lab Med.* 2007;131:1725–1727.

Drew PA, Furman J, Civantos F, et al. The nested variant of transitional cell carcinoma: an aggressive neoplasm with innocuous histology. *Mod Pathol.* 1996;9:989–994.

Holmang S, Johansson SL. The nested variant of transitional cell carcinoma—a rare neoplasm with poor prognosis. *Scand J Urol Nephrol.* 2001;35:102–105.

Huang Q, Chu PG, Lau SK, et al. Urothelial carcinoma of the urinary bladder with a component of acinar/tubular type differentiation simulating prostatic adenocarcinoma. *Hum Pathol.* 2004;35:769–773.

Lin O, Cardillo M, Dalbagni G, et al. Nested variant of urothelial carcinoma: a clinicopathologic and immunohistochemical study of 12 cases. *Mod Pathol.* 2003;16:1289–1298.

Nigwekar P, Amin MB. The many faces of urothelial carcinoma: an update with an emphasis on recently described variants. *Adv Anat Pathol.* 2008;15:218–233.

Volmar KE, Chan TY, De Marzo AM, et al. Florid von Brunn nests mimicking urothelial carcinoma: a morphologic and immunohistochemical comparison to the nested variant of urothelial carcinoma. *Am J Surg Pathol.* 2003;27:1243–1252.

Wasco MJ, Daignault S, Bradley D, et al. Nested variant of urothelial carcinoma: a clinicopathologic and immunohistochemical study of 30 pure and mixed cases. *Hum Pathol.* 2010;41:163–171.

Young RH, Oliva E. Transitional cell carcinomas of the urinary bladder that may be underdiagnosed. A report of four invasive cases exemplifying the homology between neoplastic and non-neoplastic transitional cell lesions. *Am J Surg Pathol.* 1996;20:1448–1454.

3.17–3.18

Allan CH, Epstein JI. Nephrogenic adenoma of the prostatic urethra: a mimicker of prostate adenocarcinoma. *Am J Surg Pathol.* 2001;25:802–808.

Brimo F, Herawi M, Sharma R, et al. Hepatocyte nuclear factor-1beta expression in clear cell adenocarcinomas of the bladder

and urethra: diagnostic utility and implications for histogenesis. *Hum Pathol.* 2011;42:1613–1619.

Herawi M, Drew PA, Pan CC, et al. Clear cell adenocarcinoma of the bladder and urethra: cases diffusely mimicking nephrogenic adenoma. *Hum Pathol.* 2010;41:594–601.

Mazal PR, Schaufler R, Altenhuber-Muller R, et al. Derivation of nephrogenic adenomas from renal tubular cells in kidney-transplant recipients. *N Engl J Med.* 2002;347:653–659.

Malpica A, Ro JY, Troncoso P, et al. Nephrogenic adenoma of the prostatic urethra involving the prostate gland: a clinicopathologic and immunohistochemical study of eight cases. *Hum Pathol.* 1994;25:390–395.

Oliva E, Amin MB, Jimenez R, et al. Clear cell carcinoma of the urinary bladder: a report and comparison of four tumors of müllerian origin and nine of probable urothelial origin with discussion of histogenesis and diagnostic problems. *Am J Surg Pathol.* 2002;26:190–197.

Sung MT, Zhang S, MacLennan GT, et al. Histogenesis of clear cell adenocarcinoma in the urinary tract: evidence of urothelial origin. *Clin Cancer Res.* 2008;14:1947–1955.

Tong GX, Melamed J, Mansukhani M, et al. PAX2: a reliable marker for nephrogenic adenoma. *Mod Pathol.* 2006;19:356–363.

Young RH, Scully RE. Clear cell adenocarcinoma of the bladder and urethra. A report of three cases and review of the literature. *Am J Surg Pathol.* 1985;9:816–826.

3.19

Keck B, Stoehr R, Wach S, et al. The plasmacytoid carcinoma of the bladder—rare variant of aggressive urothelial carcinoma. *Int J Cancer.* 2011;129:346–354.

Nigwekar P, Tamboli P, Amin MB, et al. Plasmacytoid urothelial carcinoma: detailed analysis of morphology with clinicopathologic correlation in 17 cases. *Am J Surg Pathol.* 2009;33:417–424.

Ricardo-Gonzalez RR, Nguyen M, Gokden N, et al. Plasmacytoid carcinoma of the bladder: a urothelial carcinoma variant with a predilection for intraperitoneal spread. *J Urol.* 2012;187:852–855.

3.20–3.22

Guo CC, Fine SW, Epstein JI. Noninvasive squamous lesions in the urinary bladder: a clinicopathologic analysis of 29 cases. *Am J Surg Pathol.* 2006;30:883–891.

Tsuzuki T, Epstein JI. Fibroepithelial polyp of the lower urinary tract in adults. *Am J Surg Pathol.* 2005;29:460–466.

3.23–3.25

Abdou NI, NaPombejara C, Sagawa A, et al. Malakoplakia: Evidence for monocyte lysosomal abnormality correctable by cholinergic agonist in vitro and in vivo. *N Engl J Med.* 1977;297:1413–1419.

Hansel DE, Nadasdy T, Epstein JI. Fibromyxoid nephrogenic adenoma: a newly recognized variant mimicking mucinous adenocarcinoma. *Am J Surg Pathol.* 2007;31:1231–1237.

Lou TY, Teplitz C. Malakoplakia: pathogenesis and ultrastructural morphogenesis. A problem of altered macrophage (phagolysosomal) response. *Hum Pathol*. 1974;5:191–207.

Smith BH. Malacoplakia of the urinary tract: a study of twenty-four cases. *Am J Clin Pathol*. 1965;43:409–417.

Smith VC, Boone TB, Truong LD. Collagen polyp of the urinary tract: a report of two cases. *Mod Pathol*. 1999;12:1090–1093.

Stanton MJ, Maxted W. Malacoplakia: a study of the literature and current concepts of pathogenesis, diagnosis and treatment. *J Urol*. 1981;125:139–146.

Stevens S, McClure J. The histochemical features of the Michaelis-Gutmann body and a consideration of the pathophysiological mechanisms of its formation. *J Pathol*. 1982;137:119–127.

Tamas EF, Epstein JI. Detection of residual tumor cells in bladder biopsy specimens: pitfalls in the interpretation of cytokeratin stains. *Am J Surg Pathol*. 2007;31:390–397.

3.26

Amin MB, Ro JY, Lee KM, et al. Lymphoepithelioma-like carcinoma of the urinary bladder. *Am J Surg Pathol*. 1994;18:466–473.

Gulley ML, Amin MB, Nicholls JM, et al. Epstein-Barr virus is detected in undifferentiated nasopharyngeal carcinoma but not in lymphoepithelioma-like carcinoma of the urinary bladder. *Hum Pathol*. 1995;26:1207–1214.

Lopez-Beltran A, Luque RJ, Vicioso L, et al. Lymphoepithelioma-like carcinoma of the urinary bladder: a clinicopathologic study of 13 cases. *Virchows Arch*. 2001;438:552–557.

Tamas EF, Nielsen ME, Schoenberg MP, et al. Lymphoepithelioma-like carcinoma of the urinary tract: a clinicopathological study of 30 pure and mixed cases. *Mod Pathol*. 2007;20:828–834.

Williamson SR, Zhang S, Lopez-Beltran A, et al. Lymphoepithelioma-like carcinoma of the urinary bladder: clinicopathologic, immunohistochemical, and molecular features. *Am J Surg Pathol*. 2011;35:474–483.

3.27

Baydar D, Amin MB, Epstein JI. Osteoclast-rich undifferentiated carcinomas of the urinary tract. *Mod Pathol*. 2006;19:161–171.

Zukerberg LR, Armin AR, Pisharodi L, et al. Transitional cell carcinoma of the urinary bladder with osteoclast-type giant cells: a report of two cases and review of the literature. *Histopathology*. 1990;17:407–411.

3.28–3.31

Alvarado-Cabrero I, Sierra-Santiesteban FI, Mantilla-Morales A, et al. Micropapillary carcinoma of the urothelial tract. A clinicopathologic study of 38 cases. *Ann Diagn Pathol*. 2005;9:1–5.

Comperat E, Roupret M, Yaxley J, et al. Micropapillary urothelial carcinoma of the urinary bladder: a clinicopathological analysis of 72 cases. *Pathology*. 2010;42:650–654.

Council L, Hameed O. Differential expression of immunohistochemical markers in bladder smooth muscle and myofibroblasts, and the potential utility of desmin, smoothelin, and vimentin in staging of bladder carcinoma. *Mod Pathol*. 2009;22:639–650.

Jimenez RE, Keane TE, Hardy HT, et al. pT1 urothelial carcinoma of the bladder: criteria for diagnosis, pitfalls, and clinical implications. *Adv Anat Pathol*. 2000;7:13–25.

Larsen MP, Steinberg GD, Brendler CB, et al. Use of ulex europaeus agglutinin I (UEAI) to distinguish vascular and "pseudovascular" invasion in transitional cell carcinoma of bladder with lamina propria invasion. *Mod Pathol*. 1990;3:83–88.

Lotan TL, Ye H, Melamed J, et al. Immunohistochemical panel to identify the primary site of invasive micropapillary carcinoma. *Am J Surg Pathol*. 2009;33:1037–1041.

Miyamoto H, Sharma RB, Illei PB, et al. Pitfalls in the use of smoothelin to identify muscularis propria invasion by urothelial carcinoma. *Am J Surg Pathol*. 2010;34:418–422.

Paner GP, Brown JG, Lapetino S, et al. Diagnostic use of antibody to smoothelin in the recognition of muscularis propria in transurethral resection of urinary bladder tumor (TURBT) specimens. *Am J Surg Pathol*. 2010;34:792–799.

Paner GP, Ro JY, Wojcik EM, et al. Further characterization of the muscle layers and lamina propria of the urinary bladder by systematic histologic mapping: implications for pathologic staging of invasive urothelial carcinoma. *Am J Surg Pathol*. 2007;31:1420–1429.

Paner GP, Shen SS, Lapetino S, et al. Diagnostic utility of antibody to smoothelin in the distinction of muscularis propria from muscularis mucosae of the urinary bladder: a potential ancillary tool in the pathologic staging of invasive urothelial carcinoma. *Am J Surg Pathol*. 2009;33:91–98.

Ramani P, Birch BR, Harland SJ, et al. Evaluation of endothelial markers in detecting blood and lymphatic channel invasion in pT1 transitional carcinoma of bladder. *Histopathology*. 1991;19:551–554.

Reuter VE. Lymphovascular invasion as an independent predictor of recurrence and survival in node-negative bladder cancer remains to be proven. *J Clin Oncol*. 2005;23:6450–6451.

Samaratunga H, Khoo K. Micropapillary variant of urothelial carcinoma of the urinary bladder; a clinicopathological and immunohistochemical study. *Histopathology*. 2004;45:55–64.

Sangoi AR, Beck AH, Amin MB, et al. Interobserver reproducibility in the diagnosis of invasive micropapillary carcinoma of the urinary tract among urologic pathologists. *Am J Surg Pathol*. 2010;34:1367–1376.

3.32

Baker PM, Young RH. Radiation-induced pseudocarcinomatous proliferations of the urinary bladder: a report of 4 cases. *Hum Pathol*. 2000;31:678–683.

Chan TY, Epstein JI. Radiation or chemotherapy cystitis with "pseudocarcinomatous" features. *Am J Surg Pathol*. 2004;28:909–913.

Lane Z, Epstein JI. Pseudocarcinomatous epithelial hyperplasia in the bladder unassociated with prior irradiation or chemotherapy. *Am J Surg Pathol*. 2008;32:92–97.

3 BLADDER

3.33

Tavora F, Fajardo DA, Lee TK, et al. Small endoscopic biopsies of the ureter and renal pelvis: pathologic pitfalls. *Am J Surg Pathol.* 2009;33:1540–1546.

3.34–3.37

Abenoza P, Manivel C, Fraley EE. Primary adenocarcinoma of urinary bladder. Clinicopathologic study of 16 cases. *Urology.* 1987;29:9–14.

Ashley RA, Inman BA, Sebo TJ, et al. Urachal carcinoma: clinicopathologic features and long-term outcomes of an aggressive malignancy. *Cancer.* 2006;107:712–720.

Chen YB, Epstein JI. Primary carcinoid tumors of the urinary bladder and prostatic urethra: a clinicopathologic study of 6 cases. *Am J Surg Pathol.* 2011;35:442–446.

Cheng L, Montironi R, Bostwick DG. Villous adenoma of the urinary tract: a report of 23 cases, including 8 with coexistent adenocarcinoma. *Am J Surg Pathol.* 1999;23:764–771.

Clement PB, Young RH. Endocervicosis of the urinary bladder. A report of six cases of a benign mullerian lesion that may mimic adenocarcinoma. *Am J Surg Pathol.* 1992;16:533–542.

Comiter CV. Endometriosis of the urinary tract. *Urol Clin North Am.* 2002;29:625–635.

el-Mekresh MM, el-Baz MA, Abol-Enein H, et al. Primary adenocarcinoma of the urinary bladder: a report of 185 cases. *Br J Urol.* 1998;82:206–212.

Grignon DJ, Ro JY, Ayala AG, et al. Primary adenocarcinoma of the urinary bladder. A clinicopathologic analysis of 72 cases. *Cancer.* 1991;67:2165–2172.

Jacobs LB, Brooks JD, Epstein JI. Differentiation of colonic metaplasia from adenocarcinoma of urinary bladder. *Hum Pathol.* 1997;28:1152–1157.

Roy S, Parwani AV. Adenocarcinoma of the urinary bladder. *Arch Pathol Lab Med.* 2011;135:1601–1605.

Seibel JL, Prasad S, Weiss RE, et al. Villous adenoma of the urinary tract: a lesion frequently associated with malignancy. *Hum Pathol.* 2002;33:236–241.

3.38

Cheng L, Leibovich BC, Cheville JC, et al. Paraganglioma of the urinary bladder: can biologic potential be predicted? *Cancer.* 2000;88:844–852.

Zhou M, Epstein JI, Young RH. Paraganglioma of the urinary bladder: a lesion that may be misdiagnosed as urothelial carcinoma in transurethral resection specimens. *Am J Surg Pathol.* 2004;28:94–100.

3.39

Agoff SN, Lamps LW, Philip AT, et al. Thyroid transcription factor-1 is expressed in extrapulmonary small cell carcinomas but not in other extrapulmonary neuroendocrine tumors. *Mod Pathol.* 2000;13:238–242.

Abrahams NA, Moran C, Reyes AO, et al. Small cell carcinoma of the bladder: a contemporary clinicopathological study of 51 cases. *Histopathology.* 2005;46:57–63.

Cheng L, Pan CX, Yang XJ, et al. Small cell carcinoma of the urinary bladder: a clinicopathologic analysis of 64 patients. *Cancer.* 2004;101:957–962.

Jones TD, Kernek KM, Yang XJ, et al. Thyroid transcription factor 1 expression in small cell carcinoma of the urinary bladder: an immunohistochemical profile of 44 cases. *Hum Pathol.* 2005;36:718–723.

Koay EJ, Teh BS, Paulino AC, et al. A surveillance, epidemiology, and end results analysis of small cell carcinoma of the bladder: epidemiology, prognostic variables, and treatment trends. *Cancer.* 2011;117:5325–5333.

Wang X, MacLennan GT, Lopez-Beltran A, et al. Small cell carcinoma of the urinary bladder—histogenesis, genetics, diagnosis, biomarkers, treatment, and prognosis. *Appl Immunohistochem Mol Morphol.* 2007;15:8–18.

3.40

Dirnhofer S, Koessler P, Ensinger C, et al. Production of trophoblastic hormones by transitional cell carcinoma of the bladder: association to tumor stage and grade. *Hum Pathol.* 1998;29:377–382.

Iles RK, Persad R, Trivedi M, et al. Urinary concentration of human chorionic gonadotrophin and its fragments as a prognostic marker in bladder cancer. *Br J Urol.* 1996;77:61–69.

Sievert K, Weber EA, Herwig R, et al. Pure primary choriocarcinoma of the urinary bladder with long-term survival. *Urology.* 2000;56:856.

3.41

Cheng L, Zhang S, Alexander R, et al. Sarcomatoid carcinoma of the urinary bladder: The final common pathway of urothelial carcinoma dedifferentiation. *Am J Surg Pathol.* 2011;35:e34–e46.

Ikegami H, Iwasaki H, Ohjimi Y, et al. Sarcomatoid carcinoma of the urinary bladder: a clinicopathologic and immunohistochemical analysis of 14 patients. *Hum Pathol.* 2000;31:332–340.

Jones EC, Young RH. Myxoid and sclerosing sarcomatoid transitional cell carcinoma of the urinary bladder: a clinicopathologic and immunohistochemical study of 25 cases. *Mod Pathol.* 1997;10:908–916.

Lopez-Beltran A, Pacelli A, Rothenberg HJ, et al. Carcinosarcoma and sarcomatoid carcinoma of the bladder: clinicopathological study of 41 cases. *J Urol.* 1998;159:1497–1503.

Wang J, Wang FW, Lagrange CA, et al. Clinical features of sarcomatoid carcinoma (carcinosarcoma) of the urinary bladder: analysis of 221 cases. *Sarcoma.* 2010; 2010 (epub).

Young RH, Wick MR, Mills SE. Sarcomatoid carcinoma of the urinary bladder. A clinicopathologic analysis of 12 cases and review of the literature. *Am J Clin Pathol.* 1988;90:653–661.

3.42–3.44

Harik LR, Merino C, Coindre JM, et al. Pseudosarcomatous myofibroblastic proliferations of the bladder: a clinicopathologic study of 42 cases. *Am J Surg Pathol.* 2006;30:787–794.

Hirsch MS, Dal Cin P, Fletcher CD. ALK expression in pseudosarcomatous myofibroblastic proliferations of the genitourinary tract. *Histopathology.* 2006;48:569–578.

Martin SA, Sears DL, Sebo TJ, et al. Smooth muscle neoplasms of the urinary bladder: a clinicopathologic comparison of leiomyoma and leiomyosarcoma. *Am J Surg Pathol.* 2002;26:292–300.

Montgomery EA, Shuster DD, Burkart AL, et al. Inflammatory myofibroblastic tumors of the urinary tract: a clinicopathologic study of 46 cases, including a malignant example inflammatory fibrosarcoma and a subset associated with high-grade urothelial carcinoma. *Am J Surg Pathol.* 2006;30:1502–1512.

Lee TK, Miyamoto H, Osunkoya AO, et al. Smooth muscle neoplasms of the urinary bladder: a clinicopathologic study of 51 cases. *Am J Surg Pathol.* 2010;34:502–509.

Proppe KH, Scully RE, Rosai J. Postoperative spindle cell nodules of genitourinary tract resembling sarcomas. A report of eight cases. *Am J Surg Pathol.* 1984;8:101–108.

Ro JY, el-Naggar AK, Amin MB, et al. Pseudosarcomatous fibromyxoid tumor of the urinary bladder and prostate: immunohistochemical, ultrastructural, and DNA flow cytometric analyses of nine cases. *Hum Pathol.* 1993;24:1203–1210.

Tsuzuki T, Magi-Galluzzi C, Epstein JI. ALK-1 expression in inflammatory myofibroblastic tumor of the urinary bladder. *Am J Surg Pathol.* 2004;28:1609–1614.

3.45

Wang W, Montgomery E, Epstein JI. Benign nerve sheath tumors on urinary bladder biopsy. *Am J Surg Pathol.* 2008;32:907–912.

4

Testis

	Normal Spermatogenesis	Hypospermatogenesis
Age	Not applicable	Postpuberty
Location	Not applicable	Usually bilateral
Symptoms	None	Infertility
Signs	Normal serum FSH, LH, testosterone, and prolactin	Normal serum FSH, LH, testosterone, and prolactin
Etiology	None	Iatrogenic (chemotherapy or radiation), alcoholism, postinfectious, diabetes, cirrhosis, other endocrinopathies (hyperprolactinemia), congenital abnormalities (cryptorchidism), pesticide toxicity, and varicocele
Histology	1. Complete differentiation taking place 2. Tubules may not show complete spermatogenesis in every cross-section due to tangential sectioning at the edge of the tubule 3. Starting from the periphery of the tubule: *Spermatogonium*—small cell with pale nuclear chromatin and scant cytoplasm. *Spermatocytes*—largest and most numerous germ cells with larger nuclei and more cytoplasm. Speckled chromatin. *Spermatids*—smaller with darker dense chromatin and scant cytoplasm. *Spermatozoon*—smaller with ovoid nuclei with clearing (acrospermia) at the head. Tails not apparent on routine sections *(Figs. 4.1.1–4.1.3)* 4. Sloughing of germ cells not specific, possibly due to handling and fragile nature of the tissue 5. Normal spermatogenesis is relative to age. Men 50s and under should have approximately the same thickness with decreases as age increases 6. In order to call normal spermatogenesis, the entire biopsy should be normal	1. Complete differentiation taking place 2. Increased number of tubules may not show complete spermatogenesis in every cross-section due to tangential sectioning at the edge of the tubule 3. Full maturation through all spermatogenic stages occurs but the total number of germ cells is decreased *(Figs. 4.1.4–4.1.6)* 4. Less likely to see sloughing of germ cells 5. Should state the severity of process whether mild, moderate, or severe (i.e., only rare spermatozoa identified) 6. The percent of each pattern of spermatogenesis should be recorded (i.e., 50% normal spermatogenesis; 30% severe hypospermatogenesis; 20% Sertoli cell–only pattern)
Special studies	Not used in this differential	Not useful in this differential
Treatment	Not applicable	Directed toward inciting etiology
Prognosis	Not applicable	Fertility can be frequently achieved

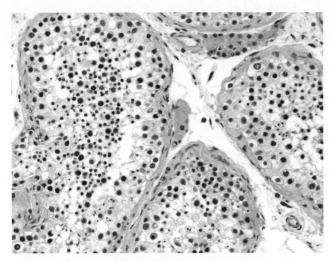

Figure 4.1.1　Normal adult seminiferous tubules showing normal spermatogenesis from spermatogonia to spermatozoa. Note the presence of primary and secondary spermatocytes and spermatids in variable proportions.

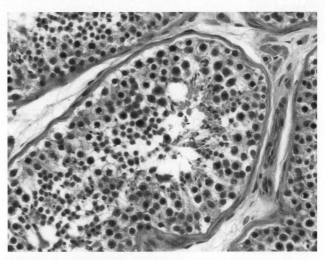

Figure 4.1.2　Normal adult seminiferous tubules showing normal spermatogenesis.

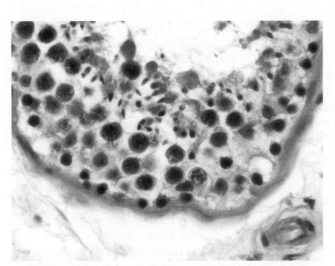

Figure 4.1.3　Normal adult seminiferous tubules showing normal spermatogenesis.

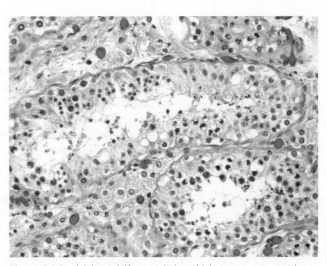

Figure 4.1.4　Adult seminiferous tubules with hypospermatogenesis. The overall total number of germ cells is decreased.

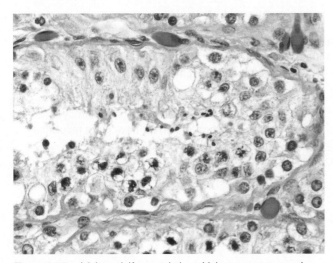

Figure 4.1.5　Adult seminiferous tubules with hypospermatogenesis.

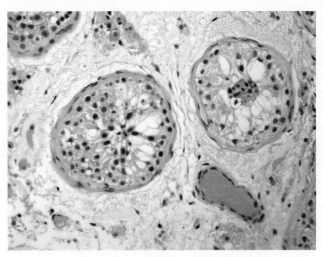

Figure 4.1.6　Adult seminiferous tubules with marked hypospermatogenesis.

	Hypospermatogenesis	Maturation Arrest
Age	Postpuberty	Postpuberty
Location	Usually bilateral	Usually bilateral
Symptoms	Infertility	Infertility
Signs	Normal serum FSH, LH, testosterone, and prolactin	Normal serum FSH, LH, testosterone, and prolactin
Etiology	Iatrogenic (chemotherapy or radiation), alcoholism, postinfectious, diabetes, cirrhosis, other endocrinopathies (hyperprolactinemia), congenital abnormalities (cryptorchidism), pesticide toxicity, and varicocele	Iatrogenic (chemotherapy, radiation, drugs, and testosterone supplementation), alcoholism, postinfectious, endocrinopathy, congenital abnormalities (cryptorchidism), and varicocele
Histology	1. Almost all tubules with complete spermatogenesis but incomplete spermatogenesis may be present in some tubules due to tangential sectioning at the edge of the tubule. Only complete cross-sections of relatively large, round tubules (i.e., sectioned through the center) should be assessed. If tangentially sectioned the tubule, can appear identical to maturation arrest 2. Full maturation through all spermatogenic stages occurs but the total number of germ cells is decreased. Critical to recognize mature spermatids to rule out maturation arrest *(Figs. 4.2.1–4.2.3)*	1. Typically, all the tubules in a biopsy will show incomplete spermatogenesis. However, this pattern may coexist with other patterns where the percent of each pattern of spermatogenesis should be recorded (i.e., 50% hypospermatogenesis; 50% maturation arrest). Should not diagnose maturation arrest on small percent of biopsy as may be an artifact 2. Spermatogenic arrest can occur at any stage of development but most commonly at the primary spermatocyte stage. Second most common pattern is spermatogenic arrest at the spermatogonia stage with very uncommon primary spermatocytes relative to spermatogonia. Spermatids are absent *(Figs. 4.2.4–4.2.6)*
Special studies	Not useful in this differential	Not useful in this differential
Treatment	Directed toward inciting etiology. Micro-TESE (microdissection testicular sperm extraction)	Directed toward inciting etiology. Micro-TESE (microdissection testicular sperm extraction) is attempted to achieve fertility
Prognosis	Fertility can be frequently achieved	Fertility can be frequently achieved. Patients with biopsies showing late (spermatocyte stage) maturation arrest have more favorable outcome

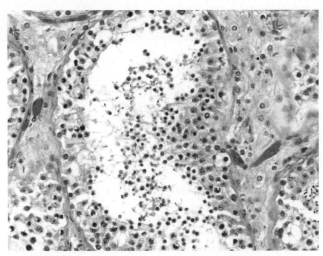

Figure 4.2.1   Adult seminiferous tubules with hypospermatogenesis. Full maturation through all spermatogenic stages occur, but the overall total number of germ cells is decreased.

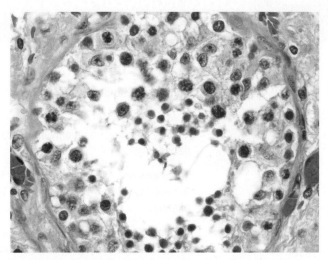

Figure 4.2.2   Adult seminiferous tubules with hypospermatogenesis.

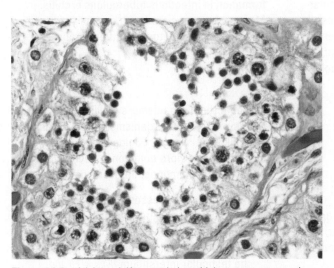

Figure 4.2.3   Adult seminiferous tubules with hypospermatogenesis.

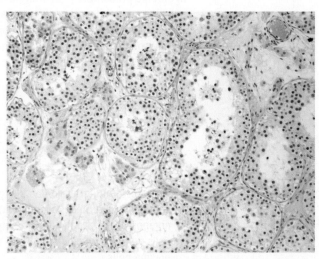

Figure 4.2.4   Adult seminiferous tubules showing maturation arrest at the secondary spermatocyte phase. Note absence of spermatid and spermatozoa.

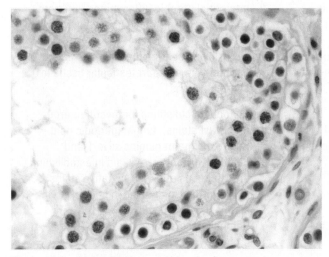

Figure 4.2.5   Adult seminiferous tubules showing maturation arrest at the secondary spermatocyte phase.

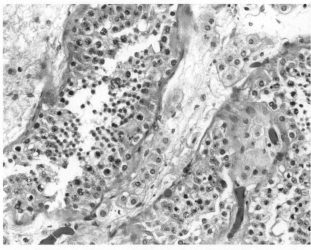

Figure 4.2.6   Adult seminiferous tubules showing maturation arrest at the spermatid phase.

4   TESTIS

	Idiopathic Granulomatous Orchitis	Infectious and Other Nonneoplastic Granulomatous Orchitis
Age	19–84 y but most commonly in fifth to seventh decades	Variable
Location	Testis and occasionally secondarily involve the epididymis and spermatic cord. Typically bilateral	More frequently initiated in the epididymis and spread to the testis in later stages. More likely to be bilateral
Symptoms	Sudden testicular pain in acute cases. Rarely fever, hematuria, dysuria, and scrotal swelling	Mild testicular enlargement may be associated with systemic symptoms such as fever and weight loss
Signs	Enlarging scrotal mass with variable pain in chronic presentation. Sudden testicular swelling and tenderness in acute cases. Ultrasound shows diffuse hypoechogenicity with associated testicular enlargement, which may raise differential of germ cell neoplasm	Testicular tenderness. Fistula and abscess formation in infectious tuberculous orchitis. Most cases associated with systemic disease and signs and symptoms in other organs
Etiology	Unknown	Mycobacterial organisms, syphilis, brucellosis, leprosy, and fungal organisms. Rarely parasitic and rickettsial agents. Etiology is unknown in sarcoidosis. More common in developing countries and immunosuppressed patients
Histology	1. Nonnecrotizing granulomas filling seminiferous tubules. Granulomas are composed of epithelioid histiocytes, giant cells admixed with lymphocytes, and plasma cells (Figs. 4.3.1–4.3.3) 2. Chronic inflammatory cells, including eosinophils infiltrate the interstitium (Fig. 4.3.4) 3. In advanced stages, seminiferous tubules become atrophic and are surrounded by fibrosis (Fig. 4.3.5)	1. In infectious processes, necrotizing and/or nonnecrotizing granulomatous inflammation composed of epithelioid histiocytes and multinucleated giant cells mainly involving the testicular interstitium (Figs. 4.3.6 and 4.3.7). The same interstitial distribution is also seen in sarcoidosis, yet nonnecrotizing granulomas are seen (Fig. 4.3.8) 2. Interstitial chronic inflammatory infiltrate composed mainly of lymphocytes 3. Fibrosis and scaring involving testicular parenchyma and paratesticular tissue in chronic lesions
Special studies	• Negative histochemical stains for mycobacterial, fungal, and bacterial organisms help exclude specific infectious granulomatous orchitis • Reticulin stains highlight intratubular architecture	• Histochemical stains for mycobacterial (acid-fast stains), fungal (periodic acid–Schiff and methenamine silver), and bacterial organisms will aid in establishing the infectious etiology. Negative stains for the organism can aid in pointing to the diagnosis of sarcoidosis • Reticulin stains demonstrate interstitial process

	Idiopathic Granulomatous Orchitis	**Infectious and Other Nonneoplastic Granulomatous Orchitis**
Treatment	Orchiectomy often performed for presumptive neoplasm. Frozen section could aid in the diagnosis and guide conservative treatment with steroids	Antibiotics to combat specific infectious agent
Prognosis	Benign inflammatory condition. Could lead to loss of spermatogenesis in the involved testis even if orchiectomy avoided	Excellent

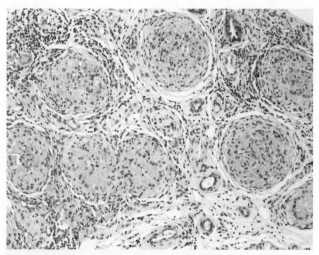

Figure 4.3.1   Idiopathic granulomatous orchitis showing nonnecrotizing granulomas filling seminiferous tubules. Granulomas are composed of epithelioid histiocytes, giant cells admixed with lymphocytes and plasma cells.

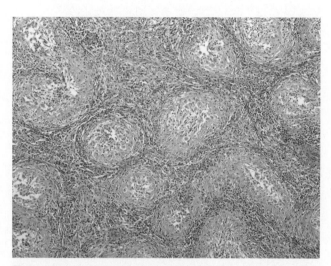

Figure 4.3.2   Idiopathic granulomatous orchitis. Granulomas are composed of epithelioid histiocytes and giant cells.

4   TESTIS

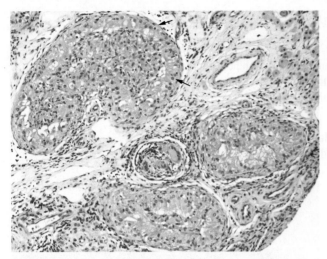

Figure 4.3.3   Idiopathic granulomatous orchitis showing nonnecrotizing granulomas filling seminiferous tubules. Residual germ cells are noted (*arrows*).

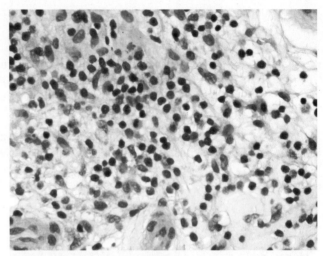

Figure 4.3.4   Idiopathic granulomatous orchitis. Associated chronic inflammation is illustrated with occasional eosinophils admixed with lymphocytes and plasma cells.

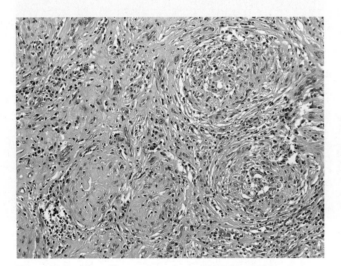

Figure 4.3.5   Idiopathic granulomatous orchitis with scarring.

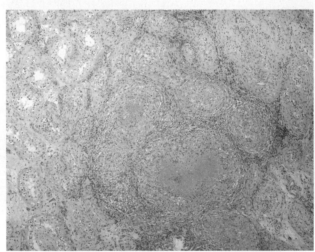

Figure 4.3.6   Mycobacterial granulomatous orchitis. Necrotizing granulomas with palisaded central necrosis is illustrated.

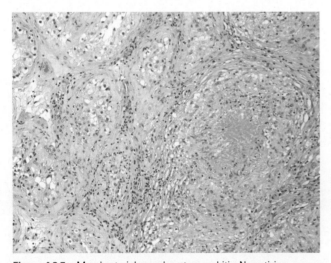

Figure 4.3.7   Mycobacterial granulomatous orchitis. Necrotizing granulomas involve the interstitium with minimal involvement of atrophic seminiferous tubules seen on the left side.

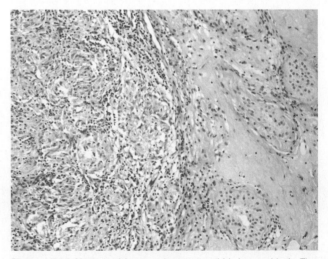

Figure 4.3.8   Nonnecrotizing granulomatous orchitis in sarcoidosis. The process primarily involves the interstitium.

	Idiopathic Granulomatous Orchitis	Intratubular Germ Cell Neoplasia Unclassified (IGCNU) with Granulomas
Age	Most commonly in fifth to seventh decades (19–84 y)	Typically 15–35 y
Location	Typically bilateral	Usually unilateral
Symptoms	Sudden testicular pain in acute cases. Rarely fever, hematuria, dysuria, and scrotal swelling	Asymptomatic
Signs	Enlarging scrotal mass with variable pain in chronic presentation. Sudden testicular swelling and tenderness in acute cases	None except for those of associated conditions such as cryptorchidism and infertility
Etiology	Unknown	Associated risk factors include cryptorchidism (4% risk) and infertility (IGCNU in 1%–2% of biopsies). Frequently adjacent to germ cell tumors
Histology	1. Seminiferous tubules filled with epithelioid histiocytes, giant cells admixed with lymphocytes, and plasma cells (Figs. 4.4.1 and 4.4.2) 2. Lacks atypical cells 3. Involved tubules may show focal spermatogenesis 4. Lymphocytes, plasma cells, and eosinophils in the interstitium	1. Intratubular epithelioid histiocytes, fewer giant cells associated with IGCNU 2. IGCNU cells are enlarged, atypical germ cells residing within seminiferous tubules as isolated cells or a single row along a usually thickened basement membrane. IGCNU cells have clear cytoplasm, irregular nuclear contours, coarse chromatin, and enlarged single or multiple nucleoli. Some IGCNU cells have mummified pyknotic enlarged hyperchromatic nuclei (Figs. 4.4.3–4.4.5) 3. Seminiferous tubules containing IGCNU usually lack active spermatogenesis and contain mostly Sertoli cells 4. Mainly lymphocytes in the interstitium
Special studies	• Negative for PLAP and OCT4 • SALL 4 and CD117 are expressed in normal adult spermatogonia	• Positive for PLAP and OCT4 (Fig. 4.4.6) • SALL4 and CD117 positive but not useful as they are not specific for IGCNU
Treatment	Orchiectomy. Frozen section could aid in the diagnosis and guide conservative treatment	If IGCNU identified on biopsy, typically just close follow-up. In some countries, contralateral biopsy performed, and if positive, then sperm banking and bilateral low-dose radiation are offered
Prognosis	Benign inflammatory condition but may lead to loss of spermatogenesis in the involved testis even if orchiectomy was avoided	Up to 50% risk of developing invasive germ cell tumor within 5 y. Risk of increased testicular germ cell tumor also in the contralateral testis

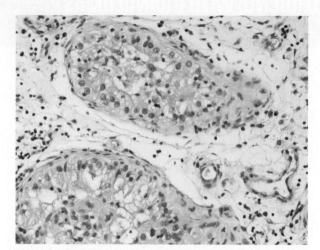

Figure 4.4.1 Idiopathic granulomatous orchitis showing nonnecrotizing granulomas filling seminiferous tubules. Note lack of cytologic atypia in Sertoli cells at periphery of the tubules.

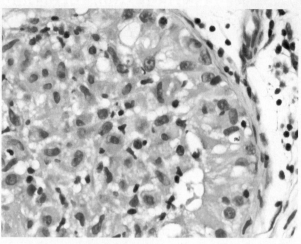

Figure 4.4.2 Idiopathic granulomatous orchitis with a seminiferous tubule filled with epithelioid histiocytes. There is a lack of atypical cells.

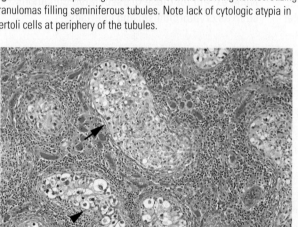

Figure 4.4.3 Some seminiferous tubules with IGCNU not involved with granulomatous response (*arrowhead*). Other tubules have granulomatous inflammation within the tubules involved by IGCNU (*arrow*).

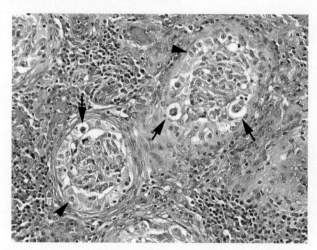

Figure 4.4.4 Nonnecrotizing granulomas involving some seminiferous tubules in association with IGCNU. Note the presence of highly atypical precursor neoplastic cells at the periphery of the tubules with typical cleared cytoplasm and coarse chromatin (*arrows*). Contrast with Sertoli cells with smaller, uniform, round-oval shape, uniform chromatin, and a single central nucleolus (*arrowheads*).

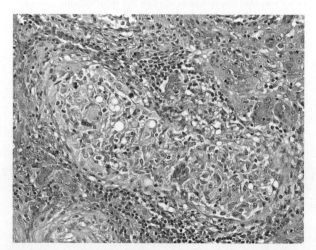

Figure 4.4.5 Nonnecrotizing granulomas in association with IGCNU (same case as in Figure 4.4.4) with extensive intratubular granulomatous reaction destroying IGCNU cells, mimicking idiopathic granulomatous orchitis.

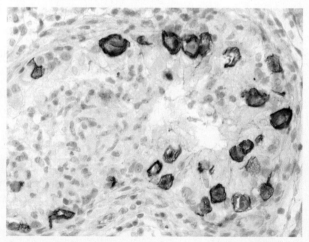

Figure 4.4.6 Nonnecrotizing granulomas in association with IGCNU highlighted by CD117.

	Granulomatous Seminoma	Infectious and Other Nonneoplastic Granulomatous Orchitis
Age	Second to fourth decades. Can also be seen in older men	Variable
Location	Usually unilateral	More frequently starts in the epididymis and spread to the testis in later stages. More likely to be bilateral
Symptoms	Painless swelling of one testicle; one-third of cases complain of scrotal heaviness or dull pain. One-tenth of cases can present with symptoms due to metastatic disease such as abdominal/back pain, cough	Mild testicular enlargement may be associated with systemic symptoms such as fever and weight loss
Signs	Usually palpable testicular nodule	Testicular tenderness, fistula, and abscess formation in infectious tuberculous orchitis
Etiology	Associated risk factors include cryptorchidism (10%), infertility, low socioeconomic status, and male genital malformations. No known reason why granulomatous response in some men. Seen in up to 50% of seminomas	Mycobacterial organisms, syphilis, brucellosis, leprosy, and fungal organisms. Rarely parasitic and rickettsial agents. Etiology remains unknown in sarcoidosis
Histology	1. Nonnecrotizing interstitial granulomatous inflammation composed of histiocytes and occasional giant cells, which when exuberant can obscure neoplastic germ cells	1. Necrotizing and/or nonnecrotizing granulomatous inflammation composed of epithelioid histiocytes and multinucleated giant cells mainly affecting the testicular interstitium. The same interstitial distribution is also seen in sarcoidosis, yet without necrotizing granulomas *(Figs. 4.5.5 and 4.5.6)*
	2. Ill-defined granulomatous inflammation, as opposed to well-formed granulomas *(Fig. 4.5.1)*	2. Granulomas tend to be well formed
	3. Lymphoplasmacytic infiltrate at times with lymphoid follicles and eosinophils are typically also present and reside in fibrovascular septae dividing the sheets of neoplastic seminoma cells	3. Interstitial chronic inflammatory infiltrate composed mainly of lymphocytes
	4. The infiltrating neoplastic seminoma cells are monotonous round-to-polygonal cleared cells with ovoid nuclei containing one or more prominent nucleoli imparting a classic "fried egg" appearance. Mitotic activity is variable. In some cases, granulomatous infiltrate so prominent almost obscuring seminoma cells *(Figs. 4.5.2 and 4.5.3)*	4. Invasive seminoma cells absent
	5. Seminiferous tubules containing IGCNU are almost invariably found in the surrounding testis	5. IGCNU absent

	Granulomatous Seminoma	**Infectious and Other Nonneoplastic Granulomatous Orchitis**
Special studies	• No need for organism stains	• Histochemical stains for mycobacterial (acid-fast stains), fungal (periodic acid–Schiff and methenamine silver), and bacterial organisms aid in establishing the infectious etiology
	• Invasive seminoma cells positive for PLAP, OCT4, CD117, and SALL4 *(Fig. 4.5.4)*	• Negative for PLAP, OCT4, CD117, and SALL4
Treatment	Stage dependent. Radical orchiectomy followed by active surveillance or adjuvant radiotherapy and/or platinum-based chemotherapy	Antibiotics to the specific infectious agent
Prognosis	Excellent prognosis with up to 90% relapse-free 5-y survival	Excellent

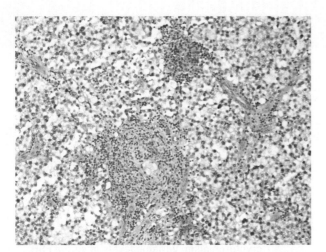

Figure 4.5.1   Focal nonnecrotizing interstitial granulomatous inflammation composed of histiocytes is seen in septae dividing sheets of seminoma cells.

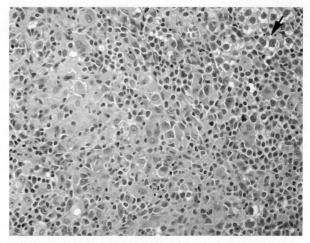

Figure 4.5.2   Rare seminoma cells (*arrow*) associated with extensive nonnecrotizing interstitial granulomatous inflammation composed of epithelioid histiocytes admixed with lymphocytes, plasma cells, and multinucleated histiocytes.

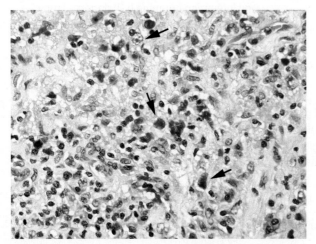

Figure 4.5.3   Rare seminoma cells (*arrows*) associated with extensive nonnecrotizing interstitial granulomatous inflammation. Some seminoma cells are very hyperchromatic where it is difficult to see nuclear detail as these cells are fragile and can show crush artifact. Others have preserved prominent nucleoli.

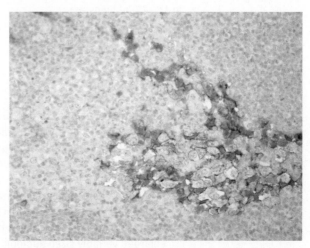

Figure 4.5.4   Seminoma cells labeled with PLAP immunostain.

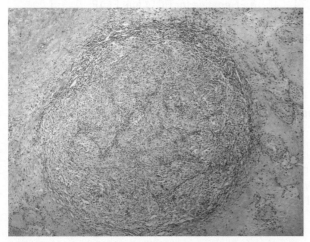

Figure 4.5.5   Nonnecrotizing granulomatous orchitis in sarcoidosis composed of well-formed granulomas. Note surrounding scarring and atrophic seminiferous tubules lacking IGCNU.

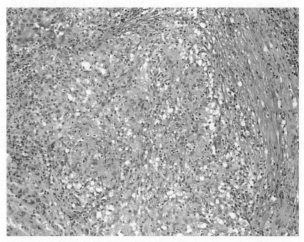

Figure 4.5.6   Mycobacterial granulomatous orchitis with discrete granuloma.

4   TESTIS

	Intratubular Germ Cell Neoplasia Unclassified (IGCNU)	Sertoli Cell–Only Pattern (Germ Cell Aplasia)
Age	15–35 y	Pre- or postpuberty
Location	Usually unilateral	Usually bilateral except when in association with the cryptorchid testis
Symptoms	Asymptomatic	Infertility
Signs	None except for those of associated conditions such as cryptorchidism and infertility	Hypogonadism in some cases. Azoospermia, cryptorchidism. Variable levels of serum FSH, LH, and testosterone depending on the etiology
Etiology	Associated risk factors include cryptorchidism (4% risk) and infertility (IGCNU in 1%–2% of biopsies)	Associated with hypogonadotropic hypogonadism due to combined deficit of FSH and luteinizing hormone (LH) during infancy; chromosomal anomalies, including 45X, 48XYYY, 46XX, and structural anomalies of chromosome Y; cryptorchidism; iatrogenic; exposure to ionizing radiation or chemotherapy; and corticosteroids. 5%–10% of male infertility cases
Histology	1. Seminiferous tubules contain IGCNU cells, which are enlarged, atypical germ cells residing as isolated cells or as a single row along a usually thickened basement membrane *(Figs. 4.6.1–4.6.3)* 2. IGCNU cells have clear cytoplasm, irregular nuclear contours, coarse chromatin, and enlarged single or multiple enlarged variably sized nucleoli 3. Seminiferous tubules containing IGCNU usually lack active spermatogenesis and contain mostly Sertoli cells. Can see contrast between Sertoli cells and IGCNU	1. Seminiferous tubules contain only Sertoli cells 2. Sertoli cells have a round-to-ovoid nucleus with a smooth outline with uniform chromatin and small uniform nucleoli *(Figs. 4.6.4–4.6.6)* 3. Uniform population of Sertoli cells
Special studies	• IGCNU cells positive for PLAP and OCT4 • IGCNU cells also positive for SALL4 and CD117 but not useful stains in this differential • Sertoli cells positive for inhibin	• Negative for OCT4 and PLAP • Nonneoplastic germ cells may be positive for SALL4 and CD117 so not useful in this differential • Sertoli cells positive for inhibin
Treatment	Typically just close follow-up. In some countries, contralateral biopsy performed, and if positive, then sperm banking and bilateral low-dose radiation are offered	Directed toward inciting etiology. Micro-TESE (microdissection testicular sperm extraction) is attempted to achieve fertility
Prognosis	Up to 50% risk of developing invasive germ cell tumor within 5 y (up to 90% risk in 7 y). Risk of germ cell tumor is also increased in the contralateral testis	Fertility can be occasionally achieved

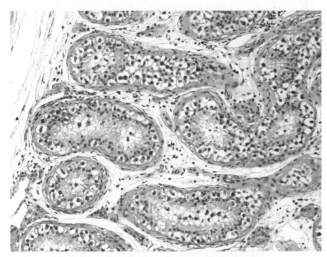

Figure 4.6.1   Seminiferous tubules contain IGCNU. Enlarged, atypical germ cells with cytoplasmic clearing in a single row along a thickened basement membrane are noted.

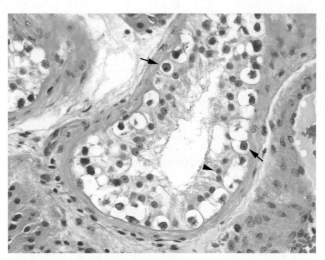

Figure 4.6.2   Seminiferous tubules contain IGCNU with enlarged hyperchromatic nuclei with coarse chromatin residing as a single row along a thickened basement membrane (*arrows*). Sertoli cell nuclei are smaller with more uniform chromatin and a single small central nucleolus (*arrowhead*).

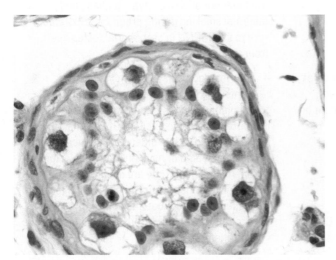

Figure 4.6.3   IGCNU cells have clear cytoplasm, irregular nuclear contours, coarse chromatin, and enlarged single or multiple enlarged variably sized nucleoli.

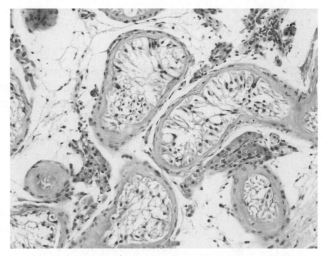

Figure 4.6.4   Seminiferous tubules contain only Sertoli cells. Cells at low power often have a wispy appearance. Peritubular fibrosis is common.

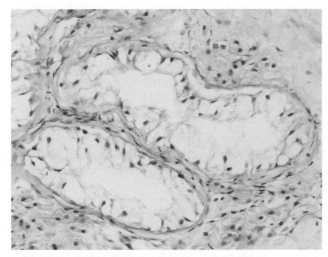

Figure 4.6.5   Seminiferous tubules contain only Sertoli cells with small bland nuclei and abundant vacuolated cytoplasm.

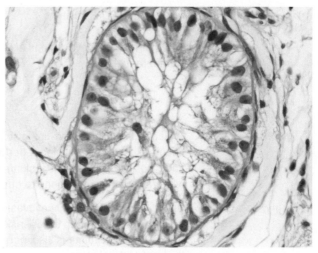

Figure 4.6.6   Seminiferous tubules contain only Sertoli cells. Nuclei are round-to-ovoid with a smooth outline, uniform chromatin and small uniform nucleoli.

4   TESTIS

	Intratubular Germ Cell Neoplasia Unclassified (IGCNU)	Prepubertal Cryptorchid Testes
Age	15–35 y	Congenital
Location	Usually unilateral	Usually unilateral but can rarely be bilateral
Symptoms	Asymptomatic	None
Signs	None except for those of associated conditions such as cryptorchidism and infertility	Congenital maldescent of one or both testes
Etiology	Associated risk factors include cryptorchidism (4% risk) and infertility (IGCNU in 1%–2% of biopsies)	Risk factors include intrauterine exposure to environmental chemicals with endocrine-disrupting properties; low birth weight; karyotypic abnormality (intersex syndrome); other genital tract malformation (i.e., hypospadias); and maternal smoking during pregnancy. Extremely rare to see IGCNU in prepubertal testes apart from an intersex disorder
Histology	1. IGCNU cells are enlarged and have clear cytoplasm, irregular nuclear contours, coarse chromatin, and enlarged single or multiple nucleoli *(Figs. 4.7.1–4.7.3)*	1. Spermatogonia have clear cytoplasm containing small size nuclei with round and regular nuclear contours, densely packed chromatin and no nucleoli. Occasionally, spermatogonia are otherwise identical, yet can be binucleated or have enlarged nuclei (giant spermatogonia). They are usually solitary in a given seminiferous tubule and can be dispersed throughout the testis *(Figs. 4.7.4–4.7.6)*
	2. Seminiferous tubules containing IGCNU usually lack active spermatogenesis and contain mostly Sertoli cells	2. Prepubertal seminiferous tubules lack active spermatogenesis
	3. IGCNU cells are within seminiferous tubules as isolated cells or as a single row along a usually thickened basement membrane	3. Sertoli cells are basally located as isolated cells along a usually thickened basement membrane
Special studies	• OCT4 and PLAP positive • Other markers not as useful in this differential	• PLAP and OCT4 negative in normal prepubertal testes • Delayed maturation in undervirilization syndromes [1] and in Down syndrome characterized by retention of fetal germ cell markers (PLAP, OCT4, CD117) but lacking typical seminoma-like morphology
Treatment	Typically just close follow-up. In some countries, contralateral biopsy performed, and if positive, then sperm banking and bilateral low-dose radiation are offered	Orchiopexy. Testicular biopsy to rule out IGCNU when cryptorchidism is associated with karyotypic abnormality or other male genital malformation
Prognosis	Up to 50% risk of developing invasive germ cell tumor within 5 y (up to 90% risk in 7 y). Risk of germ cell tumor is also increased in the contralateral testis	2%–4 % risk of developing IGCNU during adulthood. Increased risk of invasive germ cell tumor in the ipsilateral (4–7×) and contralateral testis (2–4×). Orchiopexy even before 2 y of age is not protective of subsequent neoplasia

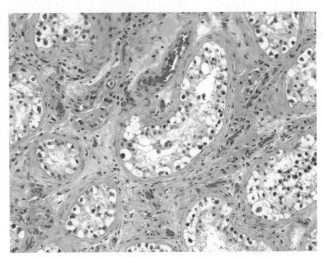

Figure 4.7.1   Seminiferous tubules contain IGCNU. Enlarged, atypical germ cells are situated as a single row along a thickened basement membrane.

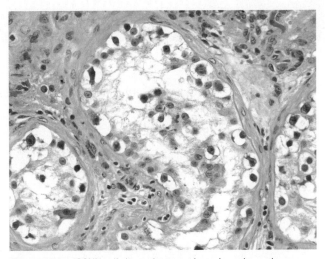

Figure 4.7.2   IGCNU cells have clear cytoplasm, irregular nuclear contours, coarse chromatin, and enlarged single or multiple enlarged variably sized nucleoli.

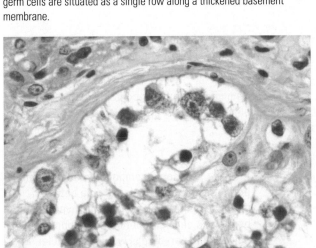

Figure 4.7.3   IGCNU cells with irregular nuclear contours and coarse chromatin.

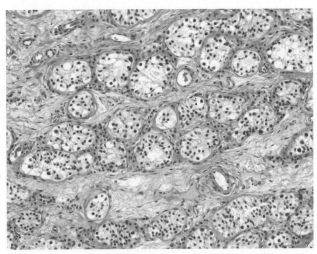

Figure 4.7.4   Spermatogonia with clear cytoplasm containing small-size nuclei with round and regular nuclear contours are seen in this prepubertal testis.

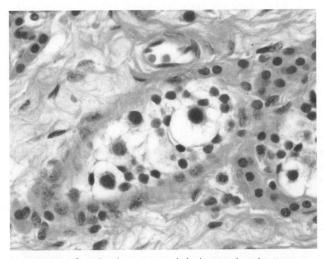

Figure 4.7.5   Occasional spermatogonia in the prepubertal testes may increase in size but maintain regular nuclear contour. The lack of atypia distinguishes these giant spermatogonia from IGCNU.

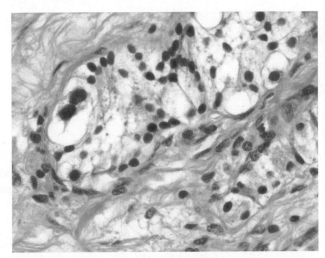

Figure 4.7.6   Spermatogonia with clear cytoplasm containing small-size nuclei with round and regular nuclear contours are seen with occasional binucleated giant spermatogonia in this prepubertal testis. The lack of nuclear atypia and prominent nucleoli are helpful features.

4 TESTIS

	Intratubular Germ Cell Neoplasia Unclassified (IGCNU)	IGCNU with Intertubular Seminoma
Age	15–35 y	Second to fourth decades
Location	Usually unilateral	Usually unilateral
Symptoms	Asymptomatic	Painless swelling of one testicle; one-third of cases complain of scrotal heaviness or dull pain. One-tenth of cases may present with symptoms due to metastatic disease such as abdominal/back pain, cough.
Signs	None except for those of associated conditions such as cryptorchidism and infertility	Usually palpable testicular nodule
Etiology	Associated risk factors include cryptorchidism (4% risk) and infertility (IGCNU in 1%–2% of biopsies)	Associated risk factors include cryptorchidism (10%), infertility, low socioeconomic status, and male genital malformations
Histology	1. IGCNU cells are enlarged, atypical germ cells residing within seminiferous tubules as isolated cells or as a single row along a usually thickened basement membrane (see Sections 4.6 and 4.7) *(Fig. 4.8.1)* 2. Lacks invasive seminoma cells 3. Lacks prominent interstitial lymphoplasmacytic infiltrate	1. Seminiferous tubules containing IGCNU are almost invariably present *(Fig. 4.8.2)* 2. Invasive seminoma component can be subtle permeating the testicular stroma between intact seminiferous tubules. The invasive neoplastic cells are monotonous round-to-polygonal cleared cells with ovoid nuclei containing one or more prominent nucleoli imparting a classic "fried egg" appearance. Mitotic activity is variable *(Figs. 4.8.3 and 4.8.4)* 3. Lymphoplasmacytic infiltrate at times with lymphoid follicles, and eosinophils are typically associated with the infiltrating seminoma. The latter is helpful in pointing to the occasionally subtle invasive intertubular seminoma component *(Figs. 4.8.5 and 4.8.6)*
Special studies	Positive for PLAP and OCT4	Intertubular infiltrating seminoma cells can be highlighted positive for PLAP and CD117, OCT4 and SALL4. Associated IGCNU positive for same markers
Treatment	Typically just close follow-up. In some countries, contralateral biopsy performed, and if positive, then sperm banking and bilateral low-dose radiation are offered	Early-stage disease typically requiring only radical orchiectomy followed by active surveillance
Prognosis	Up to 50% risk of developing invasive germ cell tumor within 5 y of diagnosis (up to 90% risk in 7 y). Risk of invasive germ cell tumor also increased in the contralateral testis	Excellent prognosis with over 90% relapse-free 5-y survival

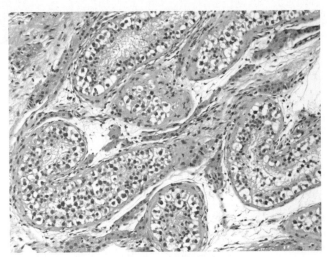

Figure 4.8.1 Seminiferous tubules contain IGCNU.

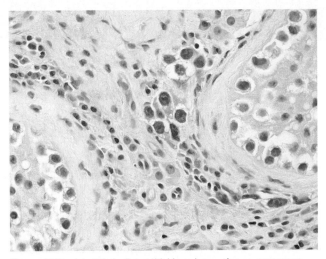

Figure 4.8.2 Intertubular/interstitial invasive seminoma component adjacent to the seminiferous tubule with IGCNU.

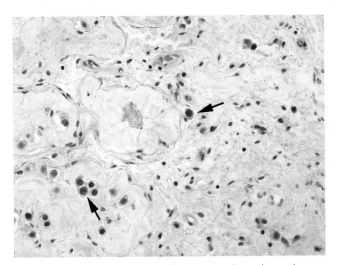

Figure 4.8.3 Intertubular/interstitial invasive seminoma (*arrows*) adjacent to sclerotic seminiferous tubules.

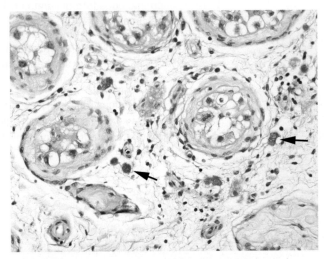

Figure 4.8.4 Intertubular/interstitial invasive seminoma (*arrows*) permeating the testicular stroma between the seminiferous tubule with IGCNU.

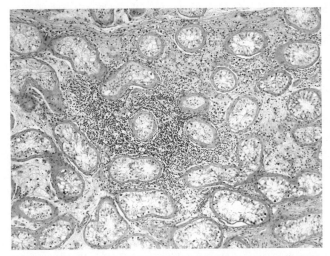

Figure 4.8.5 Associated lymphoplasmacytic infiltrate is a clue raising the suspicion for the presence of an invasive component.

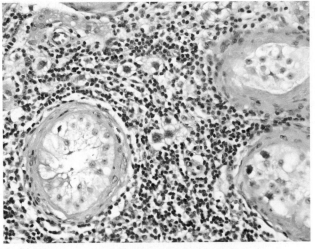

Figure 4.8.6 Same case as Figure 4.8.5 with intertubular invasive neoplastic seminoma cells in lymphoplasmacytic infiltrate.

	Seminoma, Classic Type	Spermatocytic Seminoma
Age	Second to fourth decades. Can also be seen in older men in fifth to sixth decades	Older male, typically fifth to sixth decades. Uncommonly can be seen in younger men in second to fourth decades
Location	Usually unilateral. Can occur in extratesticular midline location	Usually unilateral. No primary extratesticular counterpart exists
Symptoms	Painless scrotal swelling. In one-third of cases, scrotal heaviness or dull pain. In one-tenth of cases, symptoms due to metastatic disease	Painless testicular mass
Signs	Usually palpable testicular nodule. Occasional elevation in serum human chorionic gonadotropin (beta hCG). 2% with gynecomastia	Usually palpable testicular nodule. Negative serum tumor markers
Etiology	Associated risk factors include cryptorchidism (10%), infertility, low socioeconomic status, and male genital malformations	No association with other risk factors typical of other testicular germ cell tumors
Histology	1. Monotonous round-to-polygonal cleared cells with ovoid nuclei containing one or more prominent nucleoli *(Figs. 4.9.1 and 4.9.2)* 2. Mitotic activity is variable 3. Architecture varies from sheets, pseudoglandular/tubular, alveolar, cribriform, or intertubular *(Fig. 4.9.4)* between nonneoplastic seminiferous tubules 4. Lymphoplasmacytic infiltrate in 85% of cases. May have lymphoid follicles. Eosinophils and histiocytes typically present in fibrovascular septae *(Fig. 4.9.1)*. 5. Nonnecrotizing granulomatous response seen in up to 50% of cases (see Section 4.5) 6. Associated syncytiotrophoblastic giant cells in 10%–20% of cases (see Section 4.11) 7. IGCNU cells are almost invariably associated (80% of cases) *(Fig. 4.9.3)*	1. Three basic cell types: Predominant is round-intermediate size with eosinophilic cytoplasm and round nuclei with characteristic lacy filamentous chromatin (spiremic pattern). Second type is smaller cells with dark nuclei and scant cytoplasm, while the third type is large mononucleated or multinucleated giant cells *(Figs. 4.9.4 and 4.9.5)* 2. Mitotic activity can be brisk 3. Typical architecture sheets of neoplastic cells with areas of stromal myxoid edema imparting a pseudoglandular pattern 4. Lymphoplasmacytic infiltrate lacking 5. No associated granulomatous response 6. No associated syncytiotrophoblastic giant cells 7. Lack IGCNU cells, yet may have intratubular spermatocytic seminoma *(Fig. 4.9.6)*
Special studies	• OCT4 is negative • PLAP positive • CD117 positive • SALL4 positive • Gain of isochromosome 12p (i12p) seen in 80% of cases	• OCT4 is negative • Focal PLAP positivity may be present • CD117 positivity in 50% of cases • SALL4 may also be positive • No gain of isochromosome 12p

	Seminoma, Classic Type	**Spermatocytic Seminoma**
Treatment	Radical orchiectomy followed by active surveillance or adjuvant radiotherapy and/or platinum-based chemotherapy	Radical orchiectomy. No adjuvant radiotherapy or chemotherapy
Prognosis	Stage dependent. Overall >90% relapse-free 5-y survival	With exception of extremely rare cases associated with sarcoma at presentation, benign behavior regardless of the presence of vascular or tunical invasion

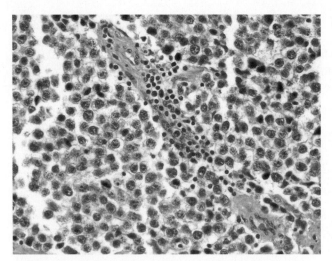

Figure 4.9.1   Classic seminoma composed of monotonous round-to-polygonal cleared cells with ovoid nuclei containing one or more prominent nucleoli with scattered interstitial lymphocytic infiltrate.

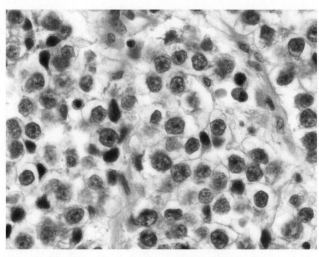

Figure 4.9.2   Monotonous round-to-polygonal cleared cells with ovoid nuclei typical of classic seminoma.

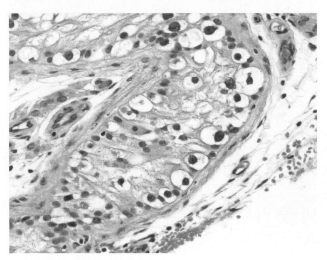

Figure 4.9.3   IGCNU is invariably present in seminiferous tubules associated with classic seminoma.

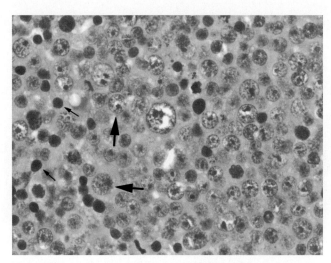

Figure 4.9.4   Spermatocytic seminoma with three cell types: (1) predominant round, intermediate-size cells with characteristic lacy filamentous chromatin (*large arrows*); (2) smaller cells with dark nuclei and scant cytoplasm (*small arrows*); and (3) large mononucleated or multinucleated giant cells (*center*). Note eosinophilic cytoplasm.

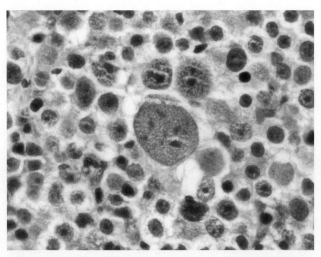

Figure 4.9.5   Spermatocytic seminoma is composed of three basic cell types. Lymphocytic host response is lacking.

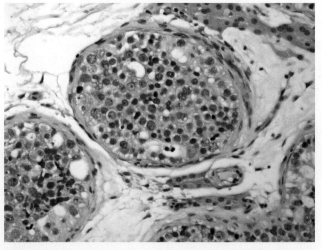

Figure 4.9.6   Intratubular spermatocytic seminoma with the same three basic cell types filling seminiferous tubules.

	Seminoma	Embryonal Carcinoma
Age	Second to fourth decades, yet can be older	Second to third decades
Location	Usually unilateral	Usually unilateral
Symptoms	Painless scrotal swelling. In one-third of cases, scrotal heaviness or dull pain. In 10% of cases, symptoms due to metastatic disease	Usually painless swelling but can present with testicular pain mimicking torsion. In 10% of cases, symptoms due to metastatic disease
Signs	Usually palpable testicular nodule. Occasional elevation in serum human chorionic gonadotropin (beta hCG) can be present. 2% with gynecomastia	Usually palpable testicular nodule
Etiology	Associated risk factors include cryptorchidism (10%), infertility, low socioeconomic status, and male genital malformations	Same as seminoma
Histology	1. Monotonous round-to-polygonal cells with ovoid nuclei containing prominent nucleoli and clear cytoplasm *(Figs. 4.10.1 and 4.10.2)*. Histologic variant with increased pleomorphism and mitotic rate in the past referred to as "anaplastic seminoma" or "high mitotic rate seminoma," which mimics embryonal carcinoma *(Fig. 4.10.3)* 2. Architecture varies from sheets, pseudoglandular/tubular, alveolar, cribriform, or intertubular *(Fig. 4.10.4)*. Pagetoid spread to the rete testis can mimic embryonal carcinoma *(Fig. 4.10.5)* 3. Cells are loosely cohesive 4. Lymphoplasmacytic infiltrate in 85% of cases 5. Nonnecrotizing granulomatous inflammation in up to 50% of cases 6. Syncytiotrophoblasts can be associated in variable distribution 7. IGCNU cells are almost invariably associated (80% of cases)	1. Large cells with abundant granular amphophilic or eosinophilic cytoplasm and large vesicular irregular nuclei with one or more irregular nucleoli. Typically, more pleomorphic compared to seminoma *(Fig. 4.10.6)*. Uncommonly can have focal clear cytoplasm *(Fig. 4.10.7)*. Mitotic activity is brisk 2. Architecture varies from solid sheets to papillary structures with clefts and gland-like structures *(Fig. 4.10.8)* 3. Cells are cohesive 4. Lymphoplasmacytic infiltrate is infrequent *(Fig. 4.10.9)* 5. Rare to see associated granulomatous inflammation 6. Syncytiotrophoblasts not as common compared to seminoma 7. IGCNU cells are almost invariably associated (80% of cases). Can also see intratubular embryonal carcinoma, which typically has very eosinophilic necrosis *(Fig. 4.10.10)*
Special studies	• CD117 positive • CD30 negative • Typically keratin negative. However, occasionally, scattered isolated loosely cohesive keratin-positive cells that are still considered seminoma	• CD117 negative • CD30 positive • Cytokeratin AE1/AE3 diffusely positive. In seminoma, if clusters of cohesive keratin-positive cells can be found on the corresponding H&E-stained slides to consist of more atypical cells, then admixed early embryonal carcinoma can be diagnosed

	Seminoma	**Embryonal Carcinoma**
Treatment	Stage dependent. Radical orchiectomy followed by active surveillance or adjuvant radiotherapy and/or platinum-based chemotherapy	Stage dependent. Radical orchiectomy followed by active surveillance, retroperitoneal lymph node dissection (RPLND), or adjuvant platinum-based chemotherapy
Prognosis	Stage dependent with more than 90% relapse-free 5-y survival	Stage dependent with over 80% relapse-free 5-y survival

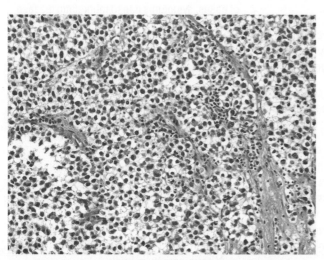

Figure 4.10.1   Classic seminoma is composed of loosely cohesive monotonous round-to-polygonal cells with clear cytoplasm.

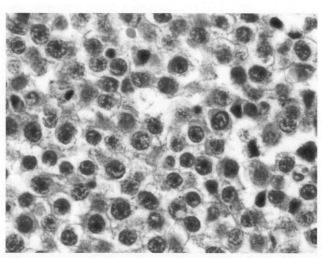

Figure 4.10.2   Relatively uniform nuclei with central prominent nucleoli.

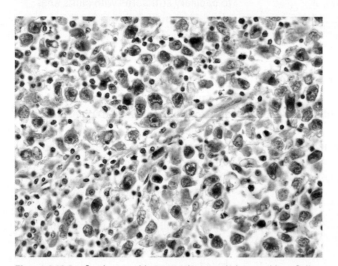

Figure 4.10.3   Seminoma with greater than usual pleomorphism. Cells are still loosely cohesive with interspersed lymphocytes.

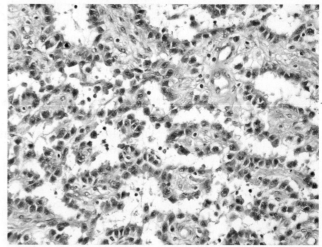

Figure 4.10.4   Seminoma with pseudoalveolar pattern. Cells are still typical of seminoma.

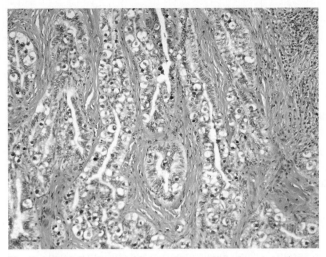

Figure 4.10.5 Seminoma with pagetoid spread into the rete testis.

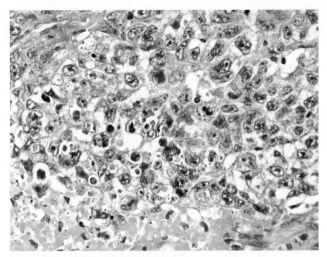

Figure 4.10.6 Embryonal carcinoma composed of large polygonal cells with abundant granular amphophilic cytoplasm and large vesicular irregular nuclei with one or more irregular nucleoli.

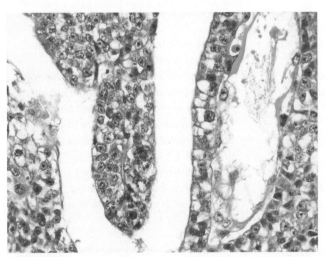

Figure 4.10.7 Embryonal carcinoma cohesive cells and focal area with clear cytoplasm.

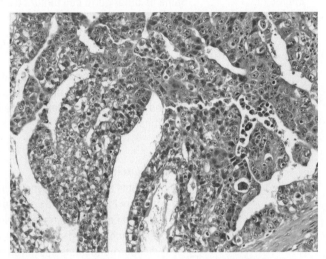

Figure 4.10.8 Embryonal carcinoma with clefts and gland-like structures.

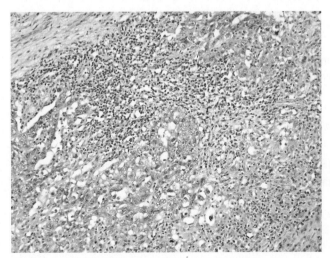

Figure 4.10.9 Unusual embryonal carcinoma with lymphocytic infiltrate. Cells are cohesive with clefts.

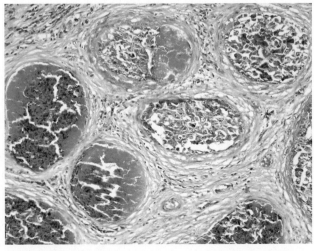

Figure 4.10.10 Intratubular embryonal carcinoma with eosinophilic necrosis.

4 TESTIS

	Seminoma with Syncytiotrophoblasts	Choriocarcinoma
Age	Second to fourth decades, yet can be older	Second to third decades
Location	Usually unilateral	Usually unilateral
Symptoms	Usually, painless scrotal swelling. 10% present with symptoms due to metastatic disease such as abdominal/back pain, cough.	Usually present with symptoms due to widespread metastases including multiorgan hemorrhage (hemoptysis, hematemesis, cerebrovascular accident, etc.)
Signs	Usually palpable testicular nodule. Syncytiotrophoblasts lead to elevation in serum beta hCG usually in the levels of 100 mIU/mL. 2% with gynecomastia	Testicular mass may not be apparent. Very high levels of serum beta hCG usually in the levels of 100,000 mIU/mL. May have gynecomastia
Etiology	Same as other germ cell tumors (see Section 4.10)	Same as other germ cell tumors (see Section 4.10)
Histology	1. Can be seen with pure seminoma or mixed germ cell tumor 2. Composed of monotonous round-to-polygonal cells with clear cytoplasm and ovoid nuclei containing one or more prominent nucleoli 3. Cells are loosely cohesive 4. Seminoma admixed with syncytiotrophoblasts, which are multinucleated cells that contain abundant basophilic cytoplasm. No cytotrophoblasts *(Fig. 4.11.1)* 5. Syncytiotrophoblasts scattered in midst of seminoma cells and tend to cluster around small blood vessels *(Figs. 4.11.2–4.11.6)* 6. Usually relatively few syncytiotrophoblasts, yet can be fairly numerous 7. Lymphoplasmacytic infiltrate common 8. Noncaseating granulomatous inflammation in up to 50% of cases 9. Vascular invasion is uncommon 10. IGCNU almost invariably associated (80% of cases)	1. Can be pure but more often mixed with other germ cell tumor elements 2. Cytotrophoblasts have pale cytoplasm surrounding an irregular, single nucleus with one or more nucleoli less prominent than in seminoma. Nuclei are usually more atypical than in seminoma *(Figs. 4.11.7–4.11.9)* 3. Cytotrophoblasts are cohesive 4. Cytotrophoblasts are intimately admixed with syncytiotrophoblasts *(Figs. 4.11.7–4.11.9)* 5. Cytotrophoblasts and syncytiotrophoblasts often associated with hemorrhage and necrosis *(Fig. 4.11.10)* 6. If in mixed germ cell tumor, usually the choriocarcinoma component is substantial, although uncommonly can be focal 7. Lymphoplasmacytic infiltrate is infrequent 8. Granulomatous reaction absent 9. Vascular invasion is common 10. IGCNU almost invariably present
Special studies	• Seminoma cells positive for OCT4 and CD117. Syncytiotrophoblasts is negative • Seminoma cytokeratin AE1/AE3 negative or at most rare positive cells. Syncytiotrophoblasts positive for AE1/AE3 • Syncytiotrophoblasts beta hCG positive	• Cytotrophoblasts and syncytiotrophoblasts negative for OCT4 and CD117 • Cytotrophoblasts and syncytiotrophoblasts positive for AE1/AE3 • Syncytiotrophoblasts beta hCG positive

	Seminoma with Syncytiotrophoblasts	**Choriocarcinoma**
Treatment	Stage dependent. Radical orchiectomy followed by active surveillance or adjuvant radiotherapy and/or platinum-based chemotherapy	Stage dependent. Radical orchiectomy followed by retroperitoneal lymph node dissection (RPLND) or adjuvant platinum-based chemotherapy
Prognosis	Syncytiotrophoblasts does not impact prognosis in otherwise classic seminoma	Typically associated with advanced stage with poor prognosis. However, stage-for-stage prognosis is comparable to other nonseminomatous germ cell tumors

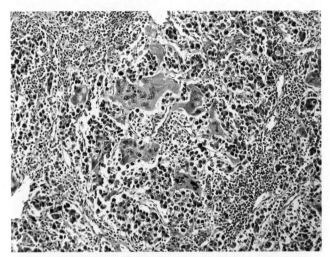

Figure 4.11.1 Seminoma admixed with syncytiotrophoblasts, which are multinucleated cells that contain abundant basophilic cytoplasm. No cytotrophoblasts are accompanied.

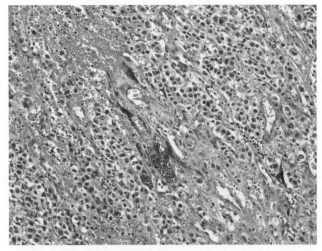

Figure 4.11.2 Syncytiotrophoblasts without associated cytotrophoblasts are seen adjacent to areas of hemorrhage in seminoma.

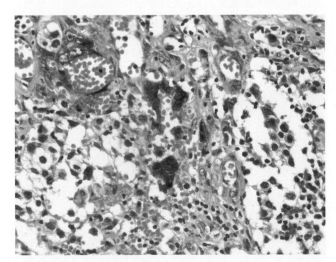

Figure 4.11.3 Syncytiotrophoblasts without associated cytotrophoblasts are seen surrounding vascular structures in seminoma.

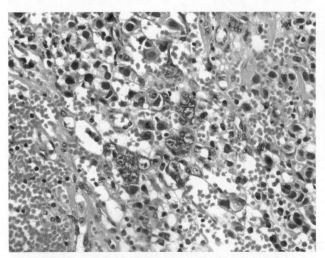

Figure 4.11.4 Syncytiotrophoblasts without associated cytotrophoblasts are seen adjacent to areas of hemorrhage in seminoma.

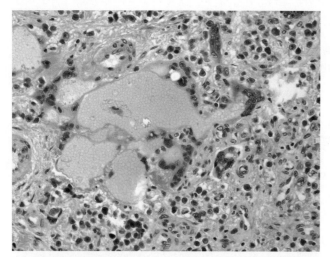

Figure 4.11.5 Syncytiotrophoblasts without associated cytotrophoblasts are seen surrounding vascular structures in seminoma.

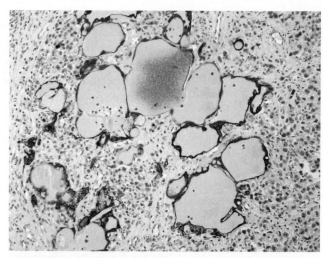

Figure 4.11.6 Same case as in Figure 4.11.5 with highlighting of syncytiotrophoblasts by HCG immunostains.

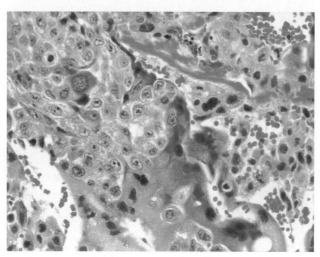

Figure 4.11.7 Cytotrophoblasts are intimately admixed with syncytiotrophoblasts in choriocarcinoma.

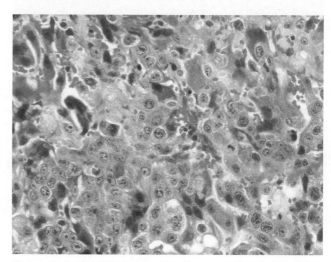

Figure 4.11.8 Cytotrophoblasts are intimately admixed with smaller syncytiotrophoblasts with amphophilic cytoplasm in choriocarcinoma. Cytotrophoblasts have paler cytoplasm surrounding an irregular, single nucleus with one or more nucleoli.

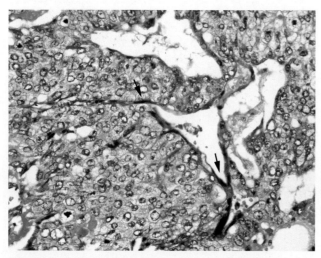

Figure 4.11.9 Choriocarcinoma with subtle syncytiotrophoblasts (*arrows*) enveloping cytotrophoblasts.

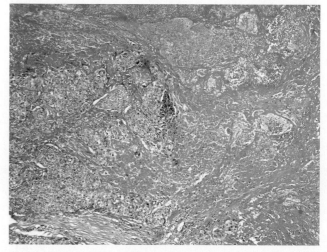

Figure 4.11.10 Choriocarcinoma with extensive hemorrhage and necrosis.

	Seminoma	Large B-Cell Lymphoma
Age	Second to fourth decades but can occur in older overlapping with lymphoma	Seventh and eighth decades, most frequent testicular tumor in this age group
Location	Usually unilateral	Over one-third of cases are bilateral
Symptoms	Painless scrotal swelling. 10% present with symptoms due to metastatic disease	Painless swelling of the scrotum or inguinal region. No associated B-cell lymphoma symptoms
Signs	Usually a palpable testicular nodule	Usually a palpable testicular/paratesticular mass
Etiology	Associated risk factors include cryptorchidism (10%), infertility, low socioeconomic status, and male genital malformations	Diffuse large B-cell lymphoma is the most common subtype (80%) in adults. Usually represents secondary involvement of the testis from the lymph node primary. Rarely, primary testicular lymphoma without nodal involvement
Histology	1. Typically a solid mass with relatively little intertubular growth that spares seminiferous tubules 2. Monotonous round-to-polygonal cleared cells with ovoid nuclei that are typically relatively uniform, although pleomorphism can be present *(Figs. 4.12.1 and 4.12.2)* 3. Cytoplasm clear 4. One or more prominent nucleoli imparting a classic "fried egg" appearance 5. Architecture varies from sheets, pseudoglandular/tubular, alveolar, cribriform, or interstitial/intertubular 6. Granulomatous inflammation in up to 50% of cases 7. Syncytiotrophoblasts present in minority of cases 8. IGCNU almost invariably present (80% of cases) 9. Does not tend to spread into adjacent adipose tissue extensively and when it extends out of the testis has more of a solid growth	1. Typically a solid mass with relatively little intertubular growth that spares seminiferous tubules *(Figs. 4.12.3–4.12.7)* 2. Predominantly large cleaved and large noncleaved atypical lymphocytes. Nuclei more irregular than seminoma *(Figs. 4.12.3, 4.12.5–4.12.7)* 3. Most cases with eosinophilic to amphophilic cytoplasm *(Figs. 4.12.3 and 4.12.7)* 4. Multiple irregular nucleoli of varying sizes 5. Diffuse sheets of cells 6. Granulomatous inflammation typically not seen in testicular lymphomas 7. Syncytiotrophoblasts not encountered 8. IGCNU typically absent 9. Can extensively involve paratesticular soft tissue with relative sparing of adipose tissue *(Fig. 4.12.8)*
Special studies	• SALL4 positive • OCT4 positive • Negative for CD45 and CD20	• SALL4 negative, except anaplastic large cell lymphoma can be positive • OCT4 not as useful in this differential as rare lymphomas positive • Positive for CD45 and CD20

	Seminoma	**Large B-Cell Lymphoma**
Treatment	Stage dependent. Radical orchiectomy followed by active surveillance or adjuvant radiotherapy and/or platinum-based chemotherapy	In vast majority of cases, orchiectomy is performed to make the diagnosis. Subsequently treated by systemic chemotherapy
Prognosis	Stage dependent with more than 90% relapse-free 5-y survival	Stage dependent with 60% 5-y tumor-free survival for early stage and 20% for advanced stage. As most patients present with advanced stage, the overall survival is 50% at 5 y. High relapse rate mainly in extratesticular location

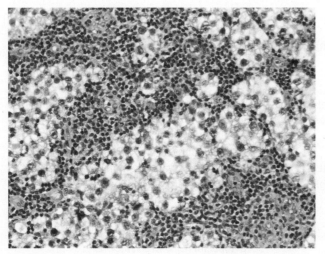

Figure 4.12.1 Classic seminoma composed of sheets of back-to-back monotonous neoplastic cells separated with associated lymphocytic infiltrate.

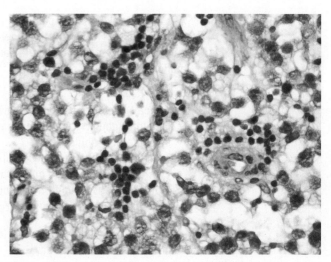

Figure 4.12.2 Classic seminoma with relatively uniform round-to-polygonal cleared cells with ovoid nuclei.

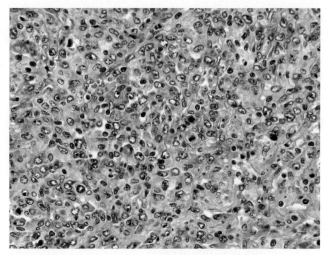

Figure 4.12.3 Large cell lymphoma with cells showing more pleomorphism than seminoma. Also the cells lack central prominent nucleoli in the majority of cells.

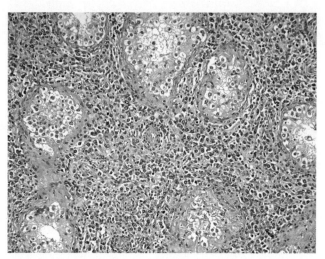

Figure 4.12.4 Lymphoma with relative preservation of testicular architecture.

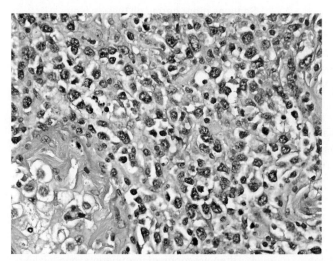

Figure 4.12.5 Large cell lymphoma with less uniformity than seminoma. Also the cells lack central prominent nucleoli in the majority of cells.

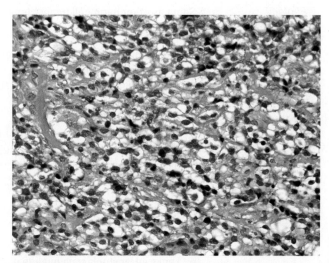

Figure 4.12.6 Lymphoma with clear cytoplasm. Cells lack vesicular nuclei with prominent nucleoli.

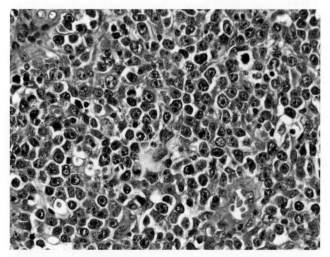

Figure 4.12.7 Lymphoma mimicking seminoma with prominent nucleoli, yet cells have amphophilic cytoplasm.

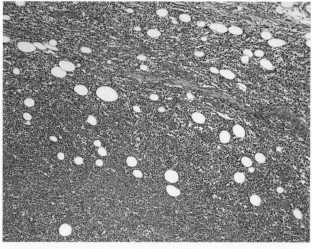

Figure 4.12.8 Lymphoma spread outside of the testis with entrapment of adipocytes.

4 TESTIS

	Seminoma	Yolk Sac Tumor, Solid Pattern
Age	Second to fourth decades, yet can be older	Two peaks: Infants/early childhood (median age 1.5 y) and postpubertal (second and third decades)
Location	Usually unilateral	Usually unilateral
Symptoms	Painless scrotal swelling. 10% present with scrotal pain and 10% with symptoms due to metastatic disease	Painless scrotal mass. Occasionally acute pain. In children, symptoms of metastatic spread (i.e., hemoptysis) at presentation in up to 10%–20% of cases
Signs	Usually palpable testicular nodule	Usually palpable testicular nodule. Serum AFP elevation in 90% of cases
Etiology	Same as other germ cell tumors (see Section 4.10)	Same as other germ cell tumors (see Section 4.10)
Histology	1. Monotonous round-to-polygonal cleared cells with ovoid nuclei containing one or more prominent nucleoli *(Fig. 4.13.1)*. Mitotic and apoptotic activity is variable 2. Cells are loosely cohesive 3. Architecture varies from sheets of back-to-back monotonous neoplastic cells, pseudoglandular/tubular, alveolar, cribriform, or interstitial/intertubular *(Figs. 4.13.2 and 4.13.3)* 4. Lacks intracytoplasmic hyaline globules 5. Lymphoplasmacytic infiltrate typically present, yet absent/minimal in 15% of cases 6. Noncaseating granulomatous reaction seen in up to 50% of cases 7. Syncytiotrophoblasts can be associated in variable distribution 8. IGCNU almost invariably associated (80% of cases)	1. Polygonal, medium-sized cells with clear to eosinophilic cytoplasm, uniform vesicular nuclei, and prominent nucleoli. Mitotic activity can be high *(Figs. 4.13.4–4.13.9)* 2. Cells are tightly cohesive 3. Solid pattern mimic seminoma *(Figs. 4.13.4–4.13.7 and 4.13.9)*. Other more common patterns include microcystic, macrocystic, glandular, papillary, myxomatous, polyvesicular vitelline, hepatoid, and endodermal sinus with Schiller-Duval bodies *(Figs. 4.13.4 and 4.13.8)* 4. Often presence of intracytoplasmic hyaline globules 5. Lymphoplasmacytic infiltrate typically absent 6. Noncaseating granulomatous reaction absent 7. Syncytiotrophoblasts less common than in seminoma but can be seen 8. IGCNU almost invariably associated in adults while absent in children
Special studies	• OCT4 positive • Glypican 3 and AFP negative • CD117 positive • Cytokeratin AE1/AE3 negative or rare cells positive	• OCT4 negative • Glypican 3 in >80% of cases. AFP expressed to a lesser extent *(Fig. 4.13.10)* • CD117 can be positive in minority of cases • Strong cytokeratin AE1/AE3 and Cam 5.2

	Seminoma	**Yolk Sac Tumor, Solid Pattern**
Treatment	Stage dependent. Radical orchiectomy followed by active surveillance or adjuvant radiotherapy and/or platinum-based chemotherapy	Stage dependent. In postpubertal patients, same therapy as other mixed germ cell tumors. With exception of cases with extratesticular spread at presentation, radical orchiectomy is followed by active surveillance in prepubertal cases
Prognosis	Stage dependent with more than 90% relapse-free 5-y survival	Stage dependent with more than 80% relapse-free 5-y survival in postpubertal patients. Prepubertal patients 95% relapse-free survival regardless of stage with a 100% relapse-free survival in stages I and II

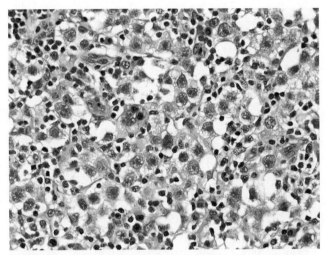

Figure 4.13.1 Classic seminoma is composed of monotonous round-to-polygonal cleared cells with lymphocytic infiltrate.

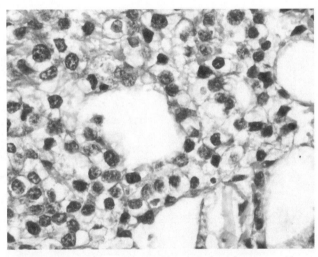

Figure 4.13.2 Classic seminoma with pseudoglandular spaces with uniform, loosely cohesive seminoma cells.

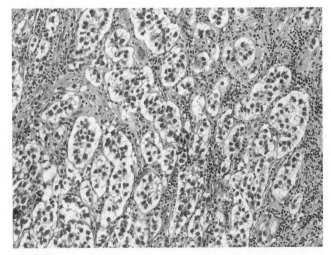

Figure 4.13.3 Classic seminoma with nesting appearance.

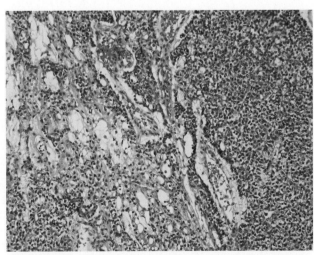

Figure 4.13.4 Yolk sac tumor composed of sheets of cells (*right*) with a more typical microcystic component (*left*).

4 TESTIS

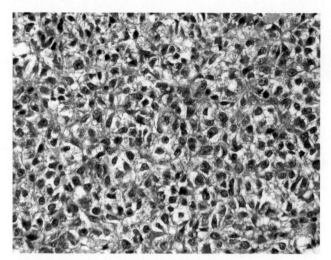

Figure 4.13.5 Same case as Figure 4.13.4 with cells mimicking seminoma, however lacking the seminoma cells' uniform shape, vesicular nuclei, and large prominent eosinophilic nucleoli.

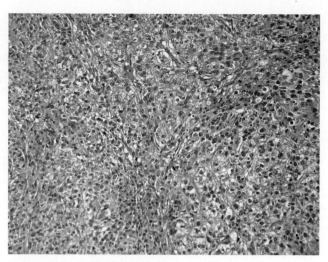

Figure 4.13.6 Solid yolk sac tumor.

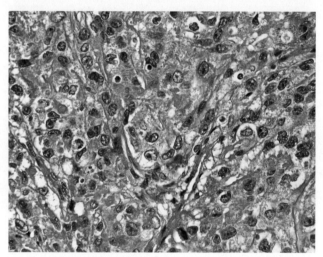

Figure 4.13.7 Same case as Figure 4.13.6 with polygonal, medium-sized, cells with clear to eosinophilic cytoplasm and variably shaped nuclei.

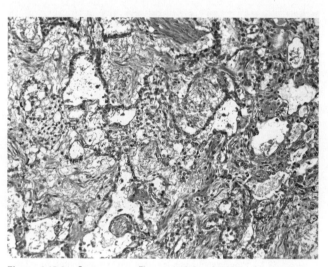

Figure 4.13.8 Same case as Figures 4.13.6 and 4.13.7 with more typical myxoid features.

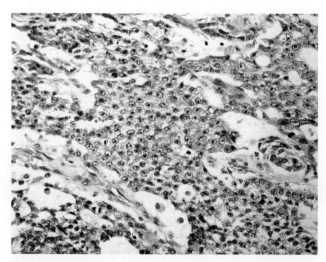

Figure 4.13.9 Solid yolk sac tumor, which is more cohesive than seminoma.

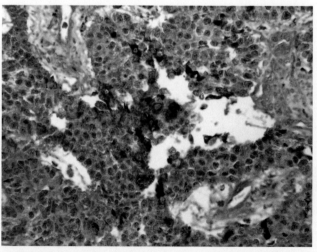

Figure 4.13.10 Same case as Figure 4.13.9 with diffuse positivity for AFP.

	Seminoma with Extensive Necrosis	Torsion
Age	Second to fourth decades, can be older	Any age but more common during childhood (two peaks: Neonatal and adolescent)
Location	Usually unilateral	Usually unilateral
Symptoms	Painless scrotal swelling. One-third of cases complain of scrotal heaviness or dull pain. One-tenth of cases may present with symptoms due to metastatic disease such as abdominal/back pain, cough.	Sudden onset severe testicular pain (76%), scrotal swelling (65%), abdominal pain, nausea, and vomiting (22%)
Signs	Usually palpable testicular nodule. Occasional elevation in serum human chorionic gonadotropin (beta hCG). 2% with gynecomastia	No palpable nodule. Spherical testicular enlargement, redness, and inflammatory scrotal signs termed "acute scrotum"
Etiology	Associated risk factors include cryptorchidism (10%), infertility, low socioeconomic status, and male genital malformations	Complicated pregnancies (prolonged labor, preeclampsia, gestational diabetes) leading to fetal stress/mechanical factors that may play a role in the pathogenesis of perinatal testicular torsion. Recently, seasonal predilection (cold temperature and humidity) has been suggested as a risk factor in childhood and adolescent cases as a result of associated hyperactive cremasteric reflex
Histology	1. Typically, does not involve the entire testis 2. Occasional seminomas can undergo extensive necrosis, yet in the center of coagulative necrosis see ghosts of seminoma cells. At edge of necrosis, may see necrotic seminoma with more cellular preservation composed of monotonous round-to-polygonal cleared cells with ovoid nuclei containing one or more prominent nucleoli *(Figs. 4.14.1–4.14.6)* 3. Nonneoplastic testis surrounding the necrotic seminoma remains viable and lacks evidence of ischemia or hemorrhage 4. Atrophic seminiferous tubules containing IGCNU may be seen in the adjacent testis 5. May see some lymphocytic infiltrate	1. Torsion occurs as a result of testicular rotation around the cord leading to interruption of blood supply and hemorrhagic infarction, such that the entire testis is affected 2. In advanced cases, complete necrosis with shadows of seminiferous tubules with basement membranes outlines can still be identified *(Figs. 4.14.9 and 4.14.10)* 3. The entire testis shows similar ischemic changes 4. No IGCNU 5. When present, inflammation is predominantly acute and composed of polymorphonuclear leukocytes
Special studies	• Positive PLAP, CD117, OCT4, and SALL4 may be maintained in necrotic seminoma *(Figs. 4.14.7 and 4.14.8)*	• PLAP, CD117, OCT4, and SALL4 negative

	Seminoma with Extensive Necrosis	Torsion
Treatment	Remains stage dependent despite regression. Radical orchiectomy followed by active surveillance or adjuvant radiotherapy and/or platinum-based chemotherapy	By the time the testis is so necrotic that it mimics necrotic seminoma, the only treatment is orchiectomy and contralateral orchiopexy
Prognosis	Stage dependent with more than 90% relapse-free 5-y survival	Diagnosis and treatment over 6 h, which would correspond to an entirely necrotic testis, have no likelihood of testicular salvage

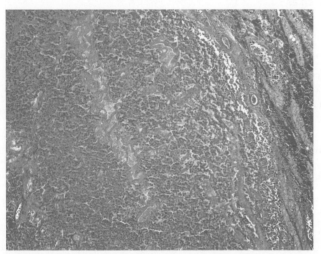

Figure 4.14.1   Seminoma with extensive necrosis. At low magnification, the lesion is very cellular and the normal testicular architecture is effaced.

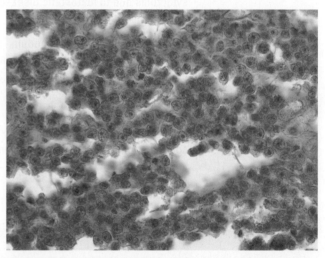

Figure 4.14.2   Higher magnification of Figure 4.14.1 with ghosts of seminoma cells, yet sufficient detail to still make out that they are seminoma cells.

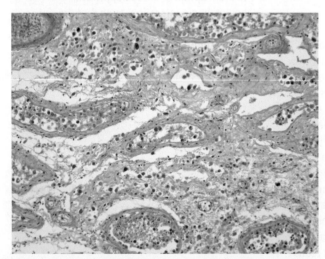

Figure 4.14.3   Seminoma with extensive necrosis. Although necrotic, the seminiferous tubules and interstitium contain large atypical hyperchromatic nuclei.

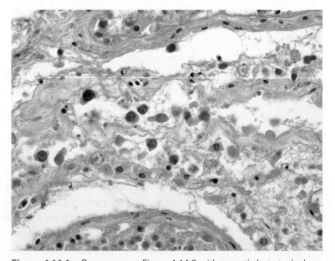

Figure 4.14.4   Same case as Figure 4.14.3 with necrotic but atypical nuclei in the interstitium.

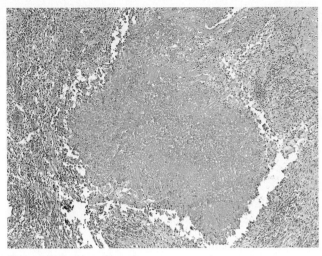

Figure 4.14.5 Necrotic seminoma.

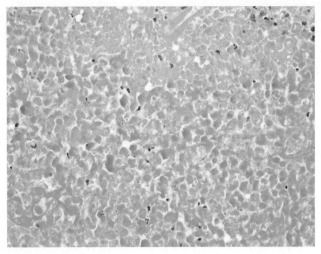

Figure 4.14.6 Same case as Figure 4.14.5 with ghosts of tumor cells lacking cytologic detail.

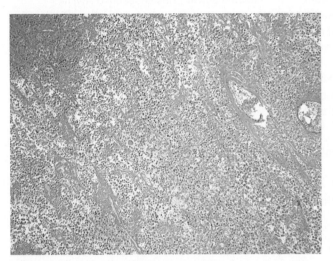

Figure 4.14.7 Necrotic seminoma demonstrating partially preserved cellular detail and classic nested architecture.

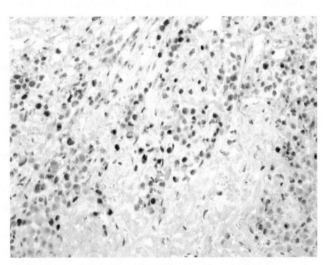

Figure 4.14.8 Same case as Figure 4.14.7 with positive nuclear staining for OCT4.

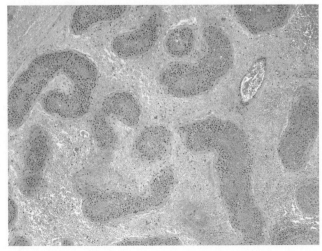

Figure 4.14.9 Testicular torsion with preservation of testicular architecture.

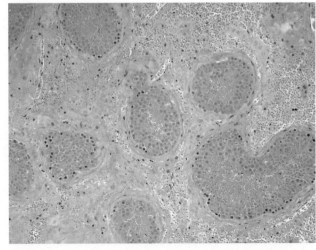

Figure 4.14.10 Same case as Figure 4.14.9 with ghost of seminiferous tubules.

4 TESTIS

	Torsion	Infarct Resulting from Vasculitis
Age	Any age but more common during childhood (two peaks: Neonatal and adolescent)	Most commonly third to fourth decades but can affect older patients
Location	Usually unilateral	Usually unilateral
Symptoms	Sudden onset severe testicular pain (76%), scrotal swelling (65%), abdominal pain, nausea, and vomiting (22%)	Testicular pain, swelling, tumor-like lesion. Extratesticular symptomatology in cases secondary to systemic vasculitis
Signs	No palpable nodule. Spherical testicular enlargement, redness, and inflammatory scrotal signs termed "acute scrotum"	No palpable nodule
Etiology	Complicated pregnancies (prolonged labor, preeclampsia, gestational diabetes) leading to fetal stress/mechanical factors that may play a role in the pathogenesis of perinatal testicular torsion. Recently, seasonal predilection (cold temperature and humidity) is suggested as a risk factor in childhood and adolescent cases as a result of associated hyperactive cremasteric reflex	Isolated polyarthritis nodosum (PAN) like in most cases. Granulomatous vasculitis more closely related to systemic vasculitis. 80% of men with PAN and 4% with Wegener granulomatosis have testicular involvement
Histology	1. Torsion occurs as a result of testicular rotation around the cord leading to interruption of blood supply and hemorrhagic infarction, such that the entire testis is affected 2. With early torsion, acute interstitial hemorrhage with a varying degree of seminiferous tubules, necrosis, and acute inflammatory response *(Fig. 4.15.1)*. After 24 h, typically complete coagulative necrosis *(Fig. 4.15.2)* 3. No evidence of vasculitis is present	1. Well-demarcated areas of testicular parenchymal infarct with varying degree of seminiferous tubules, necrosis, and acute inflammatory response. An adjacent unremarkable testis without necrosis *(Fig. 4.15.3)* 2. No interstitial hemorrhage. Necrosis limited to focal areas *(Figs. 4.15.3 and 4.15.5)* 3. Associated PAN-like vasculitis with transmural necrotizing inflammation of small- to medium-sized arteries *(Figs. 4.15.4, 4.15.6–4.15.8)*. Less frequently, necrotizing or nonnecrotizing granulomatous vasculitis and lymphocytic vasculitis *(Figs. 4.15.9 and 4.15.10)*. Affected vessels often at the edge of the testis. Vasculitis often different stages with some having fibrinoid necrosis and other organizing fibrosis. Also vasculitis often focal within a vessel. With focal testicular necrosis, in vast majority of cases, there is an associated vasculitis that should be identified histologically

	Torsion	**Infarct Resulting from Vasculitis**
Special studies	None	Histochemical stains to rule out infectious organisms in granulomatous vasculitis. Serologic immunologic studies to rule out systemic vasculitis (ANCA, rheumatoid factor, etc.)
Treatment	Testicular salvage (detorsion) and orchiopexy or orchiectomy and contralateral orchiopexy. Intraoperative biopsies can assist in treatment decision	Orchiectomy is performed as a result of a suspicion of germ cell tumor. In cases associated with systemic vasculitis, treatment is directed to specific vasculitis
Prognosis	Diagnosis and treatment earlier than 6 h increase the likelihood of testicular function salvage	Isolated testicular vasculitis cured by orchiectomy. Prognosis for cases associated with systemic vasculitis depends on severity and etiology of the vasculitis

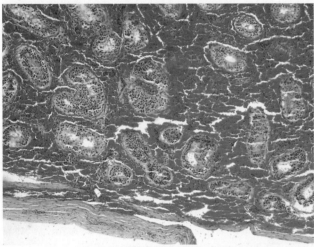

Figure 4.15.1   Testicular torsion in its early phases with diffuse hemorrhage and congestion. The entire testis was involved.

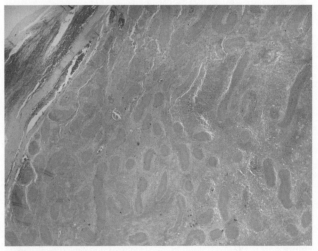

Figure 4.15.2   Ghost of ischemic seminiferous tubules in later torsion. The entire testis was involved.

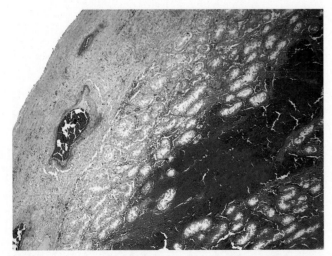

Figure 4.15.3   Infarct focally involving the testis with vasculitis in the surrounding testis.

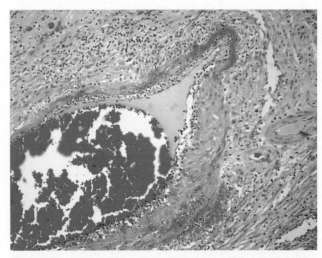

Figure 4.15.4   Same case as Figure 15.3 with vasculitis with fibrinoid necrosis of the vessel wall.

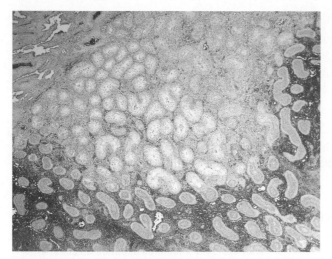

Figure 4.15.5   Focal infarct resulting from vasculitis.

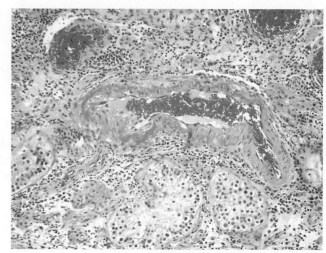

Figure 4.15.6   Subtle fibrinoid change within the vessel wall.

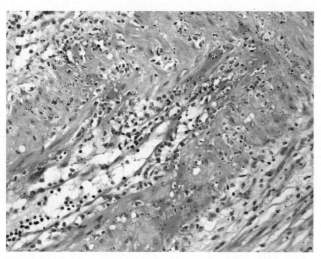

Figure 4.15.7   Vasculitis with fibrinoid necrosis and karyorrhectic debris in the vessel wall.

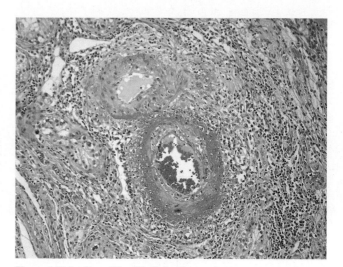

Figure 4.15.8   Vasculitis with fibrinoid necrosis.

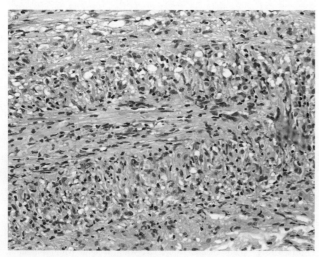

Figure 4.15.9   Granulomatous vasculitis.

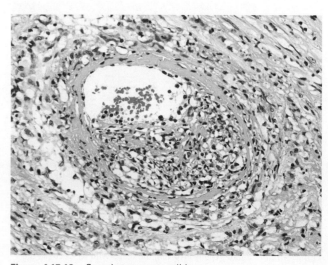

Figure 4.15.10   Granulomatous vasculitis.

	Yolk Sac Tumor, Glandular Pattern	Teratoma
Age	Two incidence peaks: Infants/early childhood (median age 1.5 y) and postpubertal (second and third decades)	Two incidence peaks: Infants/early childhood (median age 20 mo) and postpubertal (second and third decades)
Location	Usually unilateral	Usually unilateral
Symptoms	Painless scrotal mass with occasionally acute pain at presentation	Painless scrotal mass
Signs	Usually palpable testicular nodule. AFP elevation in 90% of cases	Usually palpable testicular nodular mass. HCG and AFP elevation may be seen in adult yet not prepubertal patients. Neonates may have elevated serum AFP levels
Etiology	Same as other germ cell tumors (See Section 4.10)	Same as other germ cell tumors (See Section 4.10)
Histology	1. Nonenteric patterns include microcystic, macrocystic, solid, papillary, myxomatous, endodermal sinus, polyvesicular vitelline, hepatoid, and endodermal sinus with Schiller-Duval bodies 2. Tubular or alveolar structures lined by flat to cuboidal or polygonal medium-sized cells. Neoplastic cells have clear to eosinophilic cytoplasm with uniform vesicular nuclei and conspicuous nucleoli. Subnuclear vacuoles are common *(Figs. 4.16.1–4.16.3)* 3. Absence of the muscular layer surrounding the glands 4. IGCNU almost invariably associated in adult cases while notably absent in yolk sac tumors occurring in early childhood	1. Haphazard arrangement of mature or immature embryonal or fetal-type endodermal, ectodermal, and/or mesodermal tissues. Mature or embryonal organoid structures can be seen *(Fig. 4.16.5)* 2. Glandular elements in teratoma including enteric-type glands lacking subnuclear vacuoles 3. Glands are usually surrounded by smooth muscular tissue *(Fig. 4.16.6)* 4. IGCNU is almost invariably associated in adult cases while absent in teratoma occurring in early childhood
Special studies	• Most positive for AFP and Glypican 3 *(Fig. 4.16.4)* • Most negative for EMA with 2% positive	• AFP can be positive in glands of teratoma. No data with Glypican 3 • EMA typically positive
Treatment	Stage dependent. In postpubertal patients, same therapy as other nonseminomatous germ cell tumors. With exception of cases with extratesticular spread, radical orchiectomy is followed by active surveillance in prepubertal cases. Critical to distinguish postchemotherapy metastatic glandular yolk sac tumor from teratoma: If yolk sac tumor, additional chemotherapy needed	Stage dependent. Same as other nonseminomatous germ cell tumors in postpubertal males. Prepubertal teratomas treated with orchiectomy without systemic therapy. Critical to distinguish postchemotherapy metastatic glandular yolk sac tumor from teratoma: If mature teratoma, no additional chemotherapy needed
Prognosis	Stage dependent with more than 80% relapse-free 5-y survival in postpubertal patients. Prepubertal patients 95% relapse-free survival regardless of stage with a 100% relapse-free survival in stages I and II	Stage dependent with >80% relapse-free 5-y survival in postpubertal patients. Prepubertal teratomas are benign with no reported metastasis on record

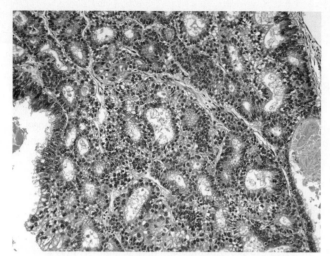

Figure 4.16.1   Yolk sac tumor with glandular pattern composed of tubular or alveolar structures lined by cuboidal cells. Glands are back to back, with lack of the surrounding muscle layer.

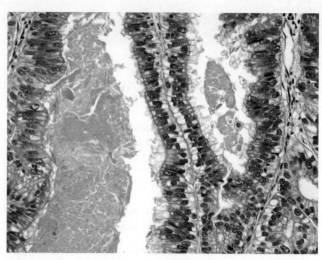

Figure 4.16.2   Same case as Figure 4.16.1 with prominent subnuclear vacuoles.

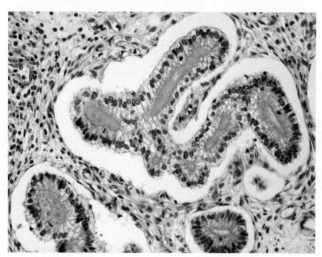

Figure 4.16.3   Yolk sac tumor with glandular pattern with lack of the surrounding muscle layer and subnuclear vacuoles.

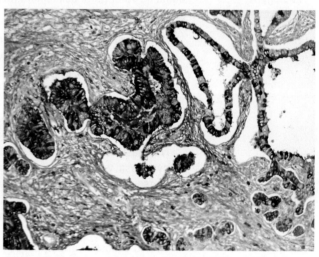

Figure 4.16.4   Same case as Figure 4.16.3 with AFP positivity.

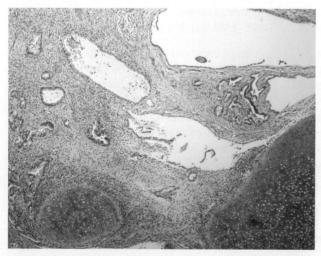

Figure 4.16.5   Teratoma with haphazard glands admixed with cartilage.

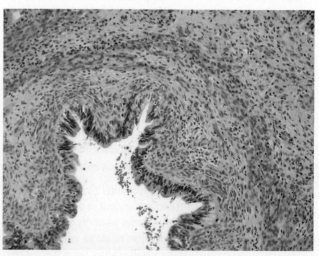

Figure 4.16.6   Teratomatous gland surrounded by smooth muscle cuff.

	Teratoma with Atypia	Teratoma with Associated Non–Germ Cell (Somatic) Malignancy
Age	Second through fourth decades	Second through fourth decades
Location	Usually unilateral	Usually unilateral
Symptoms	Painless scrotal mass	Painless scrotal mass. Abdominal symptoms of metastatic disease may occur
Signs	Usually palpable testicular nodular mass. HCG and AFP elevation may be seen	Usually palpable testicular nodular mass. In cases following chemotherapy for prior metastatic tumor, signs related to a growing abdominal mass. HCG and AFP elevation may be seen
Etiology	Atypia in teratoma not associated with specific risk factors	Seen in 3%–6% of germ cell tumors with a teratomatous component. More frequent in metastatic site following chemotherapy for a germ cell tumor
Histology	1. Haphazard arrangement of mature or immature embryonal/fetal-type endodermal, ectodermal, and/or mesodermal tissues. Focal embryonal organoid formations including nephroblastomatosis or neuroepithelial structures may be present 2. In cases of postpubertal teratoma, glands may have severe nuclear atypia and increased mitotic activity, comparable to *in situ* carcinoma, or can see atypical cartilage *(Figs. 4.17.1–4.17.3)* 3. In cases of postpubertal teratoma, can see cellular hyperchromatic stroma with increased mitotic rate often encircling teratomatous glands *(Fig. 4.17.4)*. Out of context, this stroma would be diagnostic of sarcoma, except that it does not exceed 4× field	1. Same as usual teratoma except for sheets of somatic (i.e., not germ cell tumor) elements. Somatic tumor not admixed with germ cell tumor and occupy >4× power field. More common somatic malignancies arising in teratomas are Wilms tumor, primitive neuroectodermal tumor (PNET), and rhabdomyosarcoma *(Figs. 4.17.5 and 4.17.6)* 2. Also can see sheets of various patterns of carcinoma where the glands sheet out greater than a 4× *(Figs. 4.17.7 and 4.17.8)* 3. Sarcomas arising in teratomas sheet out greater than a 4× field *(Figs. 4.17.9 and 4.17.10)*
Special studies	• Immunohistochemical stains not helpful in this differential • Gain of isochromosome 12p seen in 80% of all TGCT including adult teratoma	• Immunohistochemical stains not helpful in this differential • Gain of isochromosome 12p seen in 80% of adult teratomas. Non–germ cell malignancies arising in teratomas retain chromosomal gains in 12p and may also gain additional genetic alterations related to its somatic lineage such as t(11;22) in PNET

	Teratoma with Atypia	**Teratoma with Associated Non–Germ Cell (Somatic) Malignancy**
Treatment	The presence of areas of epithelial or mesenchymal atypia does not affect treatment of postpubertal teratoma, which is primarily stage dependent	Chemotherapy protocol specific to its somatic lineage is often used, although it is controversial whether it is superior to germ cell therapy. Best chance for cure if surgically resectable
Prognosis	The presence of areas of epithelial or mesenchymal atypia does not affect prognosis, which remains stage dependent. Overall, excellent prognosis with more than 80% relapse-free 5-y survival in postpubertal patients	Somatic malignancy in a teratoma does not alter the prognosis if confined to the testis. When a non–germ cell malignancy arises in a metastatic teratoma, the prognosis is markedly worsened with <50% patients achieving 3-y survival

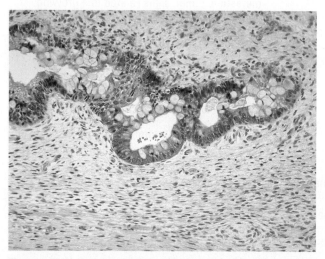

Figure 4.17.1   Postpubertal teratoma with a focal glandular component showing marked architectural and cytologic atypia approaching carcinoma *in situ.*

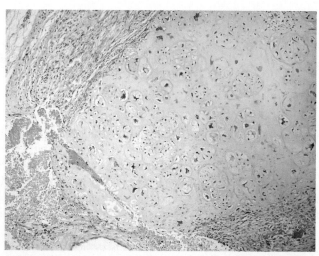

Figure 4.17.2   Postpubertal teratoma with focal cartilage with marked cytologic atypia.

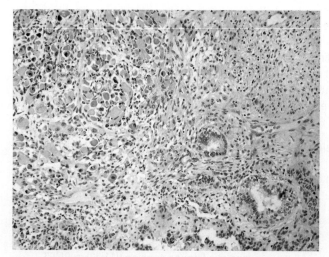

Figure 4.17.3   Teratoma with focal area of rhabdomyoblastic differentiation (*upper left*).

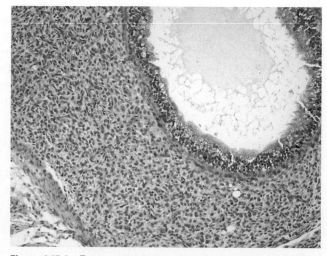

Figure 4.17.4   Teratoma gland with cuff of mitotically active stroma.

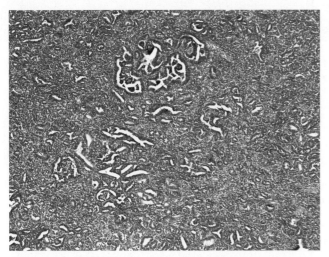

Figure 4.17.5   Postpubertal teratoma with associated non–germ cell malignancy. Expansile nodule (>4× field) of Wilms tumor.

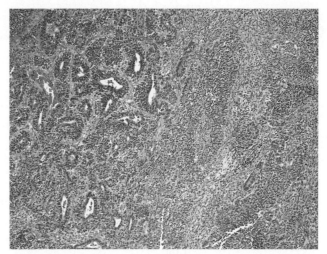

Figure 4.17.6   Postpubertal teratoma with associated non–germ cell malignancy. Expansile nodule (>4× field) of neuroectodermal proliferation indicating presence of primitive neuroectodermal tumor (PNET).

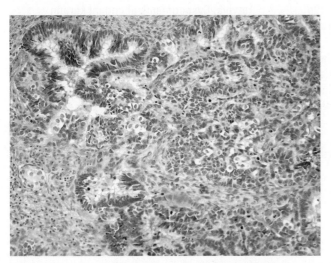

Figure 4.17.7   Postpubertal teratoma with associated non–germ cell malignancy. Glandular proliferation with complex architecture and cytologic atypia that occupied >4× field.

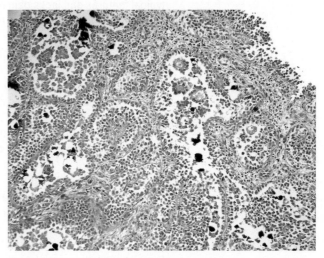

Figure 4.17.8   Postpubertal teratoma with associated non–germ cell malignancy composed of papillary adenocarcinoma.

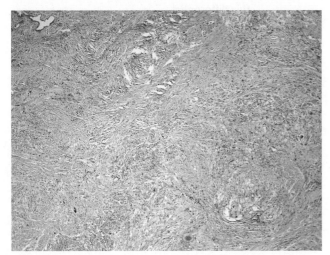

Figure 4.17.9   Postpubertal teratoma with associated non–germ cell malignancy composed of rhabdomyosarcoma occupying >4× field.

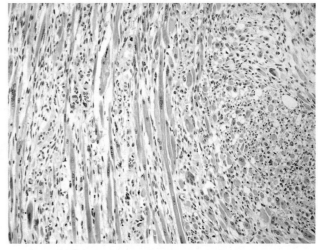

Figure 4.17.10   Same case as Figure 4.17.9 showing rhabdomyosarcoma differentiation.

4 TESTIS

	Malignant Postpubertal Teratoma	Epidermoid/Dermoid Cyst
Age	Second through fourth decades	Second through fourth decades. Mean age 24 y
Location	Usually unilateral	Usually unilateral
Symptoms	Painless scrotal mass	Painless scrotal mass
Signs	Usually palpable testicular mass. HCG and AFP elevation may be seen	Usually palpable testicular nodular mass. No elevated serum markers
Etiology	Same as other germ cell tumors (See Section 4.10)	No associated risk factors
Histology	1. Multilocular squamous-lined cysts are suspicious for malignancy, yet if no other atypical features and lacks gain of i12p could be consistent with benign teratoma *(Fig. 4.18.1)* 2. In malignant teratoma, more disordered elements. If elements other than intestinal or respiratory glands adjacent to single cyst, then should be considered malignant teratoma *(Figs. 4.18.2 and 4.18.3)* 3. May show haphazard skin adnexal structures not associated with a cyst 4. May show cytologic atypia 5. May see extensive atrophy in the uninvolved testis and/or irregular calcifications 6. IGCNU almost invariably associated (80% of cases) in adult cases while absent in teratoma occurring in early childhood	1. Unilocular cystic structure lined by mature keratinizing squamous epithelium without atypia. Cyst contains abundant keratin debris, which can rupture with associated granulomatous reaction *(Fig. 4.18.4)* 2. Can have focal adjacent intestinal, respiratory structures (often organoid surrounded by smooth muscle) or less commonly other elements next to classic epidermoid cyst *(Fig. 4.18.5)* 3. Dermoid cyst with single squamous-lined cyst surrounded by adnexal structures *(Fig. 4.18.6)* 4. No cytologic atypia 5. Lacks extensive atrophy in the uninvolved testis and/or irregular calcifications 6. IGCNU not present in the surrounding normal appearing testicular tissue
Special studies	• Immunohistochemical stains not helpful in this differential • Gain of isochromosome 12p seen in 80% of all adult teratomas	• Immunohistochemical stains not helpful in this differential • In a lesion that is not simple epidermoid or dermoid cyst would confirm benign nature with lacks of gain of isochromosome 12p
Treatment	Stage dependent. Radical orchiectomy followed by active surveillance, retroperitoneal lymph node dissection (RPLND) or adjuvant chemotherapy	Enucleation with preservation of the uninvolved testis when diagnosis is suspected based on sonographic studies and confirmed on intraoperative frozen section
Prognosis	Stage dependent with more than 80% relapse-free at 5 y	Benign behavior. Would recommend close follow-up for cases with intestinal or respiratory elements adjacent to the epidermoid/dermoid cyst as the number of reported cases and follow-up is limited

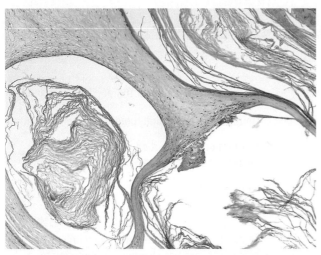

Figure 4.18.1 Multilocular squamous-lined cysts that still could benign teratoma even in a post-pubertal male if confirmed with lack of isochromosome 12p.

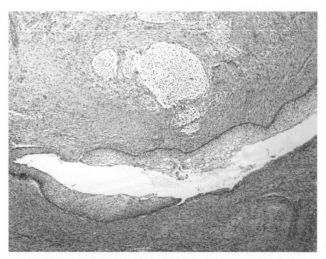

Figure 4.18.2 Malignant teratoma in a postpubertal male with a squamous cyst and adjacent neural tissue.

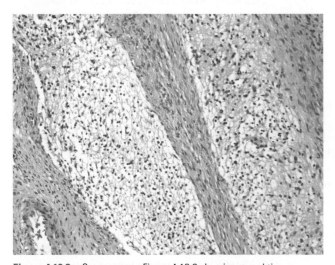

Figure 4.18.3 Same case as Figure 4.18.2 showing neural tissue.

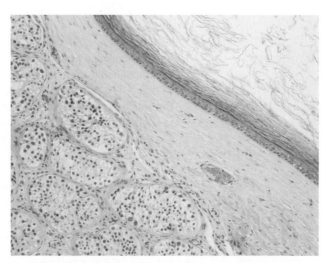

Figure 4.18.4 Epidermoid cyst composed of a unilocular cystic structure lined by mature keratinizing squamous epithelium without any atypia.

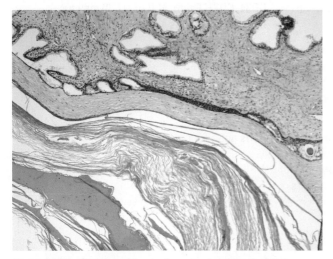

Figure 4.18.5 Presence of focal adjacent mature intestinal and respiratory structures next to classic epidermoid cyst should not exclude the diagnosis of epidermoid cyst.

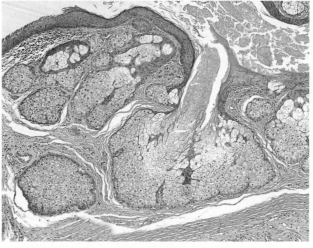

Figure 4.18.6 Testicular dermoid cyst with skin adnexal structures.

4 TESTIS

	Vascular Invasion with Germ Cell Tumors	Artifactually Displaced Tumor
Age	Usual age of germ cell tumors	Usual age of germ cell tumors
Location	In situations where it can impact stage, intratesticular	In situations where it can impact stage, intratesticular
Symptoms	None	None
Signs	None	None
Etiology	Extension into vascular spaces	Testicular germ cell tumors, especially seminoma, are very friable and common to see extensive loosely cohesive tumor cells obviously displaced on the edge of the tissue. Displaced tissue has a predilection for falling into empty spaces, including vessels, where they mimic vascular invasion
Histology	1. Tumor occupies a lymphovascular structure lined by flattened endothelial cells *(Figs. 4.19.1 and 4.19.2)* 2. The cluster will not conform to the exact shape of the vascular lumina 3. Associated fibrinous thrombosis and or mural attachment and reendothelialization *(Figs. 4.19.2 and 4.19.3)* 4. Lack of obvious background artifactual deposition of germ cell tumor cells on the tunical surface *(Fig. 4.19.4)* 5. Cluster is more cohesive and has a rounded smooth edge *(Fig. 4.19.5)* 6. Cluster looks markedly different in its architecture from the surrounding tumor	1. Tumor is within an artifactual tissue space without an endothelial lining *(Fig. 4.19.6)* 2. The cluster may conform to the exact shape of the vascular lumina 3. No evidence of thrombosis or mural attachment or reendothelialization 4. Extensive background artifactual deposition and spread of germ cell tumor cells *(Figs. 4.19.7 and 4.19.8)* 5. Cluster has an irregular appearance of loosely cohesive cells 6. Cluster looks identical to the surrounding tumor
Special studies	CD34, CD31, Factor VIII or D2/40 is positive in spaces surrounding the tumor.	CD34, CD31, Factor VIII or D2/40 may be negative in spaces surrounding the tumor.
Treatment	By itself, not treated. However, its finding can impact treatment. For example, its presence in an organ-confined germ cell tumor with <50% embryonal carcinoma removes active surveillance as an option	Does not affect treatment
Prognosis	Lymphovascular invasion categorizes a germ cell tumor as pathologic stage pT2 and is also an independent, negative prognosticator in nonseminomatous testicular germ cell tumors	Does not affect prognosis

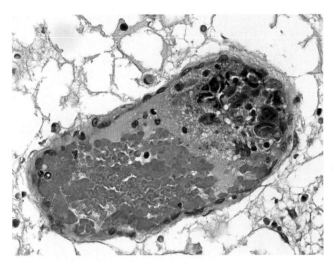

Figure 4.19.1 Embryonal carcinoma with lymphovascular invasion. Tumor nests occupy lymphovascular structures lined by flattened endothelial cells. The clusters do not conform to the exact shape of the vascular lumina, and there is associated fibrin.

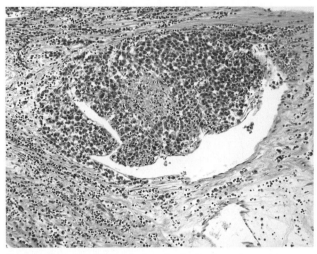

Figure 4.19.2 Lymphovascular invasion in classic seminoma. Tumor is cohesive with attachment to the vessel wall and is covered by reendothelialization.

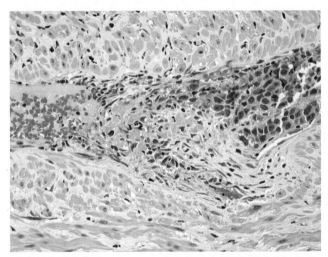

Figure 4.19.3 Vascular invasion by seminoma associated with organizing fibrin.

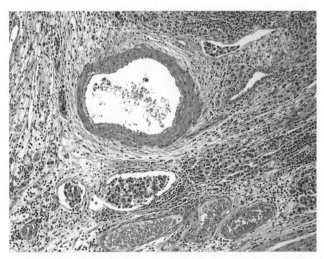

Figure 4.19.4 Vascular invasion by seminoma. There was no artifactual loose seminoma cells elsewhere.

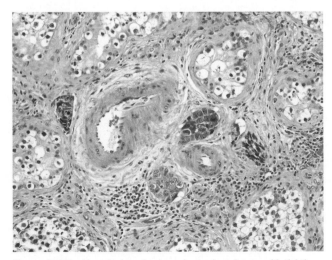

Figure 4.19.5 Vascular invasion by embryonal carcinoma with tightly cohesive tumor nests in vessels.

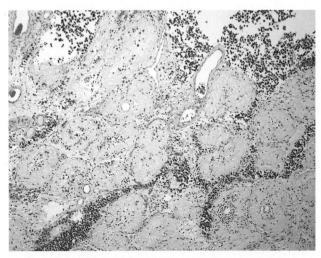

Figure 4.19.6 Irregular, loosely tight clusters of seminoma cells occupying irregular artifactual spaces at times conforming to their shape.

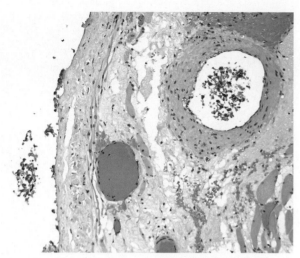

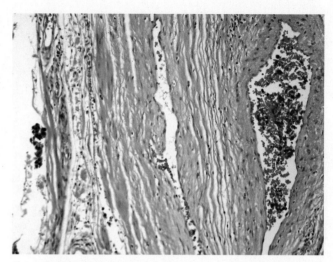

Figure 4.19.7   Artifactual spread of seminoma in the vessel. Note similar loose, detached cells on the edge of the specimen (*left*).

Figure 4.19.8   Artifactual spread of seminoma in the vessel. Note similar loose, detached cells on the edge of the specimen (*left*).

	Regressed Germ Cell Tumor	Testicular Scar
Age	Second to fourth decades	Any age
Location	Usually unilateral	Usually unilateral can be bilateral when secondary to systemic vasculitis
Symptoms	Typically symptoms related to retroperitoneal metastasis such as abdominal pain, nausea, and vomiting	None or related to triggering etiology
Signs	Rarely palpable testicular nodule. More frequently, patients present with distant metastases of germ cell tumor and are subsequently discovered to have sonographic signs of a regressed germ cell tumor	Rarely palpable testicular nodule
Etiology	Associated risk factors: same as nonregressed germ cell tumor, including cryptorchidism (10%), infertility, low socioeconomic status, and male genital malformations. All germ cell tumors at risk of regression	Trauma, infarct, systemic vasculitis, postinfectious (i.e., tuberculosis)
Histology	1. Discrete nodule of fibrous tissue at times stellate in configuration *(Figs. 4.20.1–4.20.4)* 2. Surrounding testicular parenchyma often shows atrophy with impaired spermatogenesis and tubular atrophy 3. Large, coarse calcifications within adjacent scarred tubules are seen in 50% of cases *(Fig. 4.20.5)* 4. Presence of residual IGCNU seen in 50% of cases associated with a testicular scar is diagnostic of regressed germ cell tumor. May also see intratubular embryonal carcinoma *(Fig. 4.20.6)* 5. Scar with clusters of hemosiderin-laden macrophages with lymphoplasmacytic inflammatory infiltrate	1. One or more irregular nodules of fibrous tissue 2. Surrounding testicular parenchyma usually normal, although some evidence of atrophy in partially injured tubules immediately adjacent to scar may be found *(Figs. 4.20.7 and 4.20.8)* 3. Lacks coarse calcification 4. No evidence of IGCNU in nonscarred parenchyma 5. May also show scar with clusters of hemosiderin-laden macrophages with lymphoplasmacytic inflammatory infiltrate
Special studies	Positive PLAP, OCT4, and SALL4 may help identify associated IGCNU	Absence of immunohistochemical staining with PLAP, OCT4, or SALL4 helps to rule out IGCNU
Treatment	Remains stage dependent despite regression: Radical orchiectomy followed by active surveillance or adjuvant radiotherapy and or platinum-based chemotherapy	Radical orchiectomy has usually been performed to obtain the diagnosis
Prognosis	Regression does not affect prognosis. Stage dependent	Fertility is usually preserved when the scar is unilateral

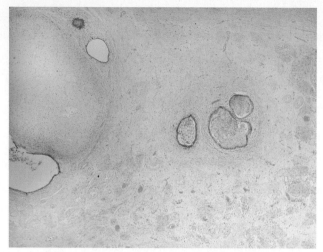

Figure 4.20.1   Partially regressed germ cell tumor with few teratoma glands and islands of cartilage in dense fibrous tissue. The patient had widespread metastases.

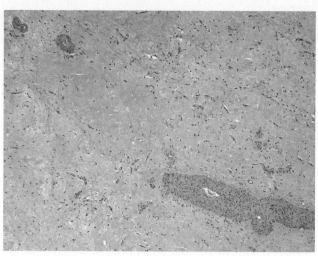

Figure 4.20.2   Regressed germ cell tumor with dense scar formation.

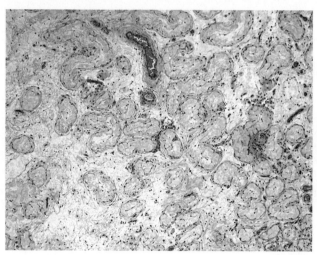

Figure 4.20.3   Same case as Figure 4.20.2 with sclerotic seminiferous tubules.

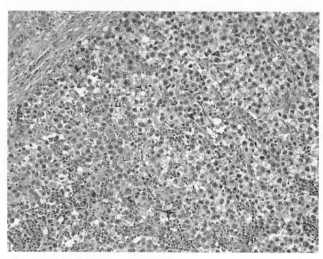

Figure 4.20.4   Same case as Figures 4.20.2 and 4.20.3 with metastatic seminoma to retroperitoneal lymph modes.

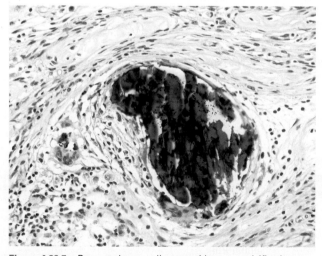

Figure 4.20.5   Regressed germ cell tumor with coarse calcifications.

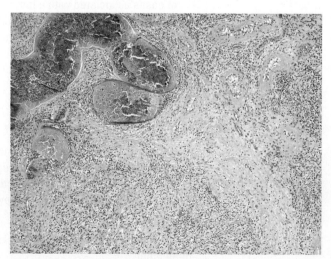

Figure 4.20.6   Regressed germ cell tumor with only residual intratubular embryonal carcinoma. The patient had metastatic embryonal carcinoma to retroperitoneal lymph modes.

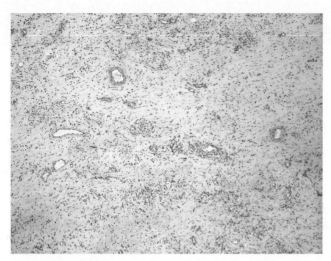

Figure 4.20.7 Irregular zones of parenchymal scarring with associated inflammation secondary to prior ischemic or inflammatory injury.

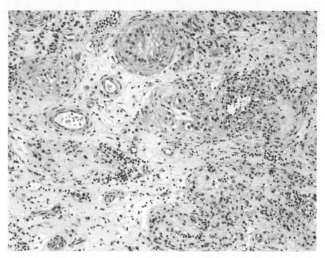

Figure 4.20.8 Same case as Figure 4.20.7 with lack of IGCNU, coarse calcifications, and dense scar formation.

4 TESTIS

	Leydig Cell Hyperplasia	Benign Leydig Cell Tumor
Age	Children and adults	Two incidence peaks in first and third decades but may occur in older adults with a mean age of 40 y
Location	Usually bilateral	Almost always unilateral
Symptoms	Isosexual precocity in children, infertility, and at times symptoms related to background etiology	Isosexual precocity in children. Gynecomastia in one-third of adult patients. Occasionally decreased libido and potency
Signs	Undescended testis, signs of Klinefelter syndrome, no discernable testicular mass	Testicular mass; gynecomastia
Etiology	Cryptorchidism, Klinefelter syndrome, androgen insensitivity syndrome, central sexual precocity, hCG-secreting germ cell or somatic malignancies, or often idiopathic	In up to 10% of cases, may be associated cryptorchidism. No known risk factors in remaining cases
Histology	1. Multiple enlarged clusters and small nodules of Leydig cells interspersed among preexisting, frequently atrophic seminiferous tubules (*Figs. 4.21.1–4.21.4*) 2. Although some nodules may be dominant, surrounding the interstitium shows varying degrees of Leydig cell hyperplasia 3. Identical cytology to benign Leydig cell tumor 4. Sheets of Leydig cells 5. May see Leydig cells around nerves in the hilum of the testis (*Figs. 4.21.5 and 4.21.6*)	1. Fairly well-circumscribed but unencapsulated mass measuring 3–5 cm in diameter. Minimal entrapped seminiferous tubules are present; may be seen at the periphery of the nodule (*Figs. 4.21.7 and 4.21.8*) 2. Surrounding the interstitium with normal or decreased Leydig cells 3. Neoplastic cells are polygonal in shape with characteristic abundant granular eosinophilic cytoplasm. Lipochrome pigment and Reinke crystals may be present in 15% and 30% of cases, respectively. Tumor cell nuclei are usually round with conspicuous nucleoli (*Figs. 4.21.5–4.21.8*) 4. Usually diffuse sheets with less frequently cord-like, pseudoglandular, small vacuolar with lipid, microcystic, and spindle cell morphology 5. Would not see extension out of the testis with perineural invasion with an otherwise benign Leydig cell tumor
Special studies	Not helpful in this differential diagnosis	Not helpful in this differential diagnosis
Treatment	Radical orchiectomy is usually performed by the time the diagnosis is made	Radical orchiectomy is usually performed by the time the diagnosis is made
Prognosis	Related to the associated etiology	Benign

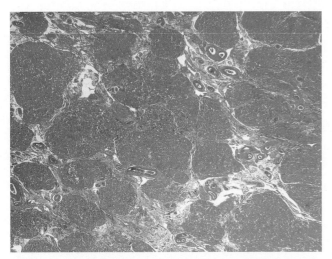

Figure 4.21.1   Multiple enlarged clusters and small nodules of Leydig cell hyperplasia interspersed among preexisting, frequently atrophic seminiferous tubules in a patient with Klinefelter syndrome.

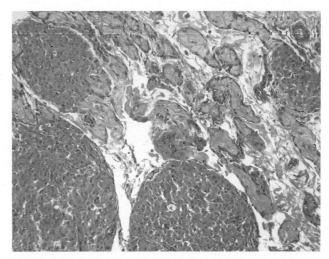

Figure 4.21.2   Same case as Figure 4.21.1.

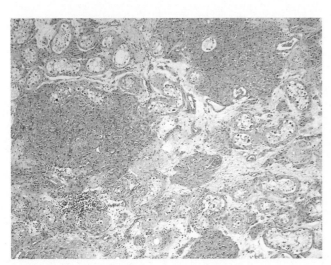

Figure 4.21.3   Multiple enlarged clusters and small nodules of Leydig cell hyperplasia.

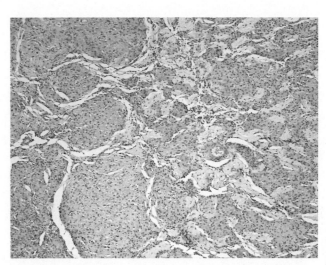

Figure 4.21.4   Multiple enlarged clusters and small nodules of Leydig cell hyperplasia with a somewhat more diffuse growth.

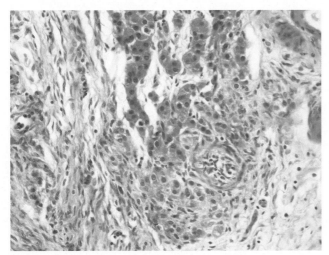

Figure 4.21.5   Leydig cells around nerves in the hilum of the testis.

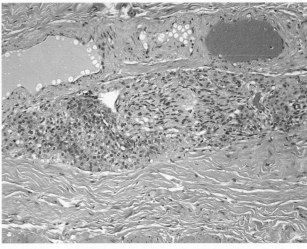

Figure 4.21.6   Leydig cells around nerves in the hilum of the testis.

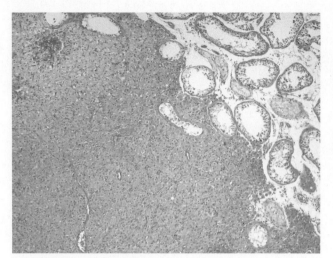

Figure 4.21.7 Benign Leydig cell tumor with minimal entrapment of surrounding seminiferous tubules.

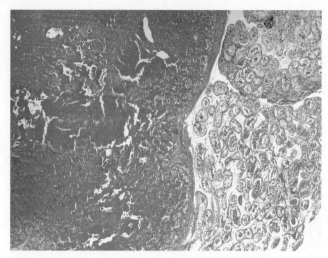

Figure 4.21.8 Benign well-circumscribed Leydig cell tumor.

	Benign Leydig Cell Tumor	Malignant Leydig Cell Tumor
Age	Two incidence peaks in first and third decades but may occur in older adults with a mean age of 40 y	Older adults with a mean age of 63 y
Location	Almost always unilateral	Almost always unilateral
Symptoms	Isosexual precocity in children. Gynecomastia in one-third of adult patients. Occasionally decreased libido and potency	Only rare endocrine manifestations (i.e., gynecomastia). Symptomatology due to retroperitoneal or visceral metastasis in 20% of cases at the time of diagnosis
Signs	Testicular mass, gynecomastia	Testicular mass
Etiology	In up to 10% of cases, associated with cryptorchidism. More common in Whites than African Americans and Asians	Approximately 10% of all Leydig tumors. More common in Whites than African Americans and Asians
Histology	1. Usually <5 cm (average 2.7 cm) 2. Fairly well-circumscribed yet unencapsulated mass that may show minimal infiltration between surrounding seminiferous tubules *(Fig. 4.22.1)* 3. Usually a diffuse sheet-like architecture but may be nodular, trabecular, cord-like, pseudoglandular, small vacuolar with lipid, and microcystic 4. Cells are polygonal with abundant granular eosinophilic cytoplasm. Lipochrome pigment and Reinke crystals present in 15% and 30 % of cases, respectively *(Fig. 4.22.2)* 5. Nuclei usually round with conspicuous nucleoli. Scattered larger cells may be seen 6. Lacks nuclear hyperchromasia 7. Lacks necrosis or lymphovascular invasion 8. No or low (<3 per 10 HPF) mitotic activity 9. If no worrisome histologic features (see Malignant Leydig cell tumor) are present, diagnose as "benign Leydig cell tumor." If only a few atypical features are present (i.e., larger size but otherwise benign), then diagnose "Leydig cell tumor of uncertain malignant potential." If only one atypical feature present, add that a favorable prognosis is likely	1. Usually larger than 5 cm (average 6.9 cm) 2. Can be more diffusely infiltrative between surrounding seminiferous tubules *(Fig. 4.22.3)* 3. Usually a diffuse sheet-like architecture but may be nodular, trabecular, cord-like, pseudoglandular, small vacuolar with lipid, and microcystic 4. Cells are polygonal with abundant granular eosinophilic cytoplasm. Lipochrome pigment and Reinke crystals present in 15% and 30% of cases, respectively 5. Nuclei may be round or more irregular with conspicuous nucleoli *(Figs. 4.22.4–4.22.6)* 6. Nuclear hyperchromasia prominent 7. May have associated necrosis or lymphovascular invasion 8. Often shows increased mitotic activity (>3 per 10 HPF) *(Figs. 4.22.7 and 4.22.8)* 9. Most malignant Leydig cell tumors having at least 4 of the following characteristics: >5 cm; nuclear hyperchromasia and pleomorphism, increased mitoses, vascular invasion, widespread invasion into surrounding the testis, and necrosis
Special studies	Not helpful in this differential	Not helpful in this differential

	Benign Leydig Cell Tumor	**Malignant Leydig Cell Tumor**
Treatment	Radical orchiectomy is usually performed by the time the diagnosis is made. No additional therapy is required	Radical orchiectomy usually performed followed by retroperitoneal lymph node resection. Chemotherapy is of no value
Prognosis	Benign	Most patients die within 5 y of diagnosis. Common metastatic sites are the retroperitoneal lymph nodes, lung, liver, and bone in decreasing frequency

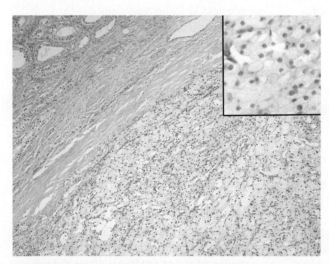

Figure 4.22.1   Benign Leydig cell tumor with a well-circumscribed but unencapsulated border. The cytoplasm is finely vacuolated with lipid. Nuclei are round and uniform **(inset)**.

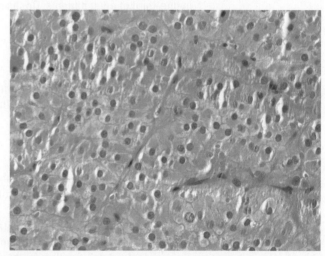

Figure 4.22.2   Benign Leydig cell tumor with abundant granular eosinophilic cytoplasm. Nuclei are round and uniform.

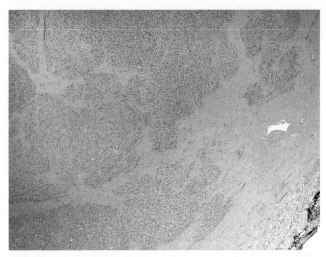

Figure 4.22.3 Malignant Leydig cell tumor showing irregular infiltrative border.

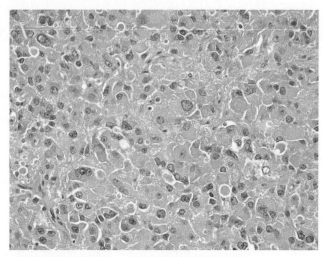

Figure 4.22.4 Malignant Leydig cell tumor showing nuclear pleomorphism.

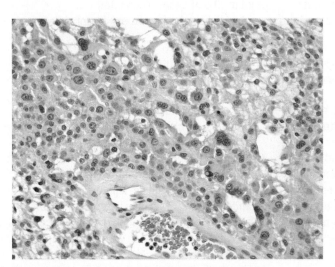

Figure 4.22.5 Malignant Leydig cell tumor showing nuclear pleomorphism.

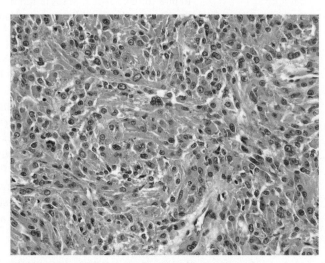

Figure 4.22.6 Malignant Leydig cell tumor showing nuclear pleomorphism and architectural disorganization.

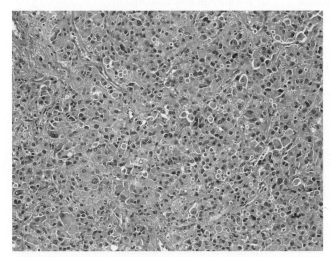

Figure 4.22.7 Malignant Leydig cell tumor showing architectural disorganization at low magnification.

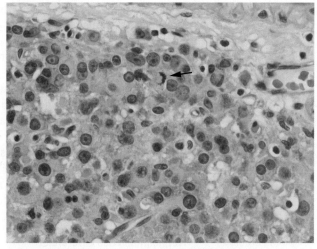

Figure 4.22.8 Same case as Figure 4.22.7 with increased mitotic activity (*arrow*).

	Large Cell Calcifying Sertoli Cell Tumor	Leydig Cell Tumor
Age	Children and adulthood (2–50-year-old range) with a mean age of 21 y	Two incidence peaks in first and third decades but may occur in older adults with a mean age of 40 y
Location	Majority unilateral but 20%–30% bilateral	Almost always unilateral
Symptoms	Testicular swelling. Additional symptoms related to associated conditions such as acromegaly, hypercortesolimea, gynecomastia, sexual precocity (see below)	Isosexual precocity in children. Gynecomastia in one-third of adult patients. Occasionally decreased libido and potency
Signs	Testicular mass	Testicular mass, gynecomastia
Etiology	In one-third of cases, association with Peutz-Jeghers syndrome or Carney syndrome is present	In up to 10% of cases associated cryptorchidism. No known risk factors in remaining cases
Histology	1. Usually a well-circumscribed mass measuring up to 4 cm in diameter (average 2 cm) 2. Tumor cells are arranged in sheets, nests/solid tubules, or trabeculae separated by myxoid to hyalinized fibrous stroma 3. Tumor cells are typically large round but occasionally cuboidal/columnar. Contain abundant granular eosinophilic cytoplasm and round nuclei with moderate-sized one to two nucleoli. Mitoses are rare in benign lesions 4. Large laminated/psammomatous calcifications with focal ossification (Figs. 4.23.1–4.23.3) 5. Intratubular hyalinizing Sertoli cell nodule may be seen, associated with Peutz-Jeghers syndrome (Fig. 4.23.4) 6. In the setting of Peutz-Jeghers syndrome, some tumors resemble sex cord tumors with annular tubules (SCTAT) 7. Approximately 15% are malignant. Patients are usually older (average age 39 vs. 17 y). Features associated with malignancy include: >4 cm, marked nuclear pleomorphism and hyperchromasia, increased mitoses (>3 per 10 HPF), extratesticular spread, necrosis, and lymphovascular invasion (≥2 features diagnostic of malignant)	1. Usually a well-circumscribed mass measuring 3–5 cm in diameter 2. Some tumors may acquire a nodular to trabecular architecture introduced by a more prominent fibrous stroma 3. Neoplastic cells are polygonal in shape with characteristic abundant granular eosinophilic cytoplasm. Lipochrome pigment and Reinke crystals may be present in 15% and 30% of cases, respectively. Tumor cell nuclei are usually round with conspicuous nucleoli (Figs. 4.23.5 and 4.23.6) 4. No calcifications are seen 5. No intratubular component 6. Sex cord tumors with annular tubular morphology not present 7. See Section 4.21 for benign vs. malignant Leydig cell tumor
Special studies	Not helpful in this differential	Not helpful in this differential

	Large Cell Calcifying Sertoli Cell Tumor	**Leydig Cell Tumor**
Treatment	Radical orchiectomy is usually performed by the time the diagnosis is made. When tumors are multifocal/bilateral, a conservative approach is necessary given their usual benign course. In cases with a significant risk for malignant behavior, retroperitoneal lymph node resection may be required	Radical orchiectomy is usually performed by the time the diagnosis is made. In cases that are deemed to have a significant risk for malignant behavior, retroperitoneal lymph node resection is required
Prognosis	If malignant, associated with a poor prognosis. Otherwise cured	Most patients with malignant Leydig cell tumor die within 5 y of diagnosis

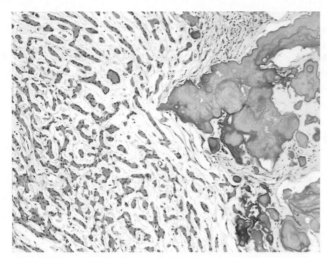

Figure 4.23.1 Large cell calcifying Sertoli cell tumor with large laminated/psammomatous calcifications with focal ossification and myxoid stroma.

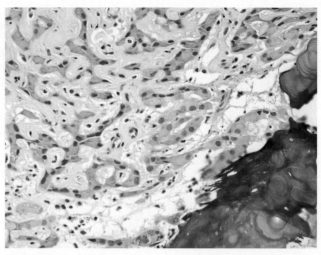

Figure 4.23.2 Same case as Figure 4.23.1 with large round-to-cuboidal cells with abundant granular eosinophilic cytoplasm.

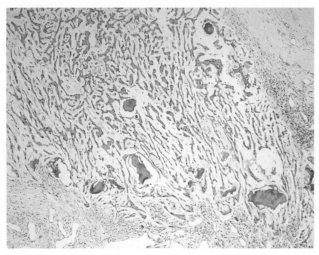

Figure 4.23.3 Large cell calcifying Sertoli cell tumor with mostly Sertoli cell tumor cells and smaller calcifications.

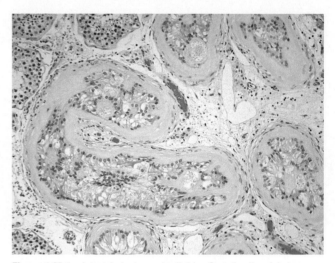

Figure 4.23.4 Intratubular tumor hyalinizing Sertoli cell nodule in a case of large cell calcifying Sertoli cell tumor. Seminiferous tubules contain large Sertoli cells with vacuolated to eosinophilic cytoplasm and a markedly thickened peritubular basement membrane with intratubular deposits of the same hyalinized material.

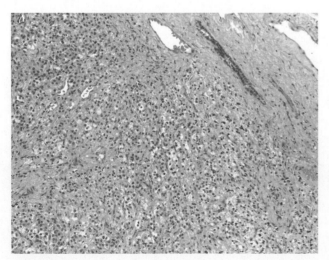

Figure 4.23.5 Benign Leydig cell tumor with a well-circumscribed but unencapsulated border.

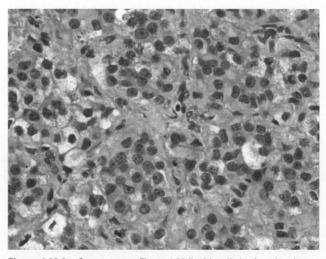

Figure 4.23.6 Same case as Figure 4.23.5 with cells having abundant granular eosinophilic cytoplasm and bland nuclei with visible nucleoli.

	Sertoli Cell Nodule	Benign Sertoli Cell Tumor
Age	Any age	Almost exclusively in adult patients (average age 46 y)
Location	Almost always unilateral	Unilateral
Symptoms	Related to associated lesion. Testicular swelling when encountered in the setting of testicular germ cell tumor. Undescended testis in the setting of cryptorchidism	Testicular swelling. Usually no endocrine manifestation
Signs	No identifiable palpable mass	Testicular mass
Etiology	Typically encountered incidentally resected cryptorchid testes. Up to one-fifth of resected normally descended testes may contain Sertoli cell nodules microscopically when examined for other etiology	None
Histology	1. Only rarely the small nodules can be grossly seen. Usually identified microscopically as nonencapsulated nodule measuring <1 cm. in largest diameter 2. Lacks bands of eosinophilic collagen 3. Two patterns: (1) Tubules lined by immature Sertoli cells that lack atypia and contain luminal hyaline material, which in some cases form laminated calcifications (*Fig. 4.24.1*); (2) crowded small Sertoli cell tubules, resembling fetal tubules (*Figs. 4.24.2 and 4.24.3*) 4. Typically lacks lipidization of cytoplasm 5. Bland cytology and no to rare mitotic activity 6. Spermatogonia could be interspersed in some tubules. Leydig cells may also be present between the tubules 7. When found in orchiectomies performed for germ cell tumor, some of the tubules of Sertoli cell nodules may be secondarily "colonized" by IGCNU, raising the differential diagnosis of gonadoblastoma	1. Usually well-circumscribed mass usually measure <5 cm in diameter (average 3.5 cm) 2. Characteristically, at low magnification, see bands of very eosinophilic collagen dividing tumor. Sclerosing variant of a Sertoli cell tumor form approximately one-sixth of cases (15%), with extensive dense hyalinized stroma 3. Cells arranged in nests, cords, solid areas with variable number of round to elongated tubules (*Figs. 4.24.4–4.24.8*). No calcifications are seen 4. Polygonal to cuboidal cells contain abundant eosinophilic cytoplasm that may become pale or vacuolated due to lipid content 5. Bland nuclear features and rare mitotic activity are the norm 6. Lacks interspersed Leydig cells in tumor 7. Lacks IGCNU in tubules

	Sertoli Cell Nodule	**Benign Sertoli Cell Tumor**
Special studies	Not helpful in this differential diagnosis	Not helpful in this differential diagnosis. Sertoli cell tumors are usually positive for inhibin and variably focally positive for cytokeratin AE1/AE3 and S100 protein
Treatment	None	Radical orchiectomy often done as solid testicular masses are typically presumed to be malignant
Prognosis	Benign incidental lesion	Benign

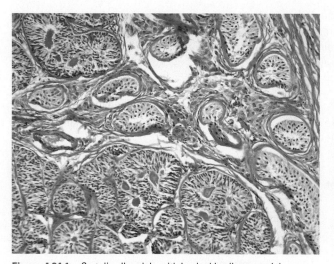

Figure 4.24.1   Sertoli cell nodule with luminal hyaline material.

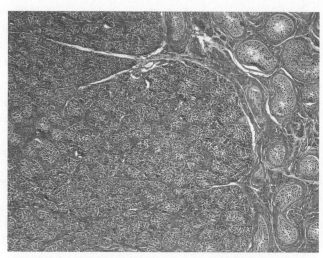

Figure 4.24.2   Sertoli cell nodule composed of crowded small Sertoli cell tubules, resembling fetal tubules.

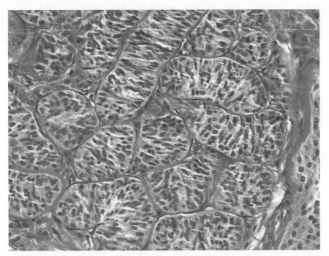

Figure 4.24.3   Higher magnification of same case as Figure 4.24.2.

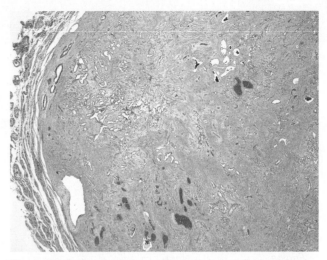

Figure 4.24.4   Sertoli cell tumor with a well-circumscribed peripheral border with extensive hyalinization.

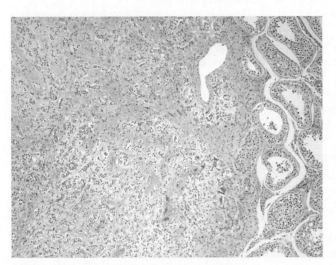

Figure 4.24.5   Sertoli cell tumor with cords of cells.

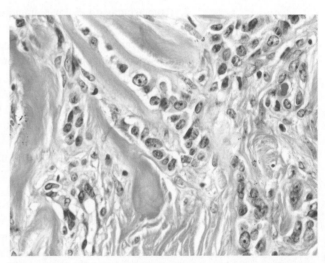

Figure 4.24.6   Higher magnification of same case as Figure 4.24.5.

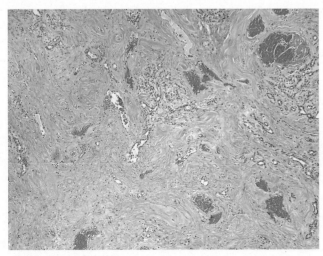

Figure 4.24.7   Sertoli cell tumor with hyalinized stroma and tubules.

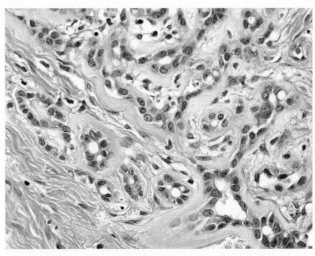

Figure 4.24.8   Higher magnification of same case as Figure 4.24.7.

	Benign Sertoli Cell Tumor	Malignant Sertoli Cell Tumor
Age	Almost exclusively in adult patients (average age 46 y)	Almost exclusively in adult patients (average age 46 y)
Location	Unilateral	Unilateral
Symptoms	Testicular swelling. No endocrine manifestation	Testicular swelling. No endocrine manifestation
Signs	Testicular mass	Testicular mass
Etiology	None	None. Around 12% of all Sertoli cell tumors
Histology	1. Usually a well-circumscribed mass *(Fig. 4.25.1)* 2. Usually measure <5 cm in diameter (average 3.5 cm) 3. Cells arranged in nests, cords, solid areas with variable number of round to elongated tubules *(Fig. 4.25.2)* 4. Polygonal-to-cuboidal cells contain abundant eosinophilic cytoplasm that may become pale or vacuolated due to lipid content 5. Bland nuclear features and rare mitotic activity are the norm 6. No necrosis 7. No lymphovascular invasion 8. Benign tumors typically have no malignant features. If only one malignant feature is seen, tumor should be diagnosed as Sertoli cell tumor of uncertain malignant potential	1. Usually well circumscribed but may infiltrate surrounding parenchyma or extend to extratesticular tissue 2. Usually measure more than 5 cm in diameter 3. Cells are arranged in round to elongated tubules. Cords and more frequent solid arrangements exist *(Figs. 4.25.3–4.25.5)* 4. Polygonal-to-cuboidal cells contain abundant eosinophilic cytoplasm that may become pale or vacuolated due to lipid content *(Fig. 4.25.6)* 5. Moderate to severe nuclear atypia and increased mitotic activity (>5 per 10 HPF) *(Figs. 4.25.7 and 4.25.8)* 6. Necrosis may be present 7. Lymphovascular invasion may be present 8. Most malignant Sertoli cell tumors demonstrate at least three of these characteristics while only rare tumors reveal one or two atypical features
Special studies	No role in predicting malignant behavior	No role in predicting malignant behavior
Treatment	Radical orchiectomy often done as solid testicular masses are typically presumed to be malignant	Radical orchiectomy. In cases that are deemed to have a significant risk for malignant behavior based on pathologic examination of primary, consideration for retroperitoneal lymph node resection should be entertained. Close clinical and radiologic observation are an alternative approach to detect early metastases and pursue them surgically. Radiation or chemotherapy is of no apparent value in metastatic cases
Prognosis	Benign	Associated with a poor prognosis

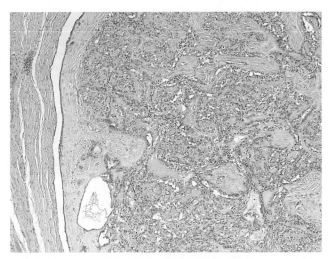

Figure 4.25.1 A well-circumscribed benign Sertoli cell tumor.

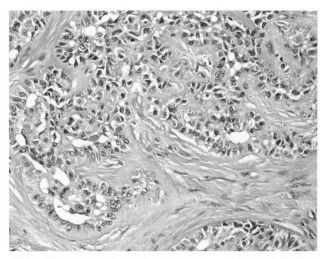

Figure 4.25.2 Same case as Figure 4.25.1 with tubules lined by benign-appearing cells lacking mitotic activity.

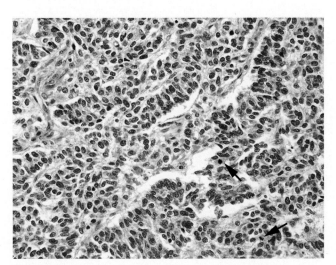

Figure 4.25.3 Malignant Sertoli cell tumor with high cellularity, overlapping nuclei, and increased mitotic activity (*arrows*).

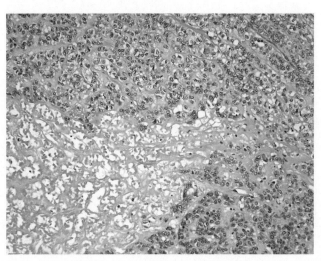

Figure 4.25.4 Malignant Sertoli cell tumor with necrosis.

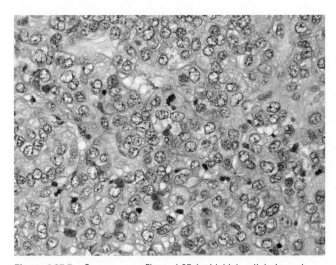

Figure 4.25.5 Same case as Figure 4.25.4 with high cellularity and mitotic figures.

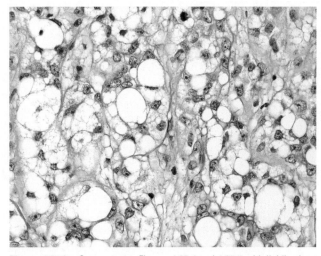

Figure 4.25.6 Same case as Figures 4.25.4 and 4.25.5 with lipidization.

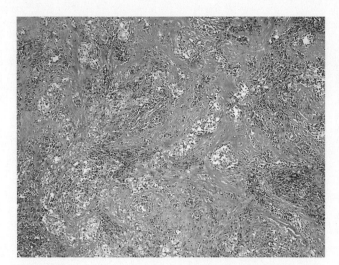

Figure 4.25.7   Malignant Sertoli cell tumor with hyalinized bands of collagen similar to that seen in benign Sertoli cell tumors.

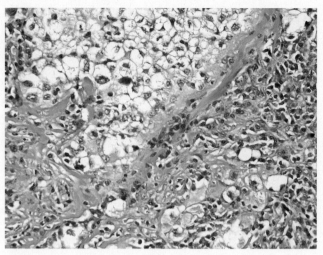

Figure 4.25.8   Same case as Figure 4.25.7 with moderate nuclear atypia.

	Benign Sertoli Cell Tumor	Carcinoid Tumor
Age	Almost exclusively in adult patients (average age 46 y)	Average age 36 y (12–65 y)
Location	Unilateral	Unilateral
Symptoms	Testicular swelling. No endocrine manifestation	Few patients present with carcinoid syndrome with diarrhea, hot flashes, and palpitations
Signs	Testicular mass	Testicular mass or swelling. May be incidentally found
Etiology	Does not occur admixed with germ cell tumors	80% are pure carcinoid tumor. Remainder associated with teratoma, epidermoid cyst, or dermoid cyst *(Fig. 4.26.6)*
Histology	1. Usually a well-circumscribed mass 2. Usually measure <5 cm in diameter (average 3.5 cm) 3. Cells arranged in nests, cords, solid areas with a variable number of round to elongated tubules *(Figs. 4.26.1–4.26.3)* 4. Nuclei with single small nucleoli *(Figs. 4.26.4 and 4.26.5)* 5. Bland nuclear features and rare mitotic activity are the norm. No necrosis 6. No lymphovascular invasion 7. Hyalinized stroma common	1. Usually well circumscribed 2. Average 2.5 cm in diameter 3. Cells are arranged in cords, ribbons, nests, and can have tubular formation *(Figs. 4.26.7–4.26.10)* 4. "Salt and pepper" nuclear chromatin *(Figs. 4.26.9 and 4.26.10)* 5. Over 90% with rare mitotic activity. Only a few cases with necrosis 6. Lymphovascular invasion absent 7. 10% of cases with desmoplastic reaction but typically not hyalinized stroma
Special studies	• Variably focally positive for cytokeratin AE1/AE3 • Usually positive for inhibin alpha (30%–90%) and calretinin • Synaptophysin can be positive in almost half of the cases with a higher rate of chromogranin staining	• Diffusely positive for cytokeratin AE1/AE3 • Negative for inhibin alpha and calretinin • Typically positive for synaptophysin with less positivity for chromogranin
Treatment	Radical orchiectomy often done as solid testicular masses are typically presumed to be malignant	Most cases are treated by radical orchiectomy. In cases with a significant risk for malignant behavior, consideration for retroperitoneal lymph node resection or close observation. Radiation and chemotherapy no value in metastatic cases
Prognosis	Benign	Most have a benign clinical course even if associated with epidermoid/dermoid cysts or teratoma. Atypical carcinoids or those associated with teratoma can occasionally exhibit metastatic spread

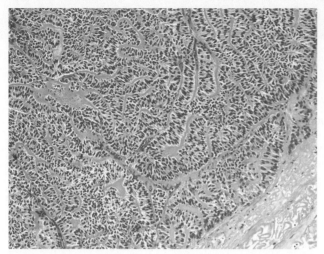

Figure 4.26.1   Sertoli cell tumor with a well-circumscribed peripheral border.

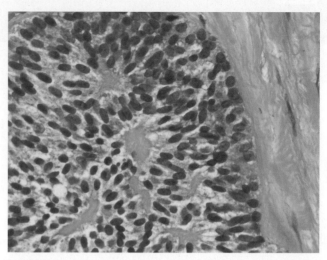

Figure 4.26.2   Same case as Figure 4.26.1 with ovoid-to-cuboidal cells arranged in a nest occasionally surround the luminal hyaline material.

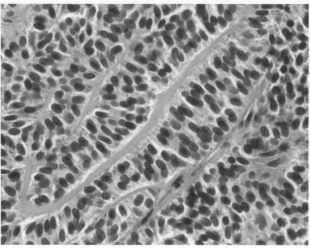

Figure 4.26.3   Same case as Figures 4.26.1 and 4.26.2 with cells arranged in cords and nests. Homogeneous chromatin pattern distinguishes the nuclei from the "salt and pepper" pattern of carcinoid nuclei.

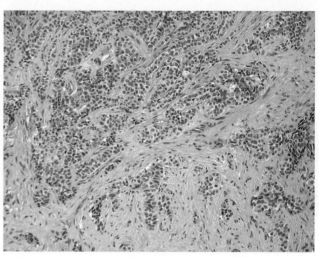

Figure 4.26.4   Sertoli cell tumor with nests and cords.

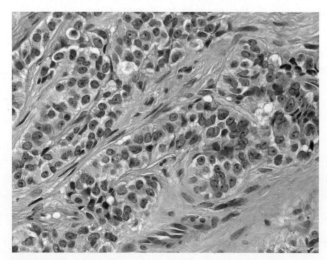

Figure 4.26.5   Same case as Figure 4.26.4 with cells having a single, small nucleolus.

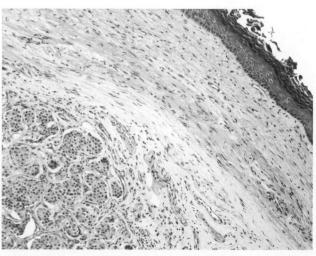

Figure 4.26.6   Carcinoid associated with teratoma.

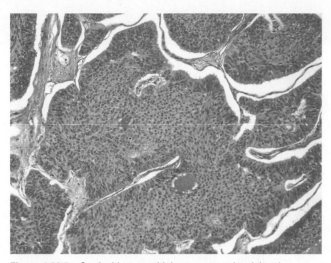

Figure 4.26.7 Carcinoid tumor with large nests and peripheral palisading.

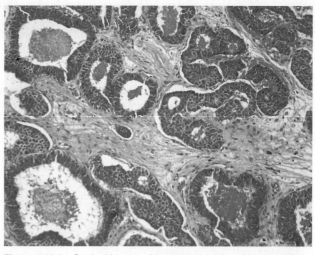

Figure 4.26.8 Carcinoid tumor with pseudoglandular tubule formation.

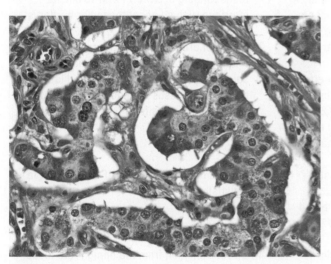

Figure 4.26.9 Carcinoid tumor with the "salt and pepper" nuclear chromatin.

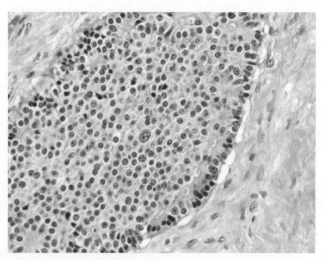

Figure 4.26.10 Carcinoid tumor with the "salt and pepper" nuclear chromatin and random nuclear atypia that does not necessarily indicate malignancy.

	Rete Testis Hyperplasia/Sertoliform Cystadenoma	Rete Testis Carcinoma
Age	Adults	Fourth to eighth decade
Location	Unilateral	Unilateral
Symptoms	Asymptomatic	Scrotal pain
Signs	Intrascrotal nodule	Tender intrascrotal nodule. May be associated with a fistula or scrotal sinus
Etiology	None	None
Histology	1. Rete testis hyperplasia: Does not form a mass. Sertoliform cystadenoma: Usually a well-circumscribed polypoid mass <3 cm often projecting into the dilated rete lumen 2. Rete hyperplasia: Increased number of rete tubules that are not well circumscribed *(Fig. 4.27.1)*. Can be seen with testicular tumors with a microcystic pattern with hyaline globules *(Fig. 4.27.2)*. Sertoliform cystadenoma: Crowded tubular structures projecting as polypoid masses at the periphery into the rete testis 3. Rete hyperplasia: Bland cuboidal cells identical to normal rete testis cells. Sertoliform cystadenoma: Lined by bland cuboidal-to-columnar cells *(Figs. 4.27.3 and 4.27.4)* 4. Sertoliform cystadenoma can involve adjacent dilated seminiferous tubules *(Fig. 4.27.5)* 5. Sertoliform cystadenoma can have fibrosis entrapping cord-like epithelial structures 6. Lacks necrosis, vascular invasion, or extension to testicular parenchyma 7. No to rare mitotic activity 8. Lesions are distinctive without the need to exclude other entities	1. Hilar mass grossly centered on the rete testis ranging between 1 and 10 cm. Its interface with adjacent testicular border is usually not well defined *(Fig. 4.27.6)* 2. Range of architectural patterns: tubuloglandular, large cellular nodules, some of which projecting into the dilated residual rete testis channels, solid sheets, retiform and kaposiform (slit like), and papillary *(Figs. 4.27.7 and 4.27.8)* 3. At least moderate degree of nuclear atypia is usually present 4. Direct transition from the benign rete testis lining to the invasive malignant neoplasm is diagnostically helpful, when present 5. Dense desmoplastic reaction is incited 6. Necrosis may be seen. Tumor usually infiltrates the adjacent testis 7. Brisk mitotic activity 8. Diagnosis based on excluding testicular tumors (germ cell or non–germ cell) or metastasis from an extratesticular primary carcinoma
Special studies	Not helpful in this differential	Differential diagnosis also includes malignant mesothelioma with immunohistochemical workup for adenocarcinoma vs. mesothelioma helpful
Treatment	Conservative excision	Wide scrotal excision (hemiscrotectomy). Chemotherapy
Prognosis	Excellent	Dismal with <1 y expected survival

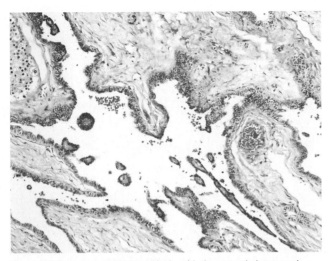

Figure 4.27.1   Rete testis hyperplasia with the expanded rete testis.

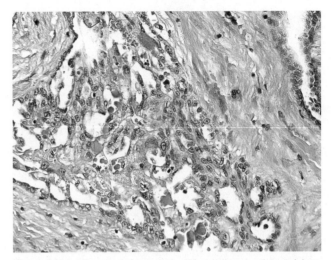

Figure 4.27.2   Rete testis hyperplasia with complex growth containing hyaline globules.

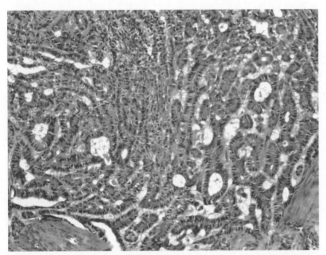

Figure 4.27.3   Sertoliform cystadenoma composed of crowded tubules lined by bland cuboidal-to-columnar cells without atypia or necrosis.

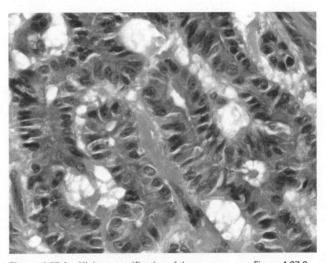

Figure 4.27.4   Higher magnification of the same case as Figure 4.27.3.

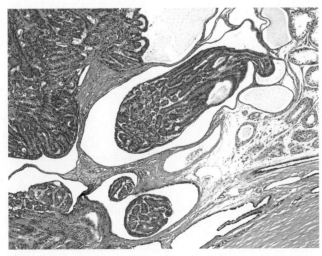

Figure 4.27.5   Same case as Figures 4.27.3 and 4.27.4 with peripheral projection into the rete testis.

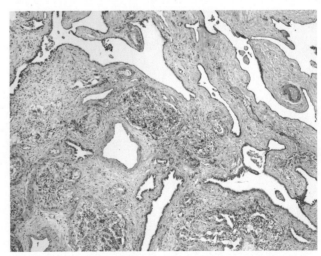

Figure 4.27.6   Rete testis carcinoma composed of infiltrative nodules and nests of epithelial cells centered on the rete testis.

4   TESTIS

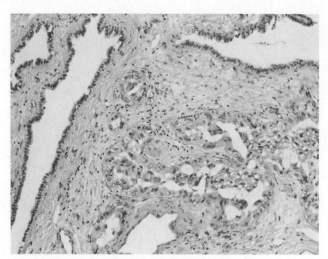

Figure 4.27.7   Same case as Figure 4.27.6 with displaying tubulopapillary architecture.

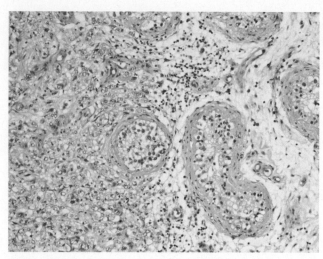

Figure 4.27.8   Same case as Figures 4.27.6 and 4.27.7 with solid nests of cells infiltrating the testis.

	Papillary Cystadenoma of the Epididymis	Metastatic Clear Cell Renal Cell Carcinoma
Age	Wide age range starting from early adulthood	Usually over 50 years old but can rarely occur at an earlier age
Location	Bilateral in one-third of patients, more commonly in von Hippel-Lindau (vHL) Syndrome	Bilateral in minority of cases
Symptoms	Mass or swelling or incidental finding. Related to von Hippel-Lindau Syndrome in familial cases	Majority has symptoms due to known primary tumors
Signs	Intrascrotal nodule	Intrascrotal mass. Majority with signs due to known primary tumors. Extremely unusual for spread to the testis or paratesticular tissue to be the presenting manifestation of renal cell carcinoma
Etiology	In 17% of vHL Syndrome patients. Mutation in the *vHL* gene (3p25 deletion) in sporadic and vHL cases	Secondary involvement from usually sporadic renal cell carcinoma via spermatic vein spread or other hematologic routes. Clear cell renal cell carcinoma in von Hippel-Lindau Syndrome patients only rarely metastasize
Histology	1. Solid and cystic mass up to 5 cm in diameter 2. Mixture in varying proportions of cystic and solid spaces (Fig. 4.28.1) 3. Tubules and papillary folds with fibrovascular cores containing colloid-like material lined by cytologically bland, clear cuboidal-to-columnar cells (Figs. 4.28.2–4.28.4) 4. In areas can have prominent subnuclear vacuoles (Fig. 4.28.5) 5. Richly vascularized 6. No evidence of necrosis or increased mitotic activity 7. No vascular invasion	1. Usually multiple nodules of variable size involving testicular, epididymal, and/or spermatic cord 2. Most metastatic tumors solid without a significant cystic component 3. Tumor is composed of sheets, nests, and acinar structures lined by clear to eosinophilic cells usually with nuclear atypia and prominent nucleoli 4. Only renal cell carcinoma with subnuclear vacuoles is clear cell papillary renal cell carcinoma which to date has not been associated with metastatic behavior 5. Richly vascularized 6. Necrosis and mitotic activity can be variable 7. Intravascular spread may be present
Special studies	• CK7 positive and AMACR negative (Fig. 4.28.6) • CD10 and RCC negative (Fig. 4.28.7) • Not helpful: Positive for cytokeratin AE1/AE3, PAX 8, CAIX (Fig. 4.28.8)	• CK 7 and AMACR negative • CD10 and RCC positive. The only kidney tumor with the same CK7 and CAIX positivity along with CD10 and RCC negativity is clear cell papillary renal cell carcinoma • Not helpful: Positive for cytokeratin AE1/AE3, PAX 8, CAIX
Treatment	Conservative excision	Surgical and systemic therapy directed to primary tumor
Prognosis	Related to vHL syndrome in familial cases	Poor

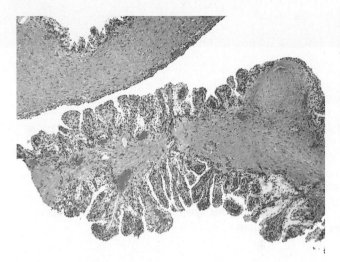

Figure 4.28.1   Papillary cystadenoma of the epididymis with papillary projection into a cyst.

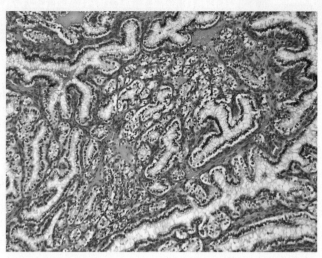

Figure 4.28.2   Papillary cystadenoma of the epididymis with branching tubules.

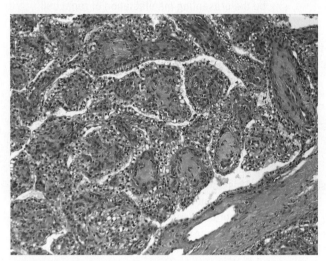

Figure 4.28.3   Papillary cystadenoma of the epididymis with papillary fronds lined by cytologically bland, clear, cuboidal-to-columnar cells.

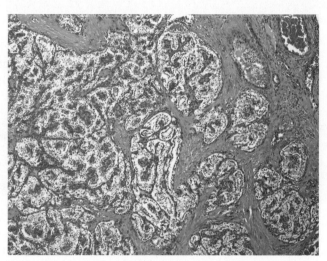

Figure 4.28.4   Papillary cystadenoma of the epididymis with complex tubulopapillary formation.

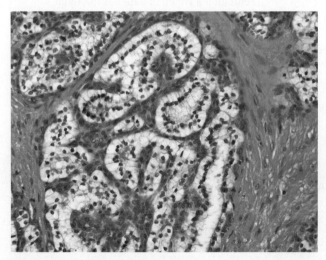

Figure 4.28.5   Papillary cystadenoma of the epididymis with prominent subnuclear vacuoles.

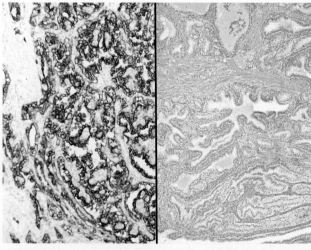

Figure 4.28.6   Papillary cystadenoma of the epididymis with positive CK7 (**left**) and negative AMACR (**right**).

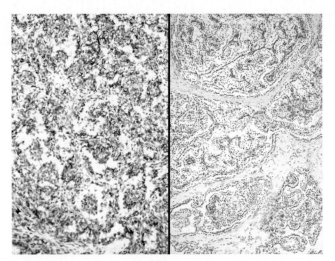

Figure 4.28.7 Papillary cystadenoma of the epididymis with positive CAIX (**left**) and negative CD10 (**right**).

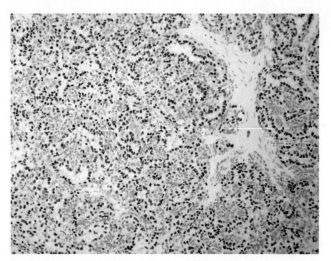

Figure 4.28.8 Papillary cystadenoma of the epididymis with positive PAX8.

	Adenomatoid Tumor of the Epididymis	Metastatic Adenocarcinoma to the Testis and Paratesticular Region
Age	Third through ninth decade (mean age 36 y)	Usually over 50 years old. Can rarely occur at an earlier age
Location	Unilateral	Bilateral in 20% of cases
Symptoms	Asymptomatic	Majority have symptoms due to known primary tumors
Signs	Intrascrotal nodule. On ultrasound, the mass is usually determined to be extratesticular. Most commonly in the epididymis but can also arise in the tunica, rete testis, and spermatic cord	Testicular or paratesticular mass. Majority with signs due to known primary tumors. Only in 6% of cases, spread to the testis is the presenting manifestation
Etiology	Mesothelial origin	Secondary spread through the vas deference (prostate adenocarcinoma), hematogenous (lung), or lymphatic (intestinal primary)
Histology	1. Usually a round-to-oval, well-circumscribed mass <2 cm but can reach 5 cm in size 2. Can focally invade the testis *(Fig. 4.29.1)* 3. Proliferation of eosinophilic focally vacuolated cells arranged in clusters, cords, and tubules *(Figs. 4.29.2–4.29.8)*. When tubules are lined by flattened cells, their appearance may mimic lymphatic structures 4. Lacks significant cytologic atypia 5. Embedded in a dense fibrous to smooth muscle stroma *(Fig. 4.29.7)* 6. In some case, can see central infarction where only a focal viable tumor is seen at the perimeter *(Figs. 4.29.9–4.29.11)* 7. Lacks perineural or intravascular invasion	1. Usually multiple nodules of variable size 2. Involves testicular, epididymal, and/or spermatic cord 3. Sheets, clusters, and glands with variable degree of glandular differentiation. Typical lineage-specific features such as goblet cells; mucinous or eosinophilic secretions, microcribriform structures may offer clue to the primary site *(Fig. 4.29.12)* 4. Significant cytologic atypia is typical although signet ring-cell adenocarcinomas may not be that pleomorphic 5. May have cellular desmoplastic stromal reaction 6. Necrosis may be seen 7. Perineural or intravascular invasion may be seen
Special studies	Calretinin expression in over 80% of cases	Metastatic adenocarcinomas negative for calretinin. Primary cell lineage could be demonstrated by expression of lineage-specific marker (i.e., PSA/NKX3.1/p501S for prostate cancer; TTF-1/napsin for lung, and CDX2 for intestinal origin)

	Adenomatoid Tumor of the Epididymis	**Metastatic Adenocarcinoma to the Testis and Paratesticular Region**
Treatment	If frozen section performed and diagnosed accurately, conservative complete excision can be performed. However, can be seen at radical orchiectomy done for presumed malignant germ cell tumor based on a solid mass involving the testis region	Systemic therapy directed to primary tumor
Prognosis	Excellent	Unless metastatic prostate cancer, prognosis is dismal

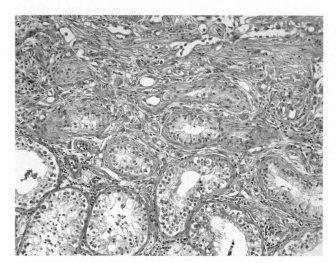

Figure 4.29.1 Adenomatoid tumor focally invading the testis.

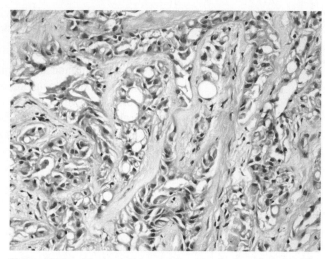

Figure 4.29.2 Adenomatoid tumor with cords of cells with eosinophilic cytoplasm and vacuoles.

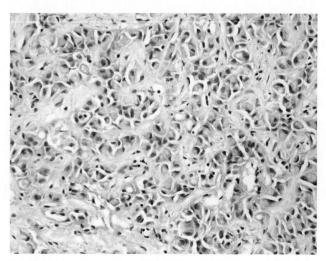

Figure 4.29.3 Same case as Figure 4.29.2 with loosely cohesive cells mimicking a signet ring-cell adenocarcinoma.

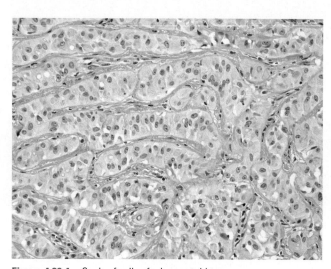

Figure 4.29.4 Cords of cells of adenomatoid tumor.

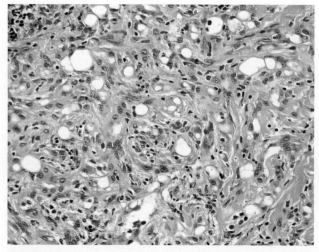

Figure 4.29.5 Adenomatoid tumor mimicking signet ring-cell adenocarcinoma.

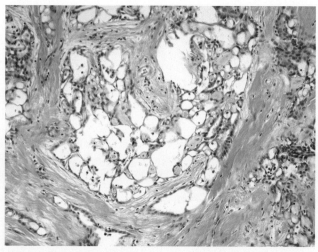

Figure 4.29.6 Adenomatoid tumor with a complex pattern mimicking cribriform carcinoma.

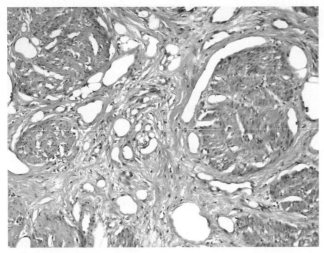

Figure 4.29.7 Adenomatoid tumor with associated smooth muscle hyperplasia.

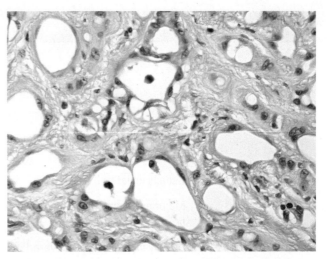

Figure 4.29.8 Same case as Figure 4.29.7 with flattened tubules.

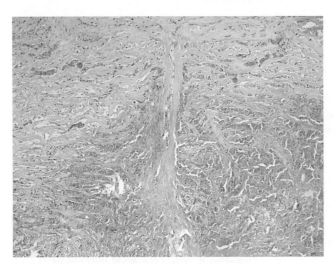

Figure 4.29.9 Adenomatoid tumor with central infarction.

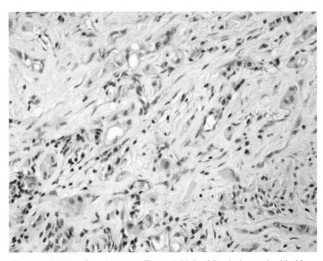

Figure 4.29.10 Same case as Figure 4.29.9 with tubules embedded in fibrous tissue at the edge of necrosis.

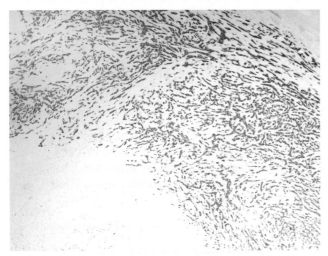

Figure 4.29.11 Same case as Figures 4.29.9 and 4.29.10 with pan-cytokeratin stain highlight the tubules around the central area of necrosis.

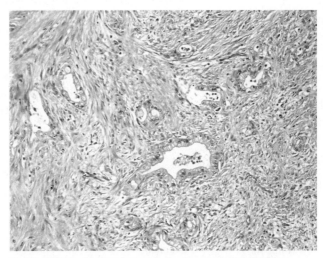

Figure 4.29.12 Metastatic pancreatic adenocarcinoma involving paratesticular tissue. Haphazard glands lined by moderately atypical cells infiltrate desmoplastic stroma.

	Vasitis Nodosa of the Spermatic Cord	Metastatic Adenocarcinoma to the Paratesticular Region
Age	Young adults in third through fifth decades (average age 36 y)	Usually over 50 years old. Can rarely occur at an earlier age
Location	Usually unilateral	Bilateral in 20% of cases
Symptoms	Majority asymptomatic but occasionally present with scrotal pain	Majority has symptoms due to known primary tumors
Signs	Usually incidentally discovered during vasovasostomy procedure. Palpable intrascrotal vas deference nodularity, 5–6 cm above the testis	Testicular or paratesticular mass. Majority with signs due to known primary tumors. Only in 6% of cases spread to the testis is the presenting manifestation
Etiology	Prior vasectomy: typically identified 1–15 y postvasectomy	Secondary spread through the vas deference (prostate adenocarcinoma), hematogenous (lung), or lymphatic (intestinal primary). Prostate is the most common to spread to this site
Histology	1. Usually a single nodule (<1 cm) in the vas deferens wall and or adventitial layer that may exude milky content on the cut section 2. A proliferation of small glands lined by cuboidal cells *(Figs. 4.30.1–4.30.4)* 3. Bland nuclei that may contain conspicuous nucleoli 4. No discernable mitotic activity 5. Benign glands may rarely show perineural and vascular invasion 6. Intraluminal sperms and associated foci of sperm granuloma (up to 70% of cases) are key differentiating features *(Figs. 4.30.5 and 4.30.6)*. Sperm granulomas often have yellow-brown ceroid pigment, which represents a degradation product of sperm	1. Usually multiple nodules of variable size involving testicular, epididymal, and or spermatic cord 2. Sheets and clusters of atypical cells with variable degree of glandular differentiation. Typical lineage-specific features such as goblet cells; mucinous or eosinophilic secretions, microcribriform structures may offer clue to the primary site 3. Typically significant cytologic atypia, yet metastatic prostate cancer may not have prominent atypia *(Figs. 4.30.7 and 4.30.8)* 4. Mitotic activity variable 5. Perineural or intravascular invasion can be seen 6. Neoplastic malignant glands do not contain intraluminal sperms. No associated foci of sperm granuloma are seen
Special studies	Keratin positive but not specific	Metastatic adenocarcinomas' primary cell lineage could be demonstrated by their lineage-specific marker expression (i.e., PSA/NKX3.1/p501S for prostate cancer; TTF-1/napsin for lung, and CDX2 for intestinal)
Treatment	Resection during vasovasostomy	Systemic therapy directed to primary tumor
Prognosis	Excellent	Dismal except for prostate cancer where hormonal therapy can give rise in some cases to prolonged remission

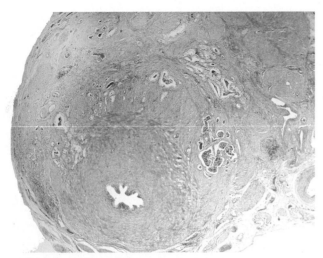

Figure 4.30.1 Vasitis nodosa showing irregular proliferation of tubular structures emanating from the central vas deferens.

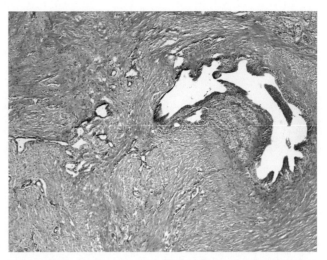

Figure 4.30.2 Vasitis nodosa showing irregular proliferation of tubules from the vas deferens.

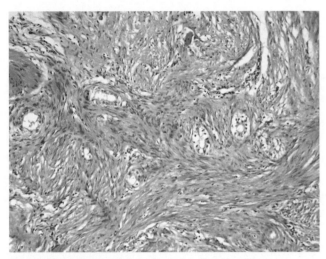

Figure 4.30.3 Ovoid-to-angulated tubules of vasitis nodosa proliferating in smooth muscle.

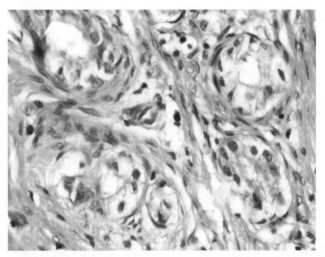

Figure 4.30.4 Vasitis nodosa tubules are lined by bland, cuboidal epithelial cells without nuclear atypia, although nucleoli may be visible.

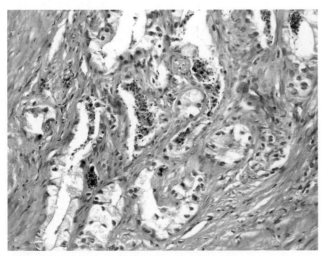

Figure 4.30.5 Vasitis nodosa with intraluminal sperm.

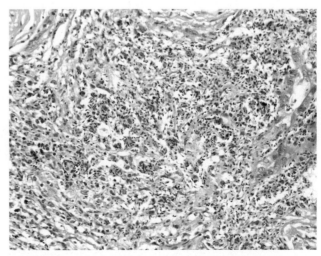

Figure 4.30.6 Same case as Figure 30.5 with sperm granuloma.

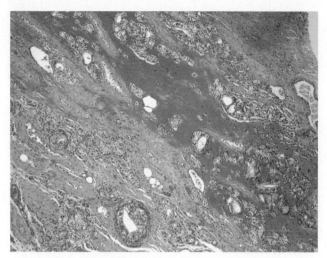

Figure 4.30.7   Metastatic prostatic adenocarcinoma secondarily involving the spermatic cord.

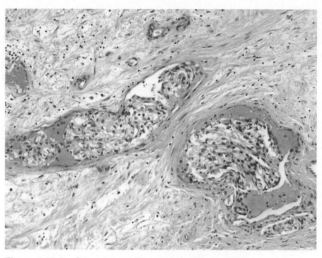

Figure 4.30.8   Same case as Figure 30.7 with prominent lymphovascular invasion.

	Paratesticular Idiopathic Smooth Muscle Hyperplasia	Normal Spermatic Cord
Age	Adults	Adults (in this differential diagnosis)
Location	Unilateral. Spermatic cord or epididymis	Not applicable
Symptoms	Discrete or ill-defined nodules or thickened or enlarged paratesticular structures	None
Signs	None	None
Etiology	Unknown but may be hamartomatous	None
Histology	1. Hyperplastic smooth muscle fascicles around ducts and vessels *(Figs. 4.31.1–4.31.5)* 2. Smooth muscle extends from vessels and ducts into the interstitium 3. Concentric proliferation of smooth muscle around the vas deferens or epididymis 4. Key to diagnosis is looking for an abnormal smooth muscle component to account for a clinical mass or abnormality. Important to diagnose to justify surgery	1. Smooth muscle around ducts and vessels normal thickness 2. Smooth muscle confined to the duct and vessels walls without extension into the interstitium 3. Normal smooth muscle around the vas deferens and epididymis *(Fig. 4.31.6)* 4. In the absence of a clinical abnormality, most likely not idiopathic smooth muscle hyperplasia
Special studies	Not helpful in this differential	Not helpful in this differential
Treatment	Excision	None
Prognosis	Excellent	Normal finding

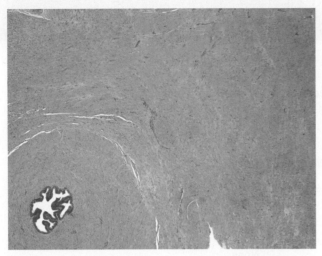

Figure 4.31.1   Paratesticular idiopathic smooth muscle hyperplasia showing marked concentric thickening around the vas deferens by proliferation of smooth muscle.

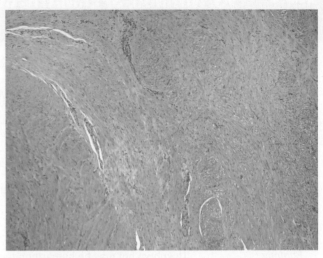

Figure 4.31.2   Same case as Figure 4.31.1 with smooth muscle surrounding the vas deferens.

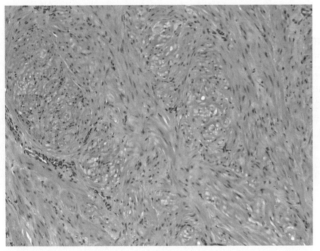

Figure 4.31.3   Same case as Figures 4.31.1 and 4.31.2 showing bland smooth muscle exterior to the vas deferens.

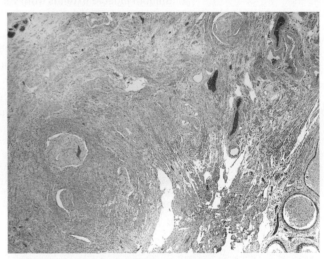

Figure 4.31.4   Paratesticular idiopathic smooth muscle hyperplasia showing proliferation of muscle around vessels.

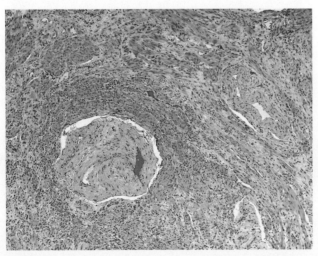

Figure 4.31.5   Higher magnification of same case as Figure 4.31.4.

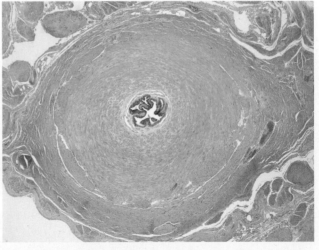

Figure 4.31.6   Normal vas deferens wall. Smooth muscle confined to the duct and vessels walls without extension into the interstitium.

	Mesothelial Hyperplasia in the Hydrocele Sac	Malignant Mesothelioma
Age	Adults	Middle-aged and elderly adults (mean age 53 y)
Location	Unilateral	Unilateral
Symptoms	Related to the associated hydrocele. Scrotal swelling	Related to the often associated hydrocele. Scrotal swelling that is misinterpreted as recurring hydrocele
Signs	Related to the associated hydrocele. Scrotal swelling, inflammatory signs in complicated hydrocele	Related to the associated hydrocele. Scrotal swelling, inflammatory signs. Occasionally, palpable ill-defined intrascrotal firm mass
Etiology	Inflammatory irritation of mesothelial lining by hydrocele content leading to reactive hyperplasia of mesothelial lining of the tunica vaginalis	Asbestos exposure present in 40% of cases
Histology	1. Grossly, no identifiable mass is noted in hydrocele sacs 2. Epithelial proliferation lacking the biphasic spindle cell pattern 3. Architecturally, simple papillary structures, tubules, and nests can be present. Solid areas and broad arborizing complex papillary structures with hyalinized fibrous core are not identified 4. Reactive proliferation remains confined to a sharply demarcated zone immediately underlying the luminal surface. Proliferating mesothelial cells typically form lines that parallel the surface of the hydrocele and fail to penetrate beyond the associated superficial zone of inflammation and fibrosis. Does not invade adipose tissue *(Figs. 4.32.1–4.32.3)* 5. Reactive cells maintain abundant cytoplasm and may contain enlarged vesicular nuclei with brisk mitotic activity in inflamed areas *(Figs. 4.32.4 and 4.32.5)* 6. Do not see invasion into the testis, scrotal tissue, or spermatic cord	1. Tumor grossly coats the tunica vaginalis. Multiple nodules can be identified 2. Approximately three-quarters of cases are epithelial in nature with the remaining cases showing a biphasic pattern 3. Architecturally, broad arborizing complex papillary and tubular structures and nests are present. May see solid areas 4. Although at times predominantly involving surface as exophytic papillary growth, at least focally, a haphazard infiltrative tubular or nested component exists. Tumor often invades adipose tissue *(Figs. 4.32.6–4.32.8)* 5. Cytologically, the neoplastic cells are relatively uniform, cuboidal with only a modest amount of eosinophilic cytoplasm. Occasionally, frank anaplasia may be demonstrated. In biphasic mesothelioma, a spindle cell component is also present 6. Tumor may infiltrate the testis, scrotal tissue, and spermatic cord connective tissue in advanced cases

	Mesothelial Hyperplasia in the Hydrocele Sac	**Malignant Mesothelioma**
Special studies	Not helpful in this differential. Glut1 is more likely to be positive in malignant mesothelioma (up to 50% of cases) compared to reactive mesothelial hyperplasia (up to 27%) but is of limited practical utility	Not helpful in this differential
Treatment	Hydrocele repair encompassing the hyperplastic lesion	Stage dependent. Radical orchiectomy with chemotherapy in metastatic setting. When skin invasion present, hemiscrotectomy is needed
Prognosis	Excellent	Overall poor with approximately half of the patients dying of disease within 2 y from diagnosis. Prognosis is significantly impacted by the extent of disease. When limited to the hydrocele sac, outcome is significantly improved with majority of patients found free of disease at 2 y follow-up in one series. Invasion into the spermatic cord, testis, or skin portends a dismal outcome with almost no survival beyond 2 y following diagnosis

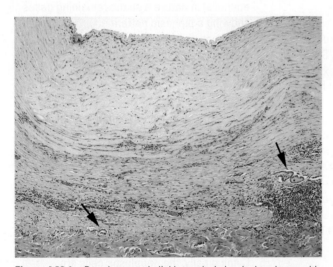

Figure 4.32.1   Reactive mesothelial hyperplasia in a hydrocele sac with proliferation of tubules (*arrows*) at interface between inflamed fibrous tissue and underlying muscle.

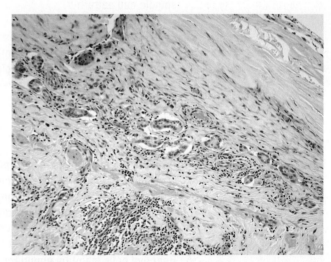

Figure 4.32.2   Same case as Figure 4.32.1 with linear mesothelial tubular proliferation.

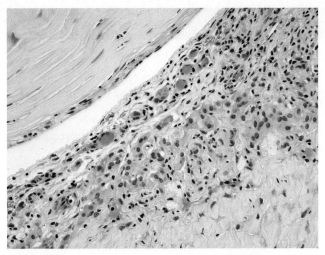

Figure 4.32.3 Reactive mesothelial hyperplasia with tubules in loose, inflamed connective tissue as opposed to infiltrating the dense acellular fibrous tissue (*top*).

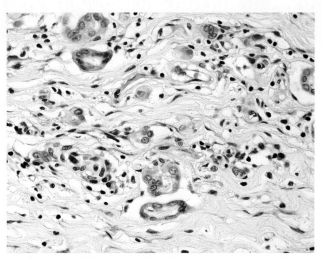

Figure 4.32.4 Reactive tubular mesothelial proliferation with hemosiderin deposition.

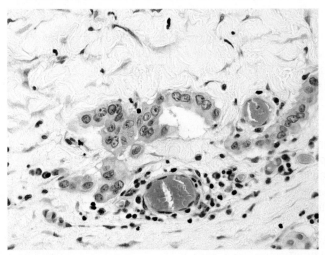

Figure 4.32.5 Reactive tubular mesothelial proliferation with visible nucleoli.

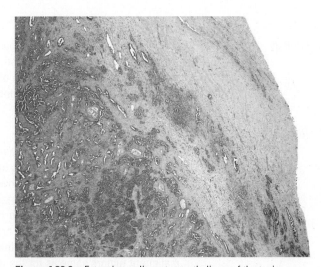

Figure 4.32.6 Extensive malignant mesothelioma of the tunica vaginalis.

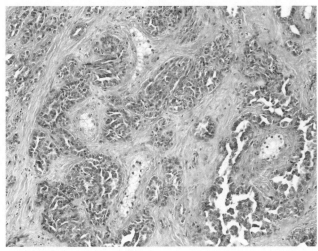

Figure 4.32.7 Same case as Figure 4.32.6 with complex tubulopapillary structures.

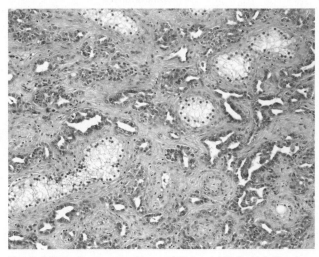

Figure 4.32.8 Same case as Figures 4.32.6 and 4.32.7 with infiltration into the testicular parenchyma.

	Paratesticular Müllerian Tumors	Metastatic Adenocarcinoma to the Testis and Paratesticular Region
Age	Mean age for paratesticular serous carcinoma is 31 y (16–42 y); 56 y for borderline serous tumors (14–77 y), and 52 y for mucinous tumors (11–69 y)	Usually over 50 years old. Can rarely occur at an earlier age
Location	Usually unilateral	Bilateral in 20% of cases
Symptoms	Dull scrotal pain and swelling	Majority have symptoms due to known primary tumors
Signs	Palpable scrotal mass with associated hydrocele. CA-125 levels may be elevated	Testicular or paratesticular mass. Majority with signs due to known primary tumors. Only in 6% of cases, spread to the testis is the presenting manifestation
Etiology	Plausible histogenesis theories for ovarian-type epithelial tumors of the paratesticular region include müllerian metaplasia of the tunica vaginalis and origin from müllerian rests	Secondary spread through the vas deference (prostate adenocarcinoma), hematogenous (lung), or lymphatic (intestinal primary)
Histology	1. The entire spectrum of histologic cell types seen in the ovary has been described. Serous and mucinous tumors of mostly borderline type are followed in frequency by endometrioid, clear cell, and transitional (Brenner) tumors. Morphologic criteria for ovarian counterparts are used. Criteria for benign, borderline, and malignant tumors same as for the ovary *(Figs. 4.33.1–4.33.7)* 2. May contain a large cystic borderline component 3. Lacks other history of tumors 4. Lacks lymphovascular invasion	1. Typical lineage-specific features such as goblet cells; mucinous or eosinophilic secretions, microcribriform structures may offer clue to primary site *(Figs. 4.33.8–4.33.10).* 2. Lacks a large cystic borderline component 3. Often the presence of clinical history of a primary tumor 4. Frequent presence of lymphovascular invasion
Special studies	Most CK7 positive	Appendiceal and metastatic colonic tumors are frequently CK7 negative. Primary cell lineage could be demonstrated by their specific marker expression (i.e., PSA/NKX3.1/p501S for prostate cancer; TTF-1/napsin for lung, and CDX2 for intestinal)
Treatment	Orchiectomy. Systemic therapy in metastatic setting	Systemic chemotherapy directed to primary tumor

	Paratesticular Müllerian Tumors	Metastatic Adenocarcinoma to the Testis and Paratesticular Region
Prognosis	The prognosis is usually excellent for completely excised borderline serous tumors. Papillary serous carcinomas are capable of recurrence and distant metastasis. Mucinous cystadenomas and mucinous tumors of borderline malignancy have demonstrated excellent prognosis including cases with microinvasion or *in situ* carcinoma. Invasive mucinous carcinoma has the potential for peritoneal spread and associated mortality	Dismal except for prostate cancer where hormonal therapy can give rise in some cases to prolonged remission

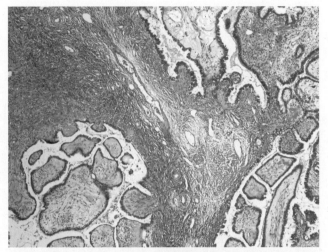

Figure 4.33.1 Müllerian-type paratesticular neoplasm equivalent to serous cystadenoma of the ovary.

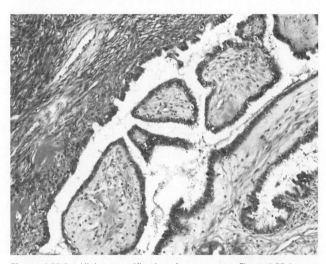

Figure 4.33.2 Higher magnification of same case as Figure 4.33.1.

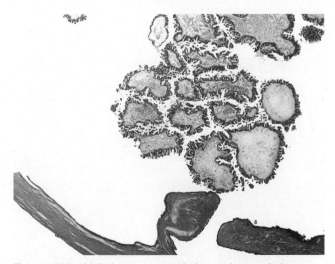

Figure 4.33.3 Müllerian-type paratesticular neoplasm equivalent to papillary serous neoplasm of borderline malignant potential of the ovary.

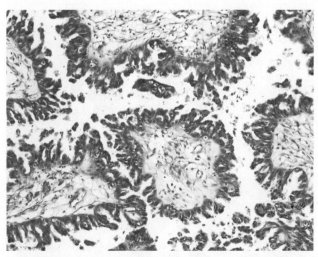

Figure 4.33.4 Higher magnification of same case as Figure 4.33.3.

4 TESTIS

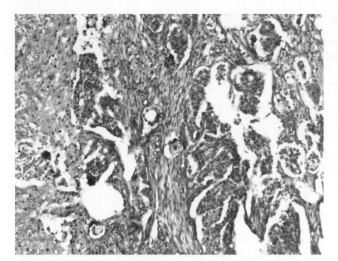

Figure 4.33.5 Müllerian-type paratesticular neoplasm equivalent to invasive papillary serous carcinoma of the ovary is shown.

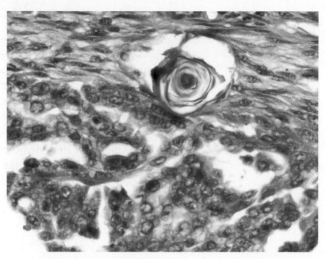

Figure 4.33.6 Higher magnification of same case as figure 4.33.5.

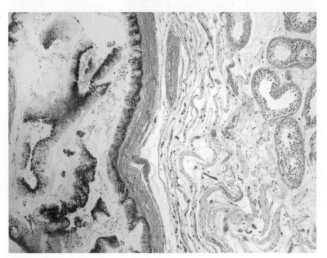

Figure 4.33.7 Müllerian-type paratesticular neoplasm equivalent to papillary mucinous neoplasm of borderline malignant potential of the ovary.

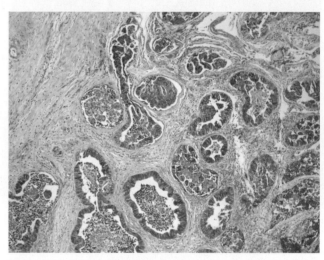

Figure 4.33.8 Metastatic colonic adenocarcinoma involving paratesticular and testicular tissue.

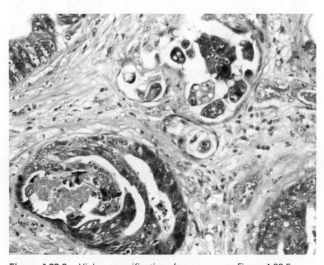

Figure 4.33.9 Higher magnification of same case as Figure 4.33.5.

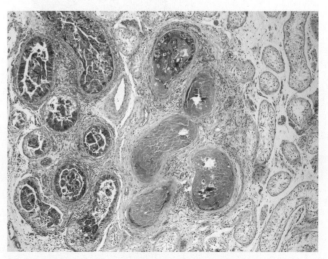

Figure 4.33.10 Same case as Figures 4.33.8 and 4.33.9 with colon carcinoma involving seminiferous tubules.

	Well-Differentiated Papillary Mesothelioma	Malignant Mesothelioma
Age	Usually young men in their second and third decades of life	Middle-aged and elderly adults (mean age 50–60s). Rarely, can be seen in children
Location	Unilateral	Unilateral
Symptoms	Related to the associated hydrocele. Scrotal swelling	Related to the associated hydrocele. Scrotal swelling that is misinterpreted as recurring hydrocele
Signs	Related to the associated hydrocele. Scrotal swelling, inflammatory sign. Occasionally an ill-defined intrascrotal mass could be palpable	Related to the associated hydrocele. Scrotal swelling, inflammatory signs. Occasionally, palpable ill-defined intrascrotal firm mass
Etiology	Unknown	Asbestos exposure present in 40% of cases
Histology	1. Single or multiple nodules can be identified in the tunica vaginalis (up to 2cm) 2. Tumor is composed of simple papillary structures lined by a single layer of cuboidal cells (Figs. 4.34.1–4.34.3). Cases with minimally more complex papillary architecture with a tubular component, focal fusion of papillae with stratification of lining cells, and focal cribriform formations have been recently designated as well-differentiated papillary mesothelioma of borderline malignant potential (Figs. 4.34.4–4.34.7) 3. Invasion is not present 4. Cytologically, the cells are bland, relatively uniform with only a modest amount of eosinophilic cytoplasm. Mitotic figures are rare if any 5. Tumors are pure epithelial without a biphasic component	1. Tumor grossly coats the tunica vaginalis. Multiple nodules can be identified 2. Architecturally, broad arborizing complex papillary and tubular structures and nests are present (Figs. 4.34.8 and 4.34.9). The papillary structures contain hyalinized fibrous cores 3. Although at times predominantly involving surface as exophytic papillary growth, at least focally, an infiltrative tubular or nested component exists. Tumor may infiltrate the testis, scrotal tissue, and spermatic cord connective tissue in advanced cases (Fig. 4.34.10) 4. Cytologically, the neoplastic cells are relatively uniform cuboidal with only a modest amount of eosinophilic cytoplasm. Occasionally, frank anaplasia may be demonstrated. Mitoses can be frequent 5. Approximately three-quarters of cases are epithelial in nature with the remaining cases maintaining a biphasic pattern
Special studies	Ki67 index typically <1%.	Ki67 index averages 25%.
Treatment	Hydrocelectomy	Stage dependent. Radical orchiectomy with chemotherapy in metastatic setting. When skin invasion present, hemiscrotectomy is needed

	Well-Differentiated Papillary Mesothelioma	**Malignant Mesothelioma**
Prognosis	Well-differentiated papillary mesothelioma behaves in a benign fashion but can recur or be multifocal. Well-differentiated papillary mesothelioma of borderline malignant potential has so far also behaved in a benign fashion but experience is limited	Overall poor with approximately half of the patients dying of their disease within 2 y of diagnosis. Prognosis is significantly impacted by the extent of disease. When limited to the hydrocele sac, outcome is significantly improved with majority of cases found to be free of disease at 2 y follow-up in one series. Invasion into the spermatic cord, testis, or skin portends a dismal outcome with almost no survival expected beyond 2 y from diagnosis

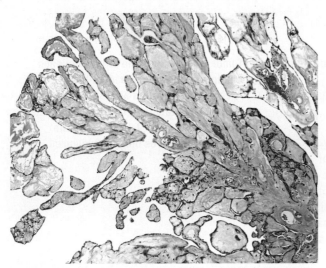

Figure 4.34.1   Well-differentiated papillary mesothelioma composed of simple papillary structures lined by a single layer of cuboidal cells.

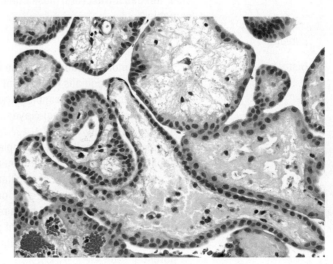

Figure 4.34.2   Same case as Figure 4.34.1.

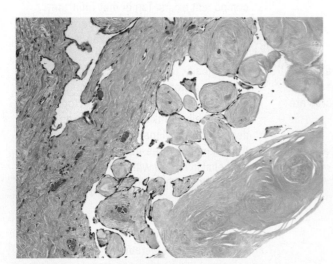

Figure 4.34.3   Well-differentiated papillary mesothelioma.

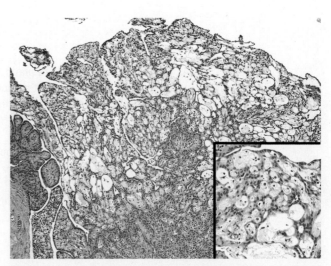

Figure 4.34.4   Well-differentiated papillary mesothelioma of borderline malignant potential with greater architectural complexity but still bland cytology and no invasion.

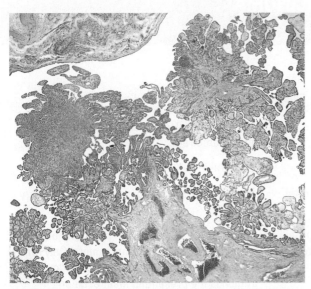

Figure 4.34.5   Well-differentiated papillary mesothelioma of borderline malignant potential.

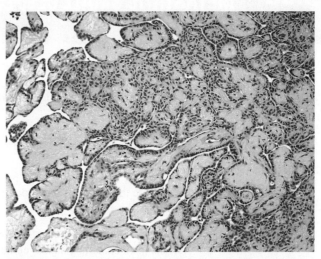

Figure 4.34.6   Same case as Figure 4.34.5. Areas are indistinguishable from well-differentiated papillary mesothelioma, and other areas are more solid.

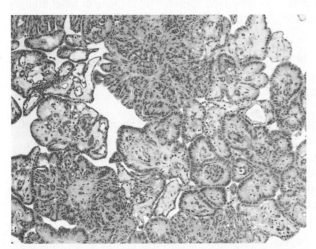

Figure 4.34.7   Well-differentiated papillary mesothelioma of borderline malignant potential with areas indistinguishable from well-differentiated papillary mesothelioma (*right*) and other areas are more complex architecturally (*top*).

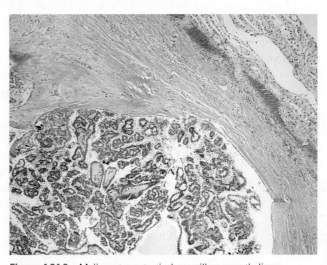

Figure 4.34.8   Malignant paratesticular papillary mesothelioma.

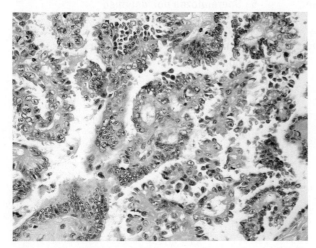

Figure 4.34.9   Higher magnification of same case as Figure 4.34.8 with overt malignant cytology.

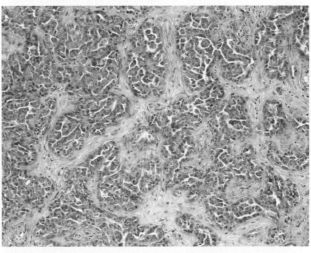

Figure 4.34.10   Malignant paratesticular papillary mesothelioma with complex tubulopapillary structures infiltrating the underling connective tissue.

4   TESTIS

	Shed Rete Testis Cells in the Hydrocele Sac	Metastatic Small Cell Carcinoma
Age	Adults	Usually over 50 years old but can rarely occur at an earlier age
Location	Unilateral	Bilateral in 20% of cases
Symptoms	Related to the associated hydrocele. Scrotal swelling	Majority has symptoms due to known primary tumors
Signs	Related to the associated hydrocele. Scrotal swelling, inflammatory sign in complicated hydrocele	Testicular or paratesticular mass. Majority with signs due to known primary tumors. Only rarely, tumor spread to the testis or paratesticular region is the presenting manifestation
Etiology	Shedding of rete testis cells with the associated artifactual change. In cases with spermatozoa, indicates that the epididymis has been nicked at surgery	Secondary spread through hematogenous or lymphatic spread from the lung or other primary sites
Histology	1. Grossly, no identifiable mass is noted in associated the hydrocele or spermatocele sacs. Reactive mesothelial proliferation may be present 2. Detached small "blue" cell clusters with focal nuclear streaming. Although the cells have bland nuclear morphology and are devoid of prominent nucleoli, the high nuclear-to-cytoplasmic ratios and hyperchromatic nature of their nuclei may raise the suspicion for small cell carcinoma (Figs. 4.35.1–4.35.5) 3. Small scattered foci 4. No mitotic figures, apoptotic bodies, or necrosis are identifiable. Clusters do not occupy lymphovascular spaces 5. Associated spermatozoa often present, although can be focal	1. Usually multiple nodules of variable size involving testicular, epididymal, and/or spermatic cord 2. Tumor composed of sheets and clusters of small-sized atypical "blue" cells with only rare prominent nucleoli. Characteristic high nuclear-to-cytoplasmic ratios and hyperchromatic molded nuclei with a typical smudgy chromatin pattern are displayed 3. Typically extensive tumor 4. Typically, very brisk mitotic activity, apoptosis, and extensive necrosis. Extensive intravascular spread is spread 5. Spermatozoa not identified
Special Studies	• Synaptophysin and chromogranin negative • CD56 is usually positive (Fig. 4.35.6) • Ki-67 index is <1%	• Synaptophysin and chromogranin usually positive • CD56 positive • Ki67 typically >50%
Treatment	Incidentally found in hydrocele or spermatocele repair	Systemic chemotherapy directed to primary tumor.
Prognosis	Excellent	Dismal

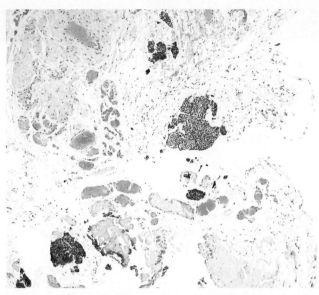

Figure 4.35.1 Detached clusters of rete testis cells acquiring a "small blue" cell morphology.

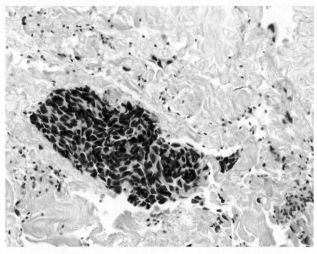

Figure 4.35.2 Small blue cells of the rete testis associated with numerous spermatozoa.

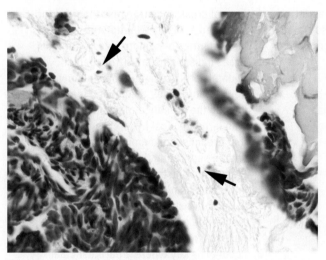

Figure 4.35.3 Crushed shed rete testis cells with rare spermatozoa (*arrows*).

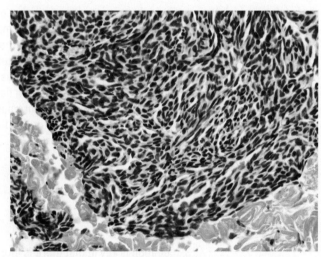

Figure 4.35.4 Rete testis cells in a hydrocele sac. Despite a high nuclear-to-cytoplasmic ratio, there are no mitoses or apoptotic bodies.

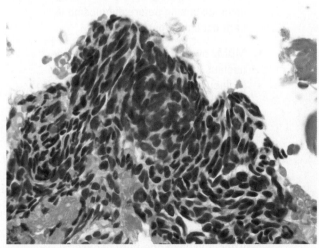

Figure 4.35.5 Crushed shed rete testis cells with bland cytology.

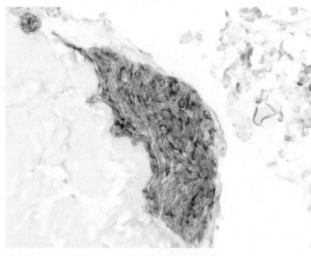

Figure 4.35.6 Shed rete testis cells stain for CD56.

4 TESTIS

	Paratesticular Lipoma	**Well-Differentiated Liposarcoma**
Age	Majority occur in adults	Majority occur in adults with a mean age of 56 y (16–90 y)
Location	Unilateral	Unilateral
Symptoms	Scrotal swelling	Scrotal swelling
Signs	Intrascrotal lobulated soft mass typically located in the upper portion of the spermatic cord, although uncommonly seen at the distal cord	Located at the base of the spermatic cord immediately adjacent to the testis. Average size 12 cm (3–30 cm)
Etiology	Some "lipomas" represent lipomatous hyperplasia of paratesticular soft tissue or just pulling down of fat in an inguinal hernia rather than true neoplasms	Unknown
Histology	1. Typical gross appearance is that of a soft lobulated, variably well-defined mass lacking areas of hemorrhage or necrosis 2. Sheets of uniform-sized adipocytes separated by thin acellular fibrous septae. The adipocytes contain flat-to-ovoid nuclei without hyperchromasia, nuclear irregularity, or mitotic activity *(Figs. 4.36.1–4.36.4)* 3. Location is key in that there is low suspicion for liposarcoma if the lesion is located in the upper inguinal region	1. Typical gross appearance is that of a soft lobulated, variably well-defined mass lacking areas of hemorrhage or necrosis 2. Areas indistinguishable from benign counterparts are not uncommon on low-power microscopy. Diagnostic features include the presence of adipose cells with large atypical hyperchromatic nuclei that are most commonly seen in fibrous septae separating the fat *(Figs. 4.36.5–4.36.8).* Classic lipoblasts with indentation by intracytoplasmic lipid vacuoles leading to a characteristic scalloping of the nuclear membrane are not always seen and not necessary for the diagnosis 3. Location is key where a paratesticular adipose lesion should be presumed to be liposarcoma with extensive sampling to look for atypical cells or do MDM2 immunostaining before diagnosing a paratesticular lipoma
Special studies	• MDM2 staining is negative • No molecular features of liposarcoma	• MDM2 overexpression yet not in every nucleus • Molecular cytogenetics: giant marker/ring chromosomes harboring amplification of the MDM2 gene region (12q13-15) are identifiable on FISH in well-differentiated liposarcoma
Treatment	Conservative lesional excision	Conservative complete excision, yet if large and adjacent to testis, typically radical orchiectomy performed
Prognosis	Benign	Favorable upon complete excision. Recurrence may occur in up to one-third of cases

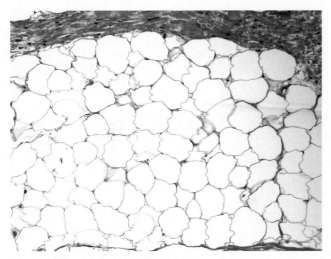

Figure 4.36.1   Spermatic cord lipoma.

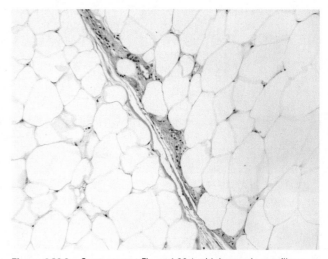

Figure 4.36.2   Same case as Figure 4.36.1 with inconspicuous fibrous septa.

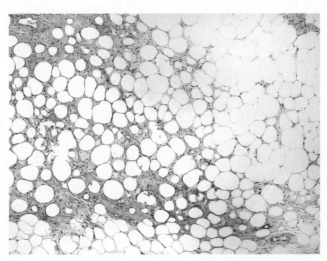

Figure 4.36.3   Spermatic cord lipoma showing focal fat necrosis and histiocytic reaction.

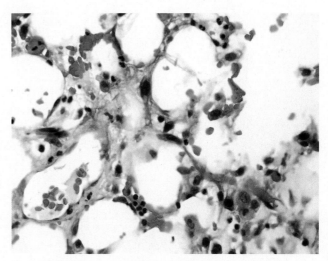

Figure 4.36.4   Same case as Figure 4.36.3 with cells with slightly enlarged nuclei in area of fat necrosis.

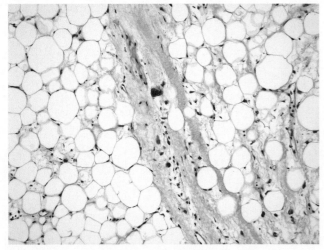

Figure 4.36.5   Well-differentiated liposarcoma of the paratesticular region. Scattered cells with markedly enlarged hyperchromatic nuclei within fibrous septae.

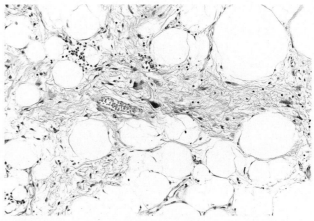

Figure 4.36.6   Paratesticular well-differentiated liposarcoma with scattered, markedly enlarged hyperchromatic nuclei within fibrous septae.

4   TESTIS

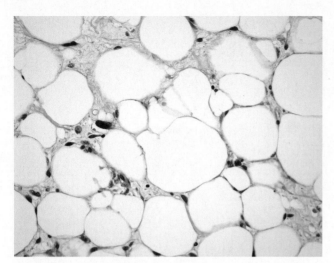

Figure 4.36.7 Paratesticular well-differentiated liposarcoma with scattered, enlarged, hyperchromatic nuclei within adipose tissue.

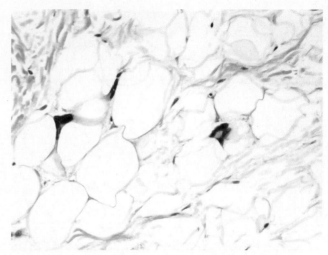

Figure 4.36.8 Paratesticular well-differentiated liposarcoma with scattered, enlarged, hyperchromatic nuclei within adipose tissue.

	Paratesticular Dedifferentiated Liposarcoma	Nonlipomatous Sarcomas
Age	Majority occur in older adults	Majority occur in older adults
Location	Unilateral	Unilateral
Symptoms	Recent enlargement of a long-standing scrotal mass	Recent enlargement of a long-standing scrotal mass
Signs	Intrascrotal firm mass with ill-defined borders. Mean size 11.5 cm (2–30 cm)	Intrascrotal firm mass with ill-defined borders. Typically large
Etiology	Dedifferentiation of well-differentiated liposarcoma (Fig. 4.37.1)	Most common paratesticular sarcoma is leiomyosarcoma
Histology	1. Most common high-grade dedifferentiated liposarcoma patterns are spindle cell NOS and malignant fibrous histiocytoma-like (Figs. 4.37.2 and 4.37.3). Other patterns include inflammatory MFH-like, myxoid, and round cell (Fig. 4.37.4). Leiomyosarcomatous and osteoid differentiation may be seen in high-grade and low-grade dedifferentiated liposarcoma (Fig. 4.37.5). Low-grade component resembling fibromatosis can be seen in high-grade dedifferentiated liposarcoma (Fig. 4.37.6) 2. Key is identifying a well-differentiated liposarcoma component. In the setting of a paratesticular pleomorphic sarcoma that is not classic in its entirely for a leiomyosarcoma, the presumption is that the tumor is a dedifferentiated liposarcoma. Areas of grossly normal fat next to the high-grade sarcoma should be thoroughly sampled to look for a low-grade component	1. Leiomyosarcoma consists of long fascicles cut in both parallel and perpendicular planes. In the vast majority of cases, even when high grade, this architecture is maintained (Figs. 4.37.9 and 4.37.10). Focal leiomyosarcomatous differentiation in a pleomorphic sarcoma is not diagnostic of leiomyosarcoma 2. If the entire lesion looks classic for leiomyosarcoma, then not necessary to extensively sample adjacent adipose tissue
Special studies	Over 90% are positive by FISH or immunohistochemistry for MDM2, with greater positivity in higher-grade dedifferentiated components (Figs. 4.37.7 and 4.37.8)	While leiomyosarcomas are negative for MDM2 in 90% of cases, approximately 40–50% of pleomorphic sarcomas also contain MDM2 amplification
Treatment	Surgical with systemic chemotherapy and or radiation	Surgical with possible systemic chemotherapy and/or radiation for high-grade lesions
Prognosis	In the largest series of 25 cases, 4 developed local recurrence, 1 local recurrence and clinical lymph node metastases, 1 systemic metastases, and 1 presented with a 15-y history of paratesticular liposarcoma and widespread metastases	Local recurrence or metastatic disease is dependent on stage and tumor grade

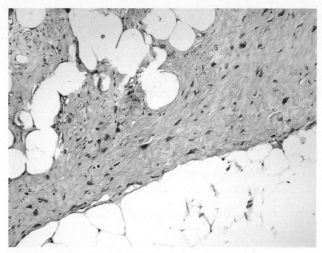

Figure 4.37.1   A well-differentiated liposarcoma component of dedifferentiated liposarcoma of the paratesticular region.

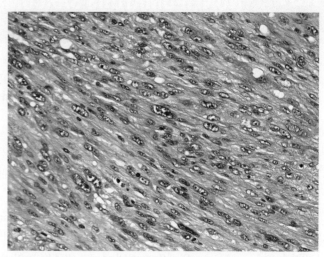

Figure 4.37.2   Spindle cell high-grade dedifferentiated liposarcoma.

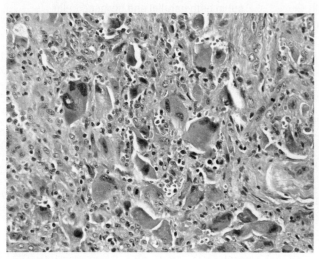

Figure 4.37.3   Malignant fibrous histiocytoma (MFH)-like high-grade dedifferentiated liposarcoma.

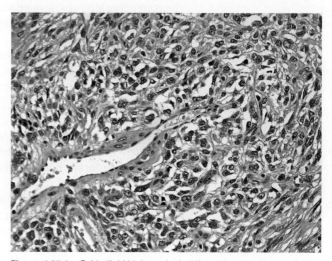

Figure 4.37.4   Epithelioid high-grade dedifferentiated liposarcoma.

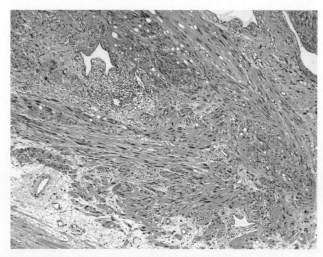

Figure 4.37.5   Focus of low-grade leiomyosarcoma in case with dedifferentiated liposarcoma elsewhere.

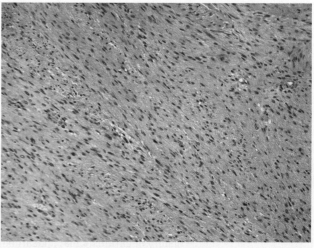

Figure 4.37.6   Fibromatosis-like low-grade dedifferentiated liposarcoma with increased cellularity yet minimal cytologic atypia.

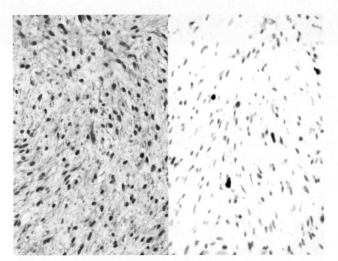

Figure 4.37.7   Scant MDM2-positive cells in low-grade dedifferentiated liposarcoma.

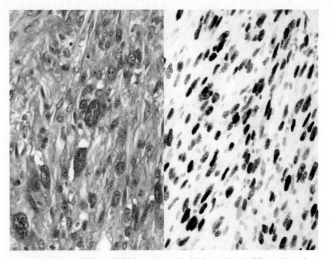

Figure 4.37.8   Diffuse MDM2 staining in high-grade dedifferentiated liposarcoma.

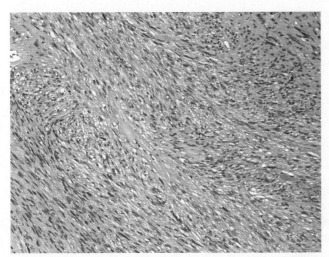

Figure 4.37.9   Leiomyosarcoma with uniform fascicles with increased cellularity containing scattered hyperchromatic nuclei seen even at lower magnification.

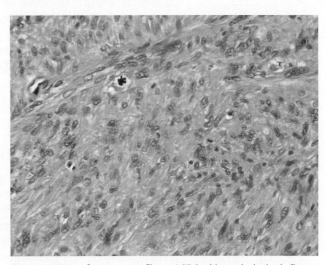

Figure 4.37.10   Same case as Figure 4.37.9 with atypical mitotic figure.

	Paratesticular Spindle Cell Rhabdomyosarcoma	Paratesticular Leiomyosarcoma
Age	Majority occur in children with mean age of 6.6 y. Only rarely in adults	Majority in men over 40 years old but can rarely occur at an earlier age
Location	Unilateral, usually in the spermatic cord	Unilateral, in the spermatic cord (80% of cases) or epididymis
Symptoms	Scrotal swelling	Scrotal swelling
Signs	Intrascrotal firm mass	Intrascrotal firm mass
Histology	1. Composed of elongated fusiform cells with light eosinophilic fibrillar cytoplasm at times arranged in fascicles, although not as prominent as in leiomyosarcoma *(Figs. 4.38.1–4.38.3)* 2. Spindle cell variant of rhabdomyosarcoma lacks necrosis. Cellularity and mitotic activity are variable. 3. Almost always a component of more conventional embryonal rhabdomyosarcoma morphology is present, characterized by the presence of primitive ovoid-to-elongate cells with uniform hyperchromatic nuclei imparting a "small blue cell" impression. Embryonal cells typically contain intense eosinophilic cytoplasm at times signaling a "rhabdoid" look. Myxoid areas are also present in the embryonal portions of the tumor	1. Fascicles of spindle cells with areas of perpendicular orientation 2. Cigar-shaped nuclei with variable degree of atypia and pleomorphism. Intracytoplasmic vacuoles may indent the pole of the ovoid nucleus. Mitotic figures are identifiable with variable frequency depending on grade *(Figs. 4.38.5 and 4.38.6)* 3. Lacks "small blue cell areas" and lacks "rhabdoid" morphology
Special studies	Positive for, myoglobin, myogenin, and MyoD1 *(Fig. 4.38.4)*	Negative for, myoglobin, myogenin, and MyoD1.
Treatment	Orchiectomy and systemic chemotherapy	Orchiectomy and systemic chemotherapy
Prognosis	One-third of paratesticular rhabdomyosarcoma patients will die of metastatic disease. The prognosis in the spindle cell variant is more favorable	Local recurrence and metastatic disease are grade dependent. One-third of patients die of metastatic disease

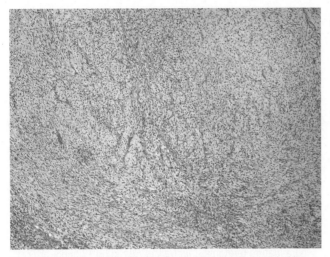

Figure 4.38.1   Paratesticular spindle cell rhabdomyosarcoma lacking the well-formed fascicles of leiomyosarcoma.

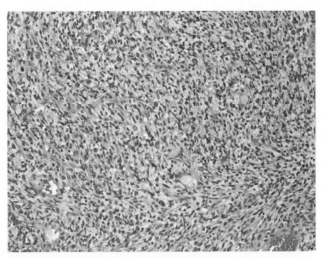

Figure 4.38.2   Same case as Figure 4.38.1 composed of elongated fusiform cells with light eosinophilic fibrillar cytoplasm.

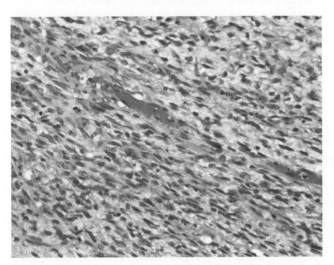

Figure 4.38.3   Same case as Figures 4.38.1–4.38.2 at higher magnification.

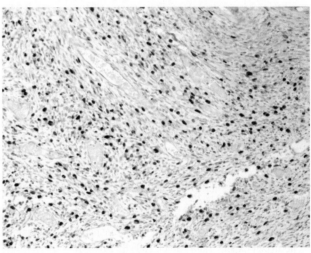

Figure 4.38.4   Same case as Figures 4.38.1–4.38.3 with myogenin positivity.

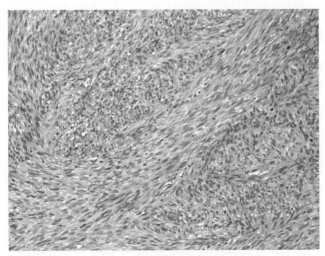

Figure 4.38.5   Paratesticular leiomyosarcoma consisting of long fascicles cut in both parallel and perpendicular planes.

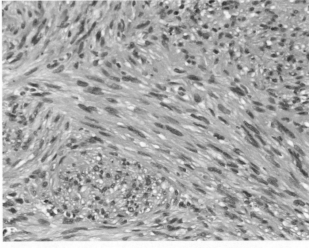

Figure 4.38.6   Same case as Figure 4.38.5 with cigar-shaped nuclei and moderate atypia.

SUGGESTED READINGS

4.1–4.4

Emerson RE, Ulbright TM. Intratubular germ cell neoplasia of the testis and its associated cancers: the use of novel biomarkers. *Pathology.* 2010;42:344–355.

Jones TD, Ulbright TM, Eble JN, et al. OCT4 staining in testicular tumors: a sensitive and specific marker for seminoma and embryonal carcinoma. *Am J Surg Pathol.* 2004;28:935–940.

Jones TD, Ulbright TM, Eble JN, et al. OCT4: a sensitive and specific biomarker for intratubular germ cell neoplasia of the testis. *Clin Cancer Res.* 2004;10:8544–8547.

Mannuel HD, Mitikiri N, Khan M, et al. Testicular germ cell tumors: biology and clinical update. *Curr Opin Oncol.* 2012;24:266–271.

4.5–4.7

Cao D, Guo S, Allan RW, et al. SALL4 is a novel sensitive and specific marker of ovarian primitive germ cell tumors and is particularly useful in distinguishing yolk sac tumor from clear cell carcinoma. *Am J Surg Pathol.* 2009;33:894–904.

Cools M, van Aerde K, Kersemaekers AM, et al. Morphological and immunohistochemical differences between gonadal maturation delay and early germ cell neoplasia in patients with undervirilization syndromes. *J Clin Endocrinol Metab.* 2005;90:5295–5303.

Eble JN, Sauter G, Epstein JI, et al. *Pathology and Genetics of Tumours of the Urinary System and Male Genital Organs.* Lyon, France: IARC Press; 2004.

Fan R, Ulbright TM. Does intratubular germ cell neoplasia, unclassified type exist in prepubertal, cryptorchid testes? *Fetal Pediatr Pathol.* 2012;31:21–24.

Iczkowski KA, Butler SL, Shanks JH, et al. Trials of new germ cell immunohistochemical stains in 93 extragonadal and metastatic germ cell tumors. *Hum Pathol.* 2008;39:275–281.

Nikolaou M, Valavanis C, Aravantinos G, et al. Kit expression in male germ cell tumors. *Anticancer Res.* 2007;27:1685–1688.

Ulbright T, Amin M, Young R. *Tumors of Testis, Adnexa, Spermatic Cord and Scrotum: Atlas of Tumor Pathology.* Armed Forces Institute of Pathology. Washington DC: IARC Press; 1999.

Wein AJ, Kavoussi LR, Novick AC, et al. *Campbell-walsh Urology.* Philadelphia, PA: Saunders; 2012.

4.8–4.10

Decaussin M, Borda A, Bouvier R, et al. Spermatocytic seminoma. A clinicopathological and immunohistochemical study of 7 cases. *Ann Pathol.* 2004;24:161–166.

Ulbright TM, Young RH. Seminoma with tubular, microcystic, and related patterns: a study of 28 cases of unusual morphologic variants that often cause confusion with yolk sac tumor. *Am J Surg Pathol.* 2005;29:500–505.

4.11–4.17

Cheng L, Zhang S, MacLennan GT, et al. Interphase fluorescence *in situ* hybridization analysis of chromosome 12p abnormalities is useful for distinguishing epidermoid cysts of the testis from pure mature teratoma. *Clin Cancer Res.* 2006;12:5668–5672.

Reuter VE. Origins and molecular biology of testicular germ cell tumors. *Mod Pathol.* 2005;18(suppl 2):S51–S60.

Sandberg AA, Meloni AM, Suijkerbuijk RF. Reviews of chromosome studies in urological tumors. III. Cytogenetics and genes in testicular tumors. *J Urol.* 1996;155:1531–1556.

Ulbright TM. Germ cell tumors of the gonads: a selective review emphasizing problems in differential diagnosis, newly appreciated, and controversial issues. *Mod Pathol.* 2005;18(suppl 2): S61–S79.

Ulbright TM. Testis risk and prognostic factors. The pathologist's perspective. *Urol Clin North Am.* 1999;26:611–626.

Ulbright TM. The most common, clinically significant misdiagnoses in testicular tumor pathology, and how to avoid them. *Adv Anat Pathol.* 2008;15:18–27.

4.18–4.38

Gordon MD, Corless C, Renshaw AA, et al. CD99, keratin, and vimentin staining of sex cord-stromal tumors, normal ovary, and testis. *Mod Pathol.* 1998;11:769–773.

Iczkowski KA, Bostwick DG, Roche PC, et al. Inhibin A is a sensitive and specific marker for testicular sex cord-stromal tumors. *Mod Pathol.* 1998;11:774–779.

Young RH, Koelliker DD, Scully RE. Sertoli cell tumors of the testis, not otherwise specified: a clinicopathologic analysis of 60 cases. *Am J Surg Pathol.* 1998;22:709–721.

5

Penis/Scrotum

	Extramammary Paget Disease	High-Grade Penile Intraepithelial Neoplasia (PeIN)
Age	Adults. Sixth to eighth decades	Younger adults
Location	Scrotum and scrotal penile junction most common locations	Shaft, glans, and perimeatal region
Symptoms	Pruritus, pain	None
Signs	Erythematous, eczematous, or ulcerated plaque-like lesion with well-defined borders	Flat to slightly raised plaque
Etiology	Unknown in majority of cases. Occasionally arise in association with underlying colorectal, urogenital, or skin adnexal carcinoma	High-risk HPV related to undifferentiated (basaloid) PeIN (most cases) and differentiated PeIN (~50% of cases)
Histology	1. Scattered more loosely cohesive atypical cells and cell clusters with abundant pale vacuolated cytoplasm in a background of normal epithelial cells *(Figs. 5.1.1 and 5.1.2)* 2. Nuclei large vesicular with prominent nucleoli 3. Vacuolated pale cytoplasm with mucinous material occasionally discernible 4. Many suprabasally located and separated from basement membranes by normal basal cells. Tends to cluster at tips of the rete ridges 5. Lacks basaloid appearance 6. Dyskeratotic cells not seen. May see mitoses and apoptosis 7. Invasion into dermis or lamina propria occasionally encountered 8. Associated hyperkeratosis, parakeratosis, and papillomatosis commonly present	1. Full-thickness cohesive atypical neoplastic cells 2. Nuclei typically not as pleomorphic in undifferentiated PeIN *(Figs. 5.1.3–5.1.6)* compared to differentiated PeIN *(Figs. 5.1.7 and 5.1.8)* 3. Cytoplasm eosinophilic identical to normal squamous cells 4. No sparing of the basal cell layer 5. Basaloid PeIN with smaller cells with high N/C ratio 6. Mitoses, individually keratinized dyskeratotic cells and apoptotic bodies seen 7. Invasion into dermis absent by definition 8. Associated surface hyperkeratosis and parakeratosis commonly present
Special studies	• Intracytoplasmic mucin on histochemical stains • CEA+, CK7+, HER2+, CAM5.2+ • Negative for high-risk HPV using in situ hybridization (ISH)	• Intracytoplasmic mucin not demonstrable on histochemical stains • Typically CEA−, CK7−, HER2−, CAM5.2− • High-risk HPV can be detected using ISH
Treatment	Wide local excision of the skin and subcutaneous tissues. Sentinel lymph node biopsy and/or regional lymphadenectomy warranted for invasive Paget disease	Complete conservative excision
Prognosis	If noninvasive, favorable prognosis. Invasion with 2-y overall survival rate approaching 50%. Depth of invasion and lymphovascular involvement prognostic	Excellent

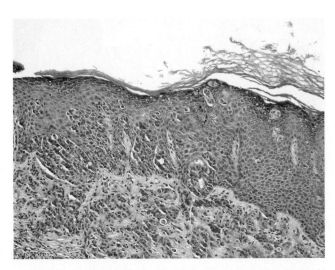

Figure 5.1.1 Extramammary Paget disease. Intraepidermal proliferation of atypical cells with abundant pale vacuolated cytoplasm. Invasion into underlying dermis is seen.

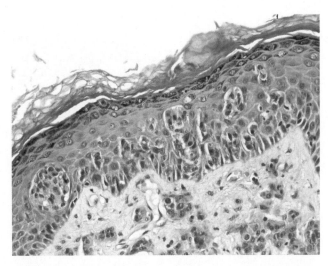

Figure 5.1.2 Same case as Figure with nest of cells with pale cytoplasm spread within otherwise normal epidermis. Invasive Paget disease is seen in the dermis (*bottom*).

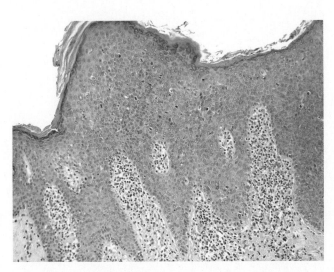

Figure 5.1.3 Undifferentiated high-grade PeIN with full-thickness proliferation of small basaloid cells.

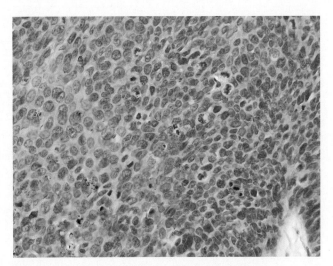

Figure 5.1.4 Same case as Figure 5.1.3 with numerous mitotic figures and dyskeratotic cells. The nuclei are smaller with high N/C ratio.

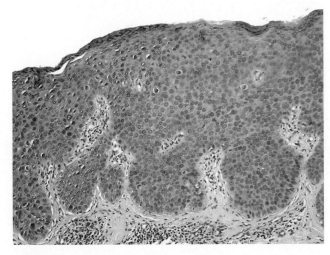

Figure 5.1.5 Undifferentiated high-grade PeIN.

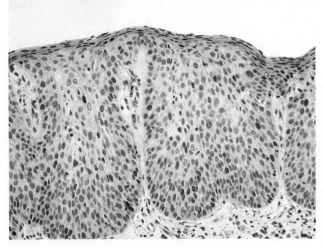

Figure 5.1.6 Undifferentiated grade PeIN.

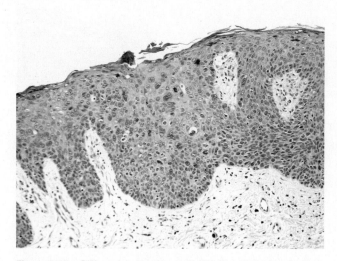

Figure 5.1.7 Differentiated high-grade PeIN with cells having significant pleomorphism and abundant cytoplasm.

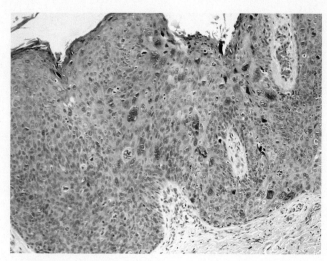

Figure 5.1.8 Differentiated high-grade PeIN.

	Pseudoepitheliomatous Squamous Cell Carcinoma	Pseudoepitheliomatous Hyperplasia
Age	Adults. Median 69 y (53–76 y)	Adults
Location	Frequently multifocal. Preferentially affects inner foreskin mucosa but also glans surface, coronal sulcus, and frenulum	Gland, coronal sulcus, and foreskin
Symptoms	None	None
Signs	Flat to slightly raised mass on inner preputial mucosa	Flat to slightly raised mass
Etiology	Majority of cases arise in association with lichen sclerosus et atrophicus (LS&A) not associated with HPV infection	Associated inflammatory dermal conditions including LS&A
Gross and Histology	1. Flat to only slightly raised, pearly whitish gray surface with irregular borders, measuring 0.4–3.5 cm (mean 2 cm) 2. Downward proliferation of very well-differentiated squamous epithelial columns and nests (Figs. 5.2.1–5.2.3) 3. Nests and columns more haphazard, deeply invasive, and irregular frequently angulated border. Abundant eosinophilic cytoplasm at the invading edge is seen with a lack of a palisaded basal layer 4. Neoplastic cells extremely well differentiated almost indistinguishable from normal epithelial cells, with only minimal atypia of basal layer 5. Adjacent flanking mucosa frequently reveals associated differentiated PeIN and LS&A	1. Flat to only slightly raised, pearly whitish gray surface with irregular borders 2. Downward proliferation of benign mature squamous epithelial columns that may give the impression of nests on cut surface 3. Columns and nests reach only a superficial level of depth ending at a linear limiting front paralleling the surface mucosa/skin. A palisaded basal layer at the interface of columns/nests with stroma is present (Figs. 5.2.4–5.2.6) 4. Hyperplastic epithelial cells indistinguishable from normal epithelial cells. Keratin pearls and individual cell keratinization not seen 5. Adjacent flanking mucosa or skin reveals changes of underlying inflammatory etiology but no PeIN
Special studies	Not helpful in differential. Both are negative for HPV on IHC and molecular studies and share similar cytokeratin profile	Not helpful in differential
Treatment	Very conservative surgical excision. At time, circumcision sufficient. Prophylactic inguinal lymphadenectomy not indicated	Directed toward underlying etiology
Prognosis	Only rare recurrence. No lymph node metastases have ever been reported	Benign

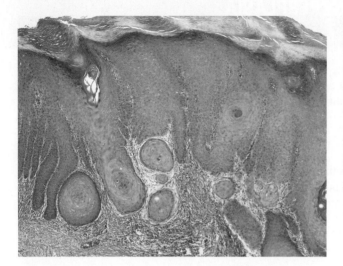

Figure 5.2.1 Pseudoepitheliomatous squamous cell carcinoma.

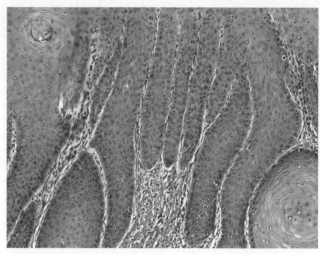

Figure 5.2.2 Same case as Figure 5.2.1 with downward proliferation of very well-differentiated squamous epithelial columns and nests.

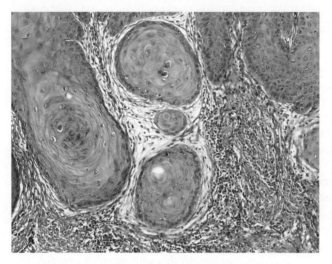

Figure 5.2.3 Nests and columns more haphazard and lack palisaded basal layer compared to hyperplasia. Also some islands have abundant eosinophilic cytoplasm at the invasive edge. Cytologic atypia is also noted (*upper right*).

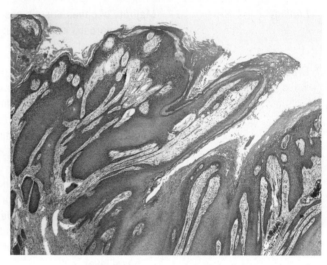

Figure 5.2.4 Pseudoepitheliomatous hyperplasia.

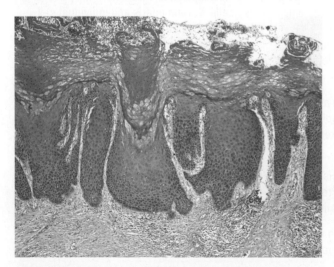

Figure 5.2.5 Same case as Figure 5.2.4 with columns and nests reaching only a superficial level of depth ending at a linear limiting front paralleling the surface mucosa/skin.

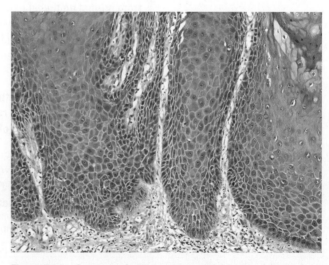

Figure 5.2.6 Same case as Figures 5.2.4 and 5.2.5 with a palisaded basal layer at the interface of columns/nests with stroma.

	Verrucous Squamous Cell Carcinoma (Verrucous SCC)	Condyloma Acuminatum
Age	Older adults. Mean age at diagnosis 70–80 y	Older adults. Mean age at diagnosis 60 y
Location	Usually unifocal. Glans or foreskin	Usually unifocal but multifocality occasionally seen. Glans, prepuce, or shaft
Symptoms	None	None
Signs	Cauliflower-like mass, slow growing	Cauliflower-like mass, soft to moderately firm slow growing
Etiology	Unknown. Not associated with HPV infection	Strongly associated with low-risk HPV infection (HPV6 and HPV11). Higher incidence in sexual partners of HPV-related cervical or anal lesions
Gross and Histology	1. Cauliflower-like large soft masses, white-gray cobblestone surface 2. Broad base bulbous papillae characterized by marked acanthosis. Fibrovascular cores very inconspicuous or absent (Fig. 5.3.1) 3. Intraepithelial keratin plugs frequently found 4. Base of papillae broad based and rounded (Fig. 5.3.2) 5. Prominent acanthosis 6. Koilocytes absent and parakeratosis ranges from mild to prominent 7. Chronic inflammatory stromal reaction, ranging from moderate to severe frequently observed. Usually only invades lamina propria and occasionally up to corpus spongiosum with infrequent extension 8. Extremely well-differentiated identical to normal squamous epithelium (Fig. 5.3.2)	1. A very small subset can reach large size (>8 cm). Grossly, cauliflower-like soft masses, white-gray cobblestone surface 2. Complex papillae with irregularly shaped prominent fibrovascular cores (Figs. 5.3.3 and 5.3.4) 3. Intraepithelial keratin plugs present 4. Base of papillae broad based and rounded 5. Prominent acanthosis 6. Extensive and prominent nuclear koilocytosis (perinuclear halo) with nuclear irregular membrane and frequent bi/multinucleation (Figs. 5.3.5 and 5.3.6). Mild dysplasia almost always present with a small subset showing focal moderate to severe dysplasia 7. Tumor base can have invaginations with inverted pushing base. Does not invade corpus spongiosum or beyond 8. Extremely well-differentiated identical to normal squamous epithelium

	Verrucous Squamous Cell Carcinoma (Verrucous SCC)	**Condyloma Acuminatum**
Special studies	IHC negative for HPV	Overall majority positive for low-risk HPV (6, 11) with only rare lesions showing other types of HPV (16, 18, 31, 32)
Treatment	Conservative surgical excision. No lymph node metastases ever been reported in pure verrucous SCC. Prophylactic inguinal lymphadenectomy not indicated	Complete conservative resection
Prognosis	Higher metastatic and recurrence rates encountered in cases with verrucous carcinoma associated with usual SCC. Generous sampling advised in verrucous SCC to rule out presence of usual SCC foci	Benign tumors even when locally destructive. A very small minority give rise to SCC

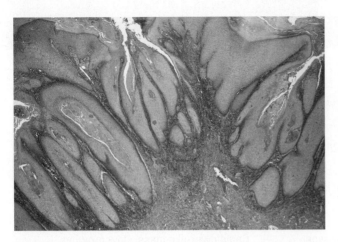

Figure 5.3.1 Verrucous squamous cell carcinoma with broad base bulbous papillae characterized by marked acanthosis. Fibrovascular cores are very inconspicuous or absent.

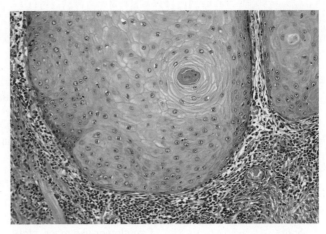

Figure 5.3.2 Same case as Figure 5.3.1 with broad base bulbous papillae and not nuclear atypia.

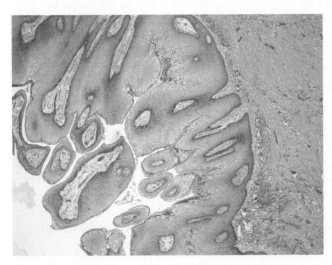

Figure 5.3.3 Condyloma acuminatum with complex papillae with irregularly shaped prominent fibrovascular cores.

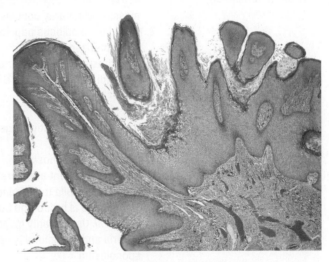

Figure 5.3.4 Condyloma acuminatum with well-formed papillae with prominent fibrovascular cores.

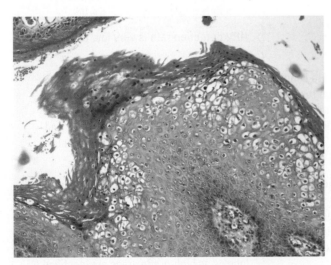

Figure 5.3.5 Condyloma acuminatum with extensive koilocytosis.

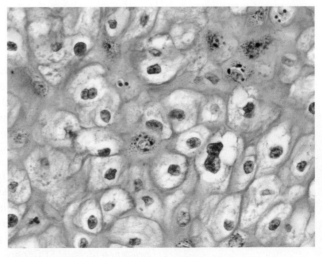

Figure 5.3.6 Same case as Figure 5.3.5 with koilocytosis, binucleated cells, and irregular nuclei.

5 PENIS/SCROTUM

	Verrucous Squamous Cell Carcinoma (Verrucous SCC)	Papillary Squamous Cell Carcinoma (Papillary SCC)
Age	Older adults. Mean age at diagnosis 70–80 y	Older adults. Mean age at diagnosis 40–50 y
Location	Usually unifocal. Glans or foreskin	Usually unifocal. Glans or foreskin
Symptoms	None	None
Signs	Cauliflower-like mass, slow growing	Cauliflower-like mass, slow growing
Etiology	Unknown. Not associated with HPV infection	Unknown. Not associated with HPV infection
Gross and Histology	1. Grossly, cauliflower-like large soft masses, white-gray cobblestone surface 2. Broad base bulbous papillae characterized by marked acanthosis. Fibrovascular cores very inconspicuous or absent (Figs. 5.4.1 and 5.4.2) 3. Intraepithelial keratin plugs frequently found 4. Prominent acanthosis 5. Koilocytes absent and parakeratosis ranges from mild to prominent 6. Tumor base is broad and pushing (Fig. 5.4.3). Usually only invades lamina propria and occasionally up to corpus spongiosum 7. Extremely well-differentiated identical to normal squamous epithelium (Fig. 5.4.4)	1. Cauliflower-like large soft masses, white-gray cobblestone surface 2. Complex papillae with irregularly shaped fibrovascular cores (Figs. 5.4.5 and 5.4.6). Tend to have some areas exhibiting condylomatous well-formed papillae and others with a more verrucous-like aspect lacking prominent fibrovascular cores 3. Intraepithelial keratin plugs not seen 4. Prominent acanthosis 5. Koilocytes absent and parakeratosis not prominent 6. Jagged tumor–stroma interface. Tends to infiltrate deeper into penile tissues compared to verrucous SCC 7. Neoplastic cells range in grade from well to moderately differentiated, with a minority of the cases poorly differentiated (Figs. 5.4.7–5.4.10)
Special studies	IHC negative for HPV	HPV detection rate is very low or even absent
Treatment	Conservative surgical excision. No lymph node metastases have ever been reported in pure verrucous SCC. Prophylactic inguinal lymphadenectomy not indicated	Managed according to penile risk-group stratification systems, taking into account histologic grade, anatomical level of maximum tumor infiltration, and the presence of vascular and perineural invasion
Prognosis	Higher metastatic and recurrence rates are encountered in cases with verrucous carcinoma associated with usual SCC. Generous sampling is advised in verrucous SCC in order to rule out the presence of usual SCC foci	Inguinal metastatic rate very low. Less than one-fifth of all patients present with inguinal involvement, and even in these cases, the mortality rate is low. Even when tumors invade penile erectile tissues, prognosis is good as long as no high-grade areas are identified

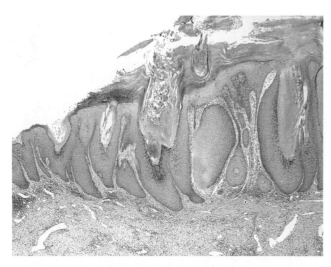

Figure 5.4.1   Verrucous squamous cell carcinoma with broad-based bulbous papillae characterized by marked acanthosis extending deeper than the adjacent benign epithelium (*left*), diagnostic of invasion.

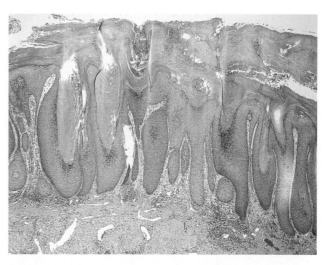

Figure 5.4.2   Same case as Figure 5.4.1 with inconspicuous or absent fibrovascular cores.

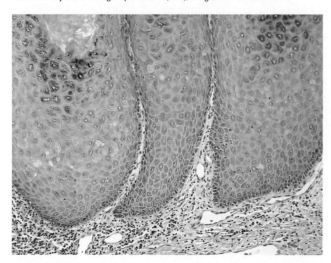

Figure 5.4.3   Same case as Figures 5.4.1 and 5.4.2 with broad-based papillae.

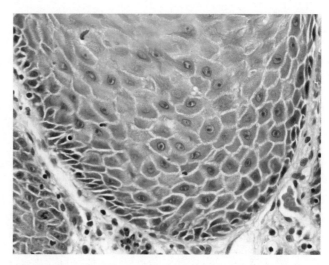

Figure 5.4.4   Same case as Figures 5.4.1 and 5.4.3 with absence of nuclear atypia.

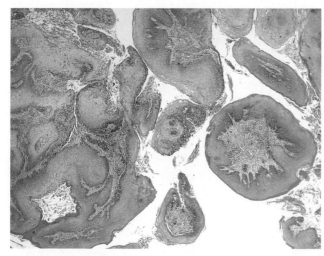

Figure 5.4.5   Papillary squamous cell carcinoma with complex papillae with irregularly shaped fibrovascular cores.

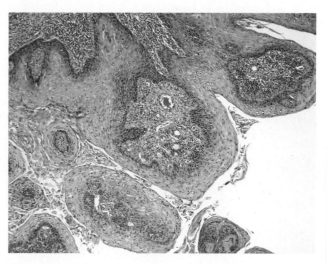

Figure 5.4.6   Another case of papillary squamous cell carcinoma with complex papillae.

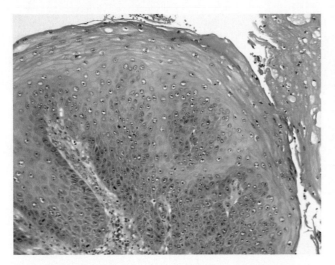

Figure 5.4.7 Same case as Figure 5.4.5 with more atypia than verrucous carcinoma. Lacks viral change seen in warty carcinoma.

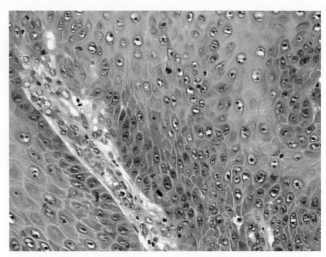

Figure 5.4.8 Same case as Figures 5.4.5 and 5.4.7 with atypia.

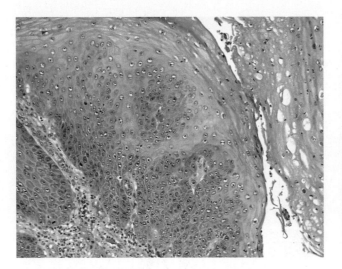

Figure 5.4.9 Same case as Figure 5.4.6 with more atypia than verrucous carcinoma.

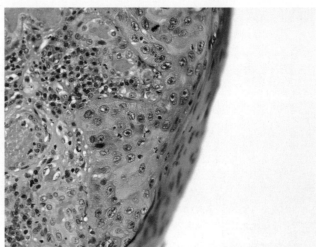

Figure 5.4.10 Same case as Figures 5.4.6 and 5.4.9 with atypia.

	Condyloma Acuminatum	Warty Squamous Cell Carcinoma (Warty SCC)
Age	Older adults. Mean age at diagnosis 60 y	Older adults. Mean age at diagnosis 60 y
Location	Usually unifocal but multifocality is occasionally seen. Glans, prepuce, or shaft	Usually unifocal. Glans
Symptoms	None	None
Signs	Cauliflower-like mass, soft to moderately firm, slow growing	Cauliflower-like mass, firm, slow growing
Etiology	Strongly associated with low-risk HPV infection (HPV6 and HPV11). Higher incidence in sexual partners of HPV-related cervical or anal lesions	Strongly associated with high-risk HPV infection
Gross and Histology	1. A very small subset can reach large size (>8 cm). Grossly, cauliflower-like soft masses, white-gray cobblestone surface 2. Complex papillae with irregularly shaped prominent fibrovascular cores 3. Intraepithelial keratin plugs present 4. Base of papillae are broad based rounded 5. Prominent acanthosis 6. Extensive and prominent nuclear koilocytosis (perinuclear halo) with nuclear irregular membrane and frequent bi/multinucleation *(Fig. 5.5.1)* 7. Mild dysplasia almost always present with a small subset showing focal moderate to severe dysplasia 8. Tumor base broad and can have invaginations with inverted pushing base. Does not invade corpus spongiosum or beyond *(Fig. 5.5.2)*	1. Cauliflower-like, firm, large mass (average 5 cm) with white-gray cobblestone surface 2. Complex papillae with irregularly shaped fibrovascular cores *(Fig. 5.5.3)* 3. Intraepithelial keratin plugs and parakeratosis with intraepithelial microabscesses 4. Tumor–stroma interface usually irregular and infiltrative, although a pushing border can rarely be seen in endophytic warty SCC *(Figs. 5.5.4 and 5.5.5)* 5. Prominent acanthosis 6. Extensive and prominent nuclear koilocytosis *(Fig. 5.5.6)* 7. Ranges in grade from well to moderately differentiated 8. Can be deeply infiltrative into corpus spongiosum and cavernosa
Special studies	• Overall majority positive for low-risk HPV (6, 11) status with only rare lesions showing other types of HPV (16, 18, 31, 32)	• High-risk HPV almost always detected using ISH

	Condyloma Acuminatum	**Warty Squamous Cell Carcinoma (Warty SCC)**
Treatment	Complete conservative resection	Managed according to penile risk-group stratification systems, taking into account histologic grade, anatomical level of maximum tumor infiltration, and the presence of vascular and perineural invasion
Prognosis	Benign tumors even when locally destructive. A very small minority of condylomas will give rise to SCC	Intermediate biologic behavior between verrucous and papillary SCC on one hand and usual-type SCC on the other. Inguinal lymph nodes metastases more frequent in deep and high-grade cases

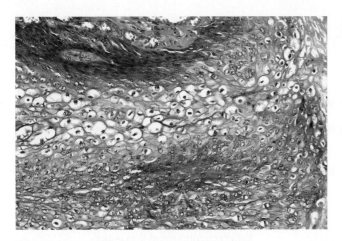

Figure 5.5.1   Condyloma acuminatum with koilocytosis.

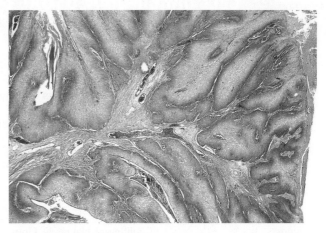

Figure 5.5.2   Same case as Figure 5.5.1 with complex growth having prominent invaginations.

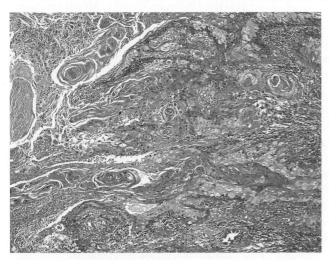

Figure 5.5.3   Warty carcinoma with complex papillae with irregularly shaped fibrovascular cores and abundant parakeratosis (surface is to the *left*).

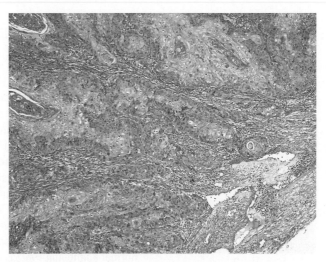

Figure 5.5.4   Same case as Figure 5.5.3 with irregular infiltrative base (*right*).

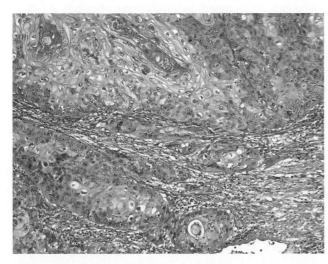

Figure 5.5.5   Same case as Figures 5.5.3 and 5.5.4 with infiltrative base composed of small irregular nests with atypia.

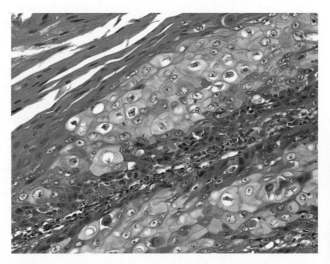

Figure 5.5.6   Same case as Figures 5.5.3 and 5.5.5 with koilocytosis and irregular crinkly nuclei.

	Verrucous Squamous Cell Carcinoma	Squamous Cell Carcinoma, Usual Type
Age	Older adults. Mean age at diagnosis 70–80 y	Adults. Mean age at diagnosis 58 y
Location	Usually unifocal. Glans or foreskin	Usually unifocal. Glans, foreskin, or coronal sulcus
Symptoms	None	None
Signs	Cauliflower-like mass, slow growing	Exophytic/ulcerated firm mass
Etiology	Unknown. Not associated with HPV infection	Unknown in majority of cases. HPV infection related in approximately 25%. More prevalent in South America, Africa, and Asia
Histology	1. Broad base bulbous papillae with marked acanthosis *(Figs. 5.6.1 and 5.6.2)*. Fibrovascular cores very inconspicuous or absent. Intraepithelial keratin plugs frequently found 2. Koilocytes absent and parakeratosis ranges from mild to prominent 3. Differentiated type PeIN (intraepithelial penile neoplasia) not present 4. Tumor base broad and pushing with a chronic inflammatory stromal reaction, ranging from moderate to severe 5. Cytologically, extremely well differentiated, indistinguishable from normal epithelium *(Fig. 5.6.3)* 6. Usually only invades lamina propria. Occasionally up to corpus spongiosum. Extension beyond infrequent 7. Should be distinguished from mixed usual-type SCC/verrucous carcinoma (hybrid verrucous SCC) where typical areas of verrucous carcinoma coexist with foci of an otherwise usual low- or high-grade SCC. Generous sampling is advised in verrucous SCC in order to rule out the presence of usual SCC foci	1. Usually lacks papillae. Can have acanthosis 2. Koilocytes absent and parakeratosis ranges from mild to prominent 3. Differentiated type PeIN (intraepithelial penile neoplasia) commonly present 4. Infiltrative base with paradoxically maturing nests and irregular sheets *(Figs. 5.6.4–5.6.10)* 5. Eosinophilic cells with little but more cytologic atypia than verrucous carcinoma, abundant cytoplasm, and prominent keratinization. More prominent degree of nuclear atypia is in basal layers of neoplastic cells 6. May only invade lamina propria with superficial involvement of corpus spongiosum. Deeply invasive examples usually seen with higher-grade lesions 7. Mixed usual-type SCC/verrucous carcinoma (hybrid verrucous SCC) occasionally encountered
Special studies	Usually not helpful in the differential diagnosis. ISH for HPV negative	ISH for HPV negative in the majority of SCC, usual type

	Verrucous Squamous Cell Carcinoma	Squamous Cell Carcinoma, Usual Type
Treatment	Conservative surgical excision. No lymph node metastases have ever been reported in pure verrucous SCC. Prophylactic inguinal lymphadenectomy not indicated	Penectomy with adjuvant radiation and chemotherapy based on depth of invasion, presence of vascular or perineural invasion, and grade. In cases where lymph node metastases are clinically suspected, inguinal lymphadenectomy is indicated
Prognosis	Minimal (<2 mm) stromal invasion (microinvasive verrucous carcinomas) not associated with nodal metastasis and prognosis is excellent, regardless of tumor size. Higher metastatic and recurrence rates encountered in hybrid verrucous SCC approaching that of SCC, usual type	Can be predicted according to penile risk-group stratification systems, taking into account histologic grade, anatomical level of maximum tumor infiltration, and the presence of vascular and perineural invasion

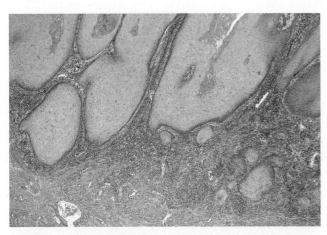

Figure 5.6.1 Verrucous squamous cell carcinoma with bulbous papillae with marked acanthosis and pushing broad base interface with chronic inflammation at the invasive front.

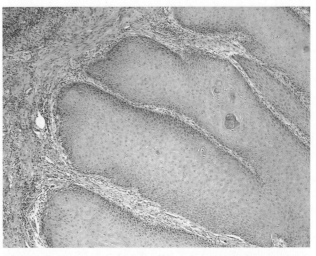

Figure 5.6.2 Verrucous squamous cell carcinoma with bulbous papillae.

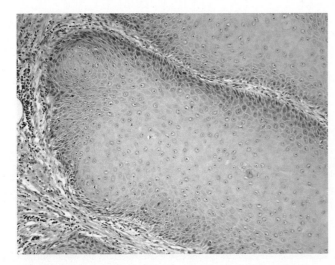

Figure 5.6.3 Same case as Figure 5.6.2 with no atypia, resembling normal squamous lining.

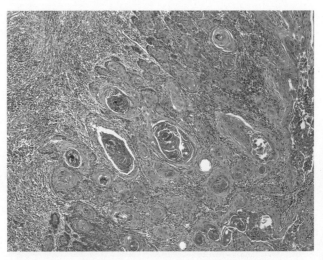

Figure 5.6.4 Squamous cell carcinoma, usual type with irregular small nests with abundant central keratinization (base of lesion is towards the *left*).

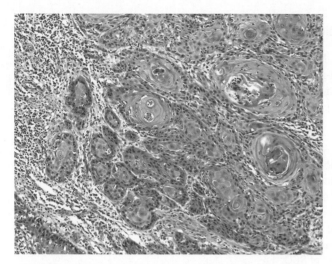

Figure 5.6.5 Higher magnification of case as Figure 5.6.4 showing abnormal maturation with squamous nests with abundant cytoplasm at the base of the lesion (*left*).

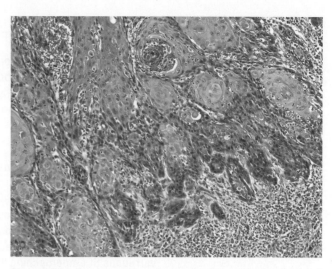

Figure 5.6.6 Squamous cell carcinoma, usual type with ragged nests of cells at the base.

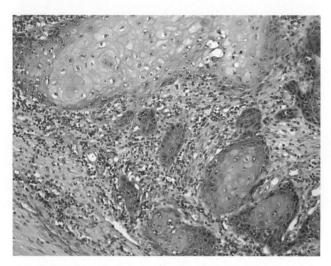

Figure 5.6.7 Squamous cell carcinoma, usual type with irregular small nests in addition to larger nests with glassy abundant cytoplasm.

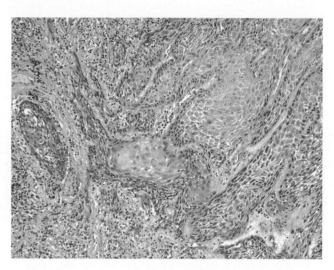

Figure 5.6.8 Squamous cell carcinoma, usual type with ragged nests of cells at the base (*left*).

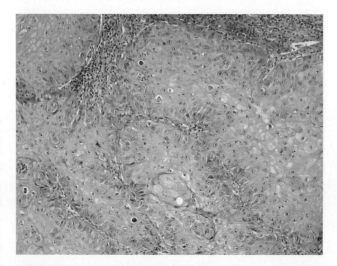

Figure 5.6.9 Squamous cell carcinoma, usual type with greater degree of cytologic atypia than verrucous carcinoma.

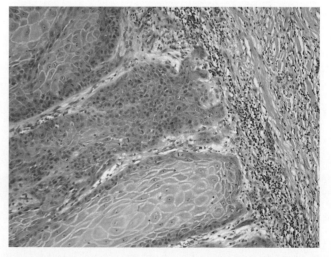

Figure 5.6.10 Squamous cell carcinoma, usual type (*top*) associated with verrucous carcinoma (*bottom*). The surface of the lesion is to the left.

	Basaloid Squamous Cell Carcinoma	**Squamous Cell Carcinoma, Usual Type**
Age	Adults. Mean age at diagnosis 50–60 y	Adults. Mean age at diagnosis 58 y
Location	Usually unifocal. Glans	Usually unifocal. Glans, foreskin, or coronal sulcus
Symptoms	None	None
Signs	Flat ulcerated firm mass	Exophytic/ulcerated firm mass
Etiology	HPV infection related. HPV16 most commonly followed by HPV18	HPV related in approximately 25%. More prevalent in South America, Africa, and Asia
Histology	1. Smaller sized basophilic cells with scant cytoplasm and distinctly high N/C ratio 2. Infiltrating round to irregular sheets, some with palisaded basal layer and separation from surrounding stroma by artifactual clefts *(Fig. 5.7.1)* 3. Usually vertical growth pattern. 4. Nuclei ovoid with inconspicuous nucleoli *(Fig. 5.7.2)* 5. Intercellular bridges not identifiable 6. Apoptotic and mitotic figures frequent (starry sky appearance) 7. Central necrosis in infiltrating nodules *(Fig. 5.7.3)* 8. May be associated with basaloid-type PeIN (intraepithelial penile neoplasia) 9. High-grade tumor by definition. Lacks significant keratinization 10. More likely to be deeply invasive 11. Mixed basaloid SCC–warty SCC occasionally encountered with koilocytic changes	1. Abundant eosinophilic cytoplasm and low N/C ratio *(Figs. 5.7.5 and 5.7.6)* 2. Infiltrating nests and irregular sheets with abundant cytoplasm. Lacks palisading 3. Majority display superficial spreading growth patterns with or without an associated vertical nodular growth component 4. Vesicular nuclei and prominent nucleoli typically present 5. Intercellular bridges typical 6. Apoptotic and mitotic figures are overall less prominent except in high-grade lesions 7. Less frequent central necrosis 8. May be associated with differentiated PeIN (intraepithelial penile neoplasia) 9. Variable grade. Grade 3 SCC shows nuclear enlargement, pleomorphism, increased mitotic activity, and little if any keratinization 10. Depth of invasion correlates with grade 11. Koilocytic changes not a feature
Special studies	Almost always positive for high-risk HPV by ISH and p16 overexpression *(Fig. 5.7.4)*	ISH for HPV and p16 negative in the majority of cases
Treatment	Total penectomy with bilateral inguinal lymph node resection. Adjuvant radiation and chemotherapy in high-stage tumors	Penectomy with or without adjuvant radiation and chemotherapy based on depth of invasion, presence of vascular or perineural invasion, and grade
Prognosis	Poor in advanced stage disease. Over half present with evidence of inguinal lymph node metastases	Dependent on risk group taking into account grade, level of infiltration, and vascular and perineural invasion

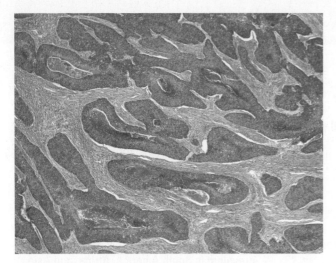

Figure 5.7.1   Basaloid squamous cell carcinoma.

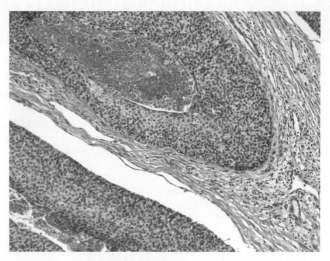

Figure 5.7.2   Same case as Figure 5.7.1 with round to irregular sheets with central necrosis, some with palisaded basal layer and separation from surrounding stroma by artifactual clefts.

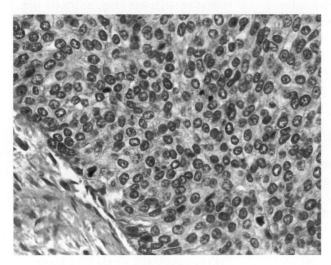

Figure 5.7.3   Same case as Figures 5.7.1 and 5.7.2 composed of smaller sized basophilic cells with scant cytoplasm and distinctly high N/C ratio.

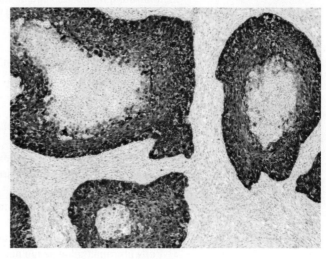

Figure 5.7.4   Same case as Figures 5.7.1–5.7.3 with strong p16 positivity.

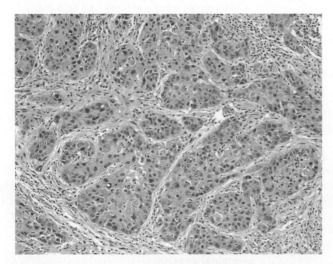

Figure 5.7.5   Moderately differentiated squamous cell carcinoma, usual type composed of nests of cells with more abundant eosinophilic cytoplasm.

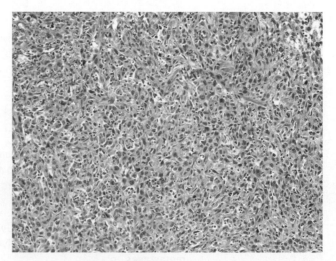

Figure 5.7.6   Poorly differentiated squamous cell carcinoma with irregular sheets of cells with more abundant eosinophilic cytoplasm.

	Aggressive Angiomyxoma	Cellular Angiofibroma (Angiomyofibroblastoma-like Tumor of the Male Genital Tract)
Age	Average age in men is 46 y (1–82 y)	Adults. Mean age at diagnosis 60 y (20s–elderly)
Location	Scrotum followed by the inguinal region, most attached to the spermatic cord. Can also occur in perineum	Superficial dermis or subcutaneous tissue of inguinal/groin or scrotal/paratesticular region
Symptoms	None	Painless slowly enlarging mass
Signs	Inguinal or scrotal mass	Inguinal or scrotal mass
Etiology	Unknown	Unknown
Gross and Histology	1. Mostly ill-defined infiltrative masses although some encapsulated. Large range in size including up to 60 cm. Cut surface smooth gray-white with soft gelatinous consistency 2. Widely scattered spindle cells with ill-defined cytoplasm in myxoid stroma rich in collagen fibers *(Figs. 5.8.1 and 5.8.2)* 3. Nuclei round to oval with inconspicuous nucleoli 4. Lacks atypia except in recurrent cases. May have numerous mast cells and lymphoid aggregates 5. Mitotic figures rare or absent 6. Variably sized vessels from small thin walled capillaries to large vessels with medial arterial hypertrophy. Can see arteries, veins, capillaries, and venules 7. Tumor can invade adipose tissue 8. Small bundles of smooth muscle cells appear to spin off of blood vessels *(Fig. 5.8.3)*	1. Well circumscribed with fibrous pseudocapsule in most cases but can in a minority of cases infiltrate into adjacent skeletal muscle *(Fig. 5.8.4)*. Wide size range with average 6.7 cm 2. Uniform, short spindle-shaped cells in edematous to fibrous stroma. Spindle cells fairly cellular usually without particular pattern *(Figs. 5.8.5 and 5.8.6)*. Occasionally fascicular with palisading. Stroma may show edema, hyalinization, short bundles of densely eosinophilic collagen 3. Nuclei ovoid to polygonal with inconspicuous nucleoli *(Fig. 5.8.7)* 4. Mild reactive atypia can be seen with inflammation 5. Usually scant mitotic figures but up to 10/10 HPF can be seen 6. Numerous small- to medium-sized thick-walled vessels. Larger vessels can be seen at the periphery. Fibrin within walls of vessel common *(Figs. 5.8.7 and 5.8.8)* 7. Lesions can contain adipose tissue *(Fig. 5.8.9)* 8. Lacks bundles of smooth muscle cells spinning off of blood vessels *(Fig. 5.8.10)*
Special studies	• Not helpful in this differential. Variable CD34. Variable SMA, desmin. ER and PR can be present	• Strong CD34 staining. Variable SMA and desmin. ER and PR positive in about 20% of cases
Treatment	Aggressive surgical excision with adjuvant hormone therapy in some cases	Simple excision
Prognosis	Locally recurs in 30% of cases. If aggressive surgical excision, fewer recurrences	Lacks local recurrence or metastases

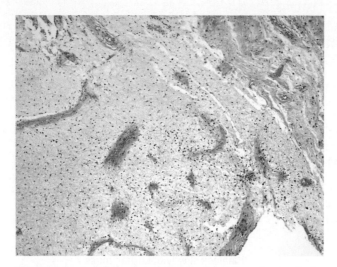

Figure 5.8.1 Aggressive angiomyxoma. Lesion was not circumscribed (not shown).

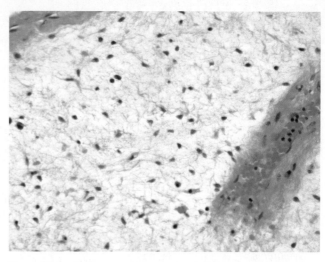

Figure 5.8.2 Same case as Figure 5.8.1 with widely scattered spindle cells with ill-defined cytoplasm in myxoid stroma.

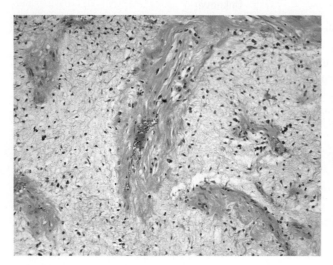

Figure 5.8.3 Same case as Figures 5.8.1 and 5.8.2 with small bundles of smooth muscle cells spinning off of blood vessels.

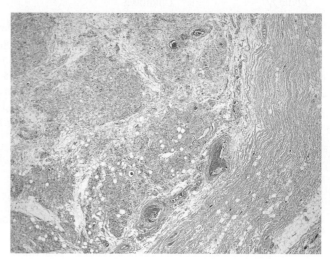

Figure 5.8.4 Well-circumscribed cellular angiofibroma.

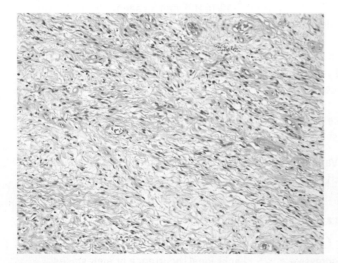

Figure 5.8.5 Cellular angiofibroma with myxoid background containing thin bundles of collagen.

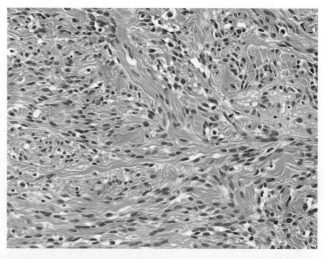

Figure 5.8.6 Cellular angiofibroma with more cellular less myxoid stroma with numerous collagen bundles.

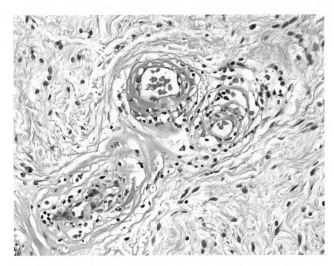

Figure 5.8.7 Cellular angiofibroma with ovoid nuclei with inconspicuous nucleoli and scant bipolar cytoplasm associated with small vessels with fibrin deposition.

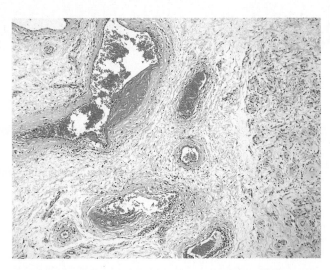

Figure 5.8.8 Cellular angiofibroma with vessels showing fibrin deposition.

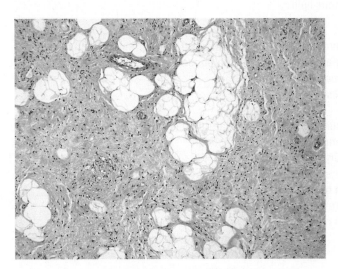

Figure 5.8.9 Cellular angiofibroma that was circumscribed containing adipose tissue, which should not be misinterpreted as infiltrative growth.

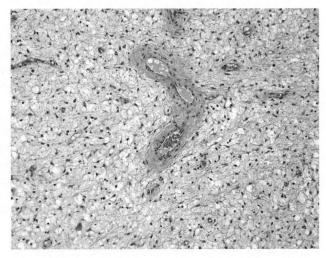

Figure 5.8.10 Cellular angiofibroma with thick-walled vessels lacking smooth muscle cells spinning off of periphery.

	Sclerosing Lipogranuloma	Well-Differentiated Liposarcoma
Age	Most men <40 y, although as old as 70 y reported	Majority occurs in adults with a mean age of 56 y (16–90 y)
Location	Dermis and subcutaneous tissue of penis and base of scrotum *(Fig. 5.9.1)*	Deep soft tissue of distal spermatic cord immediately adjacent to the testis. Lacks skin involvement
Symptoms	Variably tender masses	Scrotal swelling
Signs	Irregular hard lumpy masses	Scrotal mass, average size 12 cm (3–30 cm)
Etiology	In most cases, there is a history of injecting paraffin as a means of increasing genital size. In the rare case where such a history cannot be elicited possibly explained by endogenous lipid release from trauma	Unknown
Histology	1. Initially inflammatory with multiple small lipid vacuoles accompanied by numerous lymphocytes, histiocytes, plasma cells, and eosinophils without prominent fibrosis 2. Chronic phase with numerous fat vacuoles of various sizes ranging from minute to cystic in dense fibrosis 3. Surrounding vacuoles is dense fibrosis and often prominent foreign body giant cell reaction *(Figs. 5.9.1–5.9.7)* 4. Lacks large hyperchromatic nuclei with degenerative atypia	1. At this site, lacks prominent inflammatory component 2. Mature fat with relatively uniform size of vacuoles 3. Focal fat necrosis may be seen with multinucleated giant cells but not a prominent feature 4. In between normal-appearing fat, typically with fibrous septa are large hyperchromatic nuclei with degenerative atypia *(Figs. 5.9.8–5.9.10)*
Special studies	MDM2 overexpression not present. Lack giant marker/ring chromosomes	MDM2 immunostaining positive. Giant marker/ring chromosomes harboring amplification of the MDM2 gene region (12q13-15) are identifiable on FISH
Treatment	Conservative excision	Radical orchiectomy
Prognosis	Benign although disfiguring and embarrassing	Favorable upon complete excision. Recurrence may occur in up to one-third of cases

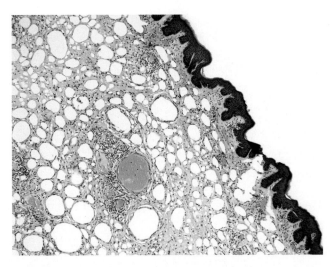

Figure 5.9.1   Sclerosing lipogranuloma extending to scrotal skin.

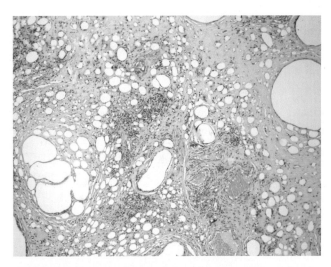

Figure 5.9.2   Sclerosing lipogranuloma with numerous fat vacuoles of various sizes ranging from minute to cystic in dense fibrosis.

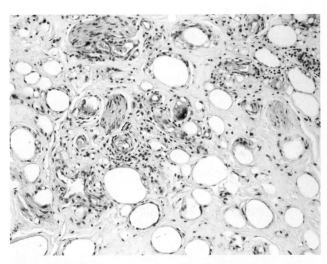

Figure 5.9.3   Sclerosing lipogranuloma with numerous fat vacuoles in dense fibrosis with scattered multinucleated giant cells.

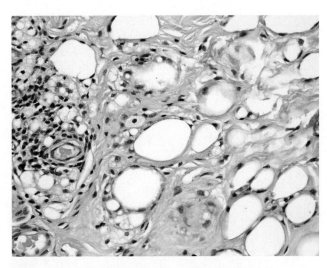

Figure 5.9.4   Sclerosing lipogranuloma with patchy chronic inflammation.

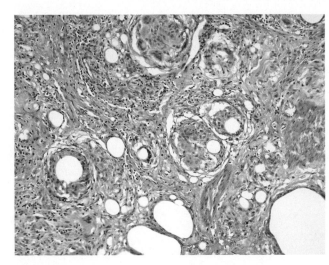

Figure 5.9.5   Sclerosing lipogranuloma with numerous foreign body giant cells.

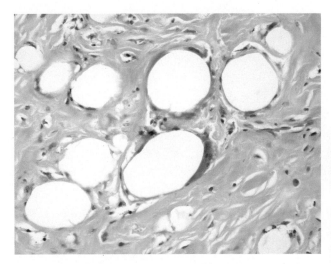

Figure 5.9.6   Sclerosing lipogranuloma with foreign body giant cell encircling a fat vacuole.

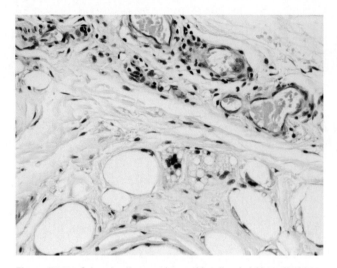

Figure 5.9.7 Sclerosing lipogranuloma with cells mimicking a lipoblast, yet lacks nuclear hyperchromasia and enlargement.

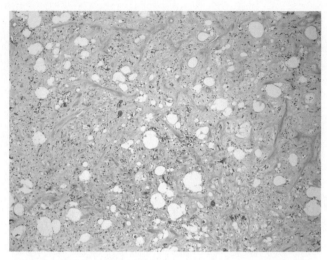

Figure 5.9.8 Well-differentiated liposarcoma showing areas of mature fat lobules within dense sclerosis.

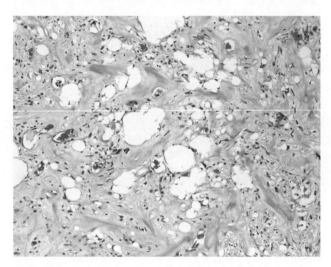

Figure 5.9.9 Same case as Figure 5.9.8 with various-sized fat vacuoles in dense fibrous tissue.

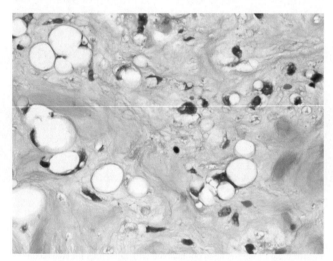

Figure 5.9.10 Same case as Figures 5.9.8 and 5.9.9 with lipoblasts with nuclear enlargement and hyperchromasia.

SUGGESTED READINGS

5.1

Bagby CM, MacLennan GT. Extramammary Paget's disease of the penis and scrotum. *J Urol.* 2009;182:2908–2909.

Hegarty PK, Suh J, Fisher MB, et al. Penoscrotal extramammary paget's disease: the University of Texas M. D. Anderson Cancer Center contemporary experience. *J Urol.* 2011;186:97–102.

5.2–5.7

Chaux A, Cubilla AL. Penile cancer: optimal management of T1G2 penile cancer remains unclear. *Nat Rev Urol.* 2013;10: 9–11.

Chaux A, Cubilla AL. Stratification systems as prognostic tools for defining risk of lymph node metastasis in penile squamous cell carcinomas. *Semin Diagn Pathol.* 2012;29:83–89.

Chaux A, Cubilla AL. The role of human papillomavirus infection in the pathogenesis of penile squamous cell carcinomas. *Semin Diagn Pathol.* 2012;29:67–71.

Chaux A, Velazquez EF, Barreto JE, et al. New pathologic entities in penile carcinomas: an update of the 2004 world health organization classification. *Semin Diagn Pathol.* 2012;29:59–66.

Chaux A, Pfannl R, Rodriguez IM, et al. Distinctive immunohistochemical profile of penile intraepithelial lesions: a study of 74 cases. *Am J Surg Pathol.* 2011;35:553–562.

Chaux A, Tamboli P, Ayala A, et al. Warty-basaloid carcinoma: clinicopathological features of a distinctive penile neoplasm. Report of 45 cases. *Mod Pathol.* 2010;23:896–904.

Cubilla AL, Lloveras B, Alejo M, et al. Value of p16(INK)(4)(a) in the pathology of invasive penile squamous cell carcinomas: a report of 202 cases. *Am J Surg Pathol.* 2011;35:253–261.

Velazquez EF, Chaux A, Cubilla AL. Histologic classification of penile intraepithelial neoplasia. *Semin Diagn Pathol.* 2012;29:96–102.

5.8–5.10

Farshid G, Weiss SW. Massive localized lymphedema in the morbidly obese: a histologically distinct reactive lesion simulating liposarcoma. *Am J Surg Pathol.* 1998;22:1277–1283.

Manduch M, Oliveira AM, Nascimento AG, et al. Massive localised lymphoedema: a clinicopathological study of 22 cases and review of the literature. *J Clin Pathol.* 2009;62:808–811.

Shon W, Ida CM, Boland-Froemming JM, et al. Cutaneous angiosarcoma arising in massive localized lymphedema of the morbidly obese: a report of five cases and review of the literature. *J Cutan Pathol.* 2011;38:560–564.

INDEX